The Prostate and Its Problems

BY

Hans R. Larsen MSc ChE
Editor, International Health News

AND

William R. Ware PhD
Emeritus Professor, University of Western Ontario

FOREWORD BY

Patrick Chambers MD

PUBLISHED BY:

INTERNATIONAL HEALTH NEWS

www.yourhealthbase.com

The Prostate and Its Problems
published by:

International Health News
1320 Point Street
Victoria BC
Canada V8S 1A5
(250) 384-2524
E-mail: editor@yourhealthbase.com

The Prostate and Its Problems does not offer medical advice. The information offered is intended to help readers make informed decisions about their health. It is not intended to be a substitute for the advice and care of a physician or other professional health care provider. The authors have endeavored to ensure that the information presented is accurate and up to date, but are not responsible for any adverse effects or consequences sustained by any reader using the information contained in this book.

First Printing – August 2006

ISBN 0-9686375-5-8

The fact you are reading this review indicates you have a need for this book. I have read other books on the prostate; however, this is one that is a must read for anyone needing help, this includes wives as well as, of course, men.

The information in The Prostate and Its Problems is without a doubt the best I have read on this subject. With the information contained in this book you are well informed to deal with most doctors on the subject of your prostate.

Please remember it is YOUR health and it is YOUR decision to make regarding treatment options. Choose wisely.
E G Beall, NC, USA

I was impressed with its comprehensiveness. I have been pleased that whenever I have a question about the prostate, I can easily find the answers I need in the book. Distinguishing the symptoms of benign prostate enlargement from those of prostate cancer has been particularly reassuring, as well as being able to understand the influences on and significance of the PSA. I keep your book handy on my bookshelf and am glad to have it to rely upon as needed.
J R Lindsley, MA, USA

The Prostate and Its Problems was recommended by an old friend. It gave me the perfect answers needed for any decision. All the answers seem to be there for me.
RT Morris, CA, USA

Heeding the popular advice for middle-aged men to have a physical exam every year, which naturally includes the prostate rectal exam and a PSA test, my doctor said that I have benign prostatic hyperplasia, or BPH. This was a few years ago, and my symptoms gradually got worse, so I did some research, and when "The Prostate and Its Problems" came out, I got a copy and read the sections on BPH, its causes and treatments.

Visits to the urologist were not comforting. When we concluded that drugs would not be the best treatment, because of side effects, I was put on a waiting list for the surgical treatment called TURP. However, my research on this and other invasive treatments caused me no little dread because of the risks, so I settled instead for what's called 'watchful waiting.'

The sections in Hans' and Bill's book on alternative treatments and therapies have given me good suggestions, and following some of these suggestions for at least a year now, the results are promising.

In my opinion, the book is written in a professional research style, as one would find in medical journals, with a description of many research studies, then a concluding section. I sometimes found it difficult to follow the descriptions, but the summaries were well-written and concise. Its thoroughness over-all is quite impressive.
B Johnston, British Columbia, Canada

Having perused several books on this subject, I can state that yours is by far the most comprehensive and readable and clarifies several aspects that I had found confusing. When I have learned all I can from it I intend to donate it to our local BC Cancer Agency storefront.
M. Marchant, British Columbia, Canada

Your book increased my knowledge immeasurably for which I am grateful beyond words.
A Encel, Australia

The Prostate and Its Problems

Contents

Foreword

With the graying of the baby boomers prostate health is looming large and concern for cancer has become an increasingly frequent topic of conversation. Unfortunately, the topic has also become increasingly complex. During more than a quarter century as a practicing pathologist, I have repeatedly been asked if, how and when to screen for prostate cancer and how to proceed if positive. As Hans Larsen and William Ware have indicated in *The Prostate and Its Problems*, these issues of screening, diagnosis and treatment are hotly debated and make prostate cancer more controversial than any other cancer. Do I request a PSA blood test and run the risk of chasing a false positive or perhaps worse, worrying about not chasing it? If the biopsy is positive, what should I do? What are my chances of ending up impotent and/or incontinent as a result of surgery or radiation? And of course, what if I don't have any insurance? While there are no absolute answers, this comprehensive work provides the most recent relevant studies impacting these decisions. Indeed much of the material is directed toward maintaining a healthy prostate and minimizing the likelihood of ever having to embark on this treacherous and tortuous path.

For a small sampling of the controversy surrounding this cancer one need look no further than PSA. Over many years the screening triple play of transrectal ultrasound, digital rectal exam and PSA has been the cornerstone of medical dogma on prostate cancer. However, from the outset the value of PSA as a screening test for prostate cancer vs. BPH has been under constant assault and the test was even proclaimed dead in 2004 by eminent urologist Professor Thomas Stamey of Stanford University Medical School. This view was based on a large autopsy study that revealed 8% of males in their twenties had prostate cancer with incidence increasing each decade until 80% had it in their seventies. Yet according to the National Cancer Institute, death due to prostate cancer in those over 65 years is only 226 per 100,000. However, it's not just PSA anymore; refinements, such as per cent free PSA (the higher the better) and PSA density (how high is it relative to size of prostate) have been added. PSA velocity (how fast is it changing) is now very much in vogue and this book has a particularly elucidating discussion of this (Chapter 4).

Once you've been determined via screening to be at risk you must decide whether to undergo biopsy. Over the past few years I have seen the incidence of low-grade prostate cancer (Gleason score less than 7) decline and it is now seen very infrequently on biopsy specimens. Whether this is because pathologists tend to err on the side of caution for medicolegal reasons is hard to say, but in any case, it tends to push the decision regarding treatment (or not) firmly back into the laps of the patient and his physician. This means that if you decide on a biopsy you are likely to face the even more daunting dilemma of treatment or not. Given the conflicting data on efficacy of surgery vs. radiation vs. watchful waiting, whether or not to even embark on this slippery slope of screening and diagnosis has come into question. This book contains all the necessary data to make an informed decision at each juncture and, as it reiterates, to always have your biopsy slides reviewed by an independent pathologist before proceeding.

Mainstream medical journal articles on both BPH and prostate cancer, many of which are financed by large pharmaceutical companies and touted as evidence-based, often fall well short of the mark on objectivity. For example, this book describes how the North American medical community has failed to embrace the well documented, evidence-based studies demonstrating the beneficial effect of saw palmetto on BPH symptoms. Saw palmetto has long been accepted by mainstream medicine in Europe as the first-line treatment for BPH; however, in North America the focus has been on surgery and finasteride despite this drug's already documented history of inducing sexual dysfunction.

The Prostate and Its Problems by Hans Larsen and William Ware tackles these thorny issues in a straightforward, easy to understand manner. The myriad questions are addressed via rigorous research translated into plain English. By sifting through all the medical literature they have presented a more balanced view, one that is both evidence-based and objective. Furthermore, unlike more traditional medical texts there is a strong emphasis on alternative, preventive strategies for avoiding inflammation, hyperplasia and cancer of the prostate. Neither author has received funding for this extraordinarily comprehensive work. Both are true scholars motivated purely by the sheer joy of learning and teaching others, and their total dedication to this goal is readily apparent in every page.

This book has appeal well beyond males. Life changing decisions on treatment for prostate cancer should be a joint decision. Oftentimes males are not prepared either emotionally or intellectually to undertake the requisite research to arrive at a well informed choice tailored to their specific situation. This then falls to their spouse. Furthermore, given that prostate and breast cancer are both hormone-dependent cancers and that men with a family history of breast cancer are more likely to get prostate cancer and women with a family history of prostate cancer are more likely to get breast cancer (Chapter 3), much of the presented preventive strategies may have equal gender appeal. Furthermore, antioxidant and anti-inflammatory strategies are of proven benefit for longevity, minimizing both cardiovascular disease and cancer in general.

If you are an informed consumer wishing to become more empowered in your healthcare decisions, then this book is for you. When made by others, many of these decisions are influenced by medicolegal and financial considerations of which you may not even be aware. Wouldn't it be better to know the most recent data and to digest them for yourself rather than to have the decision made for you? Ultimately, it's your life and your money. Hopefully, your PSA level will never become abnormal. However, if you want to become more prepared to deal with such an occurrence before the associated emotional cloud descends to color your thinking, then *The Prostate and Its Problems* by Hans Larsen and William Ware is highly recommended.

Patrick Chambers, MD
Kailua, Oahu, HI
August 2006

Patrick Chambers *received his baccalaureate degree from Princeton University in Mathematics in 1971 followed shortly thereafter by completion of medical studies at the University of California at Davis. He completed his specialty training in pathology at the Los Angeles County/University of Southern California Medical Center. After more than 25 years as a practicing pathologist and laboratory director at Torrance Memorial Medical Center he recently retired to Kailua, Hawaii, where plentiful sunlight and high vitamin D levels hopefully keep his prostate healthy and cancer free. In an annual review of 4000 American acute care hospitals Torrance Memorial was the only non-teaching hospital of any size to be named a Top 100 Hospital three years in a row (1993, 1994, 1995).*

Preface

Hans R. Larsen and William R. Ware

When we decided to join forces in the spring of 2005 to embark on the venture of writing this book, we had both for some time been following the peer-reviewed literature concerning prostate problems and in particular had done a fair amount of research into prostate cancer. One of us (WRW) had closely studied and followed developments in the diagnosis and conventional treatment of this disease, and the other (HRL) had researched alternative methods for prevention and treatment. We both had read numerous books on cancer and prostate cancer in particular and had, somewhat surprisingly, reached the conclusion that no one book covered the entire spectrum of problems. Some books written for the lay audience were excellent in explaining conventional treatment methods, others were quite comprehensive in their discussion of herbs and supplements that might prevent cancer, but none, it seemed to us, really provided the whole gamut of information necessary for a man who wants to take charge of his own health and, along with his physician, make reasoned decisions regarding diagnostic options and possible treatments of prostate problems. Prostatitis and benign prostate enlargement (BPH), although affecting millions of men, did not seem to be covered very well, perhaps because conventional treatment, certainly in the case of prostatitis, is often less than satisfactory.

So our mission was clear, to write a book that covered the three major prostate problems – prostatitis, BPH and cancer – from etiology to therapy, including both alternative and conventional measures of prevention and treatment. The intended audience includes laymen who want to be thoroughly informed and health-care professionals involved in primary care. We also agreed that all statements made in the book would be backed up with references to peer-reviewed medical journals. Another condition was that the material must include the most recent relevant published literature. Given the constraints of the cut-off date for publication, this was no small task, but you are now holding the result in your hands – over 400 pages of information documented with over 1200 references plus appendices providing additional useful information and resources.

If you have prostate problems now, the book provides a comprehensive discussion of your options and offers the opportunity to acquire the background knowledge necessary to understand the diagnosis, prognosis, and possible treatments along with the associated complications and side effects. This knowledge should enable a man to engage in a truly informed interaction with the physician or physicians involved in providing advice and treatment. Given that many of the decisions faced by a man with prostate problems are far from clear-cut, especially in the case of cancer, and that he is frequently given a choice among options, this knowledge turns out to be vital. On the other hand, if you are one of the lucky ones not yet experiencing problems, our book "The Prostate and Its Problems" may help you avoid them in the future.

This book is a thoroughly cooperative effort on the part of two authors, but it would not have been possible without the whole-hearted support of the wife of one of the authors, Judi Larsen, who was instrumental in seeing it come to fruition. Without her word processing skills, editing advice and encouragement, we could not have accomplished the task. Also acknowledged is the assistance of Hannah Koppenhoefer in connection with the artwork.

Hans R. Larsen
Victoria, BC, Canada

William R. Ware
London, ON, Canada

August 2006

INTRODUCTION

The Prostate and Its Problems

Hans R. Larsen MSc ChE

The prostate is a gland located in the pelvic area directly beneath the bladder. It surrounds the urethra (the tube that conducts urine from the bladder to the penis). The prostate is both a gland and a muscle. As a gland it produces a milky, alkaline fluid that is mixed with sperm (produced in the testicles) to produce the fluid (semen) ejaculated during sexual intercourse and masturbation. The prostate gland also contains an enzyme, 5-alpha-reductase, which converts testosterone to dihydrotestosterone. As a muscle the prostate works to propel seminal fluid through the urethra and out of the penis during ejaculation. The muscle part of the prostate also acts as a "gate" for the flow of urine. There are two shut-off valves that control urination, one (internal sphincter) at the junction of the bladder and the upper part of the prostate, the other (external sphincter) at the base (apex) of the prostate. Both are required to prevent incontinence and dribbling. The upper shut-off valve also prevents seminal fluid from "shooting backwards" into the bladder during ejaculation (retrograde ejaculation).

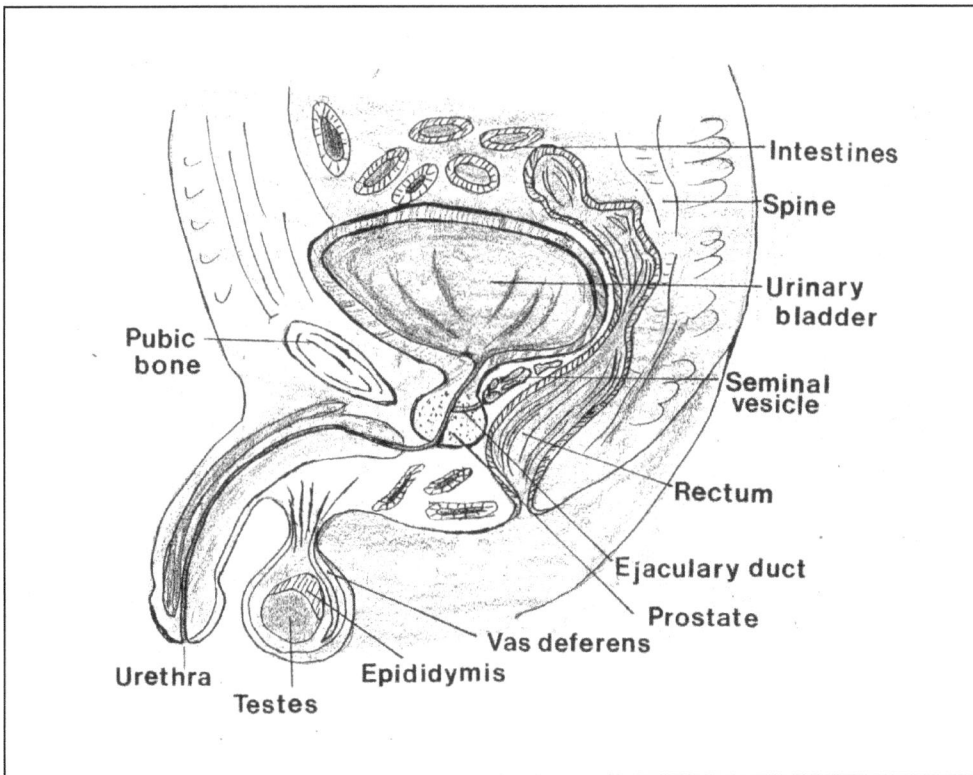

Figure 1-1. Male Pelvic Area

The prostate, prior to puberty, is quite small, about the size of a marble. It undergoes a rapid growth spurt during puberty and reaches the size of a walnut in adolescence. In middle age the prostate usually begins enlarging again and can exceed the size of a golf ball. The average weight of a normal adult prostate is 20-40 grams.

The prostate is surrounded by a dense fibrous capsule and can be divided into three zones – the peripheral zone, the central zone, and the transition zone.

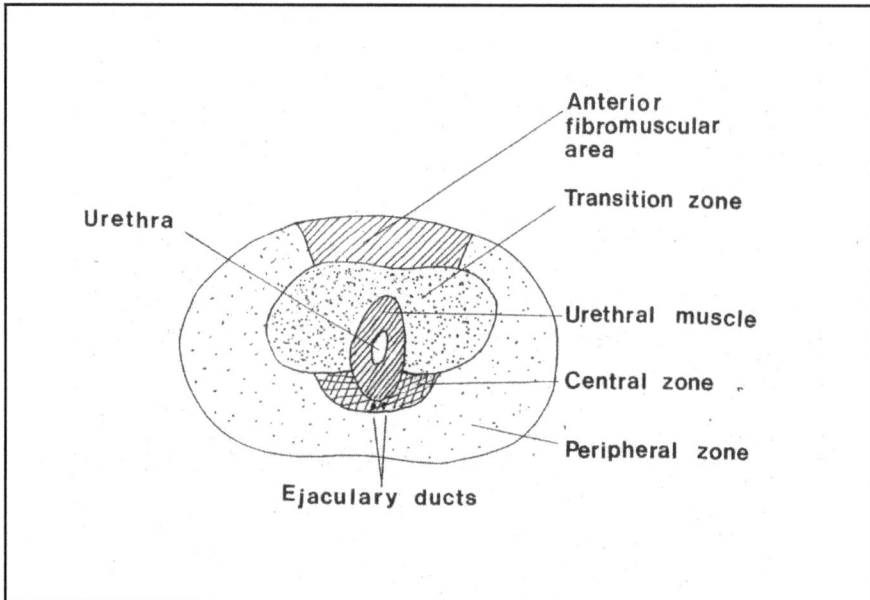

Figure 1-2. Prostate Cross-sectional View

The prostate contains three different types of cells:

- Stromal cells, which form the overall structure of the gland.
- Glandular cells, which produce a milky, alkaline fluid which, when mixed with sperm, become semen.
- Smooth muscle cells, which contract during sexual intercourse and squeeze the fluid produced by the glandular cells into the urethra. Here it mixes with semen and is then ejaculated through the penis.

As most men over the age of 50 years know only too well, the prostate is a prominent source of problems and discomfort, especially problems with urination and pain in the pelvic area. The three most common disease conditions associated with the prostate are prostatitis (inflamed prostate), prostate enlargement (benign prostatic hyperplasia or BPH), and the most feared of them all, prostate cancer. Both prostatitis and BPH usually manifest themselves through difficulties in urination (lower urinary tract symptoms or LUTS); thus it is important to understand how the urination (micturition) process works.

THE MICTURITION PROCESS

In infants, the micturition process is involuntary, in other words, it happens when it happens. However, after maturation of the nervous system the process becomes voluntary, in other words, the individual can control when and where to urinate. This control can be lost again as a result of aging, neural injury, or severe BPH. Losing control of normal bladder function is, unfortunately, very common. It is estimated that about 17 million men and women in the USA alone suffer from bladder control problems.[1]

The lower urinary tract (bladder, sphincters and urethra) is innervated by the two branches of the autonomic nervous system (ANS), the parasympathetic (vagal) branch and the sympathetic (adrenergic) branch, and also receives input from pudendal nerves originating in the somatic nervous system. These different nerves work in unison (most of the time) to control the two phases of the micturition cycle, the filling (storage) phase, and the voiding (elimination) phase. During the filling phase filtered urine flows from the kidneys through the ureter into the bladder. The bladder walls (detrusor muscle) are kept in a relaxed state by the combined action of the sympathetic and parasympathetic branches of the ANS and thus allows for filling. At the same time, sympathetic nerve activity keeps the bladder sphincter (shut-off valve) and urethra tightly closed so that leakage is avoided.

When the bladder reaches its storage capacity (about 100-150 mL or 3.5-5 ounces) a message is sent to the control center in the brain indicating that it is time for the emptying phase to begin. People without urinary dysfunction can, to a large extent, control the timing of voiding, but eventually the process must proceed. The voiding phase involves activation of vagal nerves in the bladder and expulsion of the urine through the bladder neck, sphincters and urethra. The successful voiding process needs the cooperation of the pudendal nerves and the sympathetic branch of the ANS to relax the sphincters and urethra and thus make voiding possible. It is also believed that the increased parasympathetic activity in the voiding cycle causes the release of nitric oxide, which further relaxes the outlet musculature.[2]

It is clear that the urination process is by no means simple and that things can easily go wrong. There is now evidence that some of the urinary difficulties (frequency, urgency, intermittent stream, and nocturia) involved in both prostatitis and BPH are, at least in part, due to excessive sympathetic activity which keeps the external sphincter and urethra compressed when they should be relaxed.[2,3]

The main neurotransmitter released by the nerve endings of the sympathetic branch is norepinephrine. It is well established that alpha-adrenoreceptor blockers, which inhibit the muscle-tightening effects of norepinephrine, can be helpful in dealing with prostatitis and BPH (see Chapters 1 and 2).

Sympathetic nervous system over-activity restricting urinary flow could potentially lead to a thickening of the bladder wall (development of more muscle power) in an attempt to overcome the obstruction. Obstruction of the urethra by overgrowth (BPH) can also result in the development of a thickened and overly muscular bladder wall (detrusor).

Thus, both prostatitis and BPH can affect bladder function and create a vicious feedback loop leading to a worsening of LUTS.

UNDERLYING CAUSES OF PROSTATE PROBLEMS

The three major prostate disorders, prostatitis, BPH and cancer, involve one or more of the following underlying problems:

- Uncontrolled cell growth (benign or malignant)
- Over-activity of the sympathetic nervous system (SNS)
- Bacterial infection
- Inflammation
- Neuromuscular spasm
- Severe emotional stress

Prostatitis may involve bacterial infection, inflammation, neuromuscular spasm, SNS over-activity and severe emotional stress. BPH involves SNS over-activity and benign, uncontrolled cell growth – or rather lack of controlled cell death (apoptosis). Prostate cancer involves malignant, uncontrolled cell growth and inhibited apoptosis and can, in the later stages, also involve LUTS due to pressure exerted on the urethra by the tumor.

PROSTATITIS

The name "prostatitis" is, unfortunately, somewhat misleading as neither the prostate nor an inflammation is necessarily involved. The causes, risk factors, prevention and treatment of this common disorder are discussed in detail in Chapter 1.

BENIGN PROSTATIC HYPERPLASIA (BPH)

The name "benign prostatic hyperplasia" or "enlarged prostate" is also, to some extent, a misnomer. Many cases of BPH do not involve an abnormally large prostate and are treated successfully with alpha-receptor blockers indicating that their main cause is SNS over-activity rather than overgrowth causing narrowing and pressure on the urethra. Furthermore, there is evidence that it is not really uncontrolled growth of benign cells in the transition zone (the zone bordering the urethra) that is the problem, but rather a lack of controlled cell death. The causes, risk factors, prevention and treatment of BPH are discussed in detail in Chapter 2.

PROSTATE CANCER

Prostate cancer involves the growth of abnormal (malignant) cells generally in the peripheral zone, most often close to the outer surface of the prostate. Prostate tumors thus do not, at least in the initial stages, put pressure on the urethra and thus produce no urinary symptoms. Because the tumors are on the outer part of the gland they can, however, often be felt during a digital rectal examination (DRE).

While neither prostatitis nor BPH are life-threatening in their own right, prostate cancer certainly is. Thus, the main part of this book is devoted to this disease. Chapter 3 discusses causes and risk factors. Chapter 4 covers diagnosis, and Chapter 5 is devoted to prevention. Chapter 6 and 7 discuss conventional treatment of localized and advanced cancer respectively, while Chapter 8 provides information about alternative treatments and specialized cancer clinics. Chapter 9 is devoted to a discussion of emerging trends in diagnosis, procedures and treatment for prostate problems.

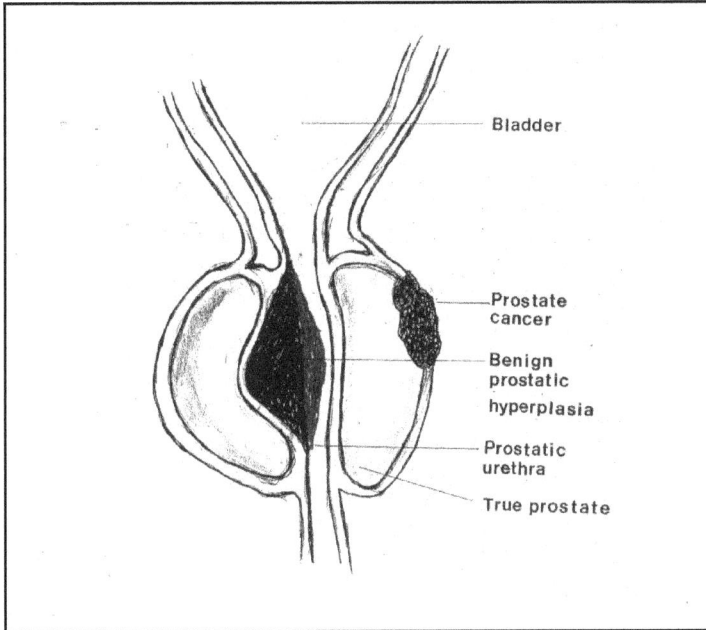

Figure 1-3. Location of BPH and Cancer

REFERENCES

1. Campbell's Urology, Saunders, Philadelphia, PA, 8th edition, 2002, p. 831
2. Campbell's Urology, Saunders, Philadelphia, PA, 8th edition, 2002, pp. 1027-1358
3. Yun, AJ and Doux, JD. Opening the floodgates: Benign prostatic hyperplasia may represent another disease in the compendium of ailments caused by the global sympathetic bias that emerges with aging. Medical Hypotheses, January 19, 2006

Chapter 1

Prostatitis

Hans R. Larsen MSc ChE

INTRODUCTION

Prostatitis is a poorly understood disease highly resistant to effective treatment. It is the most common urologic diagnosis in men below the age of 50 years and rivals BPH and prostate cancer incidence in men above the age of 50 years. More than 2 million visits to physicians in the USA every year are related to prostatitis and it is estimated that 26% of all men will have been diagnosed with prostatitis by the time they reach the age of 85 years.[1,2] The prevalence (percentage of men with the disease at any given point in time) is estimated at 10-16% in the USA, 13-14% in Europe, and about 9% in Malaysia.[3] It is clear that prostatitis not only blights the lives of many men, but also poses a significant burden on the health care system.

Prostatitis (inflammation of the prostate) is actually a misnomer as the disease may not involve inflammation and may not even be related to the prostate at all. In 1999 the National Institutes of Health agreed on standard definitions and classifications for the five different types of prostatitis found in clinical practice.[4]

NIH Classification System for Prostatitis	
Category I	Acute bacterial prostatitis
Category II	Chronic bacterial prostatitis
Category IIIA	Chronic inflammatory, nonbacterial prostatitis (symptomatic)
Category IIIB	Chronic non-inflammatory, nonbacterial prostatitis (symptomatic)
Category IV	Asymptomatic inflammatory prostatitis

CATEGORY I – ACUTE BACTERIAL PROSTATITIS

This form of prostatitis is quite rare probably accounting for only 2-5% of all cases. It is a serious condition that requires prompt treatment.[4]

SYMPTOMS AND DIAGNOSIS

Acute bacterial prostatitis involves a bacterial infection of the prostate and its main symptoms are pain in the pelvic/perineal area and frequent and painful urination. Since it is an acute infection, it is also often accompanied by fever, chills and general malaise. The diagnostic workup for patients suspected of having the condition involves physical examination (with gentle digital rectal examination), microscopic evaluation of a urine sample, a urine culture to determine the most appropriate antibiotic for treatment, and if systemic symptoms are present, cultures of blood samples. The patient's recent medical history is discussed with particular emphasis on the status of the immune system, recent urinary tract infections (UTIs), and recent medical tests such as cystoscopy, biopsies or use of catheters. The digital rectal examination (DRE) will usually reveal a tender prostate. The patient should also be assessed for urinary retention by palpating (feeling) the bladder or through an ultrasound scan.[4] The PSA (prostate specific antigen) is usually substantially elevated during the acute phase of category I prostatitis and it may take 2 to 3 months before it returns to normal even with optimum antibiotic treatment.[5] Clearly, a decision to have a prostate biopsy should not be based on a PSA value obtained within 3 months of the resolution of an acute prostatitis episode.

CAUSES AND RISK FACTORS

Category I acute bacterial prostatitis is associated with a lower urinary tract infection in most cases (65-80%) involving *Escherichia coli* (*E. coli*), a common bacteria found in the gastrointestinal tract. *Staphylococcus aureus*, *Pseudomonas* and other bacteria may also be involved.[1] It is believed that the condition is caused by an infection working its way up through the urethra and/or by reflux of infected urine into prostatic ducts.[6] The infectious bacteria can be transmitted through sexual intercourse (especially unprotected anal intercourse), from contaminated water, from swimming in a dirty pool or a contaminated lake, or from an infection elsewhere in the body. Acute prostatitis is often associated with a bladder infection.

PREVENTION

The most important preventive measure is to avoid the risk factors mentioned above and to maintain a generally good state of health, specifically a well-functioning immune system. It is also important to avoid bladder infections (cystitis) and if one does occur to eliminate it quickly. Cranberry juice or cranberry extract has been found quite effective in preventing and eliminating lower urinary tract infections.[7]

TREATMENT

If symptoms of general sepsis (fever, chills, general malaise) are present then hospitalization is frequently necessary. Treatment consists of intravenous administration of antibiotics (fluoroquinolones), intravenous hydration, and urinary drainage if urinary retention is an issue. Once the systemic symptoms are resolved treatment with antibiotics is usually continued for 3-4 weeks on an outpatient basis. As it is possible that the UTI initiating the prostatitis may be caused by stones, diverticula or anatomic abnormalities, it is also recommended that additional tests (ultrasound, CT scans, MRI) be performed in order to determine if an underlying cause can be found and eliminated.[4]

It is very important to supplement with live probiotics (*L. acidophilus, L. bifidus, L. casei,* etc.) during and for a couple of months after treatment with antibiotics, especially the broad-spectrum ones like fluoroquinolones. These antibiotics destroy the normal flora in the gut (large intestine) and their use can result in a nasty case of candidiasis, which can be very difficult to eradicate.[8]

CATEGORY II – CHRONIC BACTERIAL PROSTATITIS

The chronic form of bacterial prostatitis is also quite rare accounting for only 2-5% of all prostatitis diagnoses. Although chronic bacterial prostatitis shares many of the symptoms of the acute form, it is only rarely that category I prostatitis transforms into category II.[4]

SYMPTOMS AND DIAGNOSIS

Chronic bacterial prostatitis is a chronic or persistent infection of the prostate without the systemic involvement found in the acute form. It usually manifests itself as intermittent cystitis-like urinary symptoms (frequent and painful urination) accompanied by low level discomfort or pain in the pelvic area. A history of previous urinary tract infections is common among category II patients and should alert the physician to the diagnosis.[4]

The recommended diagnostic workup includes physical examination, medical history, urinalysis as well as referral for tests to determine potential causes of the UTIs. Urology textbooks also recommend that the Meares-Stamey localization test be performed.

The **Meares-Stamey test** is the gold standard for the diagnosis of prostatitis. The test involves the collection and analysis of three urine samples (before, during, and after prostatic massage) and one sample of prostatic secretion obtained by massage of the prostate (EPS or expressed prostatic secretion). Analysis of the samples makes it possible to determine whether bacteria and/or inflammation are present in the urethra, bladder and/or prostate.[4] The test is rarely used in today's time-constrained environment. Instead, a course of antibiotics is prescribed. If this solves the problem, then the diagnoses was probably category II prostatitis – if not, then further testing is warranted.[9,10]

CAUSES, RISK FACTORS AND PREVENTION

As in the case of acute bacterial prostatitis, category II prostatitis is caused by a bacterial infection, most often with *E. coli*. The risk factors are also similar to those for category I with special emphasis on recurrent bladder infections. Thus, the main preventive action required is to avoid such infections.

TREATMENT

The standard treatment for chronic bacterial prostatitis involves a 1-3 months course of prostate-penetrating antibiotics such as fluoroquinolones, trimethoprim-sulfamethoxazole (Septra), or trimethoprim (Protoprim). The cure rate is 60-80% with fluoroquinolones and about 30-50% with Septra and Protoprim. Overall, it is estimated that about one-third of category II patients have recurrences after a seemingly successful first treatment.[1] It is not clear why this is, but there is some speculation that stones (calculi) and other debris lodged in the ducts of the prostate may prevent the antibiotics from reaching and completely eliminating the infectious bacteria.[11]

Massage of the prostate gland, sort of an extended DRE, used to be a mainstay in the treatment of chronic prostatitis. It is possible that it may have had some beneficial effect by pushing debris and perhaps small stones out of the prostatic ducts, but it is rarely used nowadays.[10] However, there is some evidence that repetitive prostatic massage combined with antibiotic therapy may be beneficial in category II prostatitis. This approach was originally developed in the Philippines and has been evaluated by J.C. Nickel and colleagues at Queen's University in Canada. Their study involved 22 men who underwent tri-weekly prostatic massage combined with specific culture-directed antibiotic treatment for 6 to 12 weeks. The Canadian researchers conclude that 46% of the patients had a greater than 60% decrease (improvement) in symptom severity and suggest that a combination of prostatic massage and culture-specific antibiotics looks promising for the treatment of chronic bacterial prostatitis.[11]

It is possible that transurethral prostate resection (TURP) or injection of antibiotics directly into the prostate may result in a cure, but if not, lifelong medication with antibiotics in doses just high enough to prevent bladder infections may be the only option.[4]

Long-term treatment with **fluoroquinolones** such as ofloxacin (Floxin), ciprofloxacin (Cipro), and norploxacin (Noroxin) is, however, not without problems. Professor Jay S. Cohen of the University of California has identified 45 cases where patients developed serious adverse effects after taking Cipro or other fluoroquinolones. The primary reactions involved the peripheral nervous system and were manifested as numbness, twitching, spasms, tingling or burning pain. About 78% of the cases also had central nervous system involvement with symptoms such as dizziness, agitation, hallucination, and impaired cognitive function. Over 90% of the adverse reactions showed up within 2 weeks with 33% occurring within 24 hours of beginning treatment. Symptoms were often long-term in nature with 58% of patients having them for a year or more. In 40% of the cases the prescribing physician did not recognize the symptoms as a reaction to fluoroquinolones or dismissed their significance. Dr. Cohen concludes that fluoroquinolones such as Cipro are far from benign and should be used with great care. He also points out that less dangerous antibiotics such as penicillin and doxycycline are often all this is required to cure an infection.[12]

The potential problems with long-term use of fluoroquinolones are also highlighted in a study reported by a team of Dutch and British researchers. They found a significantly increased risk of Achilles tendon rupture and Achilles tendonitis in men using fluoroquinolones. The risk increased with age, dosage and concomitant use of corticosteroids (prednisone).[13] There are now also signs that some bacteria are becoming resistant to fluoroquinolones; a problem, no doubt, partly caused by the liberal prescription of the drugs for the nonbacterial types of prostatitis.[10] Antibiotics and especially fluoroquinolones can also cause nasty candida infections, both in the colon and on the head of the penis. They should not be taken without concomitant supplementation with probiotics.

CATEGORY III – NONBACTERIAL CHRONIC PROSTATITIS

Category III prostatitis, also known as **chronic pelvic pain syndrome** (CPPS), is by far the most common form and constitutes about 90-95% of all cases. It is characterized by the absence of detectable bacterial infection (Meares-Stamey test) and is further divided into two sub-categories – category IIIA where there is evidence of inflammation (presence of white blood cells in semen, post-DRE urine, and EPS), and category IIIB (also known as prostatodynia) where there is no evidence of inflammation.[14] Both categories share the characteristics of pain in the pelvic area (perineum, penis, scrotum, lower abdomen, back or groin), frequent, painful or difficult urination, and incomplete voiding of the bladder. Some patients also experience pain upon ejaculation, or erectile dysfunction.[4,15]

Although not life-threatening as such, CPPS can seriously affect quality of life. Several studies have shown that men with severe category III disease experience a quality of life comparable to that of patients with unstable angina, a recent heart attack, or Crohn's disease. Their mental outlook has been reported to be poorer than that of men with diabetes or congestive heart failure.[3] It is estimated that about 267,000 men between the ages of 25 and 84 years are diagnosed each year with category III prostatitis in the USA alone.[2]

Some treatment modalities are more applicable to category IIIA than to category IIIB. However, the two categories are usually combined in clinical studies and management recommendations. The following discussion adheres to this convention.

SYMPTOMS AND DIAGNOSIS

The most characteristic symptom of category III prostatitis is pain and this symptom is often the main distinguishing factor between prostatitis and benign prostatic hyperplasia (BPH). The pain is felt in the pelvic area specifically in the perineal area, the tip of the penis, scrotum, lower abdomen, back or groin, and may or may not originate from the prostate itself. Urinary symptoms are similar to those experienced in BPH, lower urinary tract infections (UTIs), and category I and II prostatitis. These symptoms, also known as LUTS (lower urinary tract symptoms) include frequent, difficult or painful urination, incomplete voiding of the bladder, and urgency.[2,4]

The recommended diagnostic workup for suspected category III prostatitis includes a physical examination with DRE, medical history, urinalysis and urine culture (pre and post DRE), and examination and tests to find possible causes of the UTI. The Meares-Stamey test is rarely used due to the time and effort involved in its execution. In interpreting the results of the diagnostic tests, it needs to be kept in mind that the symptoms of category III prostatitis can mimic those of lower urinary tract obstruction, bladder stones, ejaculatory duct obstruction, testicular cancer, and other chronic pain syndromes such as fibromyalgia.[4]

The initial evaluation in case of suspected category III prostatitis may also include the completion of the NIH-CPSI (National Institutes of Health Chronic Prostatitis Symptom Index) questionnaire. It includes questions designed to determine the source and severity of pain, the nature and degree of urinary difficulties, and the impact of the condition on the patient's quality of life (see Appendix D). The completed questionnaire is useful in directing treatment and measuring its benefit. [1,9,10]

There is, unfortunately, no agreement as yet as to what range of values (1-8, etc) would constitute mild, moderate, and severe prostatitis.[9,10]

Although the protocol to be followed in diagnosing men with suspected category III prostatitis is well described in urology textbooks and major review articles, it is probably rarely used in practice. It is time-consuming and expensive, so most GPs and urologists follow a more empirical approach by prescribing a 3-6 week course of antibiotics, perhaps accompanied by an anti-inflammatory and an alpha-blocker to relieve urinary symptoms. If this treatment resolves the problem then all is well – if not, then further evaluation and testing is clearly indicated. [4,9,10]

Prostatitis, PSA and LUTS
Some physicians also order a PSA (prostate specific antigen) test as part of the routine examination. This may produce misleading results in the case of suspected category III prostatitis or chronic pelvic pain syndrome (CPPS). As mentioned earlier, PSA levels can increase dramatically during the acute phase of category I prostatitis. Values as high as 50-100 ng/mL are not uncommon and it can take up to 6 months after the infection is resolved before PSA levels return to normal. [9] It is believed that inflammation disrupts the barriers that normally keep PSA within the prostate thus allowing it to escape into the blood stream resulting in higher test results.[5] Yaman *et al.* at the University of Ankara have found that PSA levels increase with increasing aggressiveness of inflammation in the prostate.[16]

The situation in case of category III prostatitis is similar, at least as far as category IIIA (inflammatory) is concerned. Caleb Bozeman and colleagues at Louisiana State University performed PSA testing on 95 men diagnosed with category IIIA prostatitis and found that they had an average PSA level of 8.48 ng/mL. The men were scheduled for biopsies, but were first given a 4-week course of antibiotics (fluoroquinolones or doxycycline) and anti-inflammatories (ibuprofen or celecoxib). At the end of the 4 weeks, 44 of the men (46.3%) had experienced a significant reduction in PSA level (to an average of 2.48 ng/mL) and their biopsies were cancelled. The researchers conclude that treatment of chronic prostatitis in men with high PSA levels can substantially reduce the need for biopsies. They also noted that PSA levels in men diagnosed with cancer following the 4-week treatment period only experienced an insignificant drop in PSA from 8.32 to 7.92 ng/mL on average.[17]

Other researchers have found average PSA values as high as 28.5 ng/mL among patients diagnosed with chronic, inflammatory prostatitis [18]. There is no indication that PSA levels are increased in non-inflammatory (category IIIB) prostatitis.

Porter *et al*. at the Virginia Mason Medical Center in Seattle determined severity of LUTS according to the American Urologic Association Symptom Score (AUAS – See Appendix E) in 569 patients who had undergone needle biopsy of the prostate guided by transrectal ultrasound (TRUS). They found a clear association between a low AUAS score (<8) and a positive biopsy result. They conclude that a low AUASS score (indicative of the absence of benign disease) is an important predictor of prostate cancer.[19] The conclusions form these studies are:

- Men with an elevated PSA level suspected of having prostatitis should undergo a 3-4 week course of antibiotics and anti-inflammatories before a decision regarding biopsy is made.

- Men with severe LUTS are less likely to have prostate cancer than are men with a low AUAS score.

CAUSES OF CHRONIC PELVIC PAIN SYNDROME

Before one can even begin to hope to understand the causes of category III prostatitis (chronic non-bacterial prostatitis), it is necessary to erase the name from one's memory and instead focus on the alternative name of the condition – **chronic pelvic pain syndrome or CPPS**. This designation corresponds much closer to reality since the pain experienced in CPPS may not originate in the prostate at all, and the condition may or may not involve inflammation.

The frustration of not knowing the cause of CPPS is shared by patient and physician alike and is aptly described in statements like the following:

"Despite its prevalence and its drain on health care resources, our understanding of the etiology, diagnosis and treatment of prostatitis has not advanced with that of other prostate diseases."[6]

"The prostatitis syndromes are some of the most prevalent conditions in urology, but also the most poorly understood."[20]

"Prostatitis is an ill-defined condition without clear-cut diagnostic criteria and treatment strategies."[21]

"By contrast, the much more common nonbacterial prostatitis and prostatodynia syndromes remain an enigma, both in etiology, appropriate work-up and therapy."[15]

"In contrast, chronic prostatitis/chronic pelvic pain syndrome (category III), which accounts for 90-95% of prostatitis cases, is of unknown etiology and is marked by a mixture of pain, urinary, and ejaculatory symptoms with no uniformly effective therapy."[4]

So in other words, we don't know what causes CPPS, we don't know how to diagnose it accurately, and we don't know how to treat it effectively.

Research into CPPS is ongoing and recent findings have shed some light on the condition. The most common symptoms of CPPS are:[2]

- Dysuria (difficult and painful urination) – 46.6%
- Perineal pain (pain in area between rectum and testicles) – 34.4%
- Frequent need to urinate – 39.2%
- Pain in the bladder/suprapubic area – 39.2%

CPPS does not necessarily involve inflammation and is perhaps more likely to be a bladder problem or a problem with the musculature of the pelvic floor (perineal bundle). Says urologist Stephen Jones MD of the Cleveland Clinic, "If the prostate is not tender on DRE then prostate inflammation is not the problem." According to Dr. Jones many of his patients actually suffer from a muscle spasm in the perineal muscle bundle, a condition that certainly would fall under the umbrella term CPPS, but has nothing to do with the prostate.[10]

Dr. Regula Doggweiler Wiygul MD, a prostatitis expert at the University of Tennessee wonders if CPPS and interstitial/painful bladder syndrome are the same disease. Dr. Wiygul also believes that neurogenic inflammation, that is, inflammation caused by the release of certain neuropeptides from sympathetic nerve endings play a role in CPPS-related inflammation. She also suggests that myofascial pain syndrome (similar to that encountered in fibromyalgia) may be involved in CPPS-related pain, particularly in the pelvic floor (perineum) muscle bundle.[22]

Drs. Michel Pontari and Michael Ruggieri at Temple University School of Medicine have studied CPPS in detail and reached the following conclusions:[14]

- There is no correlation between the number of white blood cells (an indication of inflammation) in semen, EPS or post-DRE urine and degree of pain indicating that degree of inflammation and pain are not related. This is further supported by the fact that category IV prostatitis can involve extensive inflammation, but no pain.

- It is possible that high levels of pro-inflammatory cytokines (signalling molecules) may be involved, as may inhibitors of pro-inflammatory cytokines, especially IL-10. There is some evidence that high levels of pro-inflammatory cytokines and low levels of their inhibitors are associated with pelvic pain.

- Only 33% of CPPS patients undergoing prostate biopsy are actually found to have signs of inflammation leading to the question, "Is the prostate even actually involved in the symptoms of CPPS?"

- Testosterone seems to dampen inflammation. This may be why 5-alpha reductase inhibitors such as finasteride sometimes help; presumably because they prevent the conversion of testosterone to dihydrotestosterone (DHT) thereby maintaining a higher level of testosterone.

- Mast cells (large cells located in connective tissue) when activated release, among other compounds, histamine and nerve growth factor (NGF) and NGF concentration correlates closely with pain severity.

- Psychological stress is a common feature in men with CPPS and can activate mast cells and thus indirectly increase pain. Psychological stress may also be involved in precipitating a spasm in the pelvic floor muscle bundle and thus result in pain.[10]

- Depression correlates with lower levels of IL-10, a potent inhibitor of pro-inflammatory cytokines; thus, depression could presumably indirectly result in an increase in pain level.

- It is likely that oxidative stress is involved in the process leading to pain, thus explaining why antioxidants like quercetin have been found helpful.

Drs. Pontari and Ruggieri conclude that, "The symptoms of CPPS appear to result from an interplay between psychological factors and dysfunction in the immune, neurological and endocrine systems."[14]

Researchers at the University of Washington School of Medicine have found a clear correlation between stress and subsequent pain and disability among men with CPPS.[23] Another study carried out at Queen's University in Canada confirmed a strong correlation between poor quality of life and a high level of pain in CPPS patients.[24] The results of this study prompted Richard E. Berger MD to comment, "This study suggests that better use of pain medications and antidepressive therapy may improve the quality of life in many men with pelvic pain. Perhaps our treatment would be better directed at palliating the symptoms of prostatitis rather than administering frequent ineffectual courses of antibiotics."[25]

Some researchers believe that congestion of the prostate could be involved in prostatitis[3,21]; however, others dismiss this possibility. Prostate congestion involves a feeling of fullness or pressure in the area of the prostate. It results from the build-up of semen that has not been released through ejaculation. The prostate has a built-in feedback system, which adjusts semen production to the level of sexual activity. If this level is decreased due to abstinence for extended periods of time, then the prostate can become congested with accumulated semen.

There is evidence that stones (calculi) can form in the ducts of the prostate. Cleveland Clinic researchers estimate that about 20% of men with CPPS have calculi in their prostates.[26] Bedir *et al* at the Gulhane Military Academy in Ankara, Turkey report the case of a 50-year-old man with many calculi in his prostate as indicated on DRE and x-rays. The Turkish urologists removed more than 30 stones endoscopically and analyzed their composition. They all consisted of a mixture of calcium phosphate (apatite) and calcium carbonate. After removal of the stones the patient recovered fully from the urinary retention problem that had brought him to the hospital.[27] There is also evidence that reflux of urine into the intraprostatic ducts can result in stone formation and perhaps the formation of urate crystals.[1,6] Stones or urate crystals in the ducts of the prostate could clearly lead to inflammation and pain.

It is abundantly clear from the above that CPPS is a multifactorial disease and needs to be treated as such using elements from drug therapy, phytotherapy, physical therapy, Chinese medicine and, as a last resort, surgery.

RISK FACTORS AND PREVENTION

In view of the significant pain and disability caused by CPPS, it is clearly important to know what, if any, factors might increase the risk of developing the disorder and what can be done to prevent it.

RISK FACTORS

A team of researchers from Harvard Medical School, Brigham and Women's Hospital, Harvard School of Public Health, and Massachusetts General Hospital surveyed 31,681 male American health professionals and found that 5,053 (16%) had, at some point, been diagnosed with prostatitis (category not specified). A majority of these men (57.2%) also had a history of BPH indicating that the two disorders are often coexistent (or improperly diagnosed). There was a clear indication that the probability of receiving a diagnosis of prostatitis increased with age. However, the average age of men with prostatitis was generally about 10 years younger than the average age of men with BPH. Other factors found to affect the risk of prostatitis include:[21]

- Not working full or part time
- A history of BPH
- A history of sexually transmitted disease
- A history of lower urinary tract symptoms
- A vasectomy
- A family history of prostate cancer
- Moderate alcohol consumption (1-2 drinks a day)
- Severe stress at work or at home

Most of the above factors only affected risk to a very limited degree. However, a prior history of BPH increased risk by 7.7 times and a history of severe voiding symptoms increased it by a factor of 2.8. No correlation was observed between bicycle riding and prostatitis risk; however, other researchers have noted such a correlation, as well as a correlation between prolonged sitting (nerve entrapment) and risk.[22,28]

Ja Hyeon Ku and colleagues at the Seoul National University College of Medicine in South Korea have presented a survey of known risk factors for prostatitis.[3]

- They found no significant differences in the prevalence of prostatitis among younger (less than 50 years of age) and older (more than 50 years of age) men and conclude that age, as such, is not a significant risk factor.

- The association with race and socioeconomic stage is unclear as is the possible effect of different kinds of physical activity.

- Having a sexually transmitted disease is associated with greater risk of prostatitis, but frequency of sexual intercourse is not.

- A history of BPH and urinary tract infections is associated with an increased risk of prostatitis, as is exposure to colonoscopy and severe stress at home and at work.

- Symptoms tend to be more severe during the winter months perhaps indicating that sunlight exposure or vitamin D deficiency could play a role.

A previous history of BPH and urinary tract infections are the strongest risk factors for prostatitis with stress, exposure to colonoscopy and sexually transmitted diseases being less significant factors.

PREVENTION

With the great uncertainty still surrounding the causes of CPPS and the lack of clearly-defined risk factors, except for BPH and LUTS, it is difficult to propose an effective prevention protocol. However, the following measures may be appropriate:

- Avoid prostatic congestion by avoiding sexual practices that may lead to accumulation of semen or prevent ejaculation.

- Prevent the development of BPH using the measures outlined in Chapter 2.

- Protect against sexually transmitted diseases

- Ensure an adequate intake of dietary antioxidants (vitamin A, vitamin C, vitamin E, beta-carotene, alpha-lipoic acid, selenium, resveratrol or grape seed extract) to prevent oxidative stress, which has been implicated in the etiology of CPPS.

- Treat infections of any kind promptly.

- Be alert to the symptoms of lower urinary tract infections (UTIs) and treat them promptly. Cranberry juice or capsules containing concentrated cranberry juice extract (*CranActin* or *Cran-UTI*) are quite effective in washing away bacteria clinging to the walls of the bladder and urethra.[7]

- Supplement with natural anti-inflammatories on a regular basis. Quercetin, turmeric, or Boswellia are good choices.

- There is some indication that men with CPPS have low magnesium levels in prostatic fluids[29]; however, there is no evidence that magnesium supplementation is helpful.

TREATMENT OF CHRONIC PELVIC PAIN SYNDROME

Even though the causes of CPPS are not well understood, there are pharmaceutical drugs, herbal therapies, physical treatments, minimally invasive procedures, and multimodal approaches that have proven somewhat effective in dealing with both the pain and urinary symptoms of CPPS. Some of these therapies are useful on their own, while others are used in various combinations reflecting the multi-factorial origins of CPPS.

PHARMACEUTICAL THERAPY

Although there is no evidence from clinical trials that antibiotics are effective in the treatment of CPPS which, by definition, is not caused by a bacterial infection, most GPs and urologists treating CPPS start out with a 3-6 week course of antibiotics.[1,6,9] The rationale for this is that laboratory tests may have missed the presence of bacteria, that some antibiotics may have independent anti-inflammatory properties, and that empirical evidence shows that a good proportion of CPPS patients improve if given antibiotics.[1,9] It is, of course, also possible that a large measure of the placebo effect plays a role here.[1] In any case, most physicians agree that treatment with antibiotics should not be continued if it has not proven effective at the end of 6 weeks.

Treatment with antibiotics is often combined with a dose of alpha-adrenergic receptor blocker such as tamsulosin (Flomax).[1,6,20] The rationale for this is that the alpha-blocker may improve urinary flow and thus help the antibiotics penetrate further into the prostate.[20] Some smaller trials have shown the combination to be effective, but a recent, large, randomized, double-blind trial found that neither fluoroquinolones (ciprofloxacin) nor tamsulosin nor their combination had a significant effect on pain or urinary difficulty scores (NIH-CPSI score, see Appendix D).[30] The clinical trial involved 196 men with CPPS who were treated in 10 different urology outpatient clinics. The men had suffered from CPPS for an average of 6.2 years and had a minimum NIH-CPSI score of 15. The study participants were randomized to receive a placebo, 500 mg of ciprofloxacin twice a day, 0.4 mg of tamsulosin once a day, or a combination of the two drugs. The treatment lasted for 6 weeks at which point the men were reassessed using the NIH-CPSI; they were also reassessed 9 and 12 months after beginning the treatment to evaluate long-term response. At baseline, the average total NIH-CPSI score for the men was 25 with pain score making up 12 of this, urinary score accounted for 5, and the remaining 8 related to quality-of-life. At the end of the 6-week trial period, the total score had decreased by 5 points (2 for pain, 1 for urinary difficulties, and 2 for quality-of-life). The group on ciprofloxacin scored slightly better after treatment, but the difference was not statistically significant. The percentage of men reporting marked to moderate improvement after the 6-week treatment was 22% in the placebo group, 22% in the ciprofloxacin group, 24% in the tamsulosin group, and 11% in the combination group. The researchers conclude that their data do not support the use of ciprofloxacin, tamsulosin or their combination in the treatment of men with long-standing CPPS and at least moderate symptoms according to the NIH-CPSI score.[30]

It is also common practice to prescribe NSAIDs or COX-2 inhibitors to men suffering pain from CPPS and, in many cases, they do indeed help ameliorate the pain.[1,6,9]

The use of finasteride (5-alpha-reductase inhibitor) to alleviate CPPS has also been evaluated. The rationale for this is that finasteride may improve urinary flow by shrinking the prostate and may also indirectly help reduce inflammation by maintaining higher testosterone levels. A recent clinical trial evaluated finasteride in 64 men diagnosed with CPPS. The men had all been on antibiotics previously for at least 3 weeks and 82% had also been treated with alpha-receptor blockers. The men were randomized to receive either 325 mg/day of saw palmetto or 5 mg/day of finasteride for the 1-year study period. At the end of the study, the average NIH-CPSI score had decreased from 23.9 to 18.1 in the finasteride group and from 24.7 to 24.6 in the saw palmetto group. Urinary symptoms did not improve in the finasteride group. The researchers conclude that finasteride may improve pain and quality-of-life scores in CPPS.[31]

Muscle relaxants such as baclofen and diazepam have also been suggested as means of ameliorating pain in CPPS, but there is no clinical evidence that they are effective.

There clearly is no one magic drug that will help reduce the symptoms of CPPS let alone eliminate them. However, some agents have shown promise and may help certain subgroups of men.

PHYTOTHERAPY

Because of the limited success obtained with pharmaceutical drugs, many CPPS sufferers and even the medical profession itself have investigated the possible benefits of herbal therapy. The most investigated and promising agents for the treatment of CPPS are quercetin, Cernilton (bee pollen), saw palmetto, and small-flowered willow herb (*Epilobium parviflorum*).

Quercetin is a naturally occurring bioflavonoid found in green tea, onions, and red wine. It has documented anti-inflammatory, antioxidant, and nitric oxide-inhibiting properties. Several studies have shown it to be effective in the treatment of chronic prostatitis, particularly the non-bacterial form (CPPS). Daniel Shoskes and colleagues at the University of California Medical Center evaluated the effect of supplementation with 500 mg of quercetin twice daily in a group of 30 men diagnosed with CPPS (inflammatory or non-inflammatory). The men were randomized to receive a placebo or quercetin for one month and were then re-evaluated using the NIH-CPSI score. The score decreased from 20.2 to 18.8 (not significant) in the placebo group, but decreased a very significant 38% (from 21.0 to 13.1) in the quercetin group. Two-thirds (67%) of men taking quercetin had an improvement in symptoms of at least 25% as compared to only 20% of the placebo group experiencing a 25% improvement. In a follow-up experiment, 17 patients were treated with a proprietary formulation (*Prosta-Q*) containing quercetin as well as bromelain and papain to aid in quercetin absorption. In this group, 82% experienced at least a 25% improvement in symptom score. Quercetin was particularly effective in reducing pain and improving quality-of-life score. The researchers conclude that quercetin gives significant symptomatic relief in men with non-bacterial chronic prostatitis (CPPS).[32]

Cernilton or cernitin is bee pollen gathered from the rye flower. At least two clinical trials have found it to be effective in alleviating CPPS symptoms. In 1989 Buck *et al* reported that 13 out of 15 patients with CPPS experienced complete and lasting relief or a marked improvement after supplementing with cernilton.[33] The same group later reported that cernilton also was effective in alleviating symptoms of BPH.[34] A 1993 follow-up study by Rugendorff *et al* at the University of Gottingen confirmed Buck's findings. The clinical trial involved 90 patients with CPPS who were treated with one tablet of *Cernilton N* three times daily for 6 months. The group consisted of 72 men with no complicating factors and 18 men who did have complicating factors like urethral strictures, prostatic calculi (stones), or bladder neck sclerosis. Among the 72 men with no complicating factors, 78% had a favorable response, with 36% being completely cured and 42% improving significantly. In the group with complicating factors, only one patient showed a response. Cernilton was well-tolerated by 97% of the patients.[35]

Saw palmetto is being used successfully in the treatment of BPH [36] (see Chapter 2). However, there are no clinical trials indicating that it is effective in the treatment of CPPS. As a matter of fact, one trial comparing finasteride and saw palmetto in the treatment of CPPS found no beneficial effect of saw palmetto.[31,37] Unfortunately, the authors of the trial did not specify the brand of saw palmetto used. It is well known that the effectiveness of saw palmetto extracts is highly dependent on the solvent used in the extraction process. The German prescription product *Permixon* is extracted with hexane and is the most effective and the one most often used in successful clinical trials.

Small-flowered willow herb (*Epilobium parviflorum*) is a well known folk remedy for the treatment of prostate problems, including BPH and prostatitis.[38] In 2006 Steenkamp *et al* at the University of Pretoria in South Africa evaluated 5 herbal remedies that have reputed benefits in the treatment of BPH and prostatitis, included among them were small-flowered willow herb, *pygeum africanum, Serenoa serrulata* (a form of saw palmetto), *Agathosma betulina*, and *Hypoxis hemero callidea*, two plants native to South

Africa. The researchers found that *Epilobium*, both as a tea and ethanol extract was highly effective in inhibiting the growth of E. coli in culture; the ethanol extract was substantially more effective than the water extract (tea). The ethanol extract of *Epilobium* was also very effective as both a COX-1 and COX-2 inhibitor in culture experiments and showed significant antioxidant activity. The South African researchers conclude, "Although these results support the traditional use of *Epilobium parviflorum* for treatment of BPH and prostatitis, further investigation is required for this promising plant."[39]

PHYSICAL THERAPY

Dr. Stephen Jones of the Cleveland Clinic believes that much of the pain involved in CPPS stems from a spasm or a myofascial trigger point (a specific point on a muscle at which application of pressure will elicit pain) in the perineal muscle bundle supporting the pelvic floor. He suggests hot sitz baths and sitting on a donut-shaped cushion for relief.[10] Other physical therapies mainly aimed at pain relief include acupuncture, biofeedback, high-frequency electrostimulation, and electromagnetic stimulation.

Acupuncture
Acupuncture is effective in providing pain relief and is also capable of adjusting the balance between the sympathetic and parasympathetic branches of the autonomic nervous system (ANS).[40-42] Since CPPS involves pain and likely an ANS dysfunction as evidenced by voiding difficulties, it is not surprising that acupuncture has been found effective in the treatment of prostatitis. Canadian researchers evaluated the benefits of acupuncture in 12 men with CPPS. The men had all been treated unsuccessfully with antibiotics, alpha-blockers, anti-inflammatories, and phytotherapy. They were given twice-weekly treatments for 6 weeks and were then followed for an average of 33 weeks. The treatment employed 30 needles 8 of which were electrically stimulated. At the 33-week point, average total NIH-CPSI scores had dropped from 28.2 to 8.5, pain score from 14.1 to 4.8, urinary symptoms score from 5.2 to 1.3, and quality-of-life score improved from 8.8 to 2.3. Eighty-three per cent of the patients had a sustained greater than 50% decrease in NIH-SPSI score at their final visit (average of 33 weeks). The researchers conclude that acupuncture is a safe, effective and durable therapy for CPPS.[43]

Japanese researchers have found acupuncture highly effective in treating CPPS accompanied by intrapelvic venous congestion (accumulation of blood in the veins draining the pelvic area).[44] Chinese medical researchers treated 200 patients with CPPS with acupuncture and mild moxibustion (heating of the needles with smouldering cones of herbs) and observed remarkable improvement. They conclude that acupuncture improves blood circulation in the prostate, inhibits or kills pathogenic micro-organisms, strengthens and regulates immune function, and relieves obstruction in the prostatic ducts.[45]

Biofeedback
At least two studies have evaluated the use of biofeedback in the treatment of CPPS. Ye, *et al* at the Huazhong University of Science and Technology in China treated 62 men with CPPS with biofeedback with excellent results. All the men had previously been

treated unsuccessfully with antibiotics and alpha-blockers. The patients were treated with biofeedback 5 times a week for 2 weeks (20-minute sessions). At the end of the treatments 60 patients (97%) were significantly improved or cured with no apparent side effects. Pain was relieved after 2-3 treatments and other symptoms disappeared after 4-5 treatments.[46] Clemens, *et al* at Northwestern University Medical School in Chicago believe that a pelvic floor muscle spasm may be a crucial factor in many cases of CPPS. They enrolled 19 men with CPPS in a 12-week program of bi-weekly biofeedback sessions aimed at bladder training and at relieving the spasm and preventing its recurrence. The patients were assessed using the American Urological Association (AUA) score (see Appendix D) at the beginning and end of the treatment period. Overall, AUA score decreased from 15.0 to 7.5, pain score from 5.0 to 2.0, and the average urgency score decreased from 5.0 to 2.0. Median voiding interval increased from 0.88 hours to 3.0 hours. The Chicago researchers conclude that a formalized program of neuromuscular re-education of the pelvic floor muscles together with interval bladder training can significantly and permanently improve CPPS symptoms.[47]

High-Frequency Electrostimulation

John Hubert and colleagues at the Zurich University Hospital in Switzerland have developed an electrostimulation device which markedly reduces symptoms of CPPS. The device consists of a frequency generator with two probes; one is inserted into the urethra and one is inserted into the rectum. The frequency-generator generates impulses with a frequency of 450-500 Hz and a voltage of 6 volts. The current flow can be set by the patient (between 1 and 10 mA) to a level where the patient feels a distinct, but tolerable tingling sensation in the pelvic floor (perineum). The device was tested on 14 men with non-inflammatory CPPS. They underwent twice-weekly, 30-minute sessions for 5 weeks. The overall, average NIH-CPSI score decreased from 29 prior to treatment to 14 after treatment, pain score decreased from 15 to 7, urinary complaint score from 2.5 to 1, and quality-of-life score improved from 9.5 to 5.5. The Swiss researchers conclude that the new device is effective in relieving symptoms of non-inflammatory CPPS (category IIIB). The device is technically simple and can be used by the patient at home.[48]

Low-Frequency Electromagnetic Stimulation

Urologists at St. Mary's Hospital in London, England also believe that pelvic floor spasms and exaggerated neural sensitivity are the underlying factors in many cases of CPPS. They evaluated the use of electromagnetic therapy targeting the pelvic floor (perineum) as a means of reducing the spasm and accompanying pain. Twenty-one men with CPPS were randomized to receive placebo treatments or twice-weekly electromagnetic treatments for 4 weeks using a *Neotonus* electromagnetic chair. The active treatment sessions consisted of pelvic floor stimulation for 15 minutes at 10 Hz followed by a further 15 minutes at 50 Hz. During the placebo treatments the electromagnetic pulse generator was switched off. The men were evaluated at baseline, and at 3 months and 1 year after the end of treatment. The mean pain score decreased by 45% in the active treatment group, but remained unchanged in the placebo group after 1 year. Average urinary symptoms scores decreased by 32% in the active treatment group after 3 months, but reverted to baseline after 1 year. No significant change was observed in the placebo group. The British researchers conclude that pelvic floor electromagnetic therapy may be a promising new non-invasive option for CPPS.[49]

MINIMALLY INVASIVE THERAPIES

These therapies are similar to those used in the treatment of BPH (see Chapter 2) and are considered last resorts for the treatment of CPPS. While some trials have shown positive results, there is no data indicating whether the benefits are long-term or only temporary.

Hyperthermia (heat therapy) can be delivered transrectally (via the rectum) or transurethrally (via the urethra). The heat source is usually microwave energy. It is believed that hyperthermia works by eliminating hidden bacterial infections and by destroying some sensory nerves and alpha-adrenoreceptors.[50]   Transrectal hyperthermia has not gained wide acceptance among urologists as its efficacy is limited due to the difficulty in obtaining high enough temperatures in the prostate without damaging the rectum.[50]

Transurethral thermotherapy or TUMT (see Chapter 2) has been evaluated by Nickel and Sorenson in two small studies. They found the procedure useful for the treatment of category IIIA (inflammatory) CPPS, but not for the treatment of category IIIB (non-inflammatory) CPPS. The treatment was found to elevate prostate interstitial temperature to between 45° and 60° C and resulted in significant improvement (greater than 50%) in 70% of patients.[51,52]   Choi, *et al* evaluated 78 patients with CPPS using TUMT. The study participants underwent a 1–hour session of TUMT using the *Prostatron* equipment. Complete symptom disappearance was obtained in 23% of the men and a partial response occurred in 43%.[53]

Transurethral needle ablation or TUNA (see Chapter 2) has been evaluated by Taiwanese, Korean and Finnish researchers. Results are mixed. While the Taiwanese and Korean groups found TUNA to be beneficial, the Finnish researchers found it no better than sham treatment.[54-56]

MULTIMODAL THERAPIES

Because of the relatively poor response achieved with standard conventional monotherapies, some specialized urological centers have developed protocols which encompass a series of different treatments. Daniel Shoskes and colleagues at the Cleveland Clinic in Florida report good results with a multimodal approach involving antibiotics, prostatic massage, alpha-receptor blockers, quercetin, and neuromuscular agents. A clinical trial of this approach included 53 patients with chronic prostatitis; 13% of the cases were category II, 41% were category IIIA, and the remaining 46% were category IIIB. The average (mean) age of the patients was 45 years and they had been suffering from chronic prostatitis for an average (median) of 3.5 years. Antibiotics were used first for 2-4 weeks if they had never been used before, or had proven effective for a previous episode. Prostatic massage was performed once to twice weekly in patients who had felt benefit from the first massage administered to all participants in order to obtain expressed prostatic secretions (EPS) for diagnosis. Patients who had significant urinary problems were also given tamsulosin. If the above treatment was not effective then quercetin (*Prosta-Q*) was administered and, as a last measure, neuromuscular agents such as amytriptyline and gabapentin were tried. The results of the trial were as follows:[57]

- Sixteen patients were initially treated with antibiotics because of good previous response or positive cultures. Ten of the patients also received prostatic massage and two received tamsulosin. A beneficial response was noted in 9 patients, 6 of whom had received both antibiotics and prostatic massage; however, 5 of the 9 patients experienced recurrence of their symptoms once the treatment stopped.

- Thirty patients were treated with quercetin and 6 patients were treated with quercetin and tamsulosin combined. Twenty-five (83%) of those treated with quercetin were deemed cured and required no further treatment. Three of the 6 patients (50%) on the quercetin/tamsulosin combination were also deemed cured.

- Of the 17 patients not helped by the above protocols, 10 were given tamsulosin which proved effective in 7 patients.

- Eight patients received amytriptyline alone or in combination with gabapentin and this was effective in 3 patients.

The study participants were followed for an average of 417 days at which time their NIH-CPSI score was measured and compared to their baseline score. Pain score decreased from an average of 10.4 to 5.9, urinary symptom score from 4.2 to 2.0, quality-of-life score from 8.2 to 4.7, and overall score from 22.7 to 13.2. An overall global subjective assessment concluded that 80% of the patients had improved. The researchers conclude that a step-wise approach using antibiotics, anti-inflammatories (quercetin), and neuromuscular agents can be successful in the majority of patients with long-standing chronic prostatitis.[57]

CHELATION

It is estimated that about 20% of CPPS patients have stones (calculi) in their prostates. These may contribute to inflammation and pain on their own, or prevent effective treatment by clogging up the prostatic ducts. The stones consist mainly of apatite (calcium phosphate) and are thought to be formed by reflux of nanobacteria in urine into the prostatic ducts. Nanobacteria (newly-discovered, small microorganisms with the ability to form calcium phosphate crystals at neutral pH) are also believed to be responsible for calcification of arteries.

Daniel Shoskes and his team at the Florida Cleveland Clinic recently evaluated a multimodal chelation therapy for dissolving prostatic calculi. Fifteen men who had failed all previous therapies and had evidence of prostatic calculi on transrectal ultrasound (TRUS) participated in the trial. The average age of the men was 45 years and the patients had suffered from category III prostatitis (CPPS) for an average of 6.3 years. Seven of the men had category IIIA (inflammatory) disease, while the remaining 8 had non-inflammatory CPPS.

The treatment, which was administered at bedtime for a 3-month period, included a rectal suppository containing 1500 mg of the chelating agent ethylenediaminetetraacetic acid (EDTA), 500 mg tetracycline taken orally, and a proprietary formulation called *Nanobac*. *Nanobac* contains vitamin C, selenium, EDTA, coenzyme Q10, bromelain, grapeseed extract, hawthorn berry, quercetin, l-arginine, l-lysine, l-ornithine, trypsin, papain, and vitamins B3, B6 and B9.[26] This treatment, also known as *ComET*, has been found useful in decalcification of arteries.

At the end of the treatment, the overall NIH-CPSI score had decreased from 25.6 to 13.7, pain score from 11.3 to 4.9, urinary difficulty score from 4.7 to 3.1, and quality-of-life problems score from 9.7 to 5.7. Overall, 8 patients experienced a greater than 50% improvement, 4 an improvement between 25 and 49%, and 3 patients had less than 25% improvement. Two of these 3 patients had no signs of nanobacteria in their blood or urine.

Ten patients underwent TRUS after the treatment. In 1 patient all stones had disappeared, in 5 they had decreased in number and/or size, and in 4 patients they were unchanged. The researchers conclude that the *ComET* treatment may provide significant relief in men who have failed other treatments and have signs of calculi on TRUS. They recommend larger, placebo-controlled trials to evaluate the treatment further.[26]

CONCLUSION

Category III prostatitis or chronic pelvic pain syndrome (CPPS) is a condition of multifactorial origin. There is increasing recognition that an inflamed prostate may not be the main feature of CPPS with some researchers believing that a muscle spasm or myofascial trigger point in the pelvic floor (perineum) is a major source of the pain accompanying CPPS. Precisely because of its multifactorial origin, treatment options are many and varied from antibiotics to herbal anti-inflammatories, acupuncture, and electrical or electromagnetic stimulation. It is unrealistic to expect the average GP or urologist to be aware of all these options, so it is largely up to the patient to propose to his physician that they be explored.

One very promising option that should be considered is supplementation with quercetin (500 mg twice a day). At least two studies have shown that this safe and effective natural bioflavonoid can markedly reduce symptoms in two-thirds or more of patients diagnosed with CPPS.[32,57] Quercetin is available in most health food stores and an even more effective proprietary formulation of the supplement (*Prosta-Q*) is available from Farr Laboratories, Santa Clarita, CA (www.farrlabs.com)

CATEGORY IV – ASYMPTOMATIC INFLAMMATORY PROSTATITIS

Category IV prostatitis is completely asymptomatic and its presence only noted in biopsy samples or prostatic tissue removed during treatment of BPH or cancer. Its prevalence is unknown and no treatment is necessary as long as it remains symptomless.

Chapter 2

Benign Prostatic Hyperplasia—A Not So Benign Problem

William R. Ware PhD

INTRODUCTION

Benign prostatic hyperplasia (BPH) or enlarged prostate refers to changes in the prostate that involve an overgrowth of cells (hyperplasia) which results in nodules that enlarge the gland. It is a disorder that afflicts only humans, chimpanzees and dogs. The term benign in this context means no cancer, although in general usage, according to the Oxford Dictionary, benign describes a gentle, mild or kindly condition. BPH frequently causes problems that are far from gentle or mild and in fact can be responsible for a number of *Lower Urinary Tract Symptoms* (LUTS) that range from merely bothersome to a critical emergency situation involving urinary blockage.

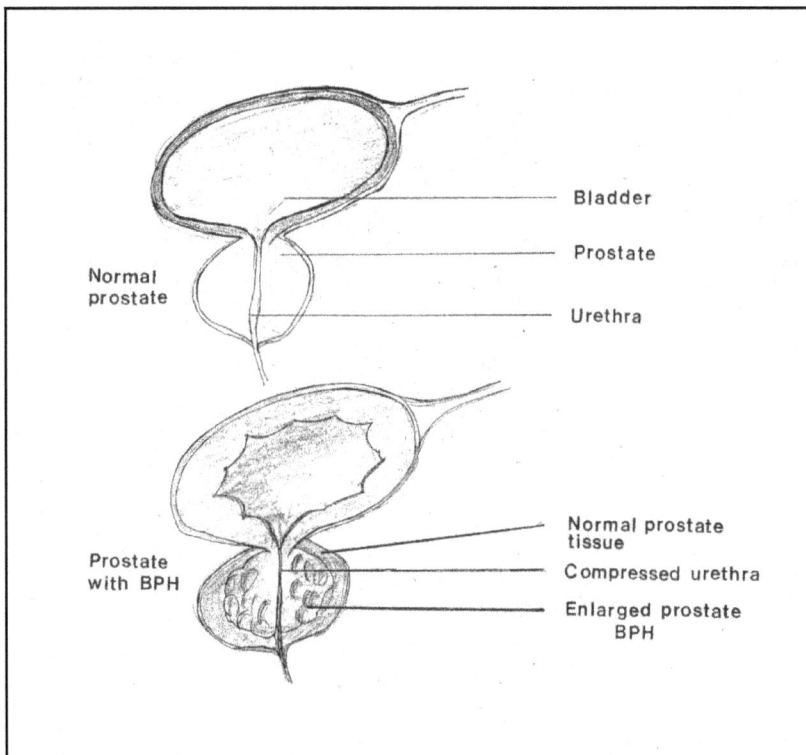

Figure 2-1. Benign Prostatic Hyperplasia

In simple terms, the urinary problems arise from the tissue of the enlarged prostate pressing against the urethra and limiting or even completely cutting off the flow. However, there is also a component of LUTS that involves the smooth muscle tone of the bladder neck and prostate mediated by stimulation of α-adrenoreceptors by the sympathetic nervous system. But what is taking place as BPH develops is somewhat more complex. First the bladder compensates for constricted outflow by building more muscle which over time thickens the bladder wall which influences its capacity to expand and store urine. The result is more frequent urination. Eventually the bladder becomes worn out and weak, a condition known as bladder decompensation [1]. Symptoms now include increased urinary urge and frequency, decreased voiding volume and flow rate, nocturia (frequent need to urinate at night), post-void dribbling and urine retention. This is an important concern for men as they age because the disorder is highly prevalent, impacts quality of life, and its incidence and severity generally increases with age, ultimately requiring surgery or other invasive interventions in a significant number of older individuals. BPH also has a negative psychological impact associated with worry over urinary symptoms, prostate cancer, and the possibility of total blockage [2]. Preventing or slowing its progression so as to avoid surgery is thus a topic of great interest.

Recorded accounts of men's urinary problems can be traced back to the 15th century BC. Hippocrates (5th century BC) described the urinary obstruction as a condition with poor prognosis and no hope for permanent relief. No significant progress in treating BPH occurred prior to the twentieth century [3]. In Victorian times men with severe urinary symptoms were known to carry catheters in hollow shafts of their walking sticks or umbrellas in order to be able to quickly deal with what has become known as *Acute Urinary Retention* (AUR). Even some cowboys were said to carry catheters in their hats [3]. By the turn of the last century surgical techniques were being used to open the urinary channel but these procedures were crude compared to modern invasive therapy, and no doubt accompanied by a high incidence of morbidity since postoperative infections were common in that era and the control of bleeding primitive. As will be discussed below, rapid and significant progress has been made in the last few decades with regard to both surgical and non-surgical treatments of BPH. Much of what has been learned regarding the natural history of this disease has in fact come from the placebo arm of drug intervention studies which allowed the close observation of untreated individuals over a number of years.

BPH is a highly prevalent disease. According to autopsy studies tissue evidence of BPH is present in 20% of men age forty, 60% of age 60 and 90% of men in their 80s [4], although some studies find lower percentages [5]. Disease progression appears to slow after 80 [6]. The severity of the problem can be judged by the observation [1] that in about 25% of all men, BPH causes urinary symptoms that are sufficiently disturbing to precipitate seeking medical advice. In a recent study it was found that there is a 45% risk of developing LUTS/BPH in a symptom-free 45 year-old man over a period of 30 years [7]. It is estimated that by 2020 over 11 million American men each year will require treatment for the symptoms of BPH and the annual cost just in the US now exceeds $8 billion [8]. An aging population is driving a rapid increase in prevalence and underlines the importance of the challenge to diagnose the disease and slow its progression at an early stage and prevent or postpone the situation where surgical intervention is required.

CAUSES OF BPH

It is a commonly held view that BPH is in part a hormone dependent disease, but the details remain unclear. In fact, the etiology of BPH is not well understood and appears multifactorial [1]. Prostate growth occurs during childhood development, but the size of the prostate remains relatively stable from puberty to middle age, after which the growth frequently resumes. Men castrated before puberty never develop BPH. Three hormones (the so-called sex steroids), testosterone (T), dihydrotestosterone (DHT) and the estrogen hormone estradiol (E2) are thought to play a role in the etiology of BPH [9]. Both T and DHT are so-called *androgens* which are hormones that stimulate the activity of male sex organs or control the development of male sex characteristics. All three of these hormones appear to be involved in cell growth within the prostate. Testosterone is converted in the prostate into the more powerful and active form DHT by the action of the enzyme 5α-reductase (there are actually two enzyme isoforms). Individuals lacking this enzyme fail to develop male sexual characteristics including a normal prostate gland, an observation which has focused attention on DHT, as has the success of the 5α-reductase inhibitors in reducing prostate size and improving the symptoms of BPH. However, studies to date seem merely to underscore the complexity of the relationship of the androgens and estrogen to the etiology of BPH.

Neuhouser *et al* [10] recently reviewed six studies examining the connection between serum steroid hormones and BPH. The results from these studies failed to present a clear or consistent picture of a relationship with comparisons between the lowest and highest quintiles generally not achieving statistical significance. However, one result was of statistical significance—a 3-fold increase in BPH risk for men in the highest vs. the lowest quintile of serum estradiol concentration. Unfortunately, serum levels do not provide a measure of prostate tissue levels. Shibata *et al* [9] found from prostate tissue analysis as a function of increasing age that intraprostatic DHT decreased with age. Intraprostatic tissue levels of T and E2 remained constant. However, Walsh *et al* earlier found no decrease of DHT prostate tissue levels with age, merely a large scatter of results, and in addition, they found that the DHT levels were the same in BPH and non-BPH prostate tissue [11]. The BPH model of Shibata *et al* involves the decreasing DHT and constant E2 tissue levels producing a "relatively estrogen-dominant status" which induces cell proliferation by some mechanism and thus yields BPH. In a recent study Roberts *et al* [12] found that in older men, there is an association between serum E2 and surrogate measures of BPH that depend on serum levels of bioavailable T. Among men with serum bioavailable T at levels above the median, E2 levels had a dose dependent positive relationship with prostate size. They point out, however, that while androgens and estrogens may act synergistically in BPH as it relates to prostate size, the precise mechanisms that underlie their effects on the maximum flow rate and other symptoms are neither simple nor clear.

Studies that implicate estradiol in the etiology of BPH have stimulated interest in intervening with aromatase enzyme inhibition which decreases the production of E2. The results have been reviewed by Sciarra and Toscano [13]. The drug Atamestane was used in both open label and randomized, controlled studies. This drug has demonstrated ability to dramatically reduce estradiol levels (40-60%). No improvement in obstructive symptoms was found in one open label and two randomized trials. A possible explanation is that the estrogen reduction is counterbalanced by the observed parallel increase in T and DHT.

This short summary of the hormone connection underscores the present uncertain state of knowledge, the probable complexity of the hormone related mechanisms, and the need for additional research, especially conducting studies that examine the complex biochemistry in the prostate itself rather than attempting to make associations with serum levels. However, this in no way decreases the importance of the observation that 5α-reductase inhibitors decrease the prostate volume and have beneficial effects on the symptoms of BPH.

A novel and fascinating alternative or companion to the hormone theory of the origin and progression of BPH has recently been advanced by Yun and Doux from Stanford University [14]. They elaborate on the hypothesis advanced and extensively developed by Yun and coworkers [15-19] that involves the autonomic nervous system as the major player in disorders associated with the aging process. The autonomic nervous system (ANS) is a primitive response system that mediates the allocation of biological effort under varying conditions. It involves both sympathetic and parasympathetic functions, which in general oppose one another and are in exquisite balance in the normal healthy individual. This nervous system operates below the conscious level and regulates functions critical to survival including heart rate, blood pressure, blood flow, tissue perfusion, sweating, hunger, satiety, body temperature, thirst and the circadian rhythms (fluctuations throughout the 24 hour period). Yun *et al* [18] believe that post-reproductive aging is an evolutionary naïve part of human life history due to the dramatic gains in average lifespan attributable to the advent of modern medicine. Because of this, the ANS has, according to their hypothesis, been rendered maladaptive and this has impacted diseases associated particularly with old age. The hypothesis of Yun and coworkers [15] is that many seemingly unrelated consequences of aging are in part manifestations of a single phenomenon which they term a sympathetic bias that is unmasked by loss of parasympathetic function during old age, as manifest by tachycardia, constipation, insomnia, erectile dysfunction, fluid retention, and systemic inflammation which in turn may contribute to type-2 diabetes, Alzheimer's disease, atherosclerosis and cancer.

Key chemicals involved in ANS activation are the adrenal hormones epinephrine and norepinephrine, and these hormones exert their effects on two types of receptors, alpha and beta. Of interest in the context of BPH is one of the two alpha-receptors which mediates vasoconstriction and smooth muscle constriction, processes that are inhibited by the so-called alpha-blocker class of drugs used to treat both BPH and hypertension. In a recent paper, Yun and Doux [14] specifically consider BPH in the context of the hypothesis that over-activity of the sympathetic nervous system (SNS) is involved in the etiology independent of androgen dysfunction. They offer the following evidence and arguments:

- The risk of BPH is associated with the risk of heart disease which they argue is a manifestation of sympathetic bias. [17,19].
- BPH risk increases with caffeine intake and decreases with alcohol consumption. This is discussed in more detail below. These opposite effects are

consistent with the known influences of caffeine and alcohol on balance in the ANS.

- Chronic heavy smoking increases the risk of BPH. Smoking is known to increase sympathetic bias.
- Animal studies support the hypothesis in that the loss of parasympathetic function produces prostate enlargement whereas surgical interruption of the prostatic sympathetic nervous system produces shrinkage.

They also point out that the beneficial effects of exercise on the risk and progression of BPH may be related to the known action of exercise on the functioning of the ANS. Yun and Doux suggest that the success of alpha-blockers in treating BPH may be in part due to an impact on autonomic balance. They predict that this viewpoint will ultimately result in novel neuromodulation therapies for this disease [14].

Additional evidence for the role of the role of the ANS is provided by recent work reported by McVary *et al* [20] who were able to correlate eight clinical measures of ANS overactivity (sympathetic bias) with the severity of lower urinary tract symptoms accompanying BPH in a group of 38 men. Stress and hostility, which increase SNS activity, have also been found to correlate positively with the extent and severity of BPH [21].

Yun and Doux highlight the role of autonomic imbalance and sympathetic bias in connection with BPH, but it has been recognized for some time that the SNS plays a significant role in the pathophysiology of BPH. The symptoms associated with BPH which are attributed to bladder outlet obstruction can be categorized as obstructive or irritative. Obstructive symptoms consist of hesitancy, poor stream, prolonged urination and feelings of incomplete emptying. Irritative symptoms include frequency, urgency, nocturia and unstable bladder contractions. BPH is also thought of in terms of a dynamic component and a static component. The latter is related to increase in prostatic mass whereas the dynamic component is related to variations in smooth muscle tone [22,23]. It is the dynamic component that is considered to be related to the SNS. Over-activity of the SNS floods the α_1-adrenoceptors (α_1-AR) with neurotransmitters leading to excessive contraction. Blocking these alpha-receptors thus produces a relaxation of smooth muscle tone and relief of the symptoms. However, what is now becoming better recognized is that some of the symptoms attributed to BPH arise from the overactive bladder syndrome that has similar pathophysiology and is characterized by bladder storage symptoms (urgency, frequency, urge incontinence and nocturia) [24,25]. This syndrome is common to both men and women and symptomatic relief is achieved for both with alpha-blockers. In fact, in men the alpha-blockers relieve not only voiding symptoms but also storage symptoms. It is also now reasonable well established [23] that a subtype AR receptor known as α_{1D}-AR is implicated in the overactive bladder symptoms and the α_{1A}-AR subtype is implicated in voiding (obstructive) symptoms. When a blocker specific to this latter receptor is used, it fails to reduce the irritative symptoms. Alpha-blockers used today either exhibit no selectivity for subtype or are specific for the A/D subtype receptors (Tamsulosin and naftopidil, an alpha blocker approved in Japan [25,26]). The use of alpha-blockers will be discussed in more detail below. They are generally considered as the first-line treatment of BPH with the 5α-reductase inhibitors generally reserved for when the alpha-blockers become ineffective or it is considered desirable to reduce the size of the prostate.

Thus for a man presenting with symptoms that include frequent urination, urgency, urge incontinence and nocturia (frequent trips to the bathroom at night) who is offered a 5α-reductase inhibitor (e.g. Proscar), it can be argued that he should question the physician as to why an alpha blocker is not being tried first, since he has the symptoms that respond to alpha-blockage for the reasons elaborated above and as indicated in clinical trials to be discussed later in this chapter.

There is growing interest in the hypothesis that inflammation is involved in the etiology of BPH [27]. In fact, Vela Navarrete *et al* [28] recently demonstrated in a pilot study that Permixon, a prescription form of the phytochemical saw palmetto used to treat the symptoms of BPH (see below), resulted in a decrease in levels of inflammation markers in prostatic tissue. The connection between prostatic inflammation and disorders in the autonomic nervous system has been discussed by Yun and Doux [14]. Other recent evidence has been reviewed by Kramer and Marberger [27]. The connection between inflammation, including systemic inflammation, and a number of prevalent diseases is currently a topic of great interest and intense research activity, and as well, a number of books for the lay audience have appeared. One of the most comprehensive and recent is by Barry Sears [29]. Finally, as will be discussed below, there is evidence that a damaged prostate vascular system may play an important role in the development of BPH [30].

POSITIVE AND NEGATIVE RISK FACTORS FOR BPH

In this context, reduction of risk is akin to protective or preventive intervention. Risk factors over which one has no control include ethnic background, age and family history. Studies conducted in a number of countries find high prevalence of moderate to severe urinary problems and while the absolute prevalence varies widely among countries, there are remarkably consistent age-related increases found in prostate volume at autopsy [5]. Based on data collected in the US, a recent study found that Asian men had the lowest risks for nocturia, physician-diagnosed BPH and surgical treatment for severe BPH. The risks for Caucasians and African Americans were similar for most measures of BPH [31]. These results are consistent with an earlier study of the influence of race and ethnicity on BPH in the Health Professionals Follow-Up [32]. The reasons for the much lower incidence found for those of Asian background is not clear, but may be due to dietary habits such as the consumption of low-fat, high-fiber diets which provide an enhanced supply of weak phytoestrogens [33].

Evidence for a genetic contribution to BPH appears quite consistent. Previous family history of either an enlarged prostate or early-onset BPH increases the risk of this disease in descendents by two to four times [34]. However, a family history of prostate cancer does not appear to confer an enhanced risk of BPH, although a family history of bladder cancer was found in to increase the risk by a factor of over two [35].

DIET

Although limited in number, recent studies support a role, albeit relatively minor, of diet in the risk of BPH. In a recent large study based on food frequency questionnaires, Suzuki *et al* [36] report the results of examining the intake of energy and macronutrients (protein, carbohydrate and various fats) on the risk of BPH. Cases were drawn from a cohort of over 51,000 individuals in the Health Professionals Follow-up Study. Four categories of BPH were used: (1) surgery for BPH; (2) high to moderate LUT symptoms; (3) total BPH consisting of the above two categories; and (4) enlarged prostate as detected by digital rectal examination. Non-cases used for comparison were defined as men who had no BPH surgery and those with a low score in a test of urinary tract symptoms. Risk, as measured by odds ratios, rose with increasing total energy intake and in a comparison of highest to lowest quintiles yielded odds ratios (ORs) of 1.29 for category (3) and 1.43 for category (2). Total protein intake (energy-adjusted) was positively associated with total BPH (OR = 1.18) and BPH surgery (OR = 1.26). Moderate increased risk was found for eicosapentaenoic (EPA), docosahexaenoic (DHA), and arachidonic (AA), all polyunsaturated fatty acids (PUFAs). All other macronutrients failed to show statistically significant associations. Food groups were not studied. The authors comment that the association with the polyunsaturated fatty acids (PUFA) should be explored further (the ORs were only marginally above 1.00. ORs less than 1.00 indicate reduced risk, whereas those above 1.00 point to increased risk) because these fatty acids have been found beneficial in the context of heart disease. In particular, the omega-3 fatty acid EPA is implicated in preventing sudden death during a heart attack. The authors also suggest that since these PUFAs are easily oxidized, their findings also suggest a possible role of oxidative stress in the etiology of BPH. The association with total calorie intake was not found in another large study reported in 2001, and in that study there was also no connection between total fat intake and BPH [37].

In 1999, Yang *et al* [38] reported a comparison between normal controls and patients with BPH, where the parameters studied included serum levels of omega-3 (n-3) and omega-6 (n-6) PUFAs. They found that the n-3 levels were significantly decreased and the n-3/n-6 PUFA ratio was lower for BPH patients relative to controls. This would be consistent with an inflammatory component to the etiology of BPH since a high ratio of n-3/n-6 is considered anti-inflammatory, but is inconsistent with the results of Suzuki *et al* [36] discussed above which was based on the PUFA content of foods reported in a food frequency questionnaire. The use of serum levels would appear to be a more direct approach to the question, but blood samples were either not available or not studied by Suzuki *et al*.

Diet from the point of view of food groups has also been investigated in relation to the risk of BPH. Bravi *et al* [39] have recently reported the results of a case control study in an Italian population involving 1369 patients treated surgically for BPH and 1451 controls admitted to the same hospitals for a wide spectrum of acute, non-neoplastic conditions. The use of a food frequency questionnaire revealed a significant trend of increasing risk with more frequent consumption of cereals, bread, poultry and eggs (odds ratios ranged from 1.39 to 1.69). Inverse (beneficial) associations were found for soups, pluses (e.g. lentils, beans etc), cooked vegetables and citrus fruit (odds ratios ranged from 0.66 to 0.82). Milk, yogurt products, coffee, tea, pasta, rice, fish, cheese, row vegetables, potatoes, fruit in general and deserts were all neutral. There are however, a number of limitations with this study. In particular, the authors point out that hospital controls may not be representative of the general population and there was the possibility of misclassification of controls. This would result in the positive risk being too low and the negative risk too high.

In a case control study of BPH patients in Athens, Greece, Lagiou *et al* [40] examined both food groups and some individual foods. They found that among the food groups, only fruits were significantly inversely associated with BPH risk. Note that Bravi *et al* also found an inverse association with citrus fruit. Increased consumption of both butter and margarine was positively associated with risk, but olive oil was neutral. Among the micronutrients studied, only zinc consumption was found to be associated with BPH risk, in this case increased risk. This might be important if confirmed because of the frequently seen recommendation to take zinc supplements for prostate health.

Additional research will be necessary to resolve these inconsistencies, but lack of agreement between studies and ORs near 1.0 suggest that diet has a rather minor role in the etiology of BPH.

ALCOHOL AND COFFEE

The connection between alcohol consumption and BPH has been the subject of several recent studies, and in one the combined effect of alcohol and coffee was examined. Neuhouser *et al* [10] have summarized the alcohol consumption studies that occurred between 1992 and 2001. Four studies found significant inverse associations with odds ratios or relative risks ranging from 0.46 to 0.72, i.e. significant protection. One study reported an OR of 0.86 that was not significant, and one found no association. In a study reported in 2004 [41], a significant beneficial trend with alcohol consumption was found with an OR of 0.71 for 3-4 drinks/day, 0.79 for 5-6, and 0.65 for ≥ 7 drinks/day. When the results were stratified according to wine, beer or liquor, the patterns of risk were similar but only marginally significant. The authors also found that the inverse relationship between alcohol and BPH was stronger in subjects with lower body mass index. They suggest an interaction between androgen levels and alcohol.

In a recently published case control study [31] involving approximately 35,000 male participants ranging in age from 55 to 74, it was also found that alcohol consumption offered significant protection from BPH. Three categories of BPH were used: (1) nocturia—10756 cases; (2) physician diagnosed BPH—526 cases; (3) surgery for BPH—973 cases. Alcohol consumption ranged from < 5 g/day (reference) to ≥ 60 g/day (a glass of table wine contains between 17 and 20 g of alcohol). ORs for low (5-15 g/day) to high consumption for categories (2) and (3) were from 0.8 to 0.6 and 0.7 to 0.4 respectively, with highly significant trends and individual ORs. These ORs indicate a moderate protective effect. Stratification by type of alcoholic beverage produced similar results, but not all ORs were statistically significant.

In one of the studies included in the summary of Neuhouser *et al* [10], the combined effects of coffee and alcohol were examined [42]. Coffee consumption was found to be rather strongly and significantly positively associated with BPH risk. When controls having no BPH were used, the ORs for BPH among coffee users was 2.20 for 1-4 cups and 2.74 for > 4 cups/day. The combined intake of one or more glasses of an alcoholic drink and 1,2 or 3 cups of coffee/day resulted in ORs well below 1.00, but only the results for one cup of coffee/day were statistically significant (OR = 0.13). Other studies that have examined the connection between coffee and BPH are inconsistent (the study by Bravi *et al* discussed above found no association) and the mechanism whereby coffee increases the BPH risk is unknown. Also, filtered coffee has a different composition than non-filtered coffee, which confuses the issue. The authors suggest that men drinking more than four cups of unfiltered coffee daily should also drink some alcohol. However, no data in this context appears available regarding the relative risks of filtered vs. unfiltered coffee.

In connection with cardiovascular disease risk, it is common to see the recommendation of up to two glasses of wine or the equivalent per day as a preventive measure for men. In fact, a recently published study found that the risk of extensive coronary calcification, a measure of atherosclerosis, was 50% lower in individuals who consumed one to two alcoholic drinks per day as compared to non-drinkers [43]. However, more than two drinks a day eliminated the benefit. Although "more than three" was not included in the data workup, three drinks a day may still be protective in this context. The studies discussed above would appear indicate that two or perhaps three alcoholic drinks such as beer or wine might also reduce the risk of BPH by around 30-50%.

SMOKING

There appears to be only one study that addresses the question of smoking and BPH, in this case cigarette smoking [44]. This was the Health Professionals Follow-Up study which involved over 29,000 men. Cases (1,813) were men reporting BPH surgery between 1986 and 1994 or men who had high lower urinary tract symptom scores between 1992 and 1994. Non-cases used for comparison had low symptom scores. It was found that current smoking was positively associated with BPH risk, but only among men who smoked 35 or more cigarettes per day. For this group the risk of BPH was statistically significantly elevated at 1.45 times that of never-smokers used for comparison. The analysis controlled for alcohol consumption and a wide range of other BPH risk factors. A potential mechanism was discussed above in connection with the hypothesis that BPH may be related to a disorder of the autonomic nervous system which can be aggravated by smoking.

MICRONUTRIENTS

The relationship between micronutrient intake and BPH risk has been the subject of only a limited number of studies. One of the most recent [45] which examined the connection with a number of micronutrients involved men who participated in the Third National Health and Nutrition Examination Survey. In this case control study the cases had three of the following four LUT symptoms, as ascertained by an interview: nocturia, hesitancy, incomplete emptying of the bladder and a weak stream. Controls were men without symptoms. Serum levels of vitamins A, C and E, α- and β-carotene, β-cryptoxanthin, lutein/zeaxanthin, lycopene and selenium were determined and compared between cases and controls. The only statistically significant lower serum levels in cases vs. controls were found for vitamin E, lycopene and selenium. When the data was examined in terms of quintiles of micronutrient concentration, there were no statistically significant trends with serum level but the odds ratios for these three micronutrients clustered around 0.5 to 0.75, suggesting that men with higher levels of circulating vitamin E, selenium and lycopene had a reduced risk of LUTS and thus presumably BPH. High serum levels of vitamin C appeared to be highly protective for current smokers (OR = 0.1, 95% confidence limits 0.02-0.67). On the other hand, for individuals who had never smoked, comparison of the highest with the lowest vitamin C quintile yielded an OR of 3.61 with 95% confidence limits of 1.10 and 11.85.   No significant associations were found with the other micronutrients studies. The authors suggest that the mechanism of action of lycopene may be associated with its ability to quench singlet oxygen and thus reduce oxidative damage. They hypothesize that the inverse association with selenium may be due to its being a constituent of glutathione peroxidase, which is a potent free radical quencher and is also know to inhibit cell growth. The positive association in non-smokers with high intakes of vitamin C was attributed to the possibility of this vitamin becoming pro-oxidative at high concentrations. No theory was offered for the protective effect observed for current smokers. It is interesting that the three micronutrients identified as possibly protective in the context of LUTS and BPH have also been implicated as protective for prostate cancer.

A number of epidemiologic, clinical and *in vitro* data suggest that phytoestrogens are involved in the pathogenesis of BPH [46].   Dietary sources include tea, fruits and vegetables and in particular soy and soy products. High phytoestrogen intake has been suggested by many observers as an explanation for the difference in incidence of BPH between Far East and Western countries. The results of a recent study [46] address this matter. Prostate tissue levels of two phytoestrogens, enterolactone and genistein, were determined in a series of men undergoing surgery to relieve the symptoms of BPH. It was found that genistein tissue levels were significantly greater in men with small prostate volumes as compared to those with large volumes. No significant correlation was found for enterolactone. Genistein is thought to be biologically the most active isoflavone in soy products. Red clover is also a good source of genistein and avoids some of the problems that may be associated with soy. The authors suggest that a possible mechanism for the influence of genistein on the incidence of BPH is that it inhibits the degradation of vitamin D, a vitamin which is implicated in prostate health. While these results do not prove a cause and effect relationship, they carry an implication of benefit in the context of BPH. A number of mechanisms have been proposed for the action of phytoestrogens in the prostate but what is clear is that there is still a lack of detained knowledge regarding the interplay of hormones, enzymes and weak estrogen-like compounds in this gland [47]. There may also be a risks associated with disturbing the hormone balance with substances having estrogenic properties.

A natural conclusion based on the above results would be that supplementation with vitamin E, selenium and lycopene and perhaps consuming modest quantities of soy containing foods might be worth considering. Unfortunately, there appear to be no randomized intervention studies that address this issue, and it may be decades before such studies are conducted, if ever.   Furthermore the amounts in the form of supplements that might be effective are unknown and the dose safety issue of some supplemental forms has never been investigated. Lycopene can be obtained from cooked tomato products, the best being tomato paste, whereas raw tomatoes are a poor source. Genistein can of course be obtained by eating soy products such as tofu (bean curd). For these two phytochemicals, food sources appear attractive and may in fact contain other beneficial substances. The selenium content of foods is highly variable since it depends on soil concentrations. Only small amounts of vitamin E are available in food compared to the amounts many individuals take in the form of supplements. Guidance regarding supplementation with these two micronutrients can perhaps be obtained from the fact that an ongoing, multicenter clinical study (the SELECT trial) of vitamin E and selenium as protective agents for prostate cancer is using supplementation of 200 micrograms of selenium as selenomethionine and 400 IU of natural vitamin E a day, amounts deemed safe for a long-term study involving over 30,000 participants. Both of these supplements are readily available at most health food stores or online.

A recent review concerning the safety of vitamins E and C should reassure individuals worried by recent media coverage of the "dangers" of taking these supplements. In this review of the scientific literature, no consistent evidence was found for adverse events among healthy individuals or those with a range of diseases for daily intakes of up to 1600 IU (equivalent to about 1000 mg of natural vitamin E) or up to 2000 mg of vitamin C [48].

BPH, DIABETES, CARDIOVASCULAR DISEASE AND THE METABOLIC SYNDROME

The hypothesis that there is an association between BPH and diabetes has been around for over 30 years but still no consensus exists. Diabetes can eventually produce bladder dysfunction which involves neuropathy. Impaired detrusor function (the muscle involved in bladder emptying) results in lower flow rates and can increase residual (post-void) urine. But BPH can also cause the same lower urinary tract symptoms even though the underlying pathology is different since BPH does not directly impair detrusor function but rather increases bladder outlet resistance and interferes with urine flow by mechanisms that are both static and dynamic. In addition, both diabetes and BPH increase with age and a fraction of patients with BPH also suffer from diabetes and vice versa. The question then is whether the incidence of comorbidity of these two diseases is greater than would be expected by chance, i.e. is diabetes an independent risk factor for BPH.

Hammarsten and Högstedt have examined this question in a direct manner by examining the correlation between the rate of prostate volume change and both non-insulin dependent diabetes mellitus, i.e. type 2 diabetes (NIDDM) and in individuals with the metabolic syndrome, a condition closely related to diabetes, and also in individuals with elevated insulin levels [49,50]. Since gland growth in BPH occurs in the transition zone (TZ), the authors used transrectal ultrasound to determine the TZ volume. They established that there was a linear and highly significant correlation between the total prostate volume and the TZ volume, and thus the former was a valid measure of BPH. Prostate growth rates were calculated assuming that the prostate had a volume of 20 mL at age 40. Prostate growth rates were obtained for 307 patients. Those with metabolic disease, NIDDM, treated hypertension, obesity and dyslipidemia (unfavorable blood cholesterol profile) all had prostate growth rates significantly greater than controls. When the fasting insulin was stratified by quartiles, those in the first quartile (< 7 mU/L) had an average annual prostate growth rate of 0.84 mL whereas in the highest quartile of plasma insulin (>13 mU/L), the rate was 1.49 mL, and this difference was statistically significant. The authors regard these results as supporting the hypothesis of a relationship between BPH and diabetes, the metabolic syndrome, and hyperinsulinemia. This hypothesis is further supported by the observation that diabetes is associated with greater BPH symptom severity even after age adjustment [51]. It is also clear from these and other studies [52] that BPH and cardiovascular disease share a common set of risk factors and thus cardio vascular disease (CVD) is probably a risk factor for BPH [37,53]. In fact, when studies segregated age-matched patient populations according to clinical signs of CVD, atherosclerosis and hypertension vs. those without [53], patients with overt vascular pathology were at a much higher risk for BPH than those where this pathology was absent, independent of age.

The relationship between diabetes and BPH progression has also recently been reported by Burke *et al* [54]. A cohort of 2115 men, 111 of whom had diabetes at baseline, was followed for 12 years. Men with diabetes had significantly greater median annual percentage change in the AUA Symptom Index and a trend toward a greater median annual percentage decrease in peak urinary flow rate compared to those without diabetes. However, there were no significant differences in prostate volume or PSA levels, a result which the authors interpret as suggesting that diabetes impacts the dynamic aspect of lower urinary tract function rather than BPH progression per se.

The question of the mechanism involved in the observed connection between diabetes, vascular disease and BPH was recently examined by Berger *et al* [30] using a novel approach. They employed computer-assisted quantification of color Doppler ultrasound to examine the patterns of blood flow in normal prostates and prostates in patients with NIDDM. The hypothesis was that diabetes related vascular damage, a well established phenomenon, might extent to the prostate. Such damage is known to reduce the available oxygen (hypoxia) and in prostate cell culture studies, hypoxia caused increased growth factor production [55,56] which could trigger prostate enlargement. The ultrasound technique permitted the examination of circulation in both the peripheral zone (PZ) and the transition zone (TZ). Significant reduced circulation was observed in the TZ of diabetic patients as compared to non-diabetic patients, whereas there were no differences in the circulation in the PZ. It will be recalled that the prostate growth in BPH occurs in the TZ. TZ circulation of patients with non-diabetic BPH as well as those with diabetes was significantly lower than controls, but no differences were found for the PZ. The authors conclude that these results indicate considerable vascular damage in the TZ of diabetic patients and this may contribute to the pathogenesis of BPH, perhaps via hypoxia. These results are inconsistent with those reported by Burke *et al* [54] described above where no correlation between the presence of diabetes and prostate volume was observed, but baseline prostate volumes were not reported and only 25% of the cohort underwent prostate volume measurement. Nevertheless, action aimed at decreasing the risk of metabolic syndrome or adult-onset diabetes (NIDDM) may be effective in reducing the risk of BPH. Obviously other health benefits would also accrue from such action.

Moyad [57] has recently reviewed the connection between obesity, physical activity and BPH. The strongest connection is with the waist-to-hip ratio (incidentally a metabolic syndrome factor), which is an indication of abdominal obesity. Abdominal fat may increase estrogen levels, providing the link to BPH. Hammarsten and Högsten in fact also observed a significant correlation between the waist-to-hip ratio and prostate growth rates [49], and Dahle *et al* [58] found that abdominal obesity was associated with a higher risk of BPH. In all the studies reviewed by Moyad, physical activity had a strong and significant impact on the risk of developing BPH. Even walking two to three hours a week resulted in a 25% reduction in the risk of BPH and in one study, men with the highest level of physical activity compared to the lowest had a 50% reduction in risk.

CONCLUSIONS

Thus if one wishes to take action to reduce the risk of BPH, the following can be considered:

- Eat lots of fruit and cooked tomato products.
- Have a limited number of alcoholic drinks each day (red wine is considered by some to be the best choice), especially if coffee is consumed.
- Adopt a lifestyle that does not lead to the metabolic syndrome, diabetes or cardiovascular disease. It is beyond the scope of this book to discuss how one goes about this! It is obviously a goal that if achieved carries benefits that extend far beyond prostate health.
- Related to the above as well as to independent evidence is the advice not to develop a "beer belly" or what some call an apple shape. That is, keep the waist in control by avoiding an accumulation of abdominal fat. Morbid examples can generally be seen at all-you-can-eat buffets.
- Exercise. It is incidentally hard to find a health problem where this is not an important recommendation. After all, we still have the genetic make-up of our ancestors who exercised almost daily while hunting and gathering.
- Consider supplementation with selenium and vitamin E using the forms discussed above. As will be discussed in Chapter 5, this may also impact the risk of prostate cancer.

The strength of the evidence backing these actions is variable, ranging from rather weak to moderately convincing. Later in this chapter both patent drug and natural remedies for BPH will be discussed in detail. It is possible that some of these substances, when taken before the growth of the prostate resumes in middle age, will prevent or delay BPH, but there is little data concerning this application. Most studies involve subjects who are already symptomatic.

DIAGNOSIS OF BPH

LOWER URINARY TRACT SYMPTOMS AND RULING OUT CANCER

The lower urinary tract symptoms (LUTS) characteristic of BPH may not in fact be due to this disease. Thus the diagnostic challenge is to differentiate between BPH and other causes of LUTS. Other causes include diabetes (LUTS by an non-BPH mechanism), Parkinson's disease, stroke, urethral stricture caused by scar tissue from catheterization or from a sexually transmitted disease such as gonorrhea, urinary tract infections, prostatitis, bladder cancer, advanced prostate cancer, and bladder stones. A recent study from the Mayo Clinic and Merck in fact identifies seventeen conditions that should be distinguished from BPH as causing LUTS. These include back surgery as well as the conditions listed above. This study also found the following percentages of men with LUTS unrelated to BPH: age 50-59, 5.4%; age 60-69, 8.5%, and age > 70, 32.8% [59]. Thus older individuals present a significant diagnostic challenge, and an oversight during the initial evaluation would result in incorrect treatment and even misclassification of subjects in clinical trials. While mild symptoms are easy to ignore, severe symptoms of LUTS such as blood in the urine, recurrent urinary tract infections, bladder stones, or trouble emptying the bladder should not be ignored, since the risk of acute urinary retention or bladder or kidney damage is elevated [1]. Correct diagnosis is critical since it determines treatment.

The American Urological Association (AUA) recommends [60] that for all patients presenting with LUTS suggestive of BPH the initial evaluation should involve a medical history, physical exam including a digital rectal exam, a urinalysis and blood tests to screen for blood and urinary tract infection. It is further recommended that symptoms be assessed with either the AUA Symptom Index or the equivalent International Prostate Symptom Score (IPSS). More extensive testing may be suggested by the results. Similar recommendations have been recently made by the European Association of Urology (EAU) [61]. The success in eliminating non-BPH causes of LUTS will depend on the skill of the diagnostician. The AUA Symptom Score (AUASS) is presented in Appendix E.

Symptoms are classified as MILD if the total score is 0-7; MODERATE for 8-18, and SEVERE from 19-35. The IPSS uses the same questions and scoring system. *This score is not necessarily diagnostic of BPH but merely indicates severity of LUTS.*

The AUA also recommends [60] that the serum prostate-specific antigen (PSA) test be *offered* under the following circumstances: (1) those with at least a 10-year life expectancy and for whom knowledge of the presence of prostate cancer would change the course or nature of the disease management; or (2) those for whom the PSA measurement may change the management of their voiding symptoms. This brings up the subject of PSA testing, an area of great controversy in urology, even in the context of BPH. The use of the word *offered* in the AUA recommendation speaks volumes.

At issue is the detection of prostate cancer (PC) in patients presenting with LUTS and the use of PSA levels in managing the treatment of BPH. The above recommendation might suggest to the reader that this test will provide an answer to the question of the presence of prostate cancer. Research in the last several years has cast serious doubt on this simple view of the PSA test and highlights the difficulties associated with the exclusion of PC when evaluating patients presenting with LUTS. Most prostate cancers occur in the peripheral zone of the gland and some are palpable, but only a portion of the surface area of the prostate is accessible via the DRE. When this exam reveals abnormalities, it is normal to pursue further the question of PC. However, the common situation is a non-suspicious DRE, and a normal or elevated PSA. But "elevated" is based on a somewhat arbitrary cut-off. A lengthy discussion of the PSA debate is not appropriate for this chapter (see Chapter 4), but the following appears important.

If the offer of a PSA test is accepted, the result will be a number ranging from the lower limit of sensitivity of the test (≈ 0.1 ng/mL) to possibly a number over 100 ng/mL. Values above 10 ng/mL are cause for alarm. The "normal" cut-off is 4 ng/mL, above which it is usual practice for physicians to suggest a biopsy. But this cut-off is not age-adjusted. However, it is now known that PC, including high-grade cancers, is not rare among men with PSA levels of less than 4.0 ng/mL. Furthermore, PSA levels between 4 and 10 ng/mL occur in men with BPH, and prostate cancer is present in only 25% of patients with PSA in this range [62]. The magnitude of the problem is illustrated by recent results reported by Thompson *et al* published in *The New England Journal of Medicine* [63]. A cohort of 2050 men with normal DRE and PSA that that had been below 4 ng/mL for seven years were enrolled and underwent biopsy at the end of the study. PC was diagnosed in 15.2% and of these, and 14.9% of PC cases had high-grade cancer. Among those with PC, the prevalence of cancer was 6.6% for the group with PSA up to 0.5 ng/ml, 10.1% for those with values between 0.6 and 1.0, 17% for those with values from 1.1 to 2.0, 23.9% for those between 2.1 and 3.0, and 26.9% for those with values between 3.1 and 4.0 ng/mL. The prevalence of high-grade cancer was 12.5% of those with PC for PSA ≤ 0.5 and 25% for PSA in the range 3.1-4.0. Tumor grade is important because if one is old enough, low-grade cancer may not pose a threat. It is well known that most men die with rather than from PC. These results point to the folly of the view that a cut-off of 4 can be used to answer the question, does this patient have cancer, and this cut-off also fails to sharply discriminate low- from high-grade tumors. In fact, if a cut-off of 2.1 had been used, it would have, on the basis of this data, missed 33% of the cancers.

Another problem involves intra-individual variations. A recent study examined this question over four years of annual check-ups. Among men with an abnormal PSA finding, a high proportion had a normal PSA finding at one or more subsequent visits. For those with a PSA greater than 4 ng/mL, i.e. a value that would trigger the recommendation of a biopsy, 44% had at least one normal value on subsequent visits. When a cutoff of 2.5 ng/mL was used similar results were obtained. Thus significant intra-individual variations must be added to the lack of specificity that characterizes this test. The authors suggest that an isolated elevated PSA level should be confirmed several weeks later before proceeding with other tests or to a biopsy [64].

Given that men with BPH have elevated PSA and that PSA tends to increase with age among the cancer free, and that as Thompson *et al* [63] demonstrated, even a PSA cut-off of 2.1 ng/mL would miss a third of cancers, it would seem that if a definitive answer regarding PC is the goal, the only solution appears to be a biopsy, *or more than one*, as some urologists suggest [1]. This appears to be the position of Dr. P. C. Walsh, the well-known urologist from Johns Hopkins Medical School who is responsible for the nerve sparing radical prostatectomy procedure [65]. Commenting on the paper by Thompson *et al,* he states "...if a patient really wants to know whether or not he has cancer, I guess we have to do a biopsy." In fact, based on the experience of Stanford University Urologists, Stamey *et al* [66] have recently taken the position that PSA is only useful in this context for estimating the size of the prostate! However, it is almost inconceivable that the recommendation would be put forward that everyone presenting with LUTS have a biopsy for PC. The term "offered" implies a discussion between patient and physician where the pros and cons and probabilities are considered, and especially what would be the next step if a certain PSA value were found. Such a discussion involves the age, health, life expectancy and attitudes of the patient and perhaps his spouse, and as well, the attitude and knowledge of the physician as regards PSA. It is important to remember that PSA is organ specific but not cancer specific.

There are other more sophisticated PSA tests that show promise for use in the differential diagnosis of BPH vs. PC. These are not routinely done and are not part of either the AUA or EAU general recommendations, but appear definitely worth considering when one is confronted with the problem of the lack of specificity of the PSA test. For example, in a recent study [67] aimed at reducing the number of biopsies in men with non-suspicious DRE and PSA between 4 and 10 ng/mL, it was found that by measuring the free PSA rather than the total PSA, and using a cut-off of $\leq 23\%$ as a criterion for biopsy, 94.4% of cancers would have been detected and 18% of biopsies yielding benign results would have been avoided. The researchers also found that PSA density, calculated from the prostate volume and total PSA, gave a similar specificity. However, PSA density requires the gland volume, which can only be reliably estimated from transrectal ultrasound or other more expensive imaging techniques. DRE generally underestimates the volume [68]. In the next few years these alternative PSA tests as well as other tests now under development will no doubt become better characterized and more commonly performed.

In spite of the problems outlined above, it appears well established that PSA has its place in the management of BPH treatment and in particular in assessing the probability of progression, an acute urinary retention episode, or the future need for surgery. A very recent consensus statement at the end of a series of papers on this subject in the *British Journal of Urology International* [69] outlines the current status of this application of PSA levels. The following points are of interest.

- Prostate volume (PV) consistently increases with age and in studies higher baseline PVs were associated with greater growth rates of the prostate. Men with a PV of ≥ 30 ml are 3.5 times more likely to have moderate to severe symptoms, 2.5 times more likely to have decreased flow rates and 3 to 4 times more likely to an AUR episode than men with lower PVs. However, the accuracy of the DRE in determining PV is limited, and MRI in general too expensive. Transrectal ultrasound provides a more accurate measure of PV, but the specialized equipment is not normally used in the physician's office environment. Thus another marker would be useful.

- PSA levels have been shown to be closely related to PV in benign glands, and even low PSA is indicative of an enlarged prostate. Eighty-nine percent of a patient group studied in Holland with PSA of at least 1.5 ng/mL had PV of > 30 mL.

- When a group of patients in the placebo arm of a drug study were examined for a correlation between PSA levels, symptom severity, and risk of AUR or surgery, those in the highest PSA quartile vs. the lowest had greater symptom severity and a higher risk for surgery to treat BPH and also higher risk of an AUR episode.

- Thus PSA appears to be a satisfactory surrogate for PV and to have utility in identifying patients with higher risk of BPH progression. The consensus group [69] concluded that men with a PSA ≥ 1.5 ng/mL should be considered at increased risk of clinically significant BPH progression and therefore should be considered for more aggressive therapy than those with PSA below this limit. For the latter, they suggest symptomatic treatment.

The suggested PSA threshold for aggressive treatment is low and would probably include many older men with BPH. But it must be pointed out that the consensus group recognizes a pharmaceutical treatment protocol is available which can reduce the size of the prostate and slow or even halt progression, and presumably the view is the earlier the better.

COEXISTENCE OF BPH AND PROSTATITIS AND RULING OUT PROSTATITIS

BPH has a high prevalence in aging men and prostatitis, while less prevalent, is nevertheless not uncommon. Thus it is not surprising that these two disorders will coexist in some patients [70]. Prostatitis has been discussed in Chapter 1. Studies that examine the prevalence of prostatitis or prostatitis-like symptoms in men with LUTS and/or BPH reveal numbers that range from 5% to 39% [70]. Differential diagnosis given the possibility that either or both diseases could be present is not simple. The prostatitis syndrome encompasses 4 categories according to the consensus definitions from the International Prostatitis Collaborative Network [71]. These are: (I) acute bacterial prostatitis; (II) chronic bacterial prostatitis; (IIIA) inflammatory chronic prostatitis/chronic pelvic pain syndrome (CP/CPPS); (IIIB) noninflammatory CP/CPPS and (IV) asymptomatic inflammatory prostatitis. More than 90% of symptomatic men have CP/CPPS [71]. The symptom that that is most useful in differentiation between prostatitis and BPH is genitourinary and pelvic pain, and the most common symptom for those with prostatitis is pain or discomfort during ejaculation. Also, perineal, penile or testicular pain experienced by some with prostatitis is not a major complaint in BPH patients, and the AUA symptom index score is generally higher for chronic prostatitis than for BPH. Bacterial prostatitis can generally be diagnosed from cultures, whereas patients with inflammatory CP/CPPS have leukocytes in their expressed prostatic secretions, post-prostate massage urine or semen. This differentiates inflammatory from noninflammatory CP/CPPS. Excess leukocyte levels in seminal fluid are also common in asymptomatic inflammatory prostatitis, which is frequently a "non-cancer" diagnosis based on histological criteria associated with a negative biopsy prompted by elevated PSA [71]. Thus it would appear to be easier to decide that prostatitis is of low probability in patients presenting with symptoms of BPH than to rule out BPH in patients presenting with symptoms of prostatitis. This is obviously a serious matter since if prostatitis is present treatment is advisable.

Prostatitis and BPH are both treated successfully in some patients with alpha-blockers, and some patients also benefit from 5α-reductase inhibitors if they have both BPH and prostatitis. Antibiotics and anti-inflammatories are also used to treat prostatitis [72], and in some studies, antibiotics are used at the start even in the absence of direct evidence of bacterial involvement [73]. Both sequential and combined therapy are being used for CP/CPPS but large randomized clinical trials have yet to report [73,74]. Readers interested in "natural" treatments of prostatitis will be interested to learn that quercetin, a bioflavonoid found in green tea, red wine and onions (and in health food stores) has been successfully used both as mono- and combined therapy for prostatitis (500 mg twice a day was used in one clinical trial [75]) [72,73]. However, as Nickel points out [70], agents such as 5α-reductase inhibitors, alpha-blockers, antibiotics, phytotherapeutic agents and anti-inflammatory drugs have been studied in connection with treating either BPH or CP/CPPS but not in patients specifically identified as having both conditions.

Thus men presenting with LUTS should expect their physician consider the possibility of prostatitis as well as its coexistence with BPH. The information presented above and in Chapter 1 is intended to assist in determining if adequate differential diagnosis has occurred.

MEDICAL TREATMENT OF BPH

The two obvious goals of medical treatment for BPH are a reduction in the severity of symptoms and the delay or elimination of progression which can ultimately lead to intolerable symptoms, acute urinary retention (AUR) and surgery.   That BPH is a progressive disease now appears well established, as is the observation that progression is associated with increasing prostate volume, in particular in the transition zone [2]. There are two standard types of prescription medication in use for the treatment of BPH, α_1-adrenoreceptor antagonists (alpha-blockers) and 5α-reductase inhibitors (5ARIs). They differ totally in their biological function and are used both as monotherapy and together in combined therapy. Both classes of drug have been rather extensively studied and the comparative side effects both within each class and between classes appear reasonably well documented. These drugs offer the potential for a conservative, non-surgical approach with minimal serious side effects and the drugs appear well tolerated. Alpha-blockers are commonly the first-choice option for the treatment of BPH.

α_1-ADRENORECEPTOR ANTAGONISTS (ALPHA-BLOCKERS)

Historically, alpha-blockers were developed for the treatment of hypertension, and their use in blood pressure treatment goes back some 30 years. Their effect on blood pressure resides in their ability to relax the smooth muscles in blood vessel walls. But it was more recently found that they also relaxed muscle tension in the prostate, bladder neck and urethra, which allowed urine to flow more freely. The older drugs, i.e. Cardura (doxazosin) and Hytrin (terazosin) act on both the prostate and the vascular system in general with associated blood pressure effects. Both must be "titrated" (a term borrowed from classical analytical chemistry) starting with a low initial dose which is then increased to achieve a minimum of adverse side effects and the reduction of BPH symptoms. These adverse effects include postural (orthostatic) hypotension (a sharp drop in blood pressure upon changing position such as standing up) as well as dizziness, fainting, and actual loss of consciousness due to diminished cerebral blood flow. These cardiovascular related side effects are a serious consideration since they can result in falls, fractures and head injuries, but proper titration to find a suitable dose level has been found to minimize these problems. There are two newer drugs, Flomax (tamsulosin) and Uroxatral (alfuzosin) that are specific in relaxing mainly the prostate and not only do they not need to be titrated to ascertain the safe dose, but their use is in general associated with a lower level of side effects. Because titration is unnecessary with these newer prostate-specific (urospecific) alpha-blockers, their use also results in a more rapid symptom improvement, although over the long term, most studies indicate that all four of these drugs are approximately equivalent in effectiveness. However, in spite of the absence of required titration of dose in the prostate-specific alpha-blockers, it has been recently pointed out that experimenting with the dosage may still be necessary to achieve optimum results, since there is at present no definitive answer to the question of either appropriate dose or for that matter, treatment duration. The same is true with the older alpha-blockers—optimum dose is a separate issue from titration by slowly building up to an effective dose to avoid adverse cardiovascular effects [76].

Milani and Djavan [77] have recently provided a comprehensive review of studies on alpha-blocker use in treating BPH with special reference to relative effectiveness, cardiovascular side effects, and the effect of alpha-blockers on blood pressure management and abnormal ejaculation. The following points are of interest.

- With regard to cardiovascular adverse events, a review of the literature indicated that the newer alpha-blockers were superior to the traditional ones when dizziness, orthostatic hypotension, and discontinuation of drug use were considered. When tamsulosin (0.4 mg) and alfuzosin (10 mg) were directly compared, tamsulosin caused less dizziness but the incidence of syncope (unconsciousness), hypotension and discontinuations were similar. However, in elderly patients, tamsulosin caused less symptomatic orthostatic hypotension during orthostatic stress testing than did alfuzosin. Also, a comparison of studies indicated that alfuzosin might be less well tolerated in elderly patients and patients with cardiovascular comorbidity or co-medication. However, in a study recently reported by Nordling [78] a 7% incidence of dizziness was found for those on 0.4 mg of tamsulosin vs. 0% for those on 10 mg of alfuzosin. Furthermore, changes in blood pressure were less pronounced with alfuzosin vs. tamsulosin. But these effects are small, and Nordling concludes that both alfuzosin at 10 mg and tamsulosin at 0.4 mg have similar cardiovascular tolerability profile in the elderly and those taking antihypertensive drugs.

- An issue with using alpha-blockers for the treatment of BPH concerns the effect on hypertension therapy. One study indicated that tamsulosin can be administered along with several antihypertensives such as calcium antagonists, beta-blockers, and ACE inhibitors.

- Another side effect associated with alpha-blockers involves abnormal ejaculation which can take the form of retrograde ejaculation (ejaculation partially or totally into the bladder), or reduced or total absence of ejaculate volume. In placebo controlled trials, abnormal ejaculation has been reported mainly with tamsulosin. In European trials, the incidence was 4-5% whereas in US trials it was 6-11%. A direct comparison study comparing alfuzosin and tamsulosin, however, found similar percentages of patients with ejaculation failure with these two drugs, although overall, tamsulosin resulted in slightly greater incidence of abnormal ejaculation. Interestingly, tamsulosin has also been shown to slightly improve overall sexual function vs. a placebo. Studies also find that less than 1% of patients discontinue usage because of abnormal ejaculation.

The authors [77] conclude that an alpha-blocker that has a low potential to interfere with blood pressure regulation, induce cardiovascular adverse effects, or interfere with commonly used blood pressure medication should be considered a first-choice treatment option for LUTS/BPH.

The long-term efficacy and safety of the prostate-specific alpha-blocker alfuzosin has recently been reviewed by McVary [79]. Six long-term clinical trials involving a total of almost 12,000 participants were reviewed. These trials demonstrated that the beneficial effect of alfuzosin on BPH related symptoms was persistent with no evidence of decreasing response over three years. Longer term use was also associated with positive effects on quality of life and sexual functioning and these were also persistent. In addition, alfuzosin may help decrease the incidence of spontaneous acute urinary retention and other BPH complications.

An unusual side effect of the prostate-specific alpha-blocker tamsulosin has very recently been reported. Chang and Campbell [80] have provided retrospective and prospective evidence that patients taking tamsulosin are susceptible to what is termed *intraoperative floppy iris syndrome* which can cause serious problems and complications during cataract surgery. It is thought that the iris has the same α-receptors as are targeted in the prostate by tamsulosin, and it is suggested that there are both short-term and possibly long-term atrophic effects on the iris musculature. Two recent communications in *BJU International* [81,82] attempt to call urologist's attention to the problem and suggest that patients taking tamsulosin should be informed that it is necessary to suspend the use of this drug sometime prior to cataract surgery, and that ophthalmologists of course also need to be aware of the problem. While the washout time for this drug is 3-7 days, it is not clear how long a drug-free period is necessary [81]. The same problem may exist with alfuzosin which is also a prostate-specific type alpha-blocker. As discussed above, the prostate-specific alpha-blockers have become popular because they do not need dose titration. However, once a patient is at the recommended dose, they appear no better than the older systemic blockers, and the connection with the floppy iris syndrome might be one reason for choosing from among this older class. If indeed there are long-term permanent atrophic effects associated with the iris, then given the prevalence of cataracts, especially in the age group where BPH is common, this choice would remove both the potential problem and the uncertainty regarding the risk in this context. Also, by selecting an older non-specific alpha blocker, the potential problem of increased urinary symptoms leading up to cataract surgery because of the temporary termination of BPH therapy would be eliminated.

5α-REDUCTASE INHIBITORS

The enzyme 5α-reductase converts testosterone into dihydrotestosterone (DHT), the hormone thought to be involved in prostate enlargement. Inhibiting the action of this enzyme reduces the level of DHT and in fact generally significantly reduces prostate volume as well as LUTS/BPH symptoms. While alpha-blockers influence the *dynamic* aspect of BPH, inhibiting this enzyme is thought to influence the *static* component related to the size of the prostate. Inhibition improves symptoms and flow rate in part by shrinking the transition zone of the prostate [83]. At present there are only two 5α-reductase inhibitors (5ARIs) on the North American market, finasteride (Proscar) and dutasteride (Avodart). Both have now been rather extensively studied. A 1996 study by Lepor *et al* [84] indicated that finasteride failed to alleviate BPH symptoms, and a second placebo-controlled randomized trial also found no benefit of finasteride [85]. It has been suggested that the these studies failed because of low prostate volume in the subjects and that as well, insufficient time was allowed for finasteride to reach complete effectiveness [83,86]. The Lepor *et al* study is the only one cited with regard to Proscar in a book on prostate health [87] published in 2005, where the position is taken that Proscar "does not relieve any symptoms." In fact, both earlier and recent studies have found this drug to be effective. Indeed, the landmark Proscar Long-term Efficacy and Safety Study (PLESS) which involved 3000 men and extended over a four-year period, found that finasteride was as effective as alpha-blockers for symptom relief and was more effective than alpha-blockers in preventing acute urinary retention and the need for surgery [88]. Evaluation of data from this trial over an additional two years confirmed the earlier results and indicated that the use of finasteride led to a sustained decrease in the risk of acute urinary retention (AUR) and/or BPH surgery in men with BPH and enlarged prostates. Patients who switched from placebo to finasteride in the two-year trial extension had similar results to those in the continuous finasteride arm [89].

Optimal conditions for finasteride to be effective were present in another large study [90], the Medical Therapy of Prostatic Symptoms (MTOPS), where the effectiveness of finasteride alone, the alpha-blocker doxazosin alone, or both drugs in combination was investigated. The duration of the trial was five years. It was found that the combination therapy was superior in halting the progression of the disease and reducing symptoms, but finasteride was more effective than the alpha-blocker in reducing the risk of acute urinary retention or the need for surgery. The total risk of progression was reduced by 39% for doxazosin, 34% for finasteride, and 67% for the combination therapy. The risk of AUR was reduced by 35% by the alpha-blocker, 68% by finasteride and 81% by the combination, while the risk of surgery was reduced by 64% for finasteride and 67% for the combination therapy with no significant effect found with the alpha-blocker. Treatment with doxazosin alone only slightly delayed the time to acute urinary retention and did not significantly reduce the risk of invasive therapy. The authors suggest that the continued growth of the prostate during doxazosin mono-therapy overcame the reduction of prostatic urethral obstruction achieved by smooth muscle tone relaxation due to the action of the alpha-blocker alone.   However, as emphasized by Desgrandcamps in a recent paper [83] which asks the question "Who will benefit from combination therapy?" the adverse effects observed in MTOPS were found to be more or less additive in combination therapy. Desgrandchamps suggests that combination therapy be used only for patients in whom the baseline risk is high. These are generally patients with larger prostates and higher PSA values. MTOPS involved one of the older alpha-blockers.

The importance of the baseline prostate volume in connection with the success of combined therapy (finasteride plus doxazosin) vs. monotherapy is highlighted by a recently published analysis of the MTOPS data. For patients with baseline prostate volumes less than 25 mL, combination therapy was no better than doxazosin alone for decreasing the risk of clinical progression of BPH, the need for invasive intervention or improving AUA Symptom Index scores or peak urinary flow rates. For patients with either moderate size prostates (25-40 mL) or enlarged prostates (40 mL or greater), combination therapy led to a benefit associated with the above clinical outcomes that was greater than either drug used alone. Thus to Desgrandcamps' condition of high risk for combination therapy should perhaps be added moderately or greatly enlarged gland.

In a recent study the use of finasteride was also found [91] to statistically significantly reduce the risk of BPH related surgery as compared to alpha-blocker therapy. The study covered 8 years and involved 1430 men, and all alpha-blockers commonly in use from 1994 to date were involved. These results are consistent with those reported for the MTOPS study by McConnell *et al* [90].

In an uncontrolled trial of 1000 patients the ALFIN study [92] compared the newer alpha-blocker alfuzosin (slow release) with finasteride, either alone or in combination. Those taking either the combination therapy or alfuzosin had significantly improved symptom scores, but the combination offered no additional benefit. This latter result may be due to the fact that the study followed patients for only 6 months. There do not appear to be any published studies of combination therapy using finasteride and tamsulosin. Men offered a choice between mono- and combination therapy may wish to consider the potential downside of combination therapy due to increased side effects. Long-term randomized placebo-controlled trials do not appear to have been reported for the newer alpha-blockers in combination with dutasteride (Avodart).

The 5α-reductase enzyme exists in two isoforms. Type I has been reported to be located predominantly in the skin, liver, prostate and kidney, whereas type II is found in the male genitalia and prostate. Finasteride is a type II inhibitor and typically reduces DHT by about 70%. Dutasteride, the other 5ARI currently approved by the FDA for the treatment of BPH, inhibits both isoforms. Studies have shown that dutasteride (0.4 mg) decreases DHT by over 90% [93]. Controlled studies on the efficacy and safety of long-term use of dutasteride are currently limited to three randomized, placebo-controlled phase-III clinical studies carried out over 2 years. Debruyne *et al* [94] have recently reported on these studies along with a 2-year open-label extension [95] aimed at assessing the long-term safety and efficacy of dutasteride. In a comparison between the

2-year and 4-year results, it was observed that there were continuing improvements in urinary symptoms and flow rate and a further reduction in total prostate volume in men with symptomatic BPH. In addition, the reduction in risk of AUR and BPH-related surgery which was found in the 2-year study, was durable over the 4-year treatment. The three most common side effects, impotence, decreased libido and ejaculation disorders occurred in 6.0%, 3.7% and 1.6% respectively in patients during the first year, but the incidence dropped off rapidly and dramatically after the first year to 0.4%, 0.1% and 0.1% respectively by the fourth year. Breast/nipple tenderness and breast enlargement remained more or less constant at 1% of patients. The low percentages of adverse effects after the first year suggest that dutasteride is well tolerated in long-term use. Long-term incidence of these four adverse reactions was similar in the PLESS trial of finasteride involving the open-label 2-year extension, which covered years 4 to 6. Also, for those switched from placebo to finasteride, the rate of these four side effects was similar to that seen in the first year of dutasteride use.

While both finasteride and dutasteride are obviously intended for male patients, both drugs carry warnings that women who are pregnant or may potentially become pregnant should not handle crushed or broken Proscar tablets or handle dutasteride soft-gel capsules because of the possibility of absorption of the drug through the skin. The resultant exposure, even to minute amounts, carries a potential risk of a serious abnormality in the male fetus. The seriousness of the problem is made clear by the warning in *The Physicians Desk Reference* (2005 Edition) that men treated with dutasteride should refrain from donating blood for at least six months following their last dose to prevent pregnant women from receiving the drug via blood transfusion.

Both finasteride and dutasteride have a profound effect on PSA levels with approximately a 50% reduction. This becomes an issue for those whose PSA levels are being followed for diagnostic purposes. It is now standard practice to correct PSA levels for patients taking either of these drugs in order to normalize the results with pre-treatment values or interpret absolute values. Since this is only approximate, there will be a problem for those with corrected values near a cut-off being used to decide on, for example, the advisability of a biopsy.

A study published in 2003 (The Prostate Cancer Prevention Trial--PCPT) which received considerable media attention suggested a potential new use for finasteride—the prevention of prostate cancer [96]. In a seven-year study, over 18,000 men over 55 years of age with a normal DRE and a PSA level of 3.0 or lower were randomized to 5 mg/d of Proscar or a placebo. The primary endpoint was prostate cancer during the seven-year period of study. A 24.8% reduction in prostate cancer over the seven years (confidence limits 18.6-30.6%, P<0.001) was found in men who had data for the final analysis. However, high-grade tumors were more prevalent in the finasteride group than in the placebo group (37.0% vs. 22.2%, P<0.001). This latter aspect has put a damper on what might otherwise be enthusiasm for the use of Proscar in the primary prevention of PC. However, Proscar may not actually "cause" high-grade or aggressive cancer. The authors point out that Proscar might select for high-grade tumors by selectively inhibiting low-grade tumors. The observed decrease in low-grade cancer in the Proscar group would support this explanation. An alternative explanation involves the effect of 5ARIs on prostate volume and histology, which in turn influenced the Gleason scoring. That the observation of in increase in high-grade tumors among the PCPT participants diagnosed with PC who were taking Proscar is in fact an artifact has been recently discussed by Andriole *et al* [97] who conclude that the weight of evidence supports this position. A study similar to the PCPT trial does not appear to have been conducted for dutasteride, but tissue studies suggest that treatment with this 5ARI may cause regression in some prostate cancers. One can view these results in two ways. Individuals taking Proscar for LUTS/BPH symptoms and to reduce the risk of AUR and BPH-related surgery may receive an added benefit of a lower risk of developing PC, but the risk of developing aggressive PC can be added to the "side effects" list, although it may in fact be an artifact and thus a non-issue. Life is never simple and clinical studies that are absolutely unequivocal appear rare!

The 5ARIs have the merit of reducing the prostate size, which it can be argued, represents treatment of the disease rather than treatment of symptoms. The 5ARIs also significantly retard the progression of BPH and thus delay or avoid invasive treatments for AUR or severe BPH symptoms. These characteristics distinguish the 5ARIs from the alpha-blockers which do not reduce the risk of invasive therapy. The alpha-blockers, on the on the other hand, act more rapidly and when the need for a quick response exists, they are typically the first choice.

The AUA considers the four alpha-blockers discussed above to offer appropriate treatment options for patients with LUTS secondary to BPH. The 5ARIs and combination therapy are considered appropriate for patients with demonstrable prostatic enlargement [60]. This latter recommendation is based on the observation that the 5ARIs are not effective if the prostate is not enlarged.

ALTERNATIVE TREATMENTS FOR BPH

While the alpha-blockers and the 5ARIs have rather low incidence of side effects when used long-term, there will always be interest in so-called alternative or "natural" treatments with lower or no side effects. These come under the general category of *phytotherapy* or herbal treatments. Mainstream medicine does not acknowledge the extent to which the use of some phytochemicals is in fact evidence based [1]. The American Urological Association (AUA) guidelines of 2003 state that phytotherapeutic agents and other dietary supplements cannot be recommended for treatment of BPH [60]. The EAU take a similar position—more studies are required [61]. This EAU position is surprising since the vast majority of patients in Europe with BPH are treated with phytotherapeutic agents *by physicians and by prescription*. As will be discussed below, two substances commonly used in the treatment of BPH in Europe and used as over the counter herbal remedies in North America are in fact backed by a number of randomized, placebo-controlled studies.

SERENOA REPENS (SAW PALMETTO)

The extract derived from the American dwarf palm *Serenoa repens* (saw palmetto) is unquestionably one of the most widely used phytochemicals for the treatment of the symptoms of BPH. The plant is found in swampy areas along the southeastern coast of the US and inland as far as Texas and as well in the West Indies. The ripe berries are the raw material for the extract. Historically, the dwarf palm berries were used by American Indians for genitourinary problems. Today, the extract is licensed in Germany, France and other European countries where it has the status of a prescription drug. In Germany and Austria, phytotherapy is the first line treatment for mild to moderate LUTS/BPH and represents > 90% of prescriptions for BPH [98]. In the US the popularity of saw palmetto has increased in recent years, and it is readily available in health food stores. A recent survey found that one-third of US men choosing non-surgical treatment for BPH used herbal preparations alone or in combination with prescription drugs [99].

A large number of studies aimed at evaluating the effectiveness and side effects of saw palmetto have appeared in the peer-review literature. One problem with these studies is that not all saw palmetto preparations were equal in terms of the composition of the extract, which makes comparison of results difficult. However, in Europe saw palmetto is a prescription drug (Permixon) which is standardized and subject to the quality controls normally applied to such drugs. Thus of special significance are studies that used this extract of *Serenoa repens*. Four reviews of clinical trials are of particular interest:

- Boyle *et al* [100] examined all the clinical trials using Permixon, comprising 14 randomized clinical trials and three open-label trials, involving 4280 patients. They concluded from a combined analysis that all available published trials of Permixon for treating BPH showed a significant improvement in flow rate and a reduction in nocturia as compared to a placebo.

- Gerber *et al* [101] also restricted their review of studies to those using Permixon. They reviewed both placebo-controlled studies and comparison studies with alpha-blockers and finasteride. Eighteen studies were examined. The authors summarize their results as follows: "*S. repens* extract significantly reduces the symptoms of BPH, increases urinary flow, improves the quality of life and is well tolerated. Analysis of the overall clinical database indicates that extract of *S. repens* may be considered a viable first-line therapy for treating LUTS." Comparison between Permixon and the alpha-blocker tamsulosin indicated both drugs were equally effective in treating urinary symptoms. A similar conclusion was reached regarding the comparison of Permixon and finasteride. In addition, evidence was presented that indicated the course of prostatic disease may be delayed by Permixon, especially in patients of high risk of progression. The lowest level of adverse side effects was associated with Permixon when compared to alpha-blockers and finasteride. The authors point out that the lack of Permixon induced sexual dysfunction may have been an important factor among those who prefer natural products rather than the prescription drugs.

- A comprehensive review was published in 2002 in *The Cochrane Database of Systematic Reviews* [102]. Trials were eligible for inclusion if randomized with men with BPH receiving preparations of *Serenoa repens* (alone or in combination) compared with a placebo or other BPH medication. The studies had to include clinical outcomes such as urologic symptom scales, symptoms or urodynamic measurements.   Twenty-one trials involving 3139 men were assessed.   Eighteen were double-blinded.   All were randomized.   The researchers conclude: "The evidence suggests that *Serenoa repens* provides mild to moderate improvement in urinary symptoms and flow measures. *Serenoa repens* produced similar improvement in urinary symptoms and flow compared to finasteride and is associated with fewer adverse treatment effects. The long term effectiveness, safety and ability to prevent BPH complications are not known."

- Fong *et al* [103] have reviewed studies not included in the Cochrane review [102]. In three randomized studies of the use of *Serenoa repens* for the treatment of moderately severe BPH evidence was found for efficacy in comparison to a placebo, 5α-reductase inhibitor or an alpha-blocker.   In a subset study of severe LUTS, *Serenoa repens* reduced the IPPS score by more than an alpha-blocker.

The following recent studies are also of interest:

- Djavan *et al* [103,104] found in a 3-year study that *Serenoa repens* reduced the incidence of symptomatic progression and AUR in BPH patients. Patients had mild BPH.

- Three studies that combined therapy with *Serenoa repens* and urtica extract have been reported that also found significant improvement associated with this therapy, and one was with moderate to severe cases [105-107].

- In 2002, Debruyne *et al* [108] reported on a 12-month double-blind randomized trial involving over 800 men with moderate to severe BPH. The study compare *Serenoa repens* (Permixon) with the alpha-blocker tamsulosin. It was found that Permixon and tamsulosin produced equivalent treatment results of LUTS in these patients with LUTS. Both treatments produced a 4.4-point drop in the IPPS score and as well improvements in a several other measures of LUTS.

Thus, contrary to popular belief in the medical community, there is considerable evidence, including some very recently reported, supporting the effectiveness and lack of side effects associated with the extract of *Serenoa repens* and many of relevant studies meet the often heard demand for randomized clinical trials. Noteworthy is the favorable comparison between saw palmetto and finasteride.   In the case of saw palmetto, its use as a prescription drug for decades in Europe also suggests an acceptable level of long-term safety.

Nevertheless, a study by Bent *et al* which achieved publication in the *New England Journal of Medicine* (NEJM, February 9, 2006) and which received immediate media attention, reported null results for a randomized clinical trial (225 men) of saw palmetto for the treatment of BPH [109]. Some might wonder if this paper would have been accepted by the NEJM if the results had been positive. In view of the very large number of randomized trials, many placebo controlled, that have showed benefit, generally equal to that of finasteride or alpha blockers, the results of this study may appear surprising. The authors fail to emphasize in their conclusions that their results apply only to individuals with moderately severe to severe BPH as judged by AUA scores, whereas saw palmetto is frequently used for mild to moderately severe disease. However, the study by Debruyne *et al* [108] discussed above involved patients with similar severity of disease, and saw palmetto alone produced dramatic improvements in LUTS symptoms which were equivalent to the alpha blocker. The authors only compare their results with the meta-analysis from Cochrane Database study [102] which covered the literature only up to 1997 and, as indicated above, found in favor of saw palmetto. Thus they choose to ignore a number of studies (see above) post-dating that review which also disagree strongly with their results. Many readers of the NEJM will not be sufficiently familiar with the saw palmetto literature to pick up this omission, although two of the omitted studies are mentioned in an accompanying editorial [110].

This single study by Bent *et al* has been heralded as proof that saw palmetto simply does not work for anyone (e.g. editorial comment in *Journal Watch,* published by the NEJM, March 1, 2006). Do the authors of this study and those who are providing editorial comment really believe that the European medical community has been *prescribing* saw palmetto for many years as the first-line treatment of BPH when in fact it does not work at all? There is a point where even anecdotal evidence from foreign countries must carry some weight! Phytopharmaceuticals in fact represent up to 80% of all European prescriptions for BPH! As elaborated above, there is now a quite considerable body of data from randomized trials, many placebo controlled, that support this widespread European use of saw palmetto as a treatment for BPH, and Bent *et al* need to explain why almost all of these trials universally and significantly contradict their results and conclusions. Their arguments involving the effectiveness of blinding in some of the studies reviewed in the Cochrane Database study appear to be a very weak response to this quite considerable body of results involving several thousand men that compare unfavorably to their study. Whether or not there are problems associated with the saw palmetto product used as compared to the European pharmaceutical grade saw palmetto (Permixon) used in most studies is not clear [110].

While the biological mechanism of the action of saw palmetto is not well understood, there have been a number of studies addressing this subject which have produced several hypotheses [111]. Saw palmetto appears to have 5α-reductase inhibitory properties, as judged by the decrease in DHT and the increase in testosterone seen in prostate tissue samples when individuals taking the extract are compared to controls [112]. The results were similar to those produced by finasteride. A number of cell and tissue culture studies also suggest this [111]. Most of the components of the extract have been isolated and identified. The extract is predominantly composed of fatty acids. When these were tested in cell culture for 5α-reductase inhibitory activity, the oleic, linolenic, lauric and myristic acid fractions were all found to have this property [113]. Saw palmetto also appears to preferentially reduce DHT in the transition zone [114] and studies of gene expression suggest that saw palmetto shifts the balance between proliferation and programmed cell death (apoptosis) with resultant tissue growth inhibition [115].

The possible connection between inflammation, BPH and Permixon treatment has been investigated. In a recent study, Vavarrete *et al* [116] examined prostate tissue obtained during surgery from patients given either Permixon or no treatment for three months prior to the operation. Two biological markers for inflammation, Tumor Necrosis Factor-alpha and Interlukin-1-beta were both dramatically lower in the tissue of the treated group. Treatment was accompanied by a significant reduction in the IPSS score in the three months prior to surgery. These results are consistent with the commonly observed presence of inflammation related mono-nuclear cells in BPH tissue that are absent in normal prostate tissue. The authors speculate that Permixon modifies the inflammatory status of the prostate through cytokine regulation.

Finally, studies consistently report that saw palmetto has little or no influence on prostate volume nor does it decrease the PSA level [111,112]. Thus, while 5α-reductase inhibition appears to be part of the action of this extract, there are mechanistic differences as compared to the synthetic 5α-reductase inhibitors such as finasteride. While saw palmetto does not interfere with the use of PSA in the context of PC, it may be less successful in the long term in halting progression of BPH than the synthetic 5α-reductase inhibitors because it fails to reduce the prostate volume. Saw palmetto also does not act as fast as the new prostate-specific alpha-blockers in relieving symptoms of BPH. In addition, adding saw palmetto to alpha-blocker (tamsulosin) therapy does not appear to provide any additional benefit, at least in the first year [117]. However, the dose of saw palmetto used in the study was only half that employed in most studies or routinely taken by many men [118].

Acquiring saw palmetto that has the amount of extract indicated on the label may be a problem in North America where Permixon is not available. The label should indicate that the capsule contains an extract that is at least 80% fatty acids, but there is no guarantee that the capsule contains the indicated amount. The dose used in many studies was 160 mg twice a day of an 80-85% preparation. Saw palmetto is frequently found combined with other phytochemicals in what are sometimes called *prostate formulas* or *prostate health* capsules.

Thus, while some will no doubt point to the recent NEJM article discussed above and claim that saw palmetto has been proven ineffective and should no longer be considered in the context of BPH, such a position obviously ignores a very large body of positive clinical evidence, most of which meets the standard demand for randomization and placebo control, and in addition, there are mechanistic studies that provide biochemical grounds for the efficacy.

PYGEUM AFRICANUM (AFRICAN PYGEUM)

An extract derived from *P. africanum* (African prune tree) is probably the second most popular phytochemical after saw palmetto used for the treatment of the symptoms of BPH. Active ingredients are extracted from the bark of this evergreen species which is found throughout Africa at altitudes above 3000 feet. Interest in its therapeutic value can be traced back to the 1700s when European travelers learned from African tribes that the bark extract could be used to treat bladder discomfort and "old man's disease" as BPH was called then. Widespread use in Europe began in the mid 1960's and it is the most commonly used remedy in France for BPH [119].

In 2000 Ishani *et al* [120] published a review of clinical studies of *P. africanum* extract. They examined 18 randomized, controlled trials involving over 1500 men that were published between 1996 and 2000. The reviewers found that *P. africanum* extract yielded significant improvement in the combined outcome of urological symptoms and flow measures. Also, subjects taking pygeum extract were more than twice as likely to report improvement in overall symptoms as compared to those taking a placebo. Nocturia was reduced by 19% and residual urine volume by 24% while peak urine flow increased by 23%. This review covers essentially the same set of studies as that reviewed in *The Cochrane Database of Systematic Reviews* in 1998, which arrived at similar conclusions [121]. Compared to saw palmetto, pygeum does not have as extensive a set of clinical studies to substantiate effectiveness, nor are the studies as large or as uniform in endpoints, but the studies that have been reported are consistent and those reviewed were randomized and placebo controlled. The popularity mentioned above in Europe and especially in France also anecdotally attests to significant effectiveness. In addition, the majority of studies report an absence of any significant adverse effects [119,120].

There has been very little research involving human subjects that has investigated possible mechanisms whereby *P. africanum* extract influences the prostate gland. However, several hypothetical mechanisms have been suggested. These have been reviewed by Levin and Das [122]. Included are (a) inhibition of various growth factors known to operate in prostate tissue; (b) a weak anti-estrogenic effect; (c) inhibition of the enzyme 5α-reductase; (d) anti-inflammatory effects. A number of other mechanisms have been investigated, mostly in an animal model of BPH, but these have emphasized effects on the bladder rather than the prostate. While a number of constituents of the pygeum extract have been isolated and identified, including the polysterol beta-sitosterol, a known anti-inflammatory agent also used in BPH phytotherapy, and alcohols that reduce the prolactin levels which might inhibit testosterone uptake by the prostate, in fact little is really known about whether one or more of the isolated constituents is an active ingredient.

African pygeum is frequently found in prostate formulations. The typical dose is 40 mg twice a day of an extract containing 13% beta-sitosterol. Preparations that fail to give the percentage of sitosterol should be viewed with suspicion. In addition, it is an expensive phytochemical, and there is thus motivation to short-change the consumer in order to benefit the bottom line.

BETA-SITOSTEROL (PHYTOSTEROL)

Three randomized, placebo-controlled clinical studies conducted between 1986 and 1997 which examined the effect of β-sitosterol on the symptoms of BPH have been reviewed by Wilt *et al* [123]. It was consistently found that β-sitosterol improved urologic symptoms and flow measures. In two studies, IPSS scores improved significantly as did residual urine volumes. One of the studies reviewed [124] was continued with 18 months of additional open label treatment and follow-up. It was found that the beneficial effects observed in the initial 6-month study were maintained for the additional 18 months, and patients who had been on the placebo but were switched to the β-sitosterol improved to the same extent as the treatment group. No change is prostate size was observed. These appear to be the only randomized clinical trials. However, they were of short duration and there was a lack of a standardized β-sitosterol preparation. This plant sterol is now being added to prostate formulations. The Life Extension Enhanced Natural Prostate Formula (Cat. No. 875) contains 90 mg of β-sitosterol per softgel and the recommended dose is two a day. The Whitaker formulation *Prostate Health* contains a similar amount with a comparable suggested daily dose.

URTICA DIOICA (STINGING NETTLE)

This herbal drug has been used for many years in Germany where it is believed that it is effective. However, there are no studies that appear to meet reasonable standards of acceptability that shed light on the question of how effective this herbal extract really is. When it is used in combination with saw palmetto, encouraging results are obtained but it is not possible to isolate the effects due to urtica dioica [106,107,125-127]. Thus in using stinging nettle alone, one is essentially depending on anecdotal or weak clinical evidence.

CERNILTON (CERNITIN, FLOWER POLLEN or RYE-GRASS POLLEN)

Cernilton (also called Cernitin, a proprietary preparation) is made from rye-grass pollen. It is used by millions of men worldwide for BPH and is a registered pharmaceutical throughout Western Europe, Japan, Korea and Argentina [128]. *In vitro* studies suggest that Cernilton has anti-androgenic effects, may relax urethral smooth muscle tone and increase bladder muscle contraction [128]. In reviews of clinical studies, Macdonald *et al* [128] and Wilt *et al* [129] point out that Cernilton trials were limited by their short duration, small number of participants, omissions in reported outcomes, and the unknown quality of the preparations used. However, the available evidence does suggest that Cernilton is well tolerated and modestly improves overall urological symptoms including nocturia. It does not appear to improve urinary flow measures [129]. It is clear that additional randomized controlled studies with large numbers of enrollees and significant duration are needed to evaluate the clinical effectiveness and safety of this product. Nevertheless, it is included in prostate formulations such as Dr. Julian Whitaker's *Prostate Health* with a recommended dose of 200-400 mg/day. Life Extension prostate formulations also contain Cernilton.

OTHER PHYTOTHERAPY

The phytoestrogens daidzein and genistein found in soy and red clover are commonly promoted for the prevention or treatment of BPH, but these substances exert estrogenic effects that may pose risks by disturbing the hormonal balance [130]. An herbal tea made from the Small-flowered Willow also has a following based on anecdotal evidence (see www.maria-treben.biz/prostate.htm).

Part of the folklore of prostate phytotherapy is the use of pumpkin seed or extract for BPH. There appears to be only one study reported in the literature in the past 10 years that provides some evidence [131]. In this study 2245 men with mild to moderate BPH were given a European pumpkin seed extract (*Prosta Fink Forte* capsules—1-2 per day) for 3 months. The symptom scores decreased by 41.4% and the quality of life improved by 46.1% with more than 96% of men reporting no undesirable side effects. Dr. Julian Whitaker's *Prostate Health* formulation contains 200 mg of pumpkin seed oil per 2 softgels with a daily dose recommendation of 2-4 capsules. This appears comparable to *Prosta Fink Forte* which has 500 mg of an extract containing 92% fats.

CONCLUSIONS

Men electing to treat BPH with phytochemicals may wish to consider combined therapy such as is provided by prostate formulations that contain most of the substances discussed above that were found beneficial. In Europe, combined therapy has been used for some time including treatment in cases of moderate to severe BPH. While combined therapy has not had the extensive testing that the individual components have received, reports are starting to appear, including one that involved moderate to severe cases [105-107]. All of these studies were randomized and placebo controlled and found statistical significant benefits accrued from the combined therapy, which in all cases involved saw palmetto plus urtica extract.

INVASIVE TREATMENTS FOR BPH

Historically, surgery was the most common treatment for BPH, but surgery is on the decline because of the increased use of medications and the use of less invasive therapy. However, when drug therapy fails or if symptoms worsen to the point where they severely affect normal living, invasive treatment may become necessary. Repeated acute urinary retention episodes, repeated bleeding in the urine, bladder stones, or recurrent urinary tract infections may prompt the consideration of an invasive or surgical solution to the problem. These procedures are designed to either physically remove, "vaporize" or kill prostate tissue. Dead tissue which remains after the procedure sloughs off over a period of time. Descriptions of invasive procedures for relieving the severe results and complications of BPH should stimulate a strong interest in prevention!

Minimally invasive procedures for treating BPH are of fairly recent origin. Comparison studies both within this group and between these procedures and conventional surgery are limited. Comparisons are also difficult because of the variations and evolution of techniques and equipment and variations in the level of training and skill of those doing the operations, important variables which are difficult to quantify and take into account.

TRANSURETHRAL RESECTION OF THE PROSTATE (TURP)

This surgical procedure is also colloquially known at the "Roto-Rooter" operation. It accounts for 95% of the surgical procedures done to relieve the symptoms of BPH. Increased use of medical therapy has reduced the number of TURPs by 60% in the past decade, but it is still one of the most commonly performed operations in the US [1]. The operation is done under general anesthesia or a spinal block. The surgeon threads a narrow instrument into the urethra and employs small cutting tools to remove excess prostate tissue and a small electrical loop to cauterize the wound. The so-called internal urinary sphincter at the base of the bladder is generally removed in this operation, leaving only the external urinary sphincter at the exit end of the prostate for urinary control. The tissue recovered is normally examined by a pathologist and it is not uncommon to discover histological evidence of prostate cancer. In his recent book [1], Dr. Peter Scardino provides the following statistics regarding side effects and complications, statistics presumably based in part on the experiences at Memorial Sloan-Kettering Cancer Center, where he is, at this writing, chair of urology. Bleeding that may require transfusion—4% of cases; acute urinary retention—6 to 7%, infections—2%, urinary stricture—5%, incontinence—1%. Erectile dysfunction is reported in about 13% of cases, but Scardino claims that a properly performed TURP should not cause this side effect. Over 50% of men develop retrograde ejaculation (ejaculation partially or totally into the bladder due to the absence of the internal urinary sphincter) with resultant partial or complete infertility. The durability of the treatment is indicated by the fact that on average only about 1-2% per year experience recurrence requiring additional treatment. There is also what is known as TURP syndrome caused by the irrigating solution being absorbed into the blood stream which can result in symptoms of mental confusion, visual and digestive disturbances and cardiac symptoms. Presumably, the risk of complications and side effects increases when the surgery is performed by less experienced or less skilled surgeons. Scardino suggests that it is "always wise to put yourself in the best possible hands" but many, even perhaps most patients do not have the option or the opportunity of searching out and selecting the ideal solution.

In a review published in early 2006, Lynch and Anson [132] summarize what in their view is the current status of this surgical procedure: "Whilst our attention has been distracted by the many alternative treatments brought to the market over the past decade or so, transurethral resection of the prostate has been undergoing a quiet evolution. With fine tuning of all aspects of the patient journey we can now offer a procedure with excellent long-term efficacy combined with reduced morbidity and in-patient stay." Lynch and Anson review the latest developments related to this procedure.

OPEN PROSTATECTOMY

Performed through an abdominal incision, this operation involves removal of the inner portion of the prostate while leaving the outer or peripheral portion intact. Men with very large prostates or with medical or physical problems that preclude the physical positioning required for a TURP may be offered this option. The open prostatectomy is as effective as TURP in symptom relief, but the hospital stay is generally longer and the risk of bleeding requiring transfusion greater. The risk of subsequent retrograde ejaculation is greater than in TURP, and there is a small risk of more serious surgical complications such as deep vein thrombosis, pulmonary embolism, heart attack or stroke [1].

TRANSURETHRAL INCISION OF THE PROSTATE (TUIP)

This transurethral procedure involves making one or two small incisions in the prostate near the bladder neck with an electric current or laser. This reduces the constriction. General or a spinal anesthetic is used and the procedure is sometimes done on an outpatient basis. TUIP results in less improvement in urinary flow and other symptoms and there is greater risk of recurrence and the need for additional treatment than with TURP. However, blood loss, the incidence or retrograde ejaculation, erectile dysfunction and incontinence are low [1]. The AUA guidelines [60] indicate that it should be used in cases where the prostate is only somewhat enlarged with a volume of less than 30 mL.

MINIMALLY INVASIVE THERAPIES

TRANSURETHRAL MICROWAVE THERMOTHERAPY (TUMT)

In TUMT excess prostate tissue is killed by microwave "cooking", which is more properly called coagulative necrosis. TUMT is done by inserting a microwave antenna into the urethra. The urethra is protected by a jacket through which a coolant is circulated. The probe has a balloon that inflates to close off the bladder outlet and anchor the probe. Local anesthetic is used to control pain. Urinary retention is a common temporary side effect and about 30% of TUMT treated patients need to use a urinary catheter for several days to a week and sometimes longer [133]. Other immediate complications include urgency and urinary infections. Full effects are obtained after the dead tissue sloughs off, and this can take from three to six months. Several microwave devices are currently in use in North America. The Prostatron, TherMatrx and Targis devices do not at this writing monitor the prostate tissue temperature. CoreTherm, made by Prostalund, a Swedish firm, which also uses a cooled transurethral microwave antenna, inserts a temperature probe into the prostate and monitors tissue temperature at three locations. Penile and rectal sensors are also employed to guard against unwanted tissue damage. CoreTherm uses a software-based feedback system to monitor and control in real time the temperature to which the tissue is heated which customizes the treatment to each individual patient and prevents either under treatment or excessive tissue damage. This TUMT feedback system stands out as the most distinctive treatment modality [134]. The CoreTherm procedure requires from 10 to 70 minutes, which is similar to other TUMT devices. Procedures done without actually monitoring the tissue temperature are in a sense being done blind.

Studies of the effectiveness and adverse effects compare TUMT to TURP, the so-called gold standard of non-medical treatment. There do not appear to be studies that compare head-to-head the individual devices. Hoffman *et al* [135] have reviewed six studies with a maximum follow-up of one year which compared TUMT with TURP. Five involved the Prostatron device and one employed CoreTherm. From these studies, which the authors regard as having the best available clinical data at the time (most recent study examined was published in 2001) TUMT was an effective treatment for BPH that could be delivered on an outpatient basis and had fewer adverse events than TURP. But TURP produced greater improvements in symptom scores and peak urine flow and fewer men required re-treatment. The CoreTherm based study reviewed by Hoffman *et al* has been extended with three additional years of follow-up [136]. The degree of improvement was similar to that found in the 12 month study. A small but significant difference was found for IPSS in favor of TURP, but there were no statistically significant differences in peak urine flow. There were also no differences in the quality of life between the two groups. The safety profile which favored TUMT after 12 months was preserved after 36 months. Two other recently published studies also found the CoreTherm device effective and safe in treating BPH with TUMT [137,138]. In one, prostate volume changes were measured in 33 patients and it was found that six months after TUMT, volumes dropped from an average of about 64 mL to 36 mL and after twelve months the average was 35 mL [137].

In spite of the fact that the urethra is cooled during TUMT, a recent study found extensive urethral necrosis. This observation was made on prostates available after a prostatectomy which occurred three to six weeks post-treatment (some of the patients studied had PC and were scheduled for a radical prostatectomy after TUMT). Significant necrosis was found in the bladder neck. In this study, patients were treated with the CoreTherm device. The authors comment that "this study challenges the myth that the prostatic urethra should be preserved to have effective treatment" [139].

TUMT appears to offer a number of advantages over TURP. It can be done on an outpatient basis, transfusions are not required, retrograde ejaculation is rare, and risks associated with hospitalization are avoided, In the 4 year CoreTherm study [136], impotence, urination urgency, incontinence, and urethral disorders were all significantly and dramatically lower in the TUMT group as compared to those who had a TURP. It is also an attractive option for patients with comorbidities such uncontrolled diabetes, cirrhosis of the liver, or kidney or heart disease, patients who may not be good candidates for surgery [133]. The CoreTherm device would appear to be superior to devices that do not control the tissue destruction based on actual tissue temperature measurements, but this will remain theoretical until studies involving a direct comparison are conducted.

There have been a limited number of unexpected procedure-related injuries associated with the use of TUMT, which have prompted the FDA to issue special safety recommendations (see http://www.fda.gov/cdrh/pdf/P000043b.pdf).

Compared to other minimally invasive procedures, TUMT appears to offer the soundest basis for management of BPH, since it has the longest term follow-up and the largest number of studies completed to date [140,141]. In the 2003 AUA Guidelines [60], TUMT using Prostatron, Targis, CoreTherm or TherMatrx devices was included in treatment options. The EAU guidelines [61] recommend that TUMT should be reserved for patients who prefer to avoid surgery and for high-risk patients presenting with recurrent urinary retention.

TRANSURETHRAL ELECTROVAPORIZATION (TUVP)

This is a modified TURP where a high-frequency electrical current is used to vaporize excess tissue while simultaneously cauterizing. The hospital stay is generally shorter than for TURP with less postoperative catheterization time [133]. The frequency of retrograde ejaculation and incontinence are similar to the TURP operation. About 12% of patients have blood in the urine for a few weeks after surgery [1]. In a 7-year follow-up reported by van Melick *et al* [142], no significant differences were found in subjective or objective results for patients with BPH when TUVP was compared with TURP. This is a relatively new procedure, but the operation offers the advantage of low blood loss and shorter hospitalization. Lasers can also be used as the source of energy for the tissue vaporization process. The AUA guidelines [60] take the position that long-term comparative trials are needed to determine if TUVP is superior to TURP.

TRANSURETHRAL NEEDLE ABLATION (TUNA)

In this procedure prostate tissue is heated and killed by microwave needles placed in the BPH nodules. Transrectal ultrasound is needed to insure precise needle placement. The dead tissue sloughs off slowly over days or weeks and symptom improvement is only seen after one to two months. Urine retention is common after the operation and thus a catheter must remain in place for up to a week. One-third of men develop retrograde ejaculation and there is a small risk of erectile dysfunction, but less than 1% of patients develop incontinence [1]. TUNA is regarded by the AUA as an effective treatment for partially relieving symptoms of BPH [60].

LASER-BASED PROCEDURES

The laser is merely a source of energy which can be used to coagulate, incise, vaporize, resect and dissect, all fundamentally different procedures. There are also a number of different types of lasers with different wavelengths, power, the mode of energy delivery, i.e. pulsed, continuous wave, etc., and differences in the depth of tissue penetration of the light energy (which depends on the wavelength of light). Lasers are generally more complex to maintain and operate than for example, a microwave based device. Randomized comparative studies thus far have been of short duration, have involved a very limited number of subjects and are highly dependent on the equipment employed. It is not in keeping with the general goal of this chapter to examine the various laser based procedures and how they compare with TURP or TUMT since it may be some time before laser techniques are employed on a routine basis in a large number of centers. Even then, the results will no doubt depend on the experience and skill of those doing the procedures, the specific procedure being used, and in particular the type of laser system employed. At this point, generalizations are not particularly meaningful or useful. However, in the next decade it would be reasonable to expect that laser treatments will become well established and popular if they turn out to offer some unique advantages.

EMERGING THERAPIES

The emerging therapies interstitial laser coagulation and water-induced thermotherapy are considered by the AUA as having uncertain outcomes which should be discussed with the patient, whereas they indicate that high-intensity focused ultrasound and ethanol injections are sufficiently investigational that they should not be offered outside of the framework of clinical trials.

SUMMARY

It is an understatement to say that invasive procedures are not pleasant to contemplate, nor is the required encounter with a hospital and the associated risks of antibiotic resistant infections, an overworked and perhaps stressed-out staff, and the well documented propensity to errors, sometimes fatal, associated with patient care. In addition, the presence of comorbidity can dramatically increase the risk of adverse events associated with any surgical procedure. Nevertheless, there are circumstances where this is the only alternative if BPH has progressed to the point where life is no longer bearable and medical or alternative treatments are no longer effective. There are a number of minimally invasive options, but most are relatively new and lack long-term data regarding effectiveness and side effects. The exception appears to be TUMT. Also, if one seeks out a center where a particular minimally invasive procedure is frequently carried out with a known local track record and with skill developed through experience, then some of the concerns disappear. For example, the Mayo Clinic has pioneered the use of one of the latest laser techniques which uses the KTP laser [133], and thus this would merit consideration as a potential center if one desired this particular approach.

MEDICAL VS. MINIMALLY INVASIVE TREATMENT

Finally, there is the question of the relative merits of drug treatment vs. the minimally invasive approach. Djavan *et al* have addressed this question, using TUMT as the preferred invasive treatment, partly because it is the most extensively characterized. They point out that the improvement in symptoms and voiding function is greater with TUMT than with drug therapy and the associated morbidity is low. TUMT offers long-term improvement, whereas medical treatment must be continued indefinitely. Patients with small prostates and severe baseline symptoms can be treated successfully with TUMT, whereas finasteride for example is relatively ineffective in this situation. However, they also point out that approximately 33% of patients treated with the Targis or Prostatron TUMT devices required either TURP or another intervention two to three years after TUMT [143]. Similar data for CoreTherm does not appear available, but this feedback-controlled procedure with tissue temperature monitoring might be expected to decrease the incidence of under-treatment. Djavan *et al* quote retreatment rates for TURP are by comparison about 6% over three years [134].

ACUTE URINARY RETENTION

Acute urinary retention (unrelated to surgical or other invasive intervention) represents an extreme in LUTS. The inability to urinate requires immediate emergency treatment and the longer the delay, the more painful and dangerous the episode becomes. For men who have ignored LUTS, an AUR episode provides an indication of the seriousness of the problem which cannot continue to be ignored. It is estimated that 1 in 10 men in their 70s will experience AUR over a five year interval [144]. The most common contributing factor to AUR is BPH, although the obstruction can result from prostate cancer or prostatitis. Temporary relief is generally obtained by catheterization, and surgery (the TURP operation described above) is frequently the treatment of choice for attempting a durable solution. However, there appears to be growing interest in attempting to delay, even indefinitely, the need for surgery by the use of drug therapy.

Morbidity, and especially infections, associated with catheterization depends on how long the catheter is in place, and thus any approach that minimizes this time interval is significant. Also, the risk of complications and morbidity of the TURP operation are increased when infection is present at the time of surgery. Ideally, if surgery or some other invasive procedure is required, it is much better if this is done on an elective rather than emergency basis, and thus there is interest in a protocol that allows the early removal of the catheter followed by successful voiding with the associated opportunity to delay invasive treatment and in addition to treat prior to surgery any infection that has developed [144].

While there have been case-report studies and several small randomized trials (reviewed in [144]) on the use of alpha-blockers in attempting to achieve adequate and durable voiding after the removal of the catheter in AUR (termed a successful "trial without catheter" or TWOC), there has now been reported a large, randomized, placebo controlled clinical trial. In his paper in the journal *Urology* McNeill *et al* [145] report on the results of the ALFAUR study, which used the alpha-blocker alfuzosin in an attempt to influence the outcome of a TWOC after the first episode of acute urinary retention (AUR) related to BPH. Alfuzosin is one of the newer class of α-blockers that is prostate specific and does not require titration but can be used at full strength at once without increased risk of cardiovascular side effects, an essential feature for this application. The first phase involved 360 patients who underwent emergency catheterization and were randomized to 10 mg of alfuzosin per day or a placebo for three days. Patients with a successful TWOC were then randomized in the second phase to either continue the same dose of alfuzosin or a placebo for 6 months. The primary endpoint was the need for surgery.

The motivation of the study was the desirability of delaying or eliminating the need for BPH surgery, or at least allowing the surgery to be delayed to the point where it could be scheduled in the absence of a catheter. Since bladder outlet obstruction is an important pathophysiologic mechanism of AUR, the ALFAUR study was designed to test the hypothesis that this type of alpha blocker with the well known property of relaxing the sympathetic tone at the level of the bladder neck and urethra might impact the success of the TWOC and influence the risk of and time to a second AUR episode.

In phase 1, 61% of the alfuzosin group experienced successful TWOCs compared to 47% in the placebo group. For the second phase, phase 204 patients with successful TWOCs were randomized to the alpha-blocker or placebo. In the first 3 months, 57% of the alfuzosin group required BPH surgery vs. 85% in the placebo group. Surgical risk reductions were 61%, 52% and 29% at 1, 3 and 6 months. High PSA (median post-TWOC level of 6.2 ng/mL) and high post-TWOC residual urine volume were significantly associated with increased risk of AUR relapse and BPH surgery. The 10 mg per day dose was found to be will tolerated.

The authors point out that ALFAUR is the first large, prospective, placebo-controlled study demonstrating that an alpha-blocker, in this case alfuzosin, is a useful adjunctive therapy to catheterization for the first episode of BPH-related AUR. The therapy facilitates rapid catheter removal and avoids the discomfort and potential morbidity associated with a long-term *in situ* catheter. It remains to be seen how durable the successful trials without catheter are when alfuzosin is used. From the above figures it is clear that a rather high percentage of men experiencing their first episode of AUR will have an additional episode and will need some form of invasive intervention. The 6-month risk reduction for surgery of only 29% points to the serious message that an AUR sends with the first episode. Treatment with alfuzosin provides time for the situation to be evaluated and a decision made regarding invasive intervention vs. continued medical treatment. Delay also allows the patient to consider the various treatment options in anticipation of the possibility of a second AUR episode rather than accept the treatment offered on an urgent basis.

If a TWOC has been successful, one option might be to add 5α-reductase treatment, either alone or in addition to the α-blocker, i.e. combination treatment. The merits of this option appear to be an open question and no clinical trials appear to have been reported that address the use of the 5α-reductase inhibitors in the post-AUR setting. However, this treatment protocol has been discussed above in the general context of BPH.

There is also the question of reducing the risk of a first AUR. In a recent review of AUR, Hargreave and McNeill [144] provide the following data:

- The use of finasteride compared to placebo produced a 57% lower AUR risk during a 4-year period which was then sustained over two more years.
- When dutasteride was compared with a placebo in a study that included over 4000 men, there was a 41% reduction of the risk of AUR at 2 years. Slawin *et al* [146] report similar results from a randomized controlled clinical trial with a 2-year risk reduction of AUR or surgical intervention with dutasteride therapy of 50%.
- When the combination of the alpha-blocker doxazosin and finasteride was compared with a placebo, there was a 66% reduction in the progression of symptoms which would be related to the risk of AUR.

A randomized clinical trial of 5α-reductase inhibitors or combined therapy in the TWOC setting would be interesting.

McVary [79] has very recently reviewed the success of alfuzosin in reducing the risk of or delaying the occurrence of an initial episode of AUR. The studies discussed are positive in this context but are of short-term duration. McVary also points out that in the MTOPS study, doxazosin delayed but did not prevent progression of the symptoms of BPH. Long-term prevention of AUR may require significant prostate volume reduction, or at least completely halting growth, which at present can apparently only be achieved with the 5α-reductase inhibitor class of drugs.

WATCHFUL WAITING

Watchful waiting generally implies no medical treatment. The American Urology Association (AUA) "standard" is as follows: "Patients with mild symptoms of BPH (AUA Symptom Index ≤ 7 and patients with moderate to severe symptoms (AUA Symptom Index ≥ 8) who are not bothered by their symptoms (i.e. they do not interfere with daily activities of living) should be managed using a strategy of watchful waiting." It is also suggested that information regarding the benefits and harms of BPH treatment options should be explained to patients with moderate to severe symptoms who are bothered enough to consider therapy. This "standard" highlights the dilemma associated with the natural progression of BPH and thus the question of whether to initiate medical treatment rather than watchful waiting, since it does not give guidance in the decision making process with respect to predictors of risk of progression. They are not explicitly introduced into the criteria for the option of watchful waiting. Rather, the "bothersome" nature of the symptoms is clearly the primary factor. Some would argue that there may be advantages to considering the risk of progression in selecting therapy vs. watchful waiting to alter the long-term clinical outcome of the disease [147].

Watchful waiting has been the subject of a few studies. In one type, the primary object was to determine the risk of clinical progression. In the other, the watchful waiting study was actually the placebo arm of an intervention study of either an alpha-blocker or a 5α-reductase inhibitor or both. Djavan *et al* [148] recently published a study where about 400 men were followed with examinations every 3 months for four years. All had mild LUT symptoms at baseline and were on watchful waiting. Clinical progression was defined as worsening of the IPSS with migration to the moderate or severe symptom group and an increase in IPSS of more than two points. Progression was observed in 13%, 24%, 28% and 31% of patients at 1, 2, 3, and 4 years, respectively. Nineteen (4.9%) developed acute urinary retention (AUR) during the four-year follow-up, but only 2 patients required a TURP. The study found that baseline PSA, transition zone volume (TZV) and obstructive symptom score all significantly predicted clinical progression. A baseline PSA threshold of ≥ 1.5 ng/mL and a TZV of ≥ 20mL accurately predicted clinical progression in 82% of the cohort.

In a study reported in 1995 [149] with an extended follow-up report in 1998, Flanigan *et al* [150] used the crossover from watchful waiting to TURP as a measure of failure of watchful waiting. Patients were randomly assigned to either a TURP or a watchful waiting group. The failure rate for the watchful waiting group at 5 years was 36%. Men with low baseline peak flow rates who were randomized to TURP had an 85% greater improvement in peak flow as compared to men randomized to watchful waiting who eventually crossed over and had surgery. No difference, however, was seen in adverse outcomes. The authors also note that the symptoms of some watchful waiting patients actually stabilized or regressed without treatment. It is also possible that those who regressed did not have BPH.

In a landmark study, McConnell *et al* [90] examined the long-term effect of doxazosin (alpha-blocker), finasteride (5α-reductdase inhibitor), or both on the clinical progression of BPH. The placebo arm, which was equivalent to watchful waiting, revealed the following: at 4 years, 17% experienced clinical progression, including 14 % that had a greater than 4 point increase in AUA Symptom Index score, and 2% experienced AUR. A mean increase of 2.7 points in the AUA Index was perceived by patients as a worsening of their condition, although patients with high baseline scores required only 1.2 points and those in the lowest score level needed 3.3 points to have the same perceived level of worsening. Thus the 4-point change was a significant marker. Invasive therapy due to BPH was required by 5% of the placebo group. The men were at least 50 years old, had AUA Symptom scores of 8 to 30 (moderate to severe). In this placebo group, baseline prostate volume, PSA, maximum urinary flow rate, and severity of symptoms individually predicted the risk of clinical progression.

Watchful waiting can involve so-called self-management which may improve the effectiveness of this strategy [151]. Self-management interventions include education, reassurance, fluid management, caffeine restriction, bladder retraining and avoiding if possible medication, both prescription and over-the-counter, that aggravates BPH. The principal component of reassurance involves the question of the presence or absence of prostate cancer. As pointed out above, a high level of certainty would require one or more biopsies with their attendant low but finite morbidity. Fluid management mainly involves both the quantity of fluid intake and the timing relative to daily activities and as well, timing to minimizing nocturia. Caffeine is known to aggravate the symptoms and thus should be minimized or eliminated by avoiding coffee, tea, and caffeine containing soft drinks. A large number of medications are implicated, including diuretics, antidepressants, anti-spasmodics, anti-Parkinsonian drugs, calcium channel blockers and finally, decongestants and anti-histamines which are widely available over-the-counter [151]. Consultation with a health care professional is of course essential when attempting to minimize the effects of prescription drugs on BPH. Bladder retraining involves attempting to increase the tolerance for the urgent need to urinate and this can ultimately increase the bladder capacity as well as the inter-void time. Bladder training has been shown in many studies to improve urgency, and reduce frequency and nocturia in BPH patients and as well in men and women with so-called overactive bladder [151].

From these and other studies it is clear that BPH is a progressive disease that can result in acute urinary retention episodes and invasive procedures such as TURP. However, not all individuals with mild to even moderately severe LUTS or PSA levels and prostate volume values suggesting high risk actually exhibit progression, and as indicated above, reversal or disappearance of symptoms has been observed. Thus the dilemma and the associated probability-related "numbers game." In the absence of evidence of progression, watchful waiting is obviously a winning strategy. When there is a high risk or actual evidence of progression deemed worrisome, the risk-reward question comes up since the medical treatments are not without side effect, although they appear rather low and appear to decrease with time after treatment. This is a problem that must be sorted out between the patient and his health-care provider. Since phytotherapy is generally associated with minimal or no side effects, the fact that saw palmetto (*Serenoa repens)* has been found to reduce the incidence of symptomatic progression and AUR, it is of particularly interest in this context [101,104]. Thus watchful waiting combined with either saw palmetto or a so-called prostate formula would appear to merit consideration.

Finally, buying time by either watchful waiting, medical therapy or phytotherapy will also delay when action might be necessary that involves an invasive procedure. This carries the potential benefit that over time there should be continued progress and improvement in minimally invasive procedures which may have increased effectiveness and a lower level of morbidity than present day methods.

CONCLUSIONS

BPH develops slowly starting at about 40 years of age. A clinical trial involving drug or phytochemical intervention aimed at testing a true primary preventive protocol would have to start at 35-40 and run for 20 to 40 years with periodic physical exams and questioning regarding LUTS. Half the participants would be randomized to a placebo. Such a study would be very expensive and difficult to administer over such a long period and will probably never be implemented, especially if a natural treatment is involved. Even some of the investigators might not survive for the duration of the study! Thus guidance for now must come from shorter-term studies which rely on examining the relief of symptoms and the slowing or halting of progression. Extrapolation to long-term prevention is speculative. Thus in the end, one is left with some difficult questions and related decisions. These include:

- Should phytotherapy with its apparently minimal side effects be initiated at the age of 40-50 as a preventive measure in *asymptomatic men* in the hope of slowing or stopping the renewed growth of the prostate that occurs in most men in this age group? At present, the use of phytotherapy is generally initiated when symptoms appear. In North America, it is almost always initiated by the individual whereas in Europe it is by the physician and by prescription. This early intervention in the absence of symptoms would be based on extrapolating backward the results of phytotherapy in treating symptoms and decreasing already ongoing progression. Studies are very limited that address the question of whether or not saw palmetto, for example, actually slows or stops progression. It might turn out that additional studies would not support the observed positive result. Other phytotherapeutic substances could also be considered. The uncertainty as to what to use and if it will be effective is unavoidable at this point in time.

- There is the more specific question of what to do at, say, age 40, to prevent the renewed growth of the prostate, and currently mainstream medicine appears to have no answer. The alpha-blockers treat symptoms. The 5α-reductase inhibitors probably would retard and might even prevent the resumption of prostate growth in late middle age, but the side-effects would probably not be acceptable to many asymptomatic men. An interesting but unanswered question concerns low doses of 5α-reductase inhibitors used for this purpose, but there appear to be no relevant studies. Since saw palmetto is a weak 5α-reductase inhibitor, research on its early use, as suggested above, would be of considerable interest, given the low level of side effects that thus far have been observed. At issue here is the difference between symptom relief, something that has been the main thrust of research and current practice, both in mainstream and complementary medicine, and true prevention which of necessity must involve inhibition of renewed growth of the prostate that almost invariably occurs in the age range of 40-50 and almost always cause problems in later life.

- When bothersome symptoms are present which do not immediately demand invasive intervention, what are the options? There are really only four, watchful waiting, phytotherapy, alpha-blockers and 5α-reductase inhibitors. Watchful waiting is a numbers game—there is a significant probability of progression for all men past middle age. Not everyone will progress, but any given individual has no way of knowing what will happen, only the probabilities. What does one do? The answer will depend on the individual, his tolerance for risk, his reaction to the probability of side effects, and in the case alpha-blockers or 5α-reductase inhibitors, the advice of his physician who must write the prescription. There appears to be no simple answer. Some men will elect to try phytotherapy, especially a prostate formula containing a number of active ingredients. If this fails, they probably will turn to prescription drugs. But it is likely that any of these actions will be in response to symptoms.

- Early prevention does not appear to be on the radar screen for most men and doctors are quoted as commenting that frequently the first occasion when they are asked to deal with BPH is when their patients can't "pee." It appears there is a strong tendency for men to ignore prostate problems, perhaps because they have heard that when treatment is necessary it is bad news. Visions of the roto-rooter may inhibit rational consideration of the problem and stimulate denial. But there is little doubt that waiting until an AUR forces the issue causes a man to loose a number of treatment options that, if started early enough might have prevented the episode for a long period.

- When medical treatment fails, one is faced with the decision regarding either surgery or the so-called minimally invasive treatments. A permanent catheter is obviously out of the question. Here what ultimately happens will be strongly influenced by the local urology scene, the types of treatment and equipment available, and the attitude, beliefs and ultimately the advice of the patient's urologist, who will probably be someone acquired by referral rather than selected. Some patients will have the option of shopping around at more than one urology center in search of "the best" but most will not have that luxury. Asking for a TUMT rather than a TURP will probably produce a wide spectrum of reactions from one urologist to another, but the patient should keep focused on the basic principle that it is his body that is about to be subjected to the procedure and he should have a voice in the matter. He also needs to be knowledgeable, which is what this chapter is all about.

As suggested above, life is never simple, especially when it comes to medical problems. However, the studies discussed above indicate lifestyle changes that might prove effective in preventing or delaying BPH. These include exercise, taking steps to attempt to avoid having the metabolic syndrome or adult-onset diabetes, and as well considering limited alcohol consumption. The current evidence that supplementation with vitamin E, selenium and lycopene might enhance a prevention program should also be considered. Men may also wish to consider phytotherapy as a first choice before the signs of urinary trouble appear, even in the absence of randomized trials indicating the efficacy in primary prevention.

Chapter 3

Prostate Cancer: Causes and Risk Factors

Hans R. Larsen MSc ChE

INTRODUCTION

Next to skin cancer, prostate cancer is the most common form of cancer among men. It is estimated that 230,000 new cases of prostate cancer were diagnosed in the United States during 2004 and that about 30,000 deaths due to the disease occurred during the same period[1]. In 1997 prostate cancer accounted for an estimated 28% (19,800 cases) of newly-diagnosed cancer in Canadian men and resulted in 4100 deaths[2].

The vast majority of prostate cancers are adenocarcinomas, tumors that develop in surface tissues or linings of internal organs; in other words, in the parts of the body most vulnerable to attack by carcinogens and free radicals. Prostate tumors form in the ducts of the gland and usually appear in clusters located in the peripheral zone. The development of a carcinoma (tumor) follows a specific, well-established pattern.

In the **initiation stage** DNA is attacked by a carcinogen or free radical that causes a mutation in one or more genes. Free radicals or reactive oxygen species (ROS) are formed continuously in the body as a result of normal metabolism and are an integral part of the body's defense mechanism against bacteria and viruses. Free radicals are also released during acute and chronic inflammation. It is estimated that each cell in the body receives 10,000 free radical attacks every day[3]. Cancer can be initiated when free radicals successfully attack one or more of the following three types of genes.

Oncogenes – These are the genes involved in cell growth. They are normally turned on and off to maintain equilibrium, but if mutated they may get stuck in the "on" position and allow uncontrolled cell growth.

Tumor suppressor genes – These genes act as brakes to prevent uncontrolled cell growth and the development of cancer. If disabled by free radical attacks uncontrolled cell growth can proceed unhindered.

Repair genes – These genes constantly monitor cell divisions to ensure that there are no errors in DNA replication. If they are disabled, widespread mutations can occur and perpetuate themselves.

Normally, the body's own enzyme repair mechanisms will quickly correct any genetic errors and the mutation process stops. However, once in awhile, the error goes undetected and if the mutated gene survives for five or six cell division cycles an abnormal or precancerous cell is formed. A strong immune system may still destroy these precancerous cells but if it does not then the cells enter the **promotion stage** where they start reproducing rapidly and change their properties to those characteristic of malignant cells. If the cancer cells survive the promotion stage they will enter the **progression phase** in which they grow large enough to develop their own blood supply and defense system and eventually grow into a full-blown carcinoma. If the tumor is not removed or its growth halted at this point, either by conventional or alternative means, it may, in time, spread (metastasize) to other areas of the body with usually fatal results.

The problem of uncontrolled, malignant cell growth is further exacerbated by the fact that prostate cancer cells seem to be immortal; in other words, they do not, like healthy cells, undergo programmed cell death (apoptosis) in order to make room for new cells.

Carcinoma cells also have the dubious distinction of being totally devoid of glutathione-S-transferase, the body's main endogenous defense against free radical attacks. It is not clear whether the gene responsible for glutathione production is inactivated during the early stages of cancer initiation, or whether inactivation of the gene is actually the first step in the initiation process[4]. Interestingly, glutathione-S-transferase is also absent in prostatic intraepithelial neoplasia (PIN) cells. PIN cells themselves are not cancerous but, if sufficiently atypical (high grade), may be forerunners of prostate cancer much the same way that colon polyps are not cancerous, but rather precancerous.

Another characteristic of prostate cancer cells is that they lose their ability to accumulate zinc. Normal peripheral zone prostate cells accumulate extremely high levels of zinc (3- to 10-fold greater than found in other soft tissues). However, this ability is lost in cancer cells and their zinc levels are 62-75% lower than the level in normal, healthy peripheral zone cells. The accumulation of zinc is important for three reasons:

- Zinc is a vital component in prostatic antibacterial factor, which protects the seminal fluid.
- Zinc promotes programmed cell death (apoptosis). Its loss allows proliferation of malignant cells.
- Zinc reduces the oxidation of citrate within the cell by inhibiting the enzyme m-aconitase.

Citrate is found in very high concentration in peripheral cells and is vital for the proper functioning of the prostate and reproductive system. It is normally protected from oxidation by zinc and is therefore much less available for production of energy (ATP) via the Krebs cycle. However, once zinc is lost from the cell the citrate is no longer protected and participates fully in the Krebs cycle resulting in the production of extra energy to feed the malignant cells. Some fairly recent research concludes that down regulation of the ZIP1 zinc uptake transporter may actually be the first step in the initiation of prostate cancer[5-7].

Prostate cancer comes in two varieties, **androgen-dependent** and **androgen-independent**. Androgen-dependent cancer depends on androgens (male sex hormones, primarily dihydrotestosterone) to bind to the cell's androgen receptors so as to activate genes involved in cell growth. Androgen-independent cancer, which usually occurs later in the disease progression, has developed the ability to grow without androgen receptor activation and, as a result, is more difficult to treat.

There is now also evidence that chronic inflammation and the cyclooxygenase (COX) pathway play a role in prostate cancer[8-11]. The COX pathway involves the conversion of arachidonic acid (a common unsaturated fatty acid found in animal fats) to prostaglandins. Prostaglandins come in two varieties, "good" prostaglandins and "bad" prostaglandins. The good ones are created as a normal bodily function through the action of the COX-1 enzyme and fulfill important roles in protecting the stomach lining, creating platelets for blood clotting, and ensuring proper kidney function. The bad or inflammatory prostaglandins are produced in response to an inflammatory stimulus through the action of the COX-2 enzyme and contribute to the pain, heat, and swelling accompanying an inflammation. COX-2 activity has been directly linked to prostate cancer initiation and progression and COX-2 inhibitors such as Celebrex and Vioxx have shown some promise in the prevention of prostate cancer[12].

Finally, in elucidating the mechanism of prostate cancer it has also become clear that prostate specific antigen (PSA) is not just a marker of prostate cancer, but is actually an active participant in disease progression. PSA is normally only found in the prostate itself and in seminal fluid; blood levels are extremely low or non-detectable unless prostate cancer, BPH, prostatitis, or urinary obstruction is present. However, once cancer cells develop the barrier preventing PSA from entering the blood stream starts leaking and PSA levels rise in the blood. Some researchers feel that PSA itself may be contributing to cancer progression by breaking down cell membranes facilitating further invasion of cancer cells and spreading of tumors. There is also evidence that PSA can cleave IGFBP-3 and thus release IGF-1 (insulin growth factor-1), which has been linked to prostate cancer[13,14]. Other researchers, however, feel that PSA may be beneficial based on the finding that lower levels of PSA in prostate tissue are associated with more aggressive forms of cancer [13]. So while the situation regarding PSA is not entirely clear, lower blood levels would still appear to be desirable.

It is clear that the basic cause of prostate cancer (and most other cancers) is DNA damage caused by exposure to free radicals and carcinogens. The total absence of glutathione-S-transferase and drastically reduced levels of zinc in prostate cancer cells are contributing factors. Chronic inflammation has been linked to prostate cancer development and progression and there is also some evidence that PSA may be involved in the disease process.

DEMOGRAPHIC RISK FACTORS

Everybody is continually exposed to free radicals (oxidative stress) and other carcinogens, yet only about 1 in 6 men are ever diagnosed with prostate cancer. Clearly, there must be underlying factors that increase the risk for some men. Among the more thoroughly investigated possible risk factors are the following:

- Age
- Race and nationality

- Hereditary factors
- Diet
- Occupation and exposure to toxins
- Lifestyle (BMI, cigarettes, alcohol, sex)
- Nutritional deficiencies (vitamin D, selenium)
- Hormones
- Medical history (diabetes, vasectomy, BPH, prostatitis)

AGE

Aging is associated with a substantially increased risk of prostate cancer. It is not chronological aging as such that is the culprit, but rather the cumulative effect of continuous exposure to free radical attacks (oxidative stress) over a lifetime. More than 90% of 90-year-old men have some sort of problem with the prostate, be it prostatitis, BPH or prostate cancer[1].

Sweden keeps excellent cancer records and has a prostate cancer incidence similar to that observed in North America and northern Europe. According to their statistics, the probability of being diagnosed with prostate cancer between the ages of 65 and 69 years is 0.5%/year; between the ages of 70 and 74 years it is 0.8%/year, and by age 80 years it exceeds 1.0%/year[2].

Prostate cancer statistics for the US are very similar with 4 out of 1000 men (0.4%/year) developing the disease every year in the age group 65-69 years. Corresponding numbers for the age group 70-74 years and 80-84 years are 6.5 out of 1000 (0.65%/year) and 10 out of 1000 (1.0%/year)[3]. The estimated lifetime risk of prostate cancer is 16.6% for white men and 18.1% for African-Americans with a lifetime risk of death from the disease of 3.5% and 4.3% respectively[4].

The probability of eventually being diagnosed with prostate cancer is, of course, cumulative. At age 60 years the cumulative risk is 0.45%, at age 70 years it is 3%, and by age 80 years it reaches 10%[5]. So, on the positive side, 90% of men in the general population reach the age of 80 years without being diagnosed with prostate cancer. The average (median) age at which men are diagnosed with prostate cancer is 69 years and the median age of death is 77 years.

It is estimated that it takes about 6 or 7 mutations (successful free radical attacks on DNA) to create a cancerous cell. Depending on the efficiency of the host's antioxidant defenses it can take as much as a decade before a successful mutation occurs. Add to this that it usually takes 11 or 12 years before that single cancerous cell develops into a tumor that causes a rise in PSA or a lump that can be felt during a DRE. As a matter of fact, autopsy data clearly shows that most men have latent prostate cancer when they die; that is, cancer that did not progress to the point of causing problems during their lifetime.

The fact that most prostate cancers grow very slowly leads to two observations:

(a) Unless PSA is skyrocketing or a distinct lump all of a sudden appears on a DRE examination, there is no need to panic. There is plenty of time to carefully consider the various treatment options.

(b) The possibility that dietary changes, supplementation or other measures can stop, slow down or even reverse the cancer growth is very real, except in cases of very aggressive cancers.

Thus, while aging is usually listed as THE major risk factor for cancer it is not really aging *per se* that is the problem – it is the cumulative effect of oxidative stress and this, as we shall see in Chapter 5, can be prevented or at least diminished through several different approaches.

RACE AND NATIONALITY

There are huge and important differences in the incidence of prostate cancer in various parts of the world. African-American men have an incidence rate (new cases diagnosed in a year) of 249 per 100,000 as compared to 182 per 100,000 for white Americans. Black American men who get prostate cancer are also much more likely to die from it than are white American men. Poor diet, socioeconomic realities (poorer medical care, less likelihood of seeking medical care), and the fact that black men do not generate much vitamin D from sun exposure are likely to be factors in this. However, the main culprit is clearly genetic predisposition, possibly in the form of a less favourable arrangement and number of androgen receptors on prostate cells[6].

Asian men, on the other hand, tend to have much lower rates of prostate cancer. The incidence in some parts of China, for example, is only about 2 per 100,000 or at least 100 times less than the rate experienced by African-Americans[2]. However, when Chinese men move to the United States their incidence rate goes up to eventually settle about half way between the rate found in China and that for white men in the US. Although part of the reason for the lower incidence in Asia is, no doubt, due to a much lower use of the PSA test, it is clear that there must be not only genetic differences, but also environmental and dietary differences involved.

HEREDITARY FACTORS

From 5 to 10% of all prostate cancer is believed to be directly related to inherited genetic factors. Overall, carriers of the cancer-promoting genes have a 2 to 5 times greater risk of developing prostate cancer than do men with no family history of the cancer (non-carriers).[7] Several studies have confirmed that men with a family history of prostate cancer have a substantially increased risk[2,7,8].

A study carried out in Iowa found that 4.6% of men diagnosed with prostate cancer had a father or brother similarly affected. If a father had been diagnosed, then the son would have a 2.3 times higher risk of being diagnosed; if a brother had been diagnosed, then the risk would be 4.5 times greater than that observed in the general population[5].

A team of American and Dutch researchers evaluated the results of 33 studies involving over 200,000 prostate cancer patients and found that men with a father with prostate cancer had a 2.2 times greater risk, while men with an affected brother had a 3.4 times greater risk. If two first-degree relatives (father and brother or two brothers) were affected, then the risk was 5.1 times greater than the risk in the general population. The researchers also noted that an early diagnosis (before age 65 years) in a father or brother was associated with a substantially greater risk[9].

The importance of the age at diagnosis was also observed in the original study carried out at Johns Hopkins Medical School in 1992[10]. This study found that a man whose brother had been diagnosed after the age of 65 years had a 7.7% cumulative probability of himself being diagnosed by the age of 70 years. This probability is 2.6 times higher than in the general population. However, a man whose brother had been diagnosed before the age of 53 years had a cumulative probability of 19% (6.3 times that in the general population) of himself being diagnosed by the age of 70 years. Overall, the study concluded that the cumulative probability of being diagnosed with prostate cancer at age 70 years is 3.8 times greater for a man with affected first-degree relatives than for a man without affected first-degree relatives[10].

A very large Swedish study included 182,000 fathers and 3,700 sons with medically-verified prostate cancer[11,12]. Overall, 11.6% of the prostate cancer observed was linked to inherited genes. The study concluded that a man with two or more affected first-degree relatives would have a cumulative probability of himself being diagnosed with prostate cancer by age 60 years of 5%; by age 70 years the probability would be 15% (5 times rate in general population), and by the age of 80 years it would be 30%. The risk for a son increased substantially if the father was diagnosed before the age of 70 years. In this case, the cumulative probability for a 70-year-old man would be 43%, whereas it would be only 9% if the father was diagnosed after the age of 70 years[12].

All in all, it would seem that the cumulative probability of being diagnosed with prostate cancer, if the father or one or more brothers have previously been diagnosed, is somewhere between 2.5 and 5 times the probability expected for a man with no affected first-degree relatives. The probability does, however, increase if the affected relative was diagnosed before the age of 65 years. The reason for this is that the gene (HPC1) involved in early onset (before age of 65 years) hereditary prostate cancer is much more likely to cause cancer in first-degree relatives than are the genes associated with later onset familial disease. There is some indication that the presence of HPC1 is associated with a higher Gleason score and a more advanced stage at diagnosis[8]. Fortunately, the HPC1 mutation is rare and at least one study has found that there are few clinical or pathological differences between hereditary and sporadic (not associated with genetic transmission) cancers[13]. A review of the clinical aspects of hereditary prostate cancer concluded that patients with this form of cancer should not be treated differently than those of comparable age with sporadic disease[14].

Prostate cancer and breast cancer are both hormone-dependent cancers and the familial forms share several gene abnormalities (BRCA1, BRCA2, CHEK2). Thus, men with a family history of breast cancer are more likely to get prostate cancer and women with a family history of prostate cancer are more likely to get breast cancer. The crucial point in predicting whether a daughter is at greater risk for breast cancer is the age at which the father was diagnosed with prostate cancer. If it was at an early age, i.e. before that age of 55 or 60 years, then the risk is substantially greater than if it was diagnosed at 70 years of age.

Research done in Sweden a few years ago found that women with a first-degree relative with prostate cancer had a 1.6 times greater risk of developing breast cancer than did women without such relatives. However, in families with early-onset prostate cancer, the risk for breast cancer was 4 times higher[15]. French researchers have found that women with a first-degree relative who developed early-onset prostate cancer (before the age of 55 years) had a significantly higher risk than did women whose relative had late-onset prostate cancer (diagnosed at age 75 years)[16]. It would thus appear that there is an increased risk of breast cancer among women whose father had prostate cancer, but the magnitude of this risk increase depends very much on the father's age at diagnosis.

DIET

Researchers at the University of Massachusetts Medical School have compared the mortality rate from prostate cancer in 59 countries with a variety of environmental, dietary, and socioeconomic factors. They conclude that a high overall calorie (energy) intake, a high intake of total fat and animal products (specifically milk, meat and poultry), living in an affluent society, and having good access to medical care are associated with an increased mortality from prostate cancer. On the other hand, living in relative poverty (country with low GNP), eating lots of cereals, soybeans, nuts and oilseeds, and consuming fish is strongly correlated with a lower rate of death from prostate cancer. Thus a high intake of cereals was associated with a 31.4% lower mortality and a high intake of animal products associated with a 23.8% higher mortality. Milk consumption, but not butter and cheese, was found to be very strongly related to increased prostate cancer mortality, while the consumption of soybean-based products (soymilk, tofu, tempeh and miso) was found to be strongly related to decreased mortality. Members of the *Brassica* family of vegetables (kale, cauliflower, brussel sprouts, kohlrabi and broccoli) were also found to be highly protective as were breads containing flaxseed, rye and buckwheat flour[1].

Researchers at the National Cancer Institute in Uruguay studied 175 prostate cancer patients and 233 controls. They concluded that a high total energy intake, and a high intake of total fat, red meat (beef and lamb) and desserts (rice pudding, custard, cake, marmalade and jam) were associated with an increased risk of prostate cancer. A high intake of vegetables, fruits, and vitamins C and E was found to significantly decrease the risk[2].

MEATS AND FATS

Alice Whittemore and colleagues at Stanford University School of Medicine found that men with a high intake of saturated fat (>45 grams/day), especially from red meats and dairy products, have a significantly higher risk of developing prostate cancer than do men with a lower intake (<22 grams/day). This increase in risk with increased fat intake is particularly strong for Asian-American men. The Stanford team also found that men with advanced prostate cancer were more likely to have eaten a high-fat diet than were men with less advanced cancer (except in the case of black men). The risk of developing prostate cancer was found to be unrelated to the intake of proteins, carbohydrates, alcohol, vitamin A, and carotenes[3].

Scientists at the Northwestern University School of Medicine found that men who ate red meat at least five times a week had a 2.5 times higher risk of developing prostate cancer than did men who ate red meat less than once a week. They also found that a high concentration of alpha-linolenic acid in the plasma corresponded to a 3-fold increase in the risk of developing prostate cancer. The risk increased to 8-fold in men who combined a high plasma level of alpha-linolenic acid with a low level of linoleic acid[4].

Swedish studies confirm that a high intake of fat, meat, and dairy products increases the risk of prostate cancer. Consuming fried or charcoal-grilled red meat has been clearly associated with increased risk. A high intake of alpha-linolenic acid and calcium from dairy products has both been associated with higher risk. A study found that men who consumed 600 mg/day of calcium from dairy products had a 32% greater risk than those consuming 150 mg/day or less[5].

There would seem to be little doubt that a high intake of red meat, especially if grilled or barbecued is a definite risk factor for prostate cancer. Jagadananda Ghosh and Charles Meyers at the University of Virginia Cancer Center believe they have uncovered an important clue to why red meat consumption is so damaging. They have discovered that arachidonic acid, an omega-6 fatty acid mainly found in meat and animal products, stimulates the growth of prostate cancer cells through the production of a metabolite, 5-HETE (5-hydroxyeicosatetraenoic acid). The researchers found that 5-HETE is essential for the survival of prostate cancer cells and that these cells are completely eradicated (*in vitro*) in a few hours by blocking the production of 5-HETE. They conclude that a high intake of animal fats accelerates the progression of prostate cancer and that arachidonic acid is intimately involved in this process[6].

Researchers at the Department of Public Health in North Carolina recently reported that prostate cancer patients have substantially higher levels of phytanic acid in their blood than do healthy controls. Phytanic acid is a complex fatty acid found in red meat and dairy products[7].

Other researchers believe that a high fat/meat diet provides excessive amounts of IGF-1, a hormone clearly linked to prostate cancer[8]. Just recently the US Department of Health and Human Services added heterocyclic amines to the list of likely human carcinogens. Heterocyclic amines are found in grilled and barbecued beef, pork, chicken, lamb, and fish[8].

Australian researchers have found that a high intake of preserved foods (pickled vegetables, fermented soy products, salted fish, and preserved meats) are associated with a substantially increased risk of prostate cancer[9].

CALCIUM

Several studies have implicated an excessive intake of calcium and dairy products as risk factors for prostate cancer. Edward Giovannucci and his team at Harvard Medical School have found that men with a high calcium intake have a higher risk of developing prostate cancer. Their study began in 1986 and included over 47,000 male health practitioners. The participants completed food frequency questionnaires in 1986, 1988, 1990, 1992, and 1994. Between 1986 and 1994 a total of 1792 cases of prostate cancer were diagnosed among the men with 423 of the cases being of an advanced nature. After adjusting for other factors affecting prostate cancer risk the researchers concluded that men with a calcium intake of 2000 mg/day or more have a 2.97 times higher risk of developing advanced prostate cancer and a 4.57 times higher risk of developing metastatic prostate cancer than do men with an intake of 500 mg/day or less. Both calcium from food and calcium from supplements increased the risk. Milk consumption increased the risk of prostate cancer significantly with men drinking more than two glasses per day having a 60% higher risk of advanced prostate cancer and an 80% higher risk of metastatic prostate cancer than did men who did not consume milk. The team speculates that calcium interferes with the formation of 1,25-dihydroxycholecalciferol, the biologically active form of vitamin D, which has been found to suppress the development of prostate tumors. Somewhat surprisingly, they did not find any relationship between prostate cancer risk and vitamin D intake from foods or supplements between the range of less than 150 IU/day to more than 800 IU/day. They conclude that avoidance of a high calcium intake by middle-aged and older men may reduce the risk of prostate cancer[10].

June Chan and colleagues at Harvard confirmed the correlation between calcium and an increased risk of prostate cancer. Their study involved 20,885 male American physicians who were enrolled in 1984. During 11 years of follow-up 1,012 of the men developed prostate cancer including 411 cases of advanced prostate cancer. The physicians completed food frequency questionnaires to determine their intake of calcium-containing dairy products (whole milk, skim milk, cheese and ice cream). About 57% of the calcium obtained from dairy products originated from skim milk which contains 307 mg of calcium per serving (8-oz glass). A thorough statistical analysis of the data collected showed that men who consumed more than 600 mg/day of calcium (equivalent to 2 glasses of skim milk) had a 32% greater risk of developing prostate cancer, after adjusting for other potential risk factors, than did men who consumed 150 mg/day of calcium or less[11].

Researchers at the Fox Chase Cancer Center in Philadelphia investigated the link between prostate cancer and calcium and dairy intake in a group of 3600 men participating in the first National Health and Nutrition Examination Epidemiologic Follow-up Study. Food questionnaires were given at the start of the study, when the participants were, on average, 58 years of age. The men consumed an average of 13 portions per week of dairy products, varying from 3 to 23 portions. Calcium intake was 730 mg on average and vitamin D intake was 172 IU on average (well below the officially recommended daily intake of 400 IU and substantially below the 1000 IU/day now recommended by experts in the field). Analysis showed that men in the highest third for dairy intake were 2.2 times more likely to develop prostate cancer than those in the lowest third. When each food was studied separately, risk was increased with low-fat milk but not whole milk or any other dairy food. Calcium intake also increased risk by the same amount, but in further analyses only calcium from milk was significant. Calcium supplements did not increase risk.

The authors suggest that their findings support the vitamin D suppression hypothesis. They explain that the suppressive effects of the calcium from whole milk may be countered by fortification with vitamin D, but low- fat milk has a lower vitamin-D content, as it is a fat-soluble vitamin. On the other hand, prostate cancer may simply be diagnosed more in the higher social groups that tend to drink low-fat milk and are more likely to attend screening. In conclusion, the authors state that the increased risk from dairy may occur through a calcium-related pathway. They add that the link must be clarified, as both calcium and low-fat milk may be important in avoiding osteoporosis and colon cancer[12].

Japanese researchers have combined the results of 11 studies concerning the association between milk consumption and prostate cancer risk. They conclude that milk consumption increases the risk of prostate cancer by 68%. They speculate that fat, calcium, hormones, and other factors could explain the association[13]. They are particularly suspicious of estrogen which is known to induce prostate cancer[14].

The conclusion that calcium is a risk factor for prostate cancer is, by no means, unanimous. Scientists at the Dartmouth Medical School recently reported on a trial involving 672 men who were randomly assigned to receive either placebo or 3 grams of calcium carbonate (1200 mg of elemental calcium) every day for 4 years in a trial investigating the benefit of calcium supplementation on colon cancer risk. The men were followed for a total of 12 years. The researchers conclude that calcium supplementation does not increase the risk of prostate cancer and may even have a slight protective effect[15]. Two other studies have also found little or no indication that meat and calcium are associated with an increased risk of prostate cancer[16,17].

The latest 2006 study by Edward Giovannucci and his Harvard colleagues however, again confirms that a high calcium intake increases the risk of advanced (extraprostatic) and fatal cancer. Their study involved 47,750 male health professionals who were followed for 16 years. During this time 3544 of the participants developed prostate cancer (0.5%/year). Of these cases, 533 (0.07%/year) were advanced and 312 (0.04%) were fatal. The risk of fatal cancer was 87% (RR=1.87) higher among men with a calcium intake between 1500 and 1999 mg and 143% (RR=2.43) higher among men with a daily intake above 2000 mg when compared to men with a daily intake of 500-749 mg. The researchers also observed a correlation between high calcium intakes and the risk of high-grade cancer (Gleason score equal to or above 7). There was however, no correlation between calcium intake and overall prostate cancer risk or the risk of localized disease. The study also found that a higher calcium intake was associated with a lower blood level of vitamin D ($1,25(OH)_2$ vitamin D). The researchers suggest that the lower vitamin D level may be responsible for the higher incidence of fatal prostate cancer associated with a high calcium intake[18].

Although the evidence now leans toward an association between a high calcium intake and an increased risk of advanced and fatal prostate cancer the excess risk is well below 0.1%/year. Bearing in mind that an adequate calcium intake is essential to prevent osteoporosis and colon cancer it would seem prudent to ensure the recommended daily intake of 1200 mg/day. It would also make sense to ensure an adequate daily supply of vitamin D either through regular sun exposure or through the use of supplements (400-1000 IU/day).

ALPHA-LINOLENIC ACID

There have been quite a few studies regarding the possible detrimental effect of alpha-linolenic acid (ALA) on prostate cancer initiation and progression[19-23]. Four of these suggest that more research is required before a definite conclusion can be reached, but the largest and most comprehensive study did find that an increased intake of ALA is associated with advanced prostate cancer[22].

The study involved 47,866 male American health professionals who were followed over a 14-year period beginning in 1986. The participants completed detailed food frequency questionnaires in 1986, 1990 and 1994. By the year 2000, 2965 new cases of prostate cancer had been reported with 448 of these being advanced (metastasized) or fatal. The overall incidence of new prostate cancer detected over the 14-year period was 0.5% per year.

The researchers found no correlation between ALA intake and overall prostate cancer risk, but did observe a strong association between a high ALA intake and the risk of advanced prostate cancer. Men with a high ALA intake (greater than 0.58% of energy or about 1.3 grams/day) were twice as likely to develop advanced prostate cancer as were men with a lower intake (less than 0.37% of energy or about 0.8 grams/day) even after adjusting for all other known variables that could affect the risk. The risk was slightly higher for ALA from non-animal sources than for ALA from meat and dairy sources. There was a trend for red meat, mayonnaise, margarine and creamy salad dressings to be associated with a higher risk. The intake of two other abundant fatty acids, linoleic acid and arachidonic acid, was not related to prostate cancer risk[22]. A high intake of fish oils (EPA + DHA) was associated with a 26% reduced risk of advanced prostate cancer.

Advanced prostate cancer was defined as a cancer that was fatal at the end of the follow-up or extended regionally to seminal vesicle, other adjacent organs, pelvic lymph nodes or distal organs (usually bone) at the time of diagnosis. It is, of course, important to keep in mind that the association between increased ALA intake and prostate cancer ONLY applied in the case of advanced cancer.

The increased risk of advanced prostate cancer became apparent at a daily intake above 0.2% of energy. So if total daily energy intake is about 2000 kcal then the total ALA intake above which the risk starts to increase would be 0.44 grams/day. At an intake of 1.0 gram/day the risk would double if the ALA came from non-animal sources. These intake numbers are indeed very low. To put them in perspective - the minimum daily intake of ALA for men recommended by the National Academy of Sciences in the US is 1.6 grams/day. The observed danger of advanced prostate cancer also needs to be put in perspective. The total incidence over a 14-year period was less than 1% or

0.07%/year - about 20 times less than the incidence of heart disease over a similar period (1.36%/year).

The main sources of alpha-linolenic acid are meats, seeds and vegetable oils. ALA is particularly abundant in flax seed and flax oil, but walnuts and walnut oil are also high in ALA. Almonds and hazelnuts (filberts) are very low in ALA and soy protein powder also contains very little. There is no evidence that ALA from flax seed and flax oil is associated with an increased cancer risk. As a matter of fact, there is some evidence that daily consumption of flax seed reduces PSA and cholesterol levels and may help prevent prostate cancer[24]. There is also evidence that ALA from flax seed is helpful in preventing heart disease.

It is very important to bear in mind that a connection between ALA and prostate cancer was only found in the case of ADVANCED cancer. Thus, in view of the many proven health benefits of ALA, it would seem prudent to aim at a daily intake of 1.6 grams a day as recommended by the National Academy of Sciences, but to avoid known detrimental sources of ALA in doing so.

OCCUPATION AND EXPOSURE TO TOXINS

Several occupations, including farming and working in the rubber industry, have been associated with an increased risk of prostate cancer. The data supporting an association with working in the rubber industry is not conclusive, but the association with working as a farm labourer is fairly strong and is believed to be caused by frequent exposure to pesticides and herbicides[1]. There is also evidence that exposure to diesel fumes, metal working fluids, polychlorinated biphenyls (PCBs), paint strippers, varnishes, and photographic film developers may be associated with an increased risk of prostate cancer[1,2-4].

Cadmium is a category 1 human carcinogen and several studies have found a correlation between exposure to cadmium and prostate cancer risk; other studies, however, have failed to confirm the association. Generally though, it is thought that cadmium does indeed promote prostate cancer but its effect is blunted by the presence of adequate amounts of selenium and zinc in the prostate tissue. Cadmium can be found in polluted air and water, in cigarette smoke, and in contaminated fish[1].

LIFESTYLE

BODY BUILD (ANTHROPOMETRY)

There is considerable evidence that being overweight or obese confers an increased risk of prostate cancer. An Italian study found that overweight men (BMI equal to or greater than 28) had a 4.5 times greater risk of prostate cancer than did men with a body mass index of less than 23. NOTE: Body mass index is defined as weight (in kilograms) divided by height (in meters) squared or body weight in pounds times 704 divided by height (in inches) squared. A Norwegian study reported a doubling of risk among men who were more than 30% over their desirable weight and a French study concluded that obesity was associated with a 2.5 times increased risk[1]. There have, however, been some studies that have found no correlation. There is some indication that it may be excessive muscle mass rather than fat *per se* that is the culprit. Excessive muscle mass could be a marker for an elevated lifetime exposure to androgens[1].

CIGARETTE SMOKING AND ALCOHOL CONSUMPTION

Several studies have found a strong association between cigarette smoking and the risk of developing prostate cancer, while others have failed to confirm this[5,6]. A recent study found that heavy smokers did have an increased risk and that the risk declined when smoking ceased[5,7]. While it is thus not entirely clear whether cigarette smoking may precipitate prostate cancer, there is certainly no evidence that it is protective. As a matter of fact, there is strong evidence that cigarette smoking significantly reduces survival among patients who already have prostate cancer[7-9].

A number of studies have found that heavy alcohol consumption increases the risk of prostate cancer, while others have found no association. Drinking beer and beginning to drink at an early age were found to increase risk in one study. Another study found that moderate alcohol consumption was beneficial, but that heavy consumption of hard liquor was detrimental[1]. Clearly, there is no obvious consensus on the role of alcohol consumption as a risk factor, but no evidence to indicate that a glass or two of wine a day would be detrimental. As a matter of fact, a very recent study concluded that having a glass of red wine every day reduced the risk of localized prostate cancer by about 13% and that of aggressive cancer (Gleason score >7) by almost half[10].

SEXUAL ACTIVITY

Although there are no recorded cases of prostate cancer among eunuchs, there is also no conclusive evidence that level of sexual activity or marriage itself has any significant bearing on prostate cancer risk. One study found that having sex at an early age increased risk, while another study found just the opposite. It is possible that having many different sexual partners may increase the risk since it would increase the likelihood of contracting a venereal disease, which may be a risk factor, particularly in connection with bacterial prostatitis[1].

NUTRITIONAL DEFICIENCIES

VITAMIN D

Several studies have shown that a large percentage of people living in Europe and North America are deficient in vitamin D when not exposed to sunlight during the winter months. European researchers found that 36% of elderly men and 47% of elderly women have clinically deficient blood levels of vitamin D during the winter months.[1] Michael Gloth and Jordan Tobin at Johns Hopkins School of Medicine report similar findings.[2] Researchers at the Boston University School of Medicine found that even young people (18 to 29 years of age) are likely to be vitamin D deficient towards the end of winter.[3] Canadian researchers report that people living above 42° N latitude are likely to have a pronounced vitamin D deficiency during the winter.[4,5]

Our main source of vitamin-D is sunlight. It is estimated that at least 75% of our supply comes from photochemical conversion of 7-dehydrocholesterol in the skin.[6] This conversion occurs when we are exposed to the sun's UVB rays (290-320 nm wavelength). Vitamin D itself is biologically inactive, but is converted in the liver and kidneys to 1,25-dihydroxycholecalciferol [1,25(OH)2D3] which is a powerful hormone with many functions.[7] Most foods contain very little vitamin D with the main sources being eggs, fish, and fortified milk.[6,8]

Lack of exposure to sunlight is the main cause of vitamin D deficiency. In recent years medical authorities have exhorted us to avoid the sun and apply sunscreen before we venture outside. This advice is aimed at reducing the astronomical increase in the incidence of skin cancer and melanoma. Unfortunately, although sunscreens do help prevent sunburns, they are much less effective in preventing skin cancer and melanoma; their routine use may create a false sense of security and thus be counterproductive.[9] Research has also shown that regular use of sunscreens completely eliminates the body's synthesis of vitamin D and can lead to a serious vitamin D deficiency.[10,11]

Sun avoidance by itself leads to vitamin D deficiency. Windowpanes effectively screen out UVB rays.[12] Clothing, whether it be a light cotton shirt or a heavy jogging suit, eliminates or seriously reduces the synthesis of vitamin D.[13] Air pollution (ozone and sulfur dioxide) cuts out a large portion of the sunlight needed for vitamin D synthesis and many medications (anticonvulsants, steroids) also interfere with vitamin D formation.[2,8,11,12] Vegetarians are at particular risk for vitamin D deficiency because of their high fiber intake and lack of dairy products in the diet.[14]

Health authorities have attempted to ensure that people get enough vitamin D through the diet by fortifying milk. This approach, however, is ineffective. Studies have shown that the vitamin D content of milk is highly erratic and many of the samples tested in two surveys done in Canada and the United States contained no vitamin D at all.[15,16]

The consequences of vitamin D deficiency are many and varied. Drs. Cedric and Frank Garland of the University of California suggested as early as 1980 that a lack of vitamin

D could be a major cause of colon cancer. The Garland brothers found that the incidence of colon cancer was almost three times higher in New York than in New Mexico. They attributed this to a vitamin D deficiency caused by the relative lack of sunshine in the northern United States.[17]

Vitamin D deficiencies have also been implicated in the development of breast cancer, melanoma, ovarian cancer, prostate cancer, and of course, osteoporosis and hip fractures.[2,6,18-28]

The evidence for a strong association between a vitamin D deficiency and prostate cancer is compelling. Finnish researchers, in a 13-year study of 19,000 middle-aged men, found that a low serum level of vitamin D (25-hydroxyvitamin D) is associated with a 1.7- to 3.5-fold increase in the risk of prostate cancer. The effect of a low vitamin D level was found to be particularly serious in younger men (less than 52 years of age) and was also associated with more aggressive cancer.[29] Researchers at the Boston University School of Medicine confirm the Finnish observation and conclude that, "adequate vitamin D nutrition should be a priority for men of all ages."[30]

SELENIUM

Selenium is a mineral of vital importance to both humans and animals. Not only is it a crucial antioxidant in its own right, but it is also a crucial component in the body's endogenous, primary antioxidant and free radical fighter, glutathione. Selenium enters the food chain through absorption from the soil by plants and trees. Many areas of the world have soil that is low in selenium and animals and humans, obtaining their food from these areas, are often selenium deficient.

The first indication that selenium could be important in cancer prevention probably came around 1965, but it was not until the early 1980s that the possibility of using selenium to prevent cancer began to be taken seriously. In July 1983 Walter Willett and colleagues at Harvard Medical School reported that cancer patients had significantly lower selenium levels as much as 5 years prior to diagnosis than did healthy controls. They also observed that a selenium deficiency combined with a low level of vitamins A and E increased the risk of developing cancer even further.[31]

In 1998 researchers at the Harvard School of Public Health reported that men with a high selenium level (in toenail clippings) had a 3 times lower risk of being diagnosed with advanced prostate cancer as did men with a low level. The study involved 33,737 male health professionals who provided toenail clippings in 1987. By the year 1994, 818 new cases of advanced prostate cancer had been diagnosed among the participants. After adjusting their results for family history of prostate cancer, body mass index, lycopene intake, saturated fat intake, vasectomy, and geographical location, the researchers concluded that men with an average (median) toenail level of selenium of 1.14 micrograms/g (ppm) have a 65% lower risk of advanced prostate cancer than do men with a median level of 0.66 ppm. The researchers estimate that the daily median selenium intake among men with the lowest toenail concentrations was about 86 micrograms as compared to about 159 micrograms for men with the highest toenail concentrations.[32,33]

Researchers at Stanford University and the Johns Hopkins University School of Medicine have investigated the association between blood levels of selenium and prostate cancer risk. Their study involved 52 men diagnosed with prostate cancer and 96 age-matched controls with no detectable prostate disease. The men had an average age of 69 years and were all enrolled in the Baltimore Longitudinal Study of Aging. Plasma levels of selenium measured in blood samples taken four to five years prior to the diagnosis of prostate cancer were compared for cancer patients and controls. The researchers found that men with selenium levels below 10.7 micrograms/dL had a four to five times higher incidence of prostate cancer than did men with levels above 10.7 micrograms/dL. They also noted a significant decline in selenium levels with age.[34]

Researchers at the National Cancer Institute in the US have confirmed that serum levels of selenium are inversely associated with prostate cancer risk in both white and black men. They also confirmed that the association was stronger if low selenium levels were accompanied by low levels of vitamin E.[35]

More recently, a team at Harvard Medical School weighed in with another study supporting the conclusion that low blood levels of selenium are associated with an increased risk of advanced prostate cancer. Their study involved 22,000 healthy, male physicians who were enrolled in 1982 and had blood samples taken at that time. Sufficient samples to analyze for selenium content and PSA level were available for 586 men diagnosed with prostate cancer as well as for 577 controls matched for age and smoking status. After 13 years of follow-up the researchers concluded that study participants with a plasma selenium level of 0.12-0.19 ppm had a 50% lower incidence of advanced prostate cancer than did men with a level of 0.06-0.09 ppm. The correlation was only apparent in men with a PSA level of more than 4 ng/mL and was particularly strong for those with a baseline (1982) PSA level greater than 10 ng/mL. For these men a high selenium level corresponded to a 70% decrease in the risk of advanced prostate cancer. The researchers also observed a trend for a lower incidence of localized prostate cancer with high selenium levels, but this trend was not statistically significant. They conclude that selenium is perhaps not too effective in preventing the initiation of prostate cancer, but that it is highly effective in slowing down tumor progression. They believe that selenium acts by selectively killing off cells whose DNA has been extensively damaged, by inhibiting cellular proliferation, and by its role as a key component of glutathione peroxidase, which protects cells from peroxide damage[36,37].

Dutch researchers have also reported a strong association between low toenail selenium levels and prostate cancer risk. They found that men with a high selenium level (measured 6 years prior to diagnosis) had a 30% lower risk than men with low levels. The association was particularly strong for smokers and former smokers.[38]

Although the above studies did find a strong, statistically significant association between selenium levels and the risk of prostate cancer, especially advanced cancer; other studies have found no significant associations. Canadian researchers found no correlation between selenium in toenail clippings and the risk of breast and prostate cancer, but did note an inverse association with colon cancer.[39] British researchers also found no significant correlation despite the observation that selenium levels were substantially lower than levels observed in American studies.[40] Austrian researchers examined selenium levels in newly-diagnosed prostate cancer patients and healthy controls and found no significant differences. It is, again, noteworthy that the average selenium levels in both patients and controls were substantially lower than those observed in US men.[41]

Despite these negative studies, the preponderance of evidence supports the conclusion that low body stores of selenium are associated with an increased risk of prostate cancer. The benefits of selenium have been primarily ascribed to its ability to scavenge DNA-damaging free radicals and to help in the elimination of damaged, potentially cancerous cells. Researchers at the Indiana University discovered a third possible mode by which selenium might fight cancer. They found that selenomethionine, the primary organic form of selenium, turns on a key regulatory protein, p53, which is one of the body's main initiators of DNA repair. Previous research has shown that people who have an efficient DNA repair mechanism are less likely to develop cancer.[42]

A large trial (SELECT) was recently undertaken by the National Cancer Institute in the US to evaluate the effect on prostate cancer risk of supplementation with selenium and vitamin E.

HORMONES

Hormones are chemical messenger molecules produced by glands in the body. Their function is to instruct individual cells or other hormones so as to achieve stimulation or inhibition of growth, induction or suppression of apoptosis (programmed cell death), activation or inhibition of the immune system, regulation of metabolism, control of the reproductive cycle, or induction of a new phase of life (puberty, menopause). Hormones are extremely powerful and very small quantities are required to do the job. Many diseases and disorders are associated with a deficiency or surplus of hormones and maintaining an optimal hormone level is essential for the maintenance of health. Several hormones have been associated with the risk of prostate cancer. The most important of these are:

- Insulin-like growth factor 1 (IGF-1)
- Growth hormones and enhancers
- Androgens (male sex hormones)
- Anabolic steroids
- Dehydroepiandrosterone (DHEA)

INSULIN-LIKE GROWTH FACTOR 1 (IGF-1)

IGF-1 is produced in the liver and body tissues. It is a polypeptide and consists of 70 amino acids linked together. It is mostly found in the blood bound to its carrier, IGF binding protein-3 (IGFBP-3). Only the unbound form of IGF-1 has a cancer promoting effect.

All mammals produce IGF-1 molecules very similar in structure, and human and bovine IGF-1 are completely identical. IGF-1 acquired its name because it has insulin-like activity in fat (adipose) tissue and has a structure that is very similar to that of proinsulin. The body's production of IGF-1 is regulated by the human growth hormone and peaks at puberty. IGF-1 production declines with age and is only about half the adult value at the age of 70 years. IGF-1 is a very powerful hormone that has profound effects even though its concentration in the blood serum is only about 200 ng/mL or 0.2 millionth of a gram per milliliter[1-4].

IGF-1 is known to stimulate the growth of both normal and cancerous cells[2,5]. In 1990 researchers at Stanford University reported that IGF-1 promotes the growth of prostate cells[2]. This was followed by the discovery that IGF-1 accelerates the growth of breast cancer cells[6-8]. In 1995 researchers at the National Institutes of Health reported that IGF-1 plays a central role in the progression of many childhood cancers and in the growth of tumours in breast cancer, small cell lung cancer, melanoma, and cancers of the pancreas and prostate[9]. In September 1997 an international team of researchers reported the first epidemiological evidence that high IGF-1 concentrations are closely linked to an increased risk of prostate cancer[10]. Researchers also provided evidence of IGF-1's link to breast and colon cancers[10,11].

In January 1998 June Chan and her team at Harvard confirmed the link between IGF-1 levels in the blood and the risk of prostate cancer. The effects of IGF-1 concentrations on prostate cancer risk were found to be astoundingly large - much higher than for any other known risk factor. Men having an IGF-1 level between approximately 300 and 500 ng/mL were found to have more than four times the risk of developing prostate cancer than did men with a level between 100 and 185 ng/mL. The detrimental effect of high IGF-1 levels was particularly pronounced in men over 60 years of age. In this age group men with the highest levels of IGF-1 were eight times more likely to develop prostate cancer than men with low levels. The elevated IGF-1 levels were found to be present several years before an actual diagnosis of prostate cancer was made[12].

IGF-1 promotes tumor development by stimulating cell proliferation and by inhibiting programmed cell death (apoptosis). IGF-1 also stimulates the synthesis of androgens and inhibits the formation of sex hormone-binding globulins, binding proteins that control the amount of androgens available to the prostate tissue[13]. The synthesis of IGF-1 is stimulated by insulin and there is evidence that pre-diabetics have high circulating levels of IGF-1[13]. There is also concern that IGF-1 in milk from cows treated with bovine growth hormone can increase the level of IGF-1 in humans and thus promote cancer[14].

More recently the Harvard team observed a strong association between IGF-1 and IGFBP-3 levels and the risk of advanced prostate cancer, but found no association with early stage disease. They found that men with IGF-1 levels in the highest quartile had a 5.1 times higher risk of developing advanced stage prostate cancer than did men in the lowest quartile. Men with IGFBP-3 levels in the highest quartile, on the other hand, had a 5 times lower risk of advanced stage cancer. The researchers speculate that IGF-1 not only stimulates tumour initiation and growth, but may also facilitate invasion and metastases. They conclude that measurement of IGF-1 and IGFBP-3 levels may predict the risk of advanced stage prostate cancer years before the cancer is actually diagnosed and may thus be helpful in aiding decision making about treatment[15,16].

It is clear that IGF-1 is a potent risk factor for prostate cancer and it is thus of considerable concern that people taking growth hormones are vastly increasing their IGF-1 level.

GROWTH HORMONES AND ENHANCERS

Human growth hormone (GH) is necessary for growth and a deficiency produces short people. GH does not actually stimulate growth directly, but causes the release of insulin-like growth factors, particularly IGF-1. It is IGF-1 that is responsible for growth and it stimulates the synthesis of lean muscle mass in particular.

Experiments to increase IGF-1 levels in older men through injections of recombinant (synthetic) GH produced astounding results. An 8.8% increase in lean body mass, a 14.4% decrease in fatty tissue, a 1.6% increase in vertebral bone density, and a 7.1% increase in skin thickness were reported by American medical researchers in 1990. Their trial lasted a year and although the 21 participants all remained healthy except for one who developed prostate cancer, the researchers warned that side effects such as edema, hypertension, diabetes, and enlargement of the heart could occur with prolonged use of synthetic GH. Other researchers found that GH injections in young people produced larger muscles and kidneys. More recently GH injections have become popular among athletes as a super-efficient way to increase muscle mass and strength[17,18].

Growth hormone is naturally secreted by cells in the pituitary gland and acts on the liver to produce IGF-1. IGF-1 levels are normally quite steady, but increase during periods of excessive stress, through exercise, and by consuming a diet rich in certain amino acids especially arginine, ornithine, glycine, and lysine. These amino acids act directly on the pituitary gland to stimulate the production of GH and its downstream hormone, IGF-1. Stomach acid is very tough on amino acids and only 10% or less of them actually survive long enough to get into the blood stream. This is where GH enhancers play a role. These products use a patented process to protect the amino acids in the stomach and as a result 90% or more of them are absorbed into the blood stream. It is claimed that the resulting flooding of the pituitary gland with the raw materials it needs to produce growth hormone can result in IGF-1 level increases of 200% or more. Fortunately, the body has a built- in mechanism to prevent IGF-1 levels from going too high. Somatostatin is released by the hypothalamus and its major role is to keep IGF-1 levels under control.   Unfortunately, GH enhancers also contain special peptides which suppress the natural release of somatostatin[17,19,20].

IGF-1 is a known cancer promoter, so taking growth hormone or growth hormone enhancers to increase its level is clearly not a good idea. Dr. Samuel Epstein, MD, a professor at the University of Illinois School of Public Health sums it up succinctly,

"Taking supplements to increase your IGF-1 levels is reckless, extreme, and bordering on the criminal"[21].

ANDROGENS

The main androgens (male sex hormones) are testosterone and dihydrotestosterone (DHT). DHT is formed from testosterone through the action of the enzyme 5-alpha-reductase. Androgens are synthesized from cholesterol through a pathway involving pregnenolone, progesterone, and dehydroepiandrosterone (DHEA). The main synthesis site is the Leydig cells of the testes, but smaller amounts of testosterone are also produced in the adrenal glands.

Androgens exert their influence by binding to the androgen receptors on prostate cells and signalling them to grow and replicate. There is evidence that DHT exerts a more powerful influence than does testosterone itself[22]. Unfortunately, androgens do not distinguish between healthy and cancerous cells in their growth promotion efforts and are thus believed to be largely responsible for the progression of prostate cancer. It is not entirely clear what role androgens play in the initiation of prostate cancer, but there is evidence that men castrated prior to puberty do not develop prostate cancer. It is also well established that therapy aimed at preventing androgens from causing prostate cells to grow can be very effective in halting the progression of androgen-dependent prostate cancer.

Nevertheless, the role of testosterone and DHT in prostate cancer is not without controversy. Testosterone replacement therapy (TRT) has long been used in the treatment of hypogonadism, which involves a reduced or absent secretion of androgens from the testes. There is no indication that using testosterone injections or patches to correct *bona fide* hypogonadism increases the risk of prostate cancer[22]. However, using TRT to enhance libido, build muscle mass, or alleviate depression may be another matter.

Finnish researchers studied over 16,000 men aged between 18 and 78 years and found no association between prostate cancer risk and serum levels of testosterone, sex-hormone binding globulin, and androstenedrone. They conclude that high androgen levels are not associated with an increased risk of prostate cancer in Finnish men. However, they caution that racial differences may exist in this relationship[23].

Dr. Richmond Prehn, MD of the University of Washington challenges the assumption that high androgen levels are a risk factor for prostate cancer. Dr. Prehn points out that androgen levels decline with age whereas prostate cancer incidence rises sharply. He suggests that declining androgen levels may not only lead to benign prostate hyperplasia (BPH), but may also be the initiator of uncontrolled cell growth which may ultimately lead to cancer. He further suggests that, "androgen supplementation beginning early in the middle years might, among other possible benefits, largely prevent prostate cancer." Dr. Prehn cautions that androgen supplementation may be contra-indicated in older men who already have the seeds of prostate cancer[24].

In contrast, researchers at Johns Hopkins Medical School have found a clear correlation between high levels of free (unbound) testosterone and the risk of prostate cancer[25].

Other researchers have found an association between low testosterone levels in newly diagnosed men and their risk of progressing to advanced or metastatic cancer. They speculate that low testosterone levels may increase the number of androgen receptors on prostate cells and thus result in a more virulent disease once the cancer has been initiated[26].

Clearly, the relationship between androgens and prostate cancer is controversial; however, two conclusions seem reasonably unanimous:

1. It is safe to prescribe testosterone replacement therapy in men diagnosed with hypogonadism and no signs of prostate cancer.

2. Testosterone replacement therapy should not be prescribed for men with normal levels who have been diagnosed with or are suspected of having prostate cancer. Since an accurate diagnosis of prostate cancer is difficult to achieve without at least two biopsies it is probably safest to avoid prescribing testosterone to men above the age of 55 years unless the benefits of doing so clearly outweighs the risk of prostate cancer.

ANABOLIC STEROIDS

Anabolic steroids or more correctly, anabolic-androgenic steroids are synthetic compounds designed to mimic androgens. They are available legally only by prescription and are used to treat conditions caused by abnormally low testosterone production. They can be converted into DHT through the action of 5-alpha-reductase[27].

Unfortunately, many athletes and body-builders abuse anabolic steroids in order to enhance performance and improve physical appearance. The major adverse effects of anabolic steroids include cancer, high blood pressure, a decrease in HDL cholesterol and an increase in LDL cholesterol, kidney tumors, and severe acne. Men abusing anabolic steroids have an increased risk of prostate cancer, may develop large breasts, and may experience shrinking of the testicles, infertility, increased hostility, depression, episodes of schizophrenia, and baldness[27-29].

It is likely that the adverse effects of anabolic steroid abuse may be far more serious than those uncovered in clinical trials as abusers usually consume far greater quantities than those used in trials. It is also a sobering thought that more than 3% of male grade 12 students in the US used anabolic steroids in 2004[27].

DEHYDROEPIANDROSTERONE (DHEA)

DHEA and its active metabolite DHEAS (DHEA sulfate) are hormones primarily formed in the adrenal cortex (men also generate DHEA in their testicles). DHEA and DHEAS serve as precursors for both male and female sex hormones. The output of DHEA and DHEAS is highest between the ages of 20 and 30 years and then starts declining. By age 80 years the output is only 10-20% of the peak output. This decline in DHEA with age has led to speculation that DHEA supplementation may be useful in the treatment of age-related diseases. There is now clinically substantiated evidence that DHEA replacement therapy may be useful in patients who have abnormally low levels due to chronic disease, suffer from adrenal exhaustion or have undergone therapy with corticosteroids. It may also be useful in the treatment of systemic lupus erythematosus and severe depression, can improve bone density in postmenopausal women, and has been found to combat fatigue and depression in HIV patients. Epidemiological studies have observed that low DHEA levels are associated with a higher incidence of cancer, cardiovascular disease (in men only), Alzheimer's disease, immune function suppression, and progression of HIV infections[30].

Animal experiments have shown that DHEA supplementation may slow the progression of induced prostate cancer[31]. However, there have been no human trials evaluating the effect of DHEA supplementation on initiation and progression of prostate cancer.

It is known that DHEA increases the level of free IGF-1 and decreases the level of IGFBP-1, a protein that binds IGF-1 and makes it inactive. It is also known that DHEA can be converted to testosterone and can itself bind to androgen and estrogen receptors[32-34]. These facts clearly make DHEA supplementation problematical in men diagnosed with or suspected of having prostate cancer.

In conclusion, DHEA supplementation can be highly beneficial in aging men and women with low levels of this important hormone. However, enough uncertainty surrounds the question of effects on prostate (and breast) cancer to be extremely cautious of taking it if there is the slightest suspicion of cancer. DHEA is only available by prescription in Canada and physicians are generally extremely reluctant to prescribe it. Only in the US is it still freely available over-the-counter in pharmacies and health food stores, but this may be about to change. Bill S.1137 (May 2005) has been submitted to Congress and, if approved, would classify DHEA as an anabolic steroid and thus make it available only by prescription[34].

While it is clear that IGF-1, growth hormones, and anabolic steroids are contraindicated in men diagnosed with or suspected of having prostate cancer and indeed perhaps in all men over the age of 55 years, the situation in regards to androgens and DHEA is still controversial. In view of the unreliability of prostate cancer tests, the best approach to testosterone replacement therapy and DHEA supplementation is to avoid it unless a definite deficiency has been clearly established and the therapy is closely monitored by a competent physician well aware of the potential for prostate cancer development.

MELATONIN

Melatonin is a hormone secreted by the pineal gland and is important in synchronizing the production and excretion of other hormones according to the time of day (circadian rhythm). Melatonin production is low during daylight hours and peaks between 1 and 3 AM when it is darkest.

In 1985 Christian Bartsch and colleagues at the University of Tubingen discovered that prostate cancer patients had an abnormal melatonin secretion pattern and concluded that melatonin secretion may be related to the development and growth of prostate cancer.[35]   In 1992 the same group of researchers reported that prostate cancer patients had abnormally low levels of melatonin.[36]   These findings prompted other German researchers to investigate whether people living north of the Arctic circle (many dark nights) had a lower incidence of hormone-dependent cancers, such as breast and prostate cancer. They found that this was indeed the case.[37] Moretti, *et al* at the Center for Endocrinological Oncology in Milan, Italy followed up in the laboratory and found that very small amounts of melatonin inhibited the growth of androgen-dependent prostate cancer cells in culture.[38]   The same researchers later discovered that melatonin also very significantly inhibits the growth of androgen-independent cells.[39] Chinese researchers, treating a patient with terminal, metastatic prostate cancer and rising PSA levels with 5 mg a day of melatonin (given at 8 PM), found that this therapy stabilized his disease for 6 weeks as indicated by stable PSA levels.[40] Finally, in April 2005 researchers at the University of Texas concluded that treatment of both androgen-dependent and androgen-independent prostate cancer cells with pharmaceutical doses of melatonin dramatically reduced the number of cancer cells and essentially stopped the production of new cancer cells.[41]

While it is thus clear that low melatonin levels are associated with prostate cancer and that melatonin kills both androgen-dependent and androgen-independent prostate cancer cells, it is not clear what causes low levels in the first place. Fortunately, breast cancer research provides several intriguing clues. In 1995 Molis, *et al* at Tulane University discovered that melatonin prevents the growth of breast cancer cells.[42] In October 2001 Scott Davis and colleagues at the Fred Hutchinson Cancer Research Institute reported that exposure to magnetic fields created by house wiring during the night significantly decreased melatonin production.[43] Norwegian researchers later linked exposure to magnetic fields created by residential wiring to a 58% increased risk of developing breast cancer.[44] In a controlled experiment just reported, a team of researchers from three American universities found that women exposed to relatively low magnetic fields (EMFs) of 5 and 10 mG during the night produced significantly less melatonin than women not exposed to EMFs.[45] As is common in cancer research, one recent study found no association between overall exposure to EMFs and breast cancer.[46] However, it is likely that only exposure to EMFs during the night would be detrimental.

Another important clue is the finding by Danish researchers that women who predominantly work at night have a 50% increased risk of developing breast cancer. The researchers conclude that exposure to light during the night suppresses melatonin production and hence increases the risk of cancer.[47] Jasser *et al* at Thomas Jefferson University in Philadelphia believe that the higher risk of breast cancer in industrialized countries is partly due to increased exposure to light at night.[48] Researchers at the University of Connecticut concur with this and further suggest that exposure to bright light during the day and total darkness at night is optimum.[49] Very recently the Bartsch team at the University of Tubingen in Germany concluded that, "melatonin controls not only the growth of well-differentiated cancers, but also possesses anti-carcinogenic properties". They suggest that short-term melatonin supplementation may be justified to optimize control over cancerous growth and development.[50]

There is credible evidence that a low level of melatonin is associated with an increased risk of prostate and breast cancer. It has also been demonstrated that pharmacological doses of melatonin will dramatically slow cancer progression and reintroduce appropriate cell differentiation. There is also evidence that exposure to low level electromagnetic fields created by normal (60 Hz) household electrical wiring may increase the risk of breast cancer and, by inference, prostate cancer. Finally, there is growing evidence that exposure to light during the night reduces melatonin production and thus increases cancer risk.

Hence, an inappropriately low melatonin level is a risk factor for prostate (and breast) cancer. There is evidence that a low level can be avoided by sleeping in a completely dark room at night and by ensuring that the ambient EMF level is low. Although the officially sanctioned safe continuous exposure level in the United States is 1000 mG [51], there is evidence that an exposure level of only 5 mG significantly reduces melatonin levels.[45] An obvious question is, "If low melatonin levels are detrimental, would it not make sense to supplement?" The medical literature does not contain an answer to this question. In view of the fact that melatonin is a hormone whose many and varied effects are not fully understood, continuous supplementation would probably not be wise until more information on its overall effect becomes available.[50] However, sleeping in a completely dark room with an EMF level of 1 mG or less is certainly safe and may be effective in preventing hormone-related cancers like breast and prostate cancer. It has also been suggested that supplementing with melatonin prior to a long airline flight will not only help prevent jet lag, but will also afford some protection against the ionizing radiation experienced at high altitudes.[50]

MEDICAL HISTORY

It is conceivable that medical conditions or surgical procedures affecting the prostate or the hormones controlling its growth could result in a reduced or increased risk of cancer. The following conditions and procedures have been investigated:

- Diabetes
- Metabolic syndrome
- Elevated cholesterol or triglycerides
- Benign prostatic hyperplasia (BPH)
- Prostatitis
- Transurethral resection (TURP)
- Vasectomy

DIABETES

Type 2 diabetes is the most common form of diabetes and is caused by the inability of the insulin messenger hormone to instruct cells to take in glucose. Insulin is released by the pancreas in response to the presence of sugar (glucose) in the blood stream. Glucose gets into the blood through consumption of sugar or sugar-containing foods or via the breakdown of carbohydrates into simple sugars. Insulin is a chemical messenger that acts on the walls of the cells to cause the release, from within the cell, of special protein molecules – the so-called GLUT-4 transporters. The GLUT-4 transporters rise to the cells' outer membranes where they grab hold of the glucose molecule and transport it into the interior of the cell. Here the glucose is used to produce energy and any excess is converted into fat[1]. This process functions flawlessly in non-diabetic persons resulting in a steady glucose level in the blood stream usually between 60 and 115 mg/dL (3.3 - 6.4 mmol/L) with an average of 85 mg/dL (4.7 mmol/L).

In diabetics glucose levels are not under control and can reach levels of 250 mg/dL (13.9 mmol/L) or higher. Patients with type 2 (non-insulin-dependent) diabetes usually produce an adequate amount of insulin, but for some reason the mechanism whereby the insulin summons the GLUT-4 transporters does not function. The result is that both glucose and insulin levels in the blood remain high.

High insulin levels (hyperinsulinemia) are a characteristic feature of pre-diagnosis diabetes. However, after 4 or 5 years of producing abnormally high amounts of insulin the insulin-producing beta-cells in the pancreas become exhausted and circulating insulin levels drop[2] to below those found in non-diabetic men. High insulin levels are associated with an increase in IGF-1 level, a decrease in the binding proteins that keep IGF-1 from exerting its cancer-promoting effects, and a decrease in testosterone, DHT and the proteins that bind them. IGF-1 is a strong risk factor for prostate cancer, so one might expect that diabetic men, pre-diagnosis and in the early stages of diabetes, would have a high risk of prostate cancer, while their risk after 4 or 5 years would decline to that of non-diabetic men or perhaps even lower. Several studies have found this hypothesis to be plausible.

In 1998 a team of Harvard researchers reported that men with diabetes had a 34% reduced risk of being diagnosed with prostate cancer in the 5 years following their diagnosis. After 10 years their risk was reduced by 46%[3]. Physicians at the Walter Reed Medical Center found that diabetic men had a 36% lower risk of prostate cancer than did non-diabetics. The protective effect of diabetes increased with time from a 23% reduction in the first 5 years to a 41% reduction in years 11 to 15[4].

A very large study by the American Cancer Society involving over 72,000 men concluded that diabetes was associated with an overall reduced risk of prostate cancer of 33%. However, the researchers noted that the risk was significantly increased (by 23%) in the first 3 years after diagnosis[5].

Spanish researchers recently came to a similar conclusion after studying the General Practice Research Database in the UK. This database contains data for over 2 million patients. The researchers observed that diabetic men had a 28% reduced risk of prostate cancer compared to non-diabetics. However, when studying their data further the researchers found that it was only patients who were treated with insulin or sulphonylureas that had a reduced risk (37% reduction). Untreated patients or patients treated with metformin showed no reduction in risk[6].

To further confuse the issue, there are at least three studies that have produced conflicting results. The 1959-1972 Cancer Prevention Study found a higher incidence of prostate cancer among diabetics[7]. An Italian study of diabetes and prostate cancer risk found no difference in prostate cancer incidence between diabetics and non-diabetics[8]. A recent American study found no evidence of an inverse association between a history of diabetes and the risk of recurrence of prostate cancer[9].

Thus, as in so much of the research concerning prostate cancer, there is no clear consensus as to whether diabetes is protective or if it is, whether it confers a greater risk prior to diagnosis and a reduced risk 4-5 years after diagnosis. The fact that most prostate cancers grow slowly and probably take at least 10 years from initiation to diagnosis tends to further confuse the issue.

METABOLIC SYNDROME

Metabolic syndrome encompasses a combination of hyperinsulinemia, elevated fasting glucose level, abdominal obesity, abnormal cholesterol or triglyceride levels, and hypertension. The growth of this condition has been termed epidemic and it now affects between 7 and 36% of all middle-aged men in Europe. There is no reason to believe that the incidence would be lower in North America. Over-eating and under-exercising are probably the main underlying causes of the syndrome. Metabolic syndrome is associated with an increase in the level of free, circulating IGF-1[10].

Finnish researchers report that metabolic syndrome is a definite risk factor for prostate cancer. In a 13-year study of 1880 men without cancer or diabetes at baseline they observed a 1.9-fold increase in the risk of prostate cancer among men diagnosed with metabolic syndrome. This was the case after adjusting for such confounding factors as age, alcohol consumption, physical fitness, and the intake of energy, fat, fiber, calcium, vitamin E and alpha-linolenic acid. The risk was greater among men with a BMI (body mass index) at or above 27 kg/m^2 (3-fold increase) than among lighter men (1.8-fold increase). The researchers suggest that efforts to curb the epidemic of metabolic syndrome may decrease the incidence of prostate cancer[10].

CHOLESTEROL AND TRIGLYCERIDES

Although the intake of red meat and certain fats have been associated with an increased risk of prostate cancer, it is not entirely clear whether a high cholesterol level is a risk factor as well. Two studies, which did not adjust for energy intake, found an increased risk associated with increased cholesterol levels, while one, which did adjust for energy intake, found no correlation. A more recent study performed by a group of Dutch and Swiss researchers concluded that cholesterol levels are not associated with prostate cancer risk.[11] However, a just-released study by Italian researchers conclude that high cholesterol levels do indeed increase prostate cancer risk. The team from the Instituto di Ricerche Farmacologiche Mario Negri in Milan analyzed the medical histories of 1294 men with prostate cancer and 1451 matched men with no cancer. The study participants were recruited from Italian hospitals between 1991 and 2002, and interviewed using structured questionnaires. Elevated cholesterol was defined as a total cholesterol level above 200 mg/dL (5.1 mmol/L). Participants with prostate cancer were about 50% more likely to have a high cholesterol level than were controls.

The association was somewhat stronger for men whose high cholesterol levels had been diagnosed before the age of 50 years and for men over 65, in whom there was an 80% greater likelihood of high cholesterol levels. The absence of an association between prostate cancer and 10 other medical conditions indicates that the relationship found between prostate cancer and high cholesterol is real. The researchers also found that prostate cancer patients were 26% more likely to have suffered from gallstones. The link was not statistically significant, but gallstones are often related to high cholesterol levels. Testosterone is synthesized from cholesterol, suggesting a possible biological relationship between high cholesterol and prostate cancer. Gallstones are also related to high cholesterol levels and are often composed of cholesterol. So the direct relationship found between gallstones and prostate cancer, while it was not statistically significant, suggests that a similar biological mechanism may explain the link.[12]

Thus, while there is no consensus that elevated cholesterol levels are associated with an increased risk of prostate cancer, the evidence supporting such an association is growing.

The Dutch/Swiss team did find a correlation between triglyceride levels and prostate cancer risk. They concluded that every 1 mmol/L increase in serum triglyceride level is associated with a 15% increase in risk.[11] NOTE: A desirable level of triglycerides is about 1.1 mmol/L (100 mg/dL) or less.

It is interesting that fish oils, which have been found to be protective against prostate cancer, are also highly effective in reducing triglyceride levels.[13]

BENIGN PROSTATIC HYPERPLASIA (BPH)

Conventional medical wisdom has it that men suffering from BPH are no more likely to develop prostate cancer than are men without BPH[14]. BPH may be related to prostate cancer arising in the transition rather than the peripheral zone, but it is not considered to be a precursor of prostate cancer[15].

Researchers at the National Cancer Institute recently reviewed medical data collected over a 26-year period for 87,000 Swedish BPH patients. They found that overall there was no significant difference in observed prostate cancer incidence and mortality rates among BPH patients versus the general population. However, the researchers did note a significant difference in incidence and mortality depending on the treatment received by the BPH patients. Men who received no treatment had the highest incidence (18% higher than expected); men who underwent transurethral resection (TURP) had a lower incidence, but still 10% higher than expected. Men who underwent transvesicular adenectomy (removal of entire inner core of the prostate gland) had the lowest incidence (22% lower than expected). Mortality rate for no treatment was 77% higher than expected, for TURP it was 17% lower than expected, and for transvesicular adenectomy 23% lower than expected. Unfortunately, the results of the study are likely to be significantly skewed due to the fact that the men who received no treatment were considerably older and less healthy than the men who received surgical treatment. The average age of BPH diagnosis was 74 years for patients receiving no treatment and 70 years for those receiving surgical treatment. The average age at which prostate cancer was diagnosed was 76, 77, and 78 years respectively for men undergoing no treatment, TURP and transvesicular adenectomy[16].

Swedish researchers have found that men with fast growing BPH tend to develop a more severe grade of prostate cancer than do men with slow-growing BPH[17].

It is thus not entirely clear whether there is an association between BPH and prostate cancer risk. Nevertheless, it would seem prudent to take steps to avoid the development of BPH using some of the approaches outlined in Chapter 2.

PROSTATITIS

Prostatitis may involve an acute or chronic inflammation of the prostate that can be of bacterial or unknown origin. In view of the fact that inflammation is an acknowledged risk factor for prostate cancer, it would seem plausible that long-term prostatitis would be associated with an increased risk as well. Several studies have investigated the connection but the results are ambiguous. This is partly because BPH and prostatitis often coexist and partly because of the long lead-time involved between cancer initiation and diagnosis.

Researchers at the University of Iowa found a 60% increased risk of prostate cancer among men with a history of prostatitis[18]. Mayo Clinic researchers found a strong relation between having experienced acute bacterial prostatitis and being diagnosed with prostate cancer an average of 12 years later. Chronic bacterial prostatitis was less convincingly associated and non-bacterial, chronic prostatitis (chronic pelvic pain syndrome) may not be related to prostate cancer risk at all[19]. Researchers at Johns Hopkins Medical School, on the other hand, believe that there is a link between chronic prostatitis and prostate cancer and describes the case for prostate inflammation as a cause of prostate cancer as "compelling"[20,21].

It is thus not entirely clear whether prostatitis is a risk factor for prostate cancer, but current research would tend to support the idea that it may be. It would seem prudent to avoid risk factors for prostatitis and to treat any acute or chronic incidence promptly and effectively with either conventional or alternative approaches.

TRANSURETHRAL RESECTION (TURP)

Transurethral resection is the standard surgical procedure for dealing with BPH. It involves removing parts of the prostate obstructing the urethra and causes massive trauma to the urethra and the transition zone of the prostate. A Swedish study of 87,000 BPH patients found that having undergone a TURP increased the risk of prostate cancer but reduced subsequent mortality[16]. However, a 1994 Swedish study concluded, "The results of this study suggest that neither BPH nor TURP increase the risk of developing clinical prostate cancer over the next 10 years in patients with a benign prostate gland as determined by rectal examination before TURP"[22]. A more recent Australian study reached a similar conclusion[23]. Thus, it is not entirely clear whether undergoing a TURP increases prostate cancer risk; however, there is no evidence that it increases prostate cancer mortality.

VASECTOMY

Vasectomy is a surgical operation that severs and ties the ducts (vas deferens) that connect the testes to the seminal vesicles and urethra. Although the cuts are made well away from the prostate itself, it is possible that vasectomy might increase prostate cancer risk by diminishing the secretion of prostatic fluid or by altering immune response to sperm antigens. About 500,000 vasectomies are performed annually in the US alone and it is estimated that about 12% of married men undergo a vasectomy, usually before the age of 40 years[24]. Numerous studies have been done to investigate the possible association between vasectomy and the subsequent risk of prostate cancer.

In 2002 researchers at the University of Iowa reported the results of a meta-analysis of 5 cohort studies and 17 case-control studies. Their conclusion was that men who had undergone vasectomy had a 37% greater relative risk of developing prostate cancer and that the risk increased with the length of time since vasectomy[25].

In 2005 Indian researchers compared the incidence of prostate cancer in 390 vasectomized men with that in 780 controls. They found that vasectomized men had a 1.9-fold increased risk of later developing prostate cancer compared to men who had not undergone vasectomy. The risk for men who had their vasectomy before the age of 45 years was increased 2.1-fold, while the risk for men having their procedure at a later age was 1.8 times that of controls. The risk of prostate cancer increased with time since vasectomy, with a time interval of 25 years corresponding to a 3.8-fold risk increase[26].

Johns Hopkins Medical School researchers recently reported on a study of 3330 men residing in Washington County, Maryland. They found that men who had undergone vasectomy had double the risk of developing prostate cancer than did non-vasectomized men. The risk increase was confined to low-grade cancer (a 2.9-fold risk increase). The vasectomy-associated cancer risk was higher in men who were 40 years or older at time of vasectomy (a 2.6-fold risk increase) than in men who were younger at vasectomy. The researchers also observed that the incidence of prostate cancer among vasectomized men increased significantly with time since vasectomy[24].

To put the above risk increases in perspective, it is interesting to look at the actual incidence of prostate cancer per 1000 man-years observed in the Maryland study[23].

	Incidence/1000 man-years
• Controls (no vasectomy)	2.5
• Vasectomy after age 40 years	6.5
• More than 20 years since vasectomy	4.4

In other words, the annual risk of being diagnosed with prostate cancer (during the 8-year follow-up period) was 0.25% a year for non-vasectomized men and 0.65% a year for men having a vasectomy after the age of 40 years.

Several small studies (included in the above mentioned meta-analysis) have found little or no association between vasectomy and prostate cancer[27-30], while others confirmed that vasectomy increases the risk of prostate cancer[31-33].

Overall, the evidence would tend to favor an association between vasectomy and a future (20 years or more later) risk of prostate cancer. The risk would seem to be greater the later a man has a vasectomy, although at least one study reached the opposite conclusion. It is also fairly clear that the risk increases with increasing time since the vasectomy. When all is said and done though, the real, absolute risk attributable to a vasectomy, even after age of 40, is likely less than 0.5% a year higher than the risk found among non-vasectomized men. It is certainly conceivable that this risk can be compensated for by following the prevention guidelines presented in Chapter 5.

It is of interest that Chinese researchers have found that men who have had a vasectomy have a considerably lower risk of having to contend with benign prostatic hyperplasia – an annual incidence rate of 10.8% in the vasectomy group versus 40.8% in the control group[34].

CONCLUSION

The known risk factors for prostate cancer are many and varied. While there is clearly nothing that can be done about chronological age, race, nationality and genetic make-up, there are a number of factors which, if avoided, can go a long way toward preventing the development of prostate cancer. Among the more important steps you can take are:

- Limit your intake of saturated fats, especially from red meats and dairy products.
- Limit your intake of calcium, especially from low-fat milk, to 1200 mg/day.
- Limit your intake of alpha-linolenic acid originating from mayonnaise, red meat (beef, pork and lamb), margarine, and creamy salad dressings.
- Avoid barbequed and grilled beef, pork, chicken, lamb and fish.
- Avoid preserved foods (pickled vegetables, fermented soy products, salted fish, and preserved meats).
- Avoid nutritional deficiencies, especially in regard to vitamin D and selenium.
- Avoid or limit exposure to herbicides, pesticides, diesel fumes, metal working fluids, paint strippers and varnishes.
- Maintain your ideal body weight, avoid smoking and alcohol abuse, and ensure daily sunlight exposure.

- Do not take growth hormones, growth hormone enhancers, testosterone, anabolic steroids or DHEA (dehydroepiandrosterone) except in cases of medically diagnosed deficiency where the risk associated with not taking them clearly outweighs the risk of prostate cancer.
- Ensure adequate melatonin levels by sleeping in a completely dark room at night and keep exposure to electromagnetic fields generated by house wiring as low as possible, preferably below 1 mG.
- Do whatever it takes to avoid metabolic syndrome (syndrome X) and elevated triglyceride levels.
- Do whatever is necessary to avoid elevated cholesterol and triglyceride levels.
- Do whatever it takes to avoid or at least keep BPH and prostatitis under control.
- Carefully consider the pros and cons before undergoing a vasectomy.

Chapter 4

Diagnosis and Staging of Prostate Cancer

William R. Ware PhD

INTRODUCTION

Before the blood test for prostate specific antigen (PSA) came into general use as a diagnostic tool for prostate cancer (PC), only abnormalities felt during a digital rectal exam (DRE) or symptoms suggestive of invasive cancer or metastasis such as urinary difficulties, bleeding or bone pain were available as indicators of the presence of this disease. The result was that many patients presented with non-localized or metastatic cancer, which in many cases was treatable only with palliation. In the late 1980s physicians using the new PSA blood test began detecting PC at a much earlier stage and a PSA cut-off was established above which a biopsy was indicated. Also, biopsy techniques improved and a grading system was developed for the analysis of tissue samples taken at biopsy which permitted the approximate differentiation between low-grade and perhaps biologically insignificant tumors on the one hand and potentially aggressive cancer on the other.

At present the PSA test is frequently done periodically in conjunction with physical exams and the majority of cancers now being detected are localized and viewed by many urologists as curable by the surgical removal of the prostate (radical prostatectomy) or by radiation therapy. Prognosis in general is also now more accurately established, both preoperatively and after the pathological examination of removed prostates. PSA has also become a valuable tool in detecting recurrence (also called *biochemical failure or biochemical recurrence*) after a radical prostatectomy or radiation therapy. It is also not uncommon to find evidence of PC in tissue removed during the transurethral resection operation (TURP) for benign prostatic hyperplasia, and even surgery for bladder cancer turns up unexpected PC. In spite of these advances, whether or not there has been an improvement in survival for those with PC because of the use of the PSA test remains controversial and the subject of ongoing studies. This is an important question, since surgical removal of the prostate (radical prostatectomy) or radiation treatment of PC is associated with adverse effects which can significantly and in some cases permanently decrease the patient's quality of life. As will be discussed below and in subsequent chapters, this is not a simple matter and treatment decisions are far from straight forward.

When the PSA test is done on asymptomatic individuals, generally in the course of a physical examination, this is generally termed *screening*. Both the advisability of PSA screening and the appropriate PSA cut-off level suggesting a biopsy have become what are probably the most hotly debated subjects in the history of urology, and the large number of research results and associated editorials and commentary published annually continue to fuel the debate.

This chapter will examine the screening controversy, the DRE and its shortcomings as well as utility, the various aspects of the use of PSA in diagnosis and prognosis, the biopsy techniques in current use, the histological grading system known as the Gleason Score, tumor staging and the procedures used to determine if the cancer has spread beyond the gland. The goal is to provide detailed evidence-based information so that an individual can take part in the decision making process when options are presented. It is worth mentioning that the current trend is for these options to be discussed with patients since there are serious risk-benefit considerations involved which are far from clear-cut. For example, the current guidelines of the American Urological Association for the diagnosis of benign prostatic hyperplasia (BPH) [1] indicate that the PSA test should be *offered* to patients under certain circumstances. This highlights the problems associated with this test which include coping with and responding to the positive results that may occur and implies a joint decision making process. In fact, on occasion one sees the principle stated that a diagnostic test should not be done unless it is clearly understood what action will be taken if the result is positive.

THE DIGITAL RECTAL EXAMINATION (DRE)

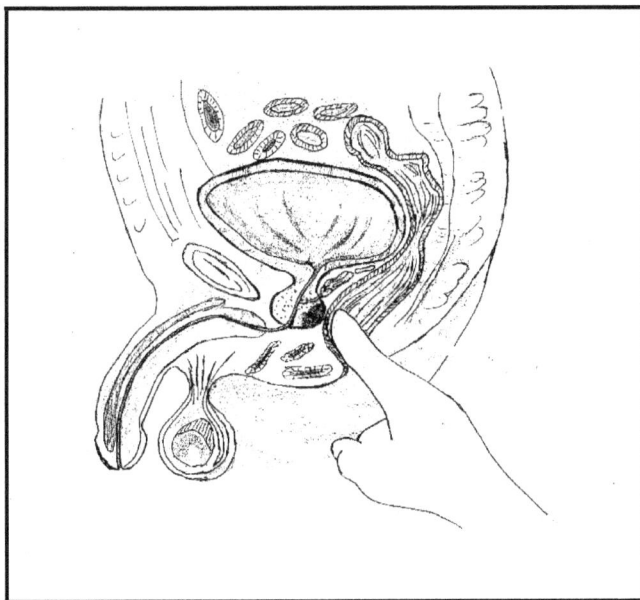

Figure 4-1. Digital Rectal Examination

The male anatomy is such that the back of the prostate is in close proximity to the front wall of the rectum. This provides the opportunity for a physician to palpate (feel) part of the surface of the gland and estimate both the prostate size and the presence or absence of abnormal growths or other features. The area that can be palpated is where carcinoma most frequently begins. Carcinomas are characteristically hard, nodular and irregular. The test also has the potential for detecting extra-prostatic tumor. At the same time, the physician can check for abnormal rectal masses indicative of possible cancer. The procedure is essentially non-invasive but may be mildly uncomfortable or distasteful. In *Dr. Peter Scardino's Prostate Book* [2], the author points out that this test is highly subjective and difficult to master. Surface irregularities such as nodules may strike one urologist as significant and another as insignificant.

The ability of the DRE to predict the presence of PC is not impressive. In a recent study of 408 consecutive patients with a mean age of 63.8 years and PSA ranging from 2.5 to 10 ng/mL, Philip *et al* [3] compared biopsy results with the observation of an abnormal DRE. Only 47% of the patients with an abnormal DRE had cancer on biopsy. There was also a poor correlation between the predicted stage and the actual pathological stage found for those that went on to have a radical prostatectomy. Also, a few patients with a normal DRE were found to have advanced cancer. The authors comment that in this study the examinations were done by two experienced urologists, and they suggest that that the accuracy might be even lower if the DREs were done by less experienced practitioners or specialist nurses.

Crawford *et al* [4] used a PSA cut-off of $\leq$ 4.0 ng/mL for normal and found in a large cohort that an abnormal DRE had a positive predictive value (percent of positives that were true positives) in the normal PSA subgroup of only about 18% based on biopsy verified cancers, but for the group with an abnormal PSA and an abnormal DRE, the predictive value of the combined abnormal indication jumped to 56%, whereas for an abnormal PSA and a normal DRE, the percentage was about 28%.

It is common practice to do both a DRE and a PSA test in the course of a physical exam. The DRE can also provide information that is useful during the biopsy. Some urologists take extra samples (cores) in areas of the prostate where the DRE indicates potential tumors [2]. A recent study suggests that the DRE is underutilized [5].

THE PSA TEST

TOTAL PSA

PSA stands for prostate specific antigen. Prior to metastasis, it is organ specific but not cancer specific. PSA is produced by cells in the prostate and released as part of the ejaculate. It was only in 1985 that the biological function of PSA was explained. After ejaculation, seminal fluid coagulates. PSA reverses this allowing sperm to achieve the required mobility. PSA is a macromolecule which cannot normally penetrate the prostate capsule nor find its way into the blood stream. Thus PSA should only be found in the prostate and in seminal fluid, and under normal circumstances only minute amounts are found in the blood. Thus significant serum levels suggest that something has gone wrong in the structural integrity of the prostate. Candidates include prostatitis, benign prostatic hyperplasia (BPH), and PC. When the prostate is successfully removed, the serum PSA level is expected to drop to near zero and remain there. However, if metastasis has occurred or if some prostate tissue has been left behind, this can result in low levels of residual PSA which may progressively increase.

When used for diagnostic purposes involving asymptomatic individuals, the PSA test is essentially a screening test. There are four outcomes, true positive, true negative, false positive and false negative. The validity of a screening test is frequently measured in terms of sensitivity and specificity. The former measures the ability of the test to correctly identify those with the disease, whereas specificity measures the success of the test in identifying subjects free of the disease. These two measures, given as percentages, are defined as follows:

Sensitivity = true positives/(true positives + false negatives)
Specificity = true negatives/(true negatives + false positives)

Too many false positives lead to poor specificity, whereas too many false negatives reduce the sensitivity. A specificity of say 50% would mean that there were as many false positives as true negatives.

The PSA test provides a continuous range of values and it is necessary to have a so-called cut-off value which defines positive and negative results. Once this cut-off is agreed upon, studies which compare the test results to the actual correct diagnosis provide a measure of the value of the test. In the case of the PSA test, for example, a positive is by definition a value above the cut-off. When no cancer exists in the patient with a value above the cut-off, this provides a false positive. Likewise, when cancer is identified in a patient with a PSA below the cut-off value, the result is a false negative. Tests with less than perfect specificity and sensitivity simply provide probabilities of having or not having the disease in question rather than an absolute yes or no answer.

In the case of prostate cancer, a biopsy is used to confirm the diagnosis, although tissue collected during surgical treatment for BPH or bladder cancer is also routinely examined for indications of cancer.   An obvious and potentially serious situation arises when evaluating the merits of a screening test if the actual confirming diagnostic procedure is not 100% accurate, which, as will be discussed below, is the case with prostate needle biopsies. An initial biopsy can miss as many as 25% of cancers, especially if it employs only six needles. Thus using only one biopsy as an indicator of the presence or absence of cancer will make the PSA test, whatever the cut-off, appear less successful than it really is. Also there is interest in the relationship between the PSA serum level and the grade or aggressiveness of the cancer. The biopsy provides important information in this context since the pathologist examines and classifies the set of cores obtained from the hollow needles used. For prostate cancer most pathologists uses a system called the *Gleason score*, which is based on the frequency of observing certain types of cells and cell patterns indicative of how advanced the cancer is. The Gleason score runs from 2 to 10, with a value of 7 or more indicating aggressive cancer. This will be discussed in detail below.   Thus the pathologist examines the biopsy cores and makes several judgments, i.e. yes, no, or not clear that there is cancer present and if cancer is found, how much of what grade is observed. The yes or no answer can then be used in studies to judge sensitivity and specificity. The connection between tumor grade or score and PSA, however, is obscured by the fact that the grading is far from perfect, and when the biopsy results are compared with actual examination of the prostate, upgrading as well as downgrading of the score are far from uncommon, especially when the Gleason score is established by pathologists who do not specialize in PC or see PC only occasionally. This will be discussed in detail when the biopsy is considered.

The cut-off of 4 ng/mL (*nanograms per milliliter is the only unit used for total PSA and therefore it will be omitted hereafter.* Incidentally, a nanogram is one billionth of a gram) was established early in the use of the PSA test and was based on data collected in a private clinic setting. A serum level of less than 4 was considered insufficient evidence in the absence of an abnormal DRE for doing a biopsy, but this was purely a probability argument since it was well known that some patients in this "normal PSA" group would in fact have positive biopsy results. The conventional wisdom dictated that many of the cancers found in this normal range presented no immediate danger. Many patients no doubt went away feeling good about their "normal" result.

While over the years since the advent of the PSA test a number of studies have addressed the question of the prevalence of PC in patients having PSA $\leq$ 4, problems with this cut-off were brought to center stage in a landmark study by Thompson *et al* [6] published in the *New England Journal of Medicine* in May of 2004. The subjects (age 62 to 91) were drawn from the placebo arm of a drug intervention clinical trial, the goal of which was to determine if Proscar (finasteride), used to treat BPH, also prevented PC. In the placebo arm, 2950 men had both a normal DRE and a PSA level $\leq$ 4.0 over a seven-year period and at the end of this period submitted to a biopsy involving a minimum of six needles. Thus the investigators were provided with tumor grading scores as well as PSA values for those in the cohort diagnosed with PC. Prostate cancer was diagnosed in 15.2% of the group and of those with PC, 14.9 % had a Gleason Score indicating advanced cancer. It needs to be emphasized that this group would not normally have been advised to undergo a biopsy if the commonly used PSA cut-off of $\leq$ 4 and a normal DRE were the criteria employed. In addition, seven years prior to the biopsy these men all had PSA < 3.0. The incidence of PC as a function of PSA measured just prior to the biopsy is of particular interest. The prevalence was 6.6% for levels up to 0.5, 10.1% for levels between 0.6 and 1.0, 17% for levels of 1.1 to 2.0, 23.9% for levels between 2.1 and 3.0, and finally 26.9% for levels between 3.1 and 4.0. For those with a diagnosis of cancer, the prevalence of high-grade cancers increased from 12.5% for the PSA range up to 0.5 to 25% for those with PSA values in the range of 3.1 to 4. These results pertain to men who during the duration of the study did not receive a biopsy nor were treated for cancer. If instead, the incidence of cancer for the entire placebo cohort is used, then for men with PSA levels of 3.0 or less and a normal DRE at the start of the trial, the incidence of cancer was 24.4% during the seven-year period, based on those diagnosed during and at the end of the trial [7].

If all the study participants with negative biopsies either during or at the end of the trial had been given a second biopsy, it is quite likely that additional cancers would have been found. As will be discussed in detail below, the six-needle biopsy can miss up to 25% of cancers. Thus the cancer prevalence results of Thompson *et al* probably in fact underestimate the true incidence. However, they only indicate that they used a minimum of six needles, which makes assessment of this aspect difficult.

Two conclusions are evident: (a) the higher the PSA in this so-called normal range of $\leq$ 4.0, the greater the probability of having prostate cancer, and the higher the PSA the greater the probability that the cancer detected is high-grade; (b) there does not appear to be a threshold for PSA levels below which the probability of having prostate cancer is negligible. Even a PSA level of between the lower limit of detectability (typically 0.1) and 0.5 corresponded to almost a 7% chance of having PC and if one is unlucky, then in addition there was a 12.5% chance that this cancer would be aggressive. The authors comment that their results run counter to the impression of many clinicians that PSA levels of 4.0 or less carry almost no risk of prostate cancer when in fact there is significant risk, including intermediate or high-grade cancer. In an editorial comment [8], Dr. Patrick Walsh of Johns Hopkins University Medical School, a very well know and respected urologist and surgeon, remarked that if a patient really wanted to know if he had PC, the study of Thompson *et al* left one with no alternative but to suggest a biopsy, since measuring PSA clearly was not the answer. What he does not mention is that more than one biopsy might be necessary to obtain a definitive answer!

TO SCREEN OR NOT TO SCREEN

Do you want at PSA test? Should I have a PSA test? These are question that may come up in the course of a physical exam. The current trend in medicine is to provide the pros and cons of screening and encourage the patient to make the decision. This in fact reflects the current status of the screening debate. Thus the patient should be armed with as much information as possible, which is in fact a tall order given the complexity of the issues. Screening for prostate cancer involves a PSA test and/or a DRE in asymptomatic men. While it is common practice to do both, the debate on the merits of screening centers on the PSA test. A number of experts have advanced arguments for and against its use. Nevertheless, as of 2002, 78% of male primary care physicians and 95% of male urologists interrogated in a national (US) sample reported having had a PSA test [9]. While the debate goes back some time into the history of this test, it is of interest to review the arguments put forward in recent reviews and editorials [10-15]. These arguments are mostly based on the use of the test for total PSA rather than recent variations such as free PSA or PSA density.

ARGUMENTS FOR SCREENING

- With the advent of widespread PSA screening in the US, the death rate from PC has declined, and in 1997 it fell below the rate recorded in 1986 when PSA was rarely measured. This is the PC-specific mortality argument. Those on both sides of the argument appear mostly to agree that the cause and effect relationship is still a hypothesis, and all await the results of ongoing trials. Preliminary results from one indicate no effect of screening on PC-related mortality [16].
- Before PSA screening, many cancers were diagnosed at a stage that could not be cured. It is generally agreed that today most cancers are identified at a much earlier stage when the cancer is localized and can be treated effectively surgically or non-surgically. This is the "higher cure rate for tumors found early" argument. Treating early cancer was not in general possible before the PSA test because there simply was no way to find it. It was organ-confined and could not be detected with the DRE.

- As a screening test for PC in general use, PSA has the highest predictive value, but only because the only other screening test in routine use is the DRE.
- The majority of cancers detected with PSA screening are clinically important. Tumors that are large enough to elevate serum PSA are mostly not the insignificant, well-differentiated microscopic tumors found at autopsy in many but not all men over that age of 50 who die from other causes.
- If one compares the incidence among cancer patients of palpable disease (positive DRE) for two periods 1983-1988 and 1999-2003, it was 92% in the pre PSA period and 17% in the recent PSA era, and the average PSA at diagnosis of PC dropped from 24 to 7.3.
- Incidence of positive lymph node and seminal vesicle disease (indicative of the spread of the cancer) is dramatically lower in the recent PSA era as compared to the earlier period. It is argued that this is due to early detection and equates to a better prognosis when the cancer is treated.
- Currently less than 10% of men have distant metastases at the time of diagnosis, which is considerably lower than was common in the pre-PSA era. Also, the percentage of men offered so-called local treatment with intent to cure (radical prostatectomy or radiation treatment) has increased significantly during the PSA era.
- The high false positive rate associated with either a 4.0 or lower cut-off can be decreased by adding %fPSA and PSA velocity (see below for a discussion of these two alternative PSA tests) to the screening protocol, thus reducing the number of biopsies that yield benign results, i.e. unnecessary biopsies.
- Some advocates of PSA screening question the argument that screening leads to over-diagnosis. The study of Etzioni *et al* [17] found that the majority of cases of PC detected by screening in the population studied (60-84 years of age in 1988) would still have had cancer detected that presented clinically within the patient lifetime.
- Some advocates of screening ask the following question. "Do those who are against PSA screening really want to return to the pre-PSA era when most of the cancers diagnosed were of an advanced stage and incurable?"

ARGUMENTS AGAINST SCREENING

- PSA screening leads to a large number of false positive results (PSA above the cut-off in cancer free individuals) which if acted upon, result in unnecessary biopsies.
- PSA screening finds insignificant cancers which would not yield clinical symptoms during the lifetime of the patient. Screening causes unwarranted treatment of slow-growing tumors. Those against screening quote such figures as 14.5% of prostate cancers removed by radical prostatectomy are clinically insignificant, but the other side points out that this means that 85.5% of patients had clinically significant tumors that were removed, many of them successfully. This is reminiscent of the two points of view where a glass is termed half-full or half-empty. Related to these observations is the comment by Epstein *et al* [18] that at Johns Hopkins, between 16 and 25% of RPs found insignificant cancer and that the incidence in recent years of truly minute

carcinoma found at RP was 5%. Epstein *et al* view this as evidence of a growing problem where potentially insignificant PC is both detected and treated.

- The decrease in mortality rate for prostate cancer seen during the PSA era is not due to screening but is the result of improved treatment including early hormone treatment and other still to be identified factors. Also, the continuous and dramatic decline over recent years of hospital autopsy rates, caused in part by both financial and legal concerns, could impact the correct assignment of prostate cancer as a cause of death, since the autopsy makes the assignment much more reliable. In fact, it is important to recognize that when a death certificate indicates the cause as prostate cancer, there is not only some uncertainty in this judgment call in the absence of an autopsy, but there is also variability in how prostate cancer caused death is actually defined. This state of affairs significantly complicates studies on cancer-specific mortality.
- A man's risk of death from prostate cancer is 3-4% whereas his lifetime risk of being diagnosed with the disease is about 17% [6]. This suggests that many prostate cancers detected in routine practice may be clinically unimportant.
- Unnecessary treatment results in unnecessary adverse effects such as impotence, incontinence and bowel disorders, and a decline in the quality of life of the treated individual. An increased risk of rectal cancer has also been recently reported associated with radiation treatment [19].
- The fear of dying from prostate cancer may be out of proportion with the real probability of death from this disease, given that approximately 250,000 US men were diagnosed with prostate cancer in 2004, but only 30,000 are expected to die from it [20].

Both the advocates and opponents of screening appear to agree that the relationship of PC-specific mortality to the advent of screening remains to be settled, but there is no disagreement as to the occurrence of a mortality decline in a number of countries [21]. When PSA was first introduced in the late 1980s, both incidence and mortality increased, but this was followed after 1991 by a decline that increased in rate. By 1997, the US PC mortality rates for white men aged < 85 had declined to levels lower than those observed in 1986. But there have been very few studies that addressed the question of cause and effect as regards the impact of screening on PC-specific mortality. There is clearly a danger slipping into the logical fallacy *post hoc ergo propter hoc* (after this, therefore because of this). There appear to be only three studies that approach or attempt to approach properly addressing the question, and they are all recent. A study conducted in Quebec found a 62% reduction in mortality when screened and unscreened populations were compared [22]. This study came under immediate criticism for design and procedural problems [23] and another interpretation of the data yielded insignificant differences [21]. In another study [24], PC-specific mortality in the Austrian state of Tyrol was compared to the rest of Austria. The motivation was that PSA screening was made more freely available in the Tyrol in 1993. While lower PC-related mortality was observed in Tyrol as compared to the rest of Austria, another explanation for this difference may be the increased proportion of patients undergoing radical prostatectomies in this state, and in fact this predated PSA screening [25]. A third study was based on the fact that PSA screening was more common in the Seattle-Puget Sound area than in the state of Connecticut and this should have translated into a lower PC-specific mortality. The results of this eleven-year study have just appeared [26] and were negative. Finally, PC mortality rates have also declined in countries where PSA screening is uncommon [27]. Confusing the issue even more is the just published case control study [28] that found the fascinating result that cholesterol lowering therapy employing the statin class of drug dramatically reduced the risk of prostate cancer (OR = 0.38, 95% confidence interval 0.21-0.69), especially more aggressive disease. A large prospective study is needed to examine this result since other studies, while not looking specifically at PC, did not find similar risk reduction. Needless to say, statin therapy is widespread and dramatically increased during the period when PSA screening was also increasing.

J.-E Damber has suggested [21] one explanation unrelated to PSA that could account for the decline in PC-specific mortality. At about the same time as PSA screening became popular, there was renewed interest in hormonal therapy, and its use then increased substantially and it became common practice to begin this therapy earlier and even employ it in combination with radiation therapy. Damber reviews several randomized clinical trials of the use of the luteinizing hormone releasing hormone agonist (e.g. goserelin) or castration along with radiation therapy which resulted in evidence of significant improvement in survival over radiation therapy alone. Even though hormonal therapy is not curative, Damber suggests that the increased use of this treatment could contribute to the observed recent decline in PC-specific mortality by delaying death from PC long enough for some patients to die from other causes.

The relevance of the mortality argument (screening is not advisable unless it has a positive effect on prostate specific mortality) should be scrutinized carefully. An individual can have metastatic PC which may go nearly to the end stage, and yet die of a stroke or heart attack, and this would not be counted as PC-specific mortality in some studies. Nevertheless, during the course of the disease, the individual would probably experience a greatly diminished quality of life associated with both the spreading cancer and its palliative treatment. The list of problems associated with advanced PC is long, but includes fatigue, depression, pain, numerous side effects associated with hormone and pain treatment, and problems once the cancer is established in other sites such as the brain, bone, lung, etc. A recent study was criticized for counting distant metastasis observed at autopsy as PC-specific death, but the authors defended this protocol by pointing out that metastatic PC was in effect a death sentence. The point is that the effect of screening on the prevalence and time to onset of metastasis is perhaps a more realistic measure of its merits than looking simply at overall PC mortality. If early detection and treatment significantly delay metastasis in those not cured, the benefit would be in some cases dying of another cause before metastasis profoundly altered the quality of life, a cause of death that would in some, perhaps even many cases be less drawn-out, debilitating, psychologically devastating and painful. There is recent evidence that screening has a significant influence on the incidence of metastatic PC [29]. In a sense, concern over cause-specific mortality is like looking at a race between the various causes of death and then basing diagnostic and therapeutic decisions on the statistics of races won and lost. Some might find this a bit simplistic, given the complexity of the end-of-life period.

Kopec *et al* have also recently addressed the issue of metastasis in the context of screening. In a study reported in 2005 based in Ontario, Canada, they performed a case control study of the screening of asymptomatic men [30]. They found that the frequency of screening as determined from medical records significantly and positively associated with a decrease in the risk of metastatic cancer with odds ratios of 0.52 for men aged 45-59 and 0.67 for those 60-84, the latter result not quite reaching statistical significance. Overall for those frequently screened, the odds ratio was 0.65 (95% confidence limits 0.45-0.93) when cases were compared to controls. Thus the case for screening impacting the risk of metastasis is gaining strength.

A recent study carried out between 1991 and 2001 involving a very large number of participants directly relates to some to the questions raised in the screening debate and in particular the suggestion to lower the PSA cut-off for triggering a biopsy [31]. Included in the study were men 45-59 years of age at baseline with PSA ≤ 2.6 and a normal DRE who complied with the screening protocol which involved periodic PSA measurements and a DRE. In this study, the indication for biopsy was PSA > 2.5 or a suspicious DRE. The six or greater needle biopsy procedure was used and not all men followed the recommendation for a biopsy. If one assumes that those refusing biopsy would have had the same cancer rate as those biopsied, then about 3% of those screened would have been found to have cancer. For those biopsied, 54% had cancer. Of these, 87% underwent a radical prostatectomy (RP) which yielded pathological characteristics of the tumor burden. Seventy-nine percent had organ confined disease, 13% possible harmless disease, and 2% possible rapidly progressing cancer. Comparison via the published literature with non-screened populations provided the following observations, *all of which favored the screened population*: (a) 80% of the cancers were non-palpable, i.e. found only by elevated PSA, (b) no tumors were clinically advanced at diagnosis; (c) 13% of tumors were judged possibly harmless i.e. low over-diagnosis compared to non-screened populations. In addition, the five-year freedom from PSA progression (biochemical failure indicating eventual metastatic cancer) was 95% which is a very good recurrence-free rate. Biochemical failure will be discussed below. The authors conclude that adherence to screening guidelines such as they employed would result in the detection of prostate cancer in most individuals that was both significant and curable.

One of the most persuasive arguments of the pro-screening advocates involves the assertion that finding PC early has a higher probability of leading to a so-called "cure." If this is true then radical prostatectomy, which is frequently the treatment of choice, should be very effective in curing cancers identified by screening. While what constitutes a cure can be debated, one option is to use the absence of post RP recurrence, so-called biochemical failure, where the PSA, after dropping to near zero, starts to increase, indicating that the disease has not been eradicated. Since 1992, at least twelve studies have addressed this question using biochemical failure as the endpoint [32,33]. While the populations studied had somewhat different characteristics, the five-year failure rate was found to be 2-20% and the 10-year rate 5-25%. Larger failure rates were associated with higher Gleason scores and higher preoperative PSA. Thus there appears to be some merit to this argument. The time lag between biochemical failure and clinical manifestation of disease may be as long as 5-8 years, followed by an additional 5-year median time to metastasis and another 5-year median time to prostate cancer specific death. Thus if biochemical failure occurs at, say, 5 years post-RP, then there would be on average about 15 years before PC-related death would be predicted. But the problem of recurrence impacts at most only to the 5-25% of individuals who had a RP, and furthermore, 75-95% were "cured." Furthermore, those with the most favorable characteristics presumably accounted for those with low recurrence rates.

A study by Antenor *et al* [34] also addresses the above issue. They followed over 2800 men with the PC stage commonly found in screening studies who were treated with a RP and then monitored prospectively to obtain the 10-year biochemical progression free survival rates. Men with preoperative PSA in the range of 2.6 to 4.0 had an 88% 10-year disease free survival rate, i.e. a 12% failure rate, whereas for a preoperative PSA level > 10, the ten-year disease free rate was only 61%. Men with a PSA level of 2.6 to 4.0 also had the greatest rate of organ-confined disease, and the lowest Gleason score found post-RP. Similar results were obtained by Freedland *et al* [35] but the disease free survival rates were lower, even at 5 years. These studies viewed together support the notion of better prognosis with early detection and treatment.

While there is also biochemical failure data available for men with screening-detected PC treated with radiation, the picture is confused by the changes over the past decade in radiation techniques and dosage, and results with the most recent protocols, including high dose, do not have extensive long-term results available. Shorter term studies with the latest protocols suggest that the disease-free survival rates are similar for RP and the current RT protocols. This will be discussed in detail in Chapter 6.

Recent studies using PC-specific mortality as an endpoint provide a similar picture as regards treatment and metastasis, but are based on comparing screening-initiated RP with a watchful waiting group where no treatment was given until palliation was required. This latter group is roughly equivalent to a pre-PSA or non-screened population. The largest difference between the RP and watchful waiting groups is seen with high-grade cancers [29,36]. One recent study with PC-specific mortality as the principal endpoint also looked at the effect of screening on subsequent distant metastasis and found the watchful waiting group at considerably greater risk than those randomized to RP [29]. Unless accidental death or a fatal comorbidity intervene, patients with distant metastasis will die of PC.

While studies that favor screening continue to appear, it is clear that this debate will not be easily resolved until a new generation of markers and procedures with a much lower level of false positives and a better indication of tumor grade are devised, tested, and approved. The wide gap between the advocates (some call them evangelists) and those against screening (called snails who keep demanding more scientific proof) is clear from the fact that American Cancer Society, the American Medical Association, and the American Urological Association favor screening with PSA and a DRE, but the U.S. Preventive Services Task Force and the American College of Physicians recommend against it. This lack of agreement has resulted in a movement to shift the decision making burden to the patient. Frequently stated advice is that the physician should discuss the pros and cons of screening with the patient and obtain input as to whether or not to proceed.

There are two trials currently on-going that may help resolve the question of the relationship between screening, the resultant early treatment, and overall PC-specific mortality. Together these two trials aim to recruit over a quarter of a million men, but the results will not be available until 2008-9 unless they report early. In fact, in a preliminary report from one of these studies [16], a favorable shift in prognostic factors was found in the screening arm of the trial, but the results failed to provide evidence that screening had an effect on PC-specific mortality. In the meantime, the mortality argument should probably be viewed with suspicion. Also, concerns have been expressed regarding one of the two studies being able to detect only a very large screening effect [9].

AGE, SCREENING, AND AGE-ADJUSTED PSA CUT-OFF

The serum level of PSA is determined by both the presence of cancer and/or BPH, and as well can be elevated by other factors discussed below. BPH increases with age and thus provides a benign cause of age-dependent PSA elevation. But the matter is complicated because the probability of cancer also increases with age. A solution, proposed by Osterling *et al* [37] in 1993, involved an age-adjusted set of PSA cut-offs, with higher PSA levels associated with more advanced age. Subsequent studies showed that the use of these cut-offs reduced the biopsy rate in men with normal DRE, but Catalona *et al* [38] demonstrated that age-specific cut-offs missed large numbers of tumors. However, this approach to the use of PSA may offer greater sensitivity for cancer detection in younger men. An examination of the literature reveals that in the past few years there has been little interest in either improving or justifying age-adjusted cut-offs as a trigger for biopsy. There appears to be no solution to the fundamental characteristic of screening tests that, no matter what the age group, decreasing the cut-off increases the sensitivity of the test but reduces the specificity with the attendant increase in false positives [27,39]. Three high-profile books for the lay audience present age-adjusted cut-off tables [2,40,41], but aside from the work of Osterling *et al*, clinical studies justifying specific numbers as offering benefit to patients appear limited. If age-adjusted cut-offs, which have cut-offs below 4 for younger men, are used in practice the motivation is presumably detecting additional cancers, especially in younger men where there PSA elevations are more likely to be due to cancer than BPH. The guidelines for triggering a biopsy from Walsh's book [41] are summarized in Table 1 and illustrate this. The first two thresholds are the same as proposed by Osterling *et al.*

Table 4-1. Age adjusted PSA thresholds for triggering the recommendation of a biopsy.

Age	PSA Threshold
40-49 years	2.5
50-59 years	3.5
≥60 years	4.0

The most significant change from the traditional cut-off of 4.0 is in the 40-49 age group. There is considerable evidence that younger men with cancer, and in particular those less than 50 years of age, initially have a greater probability of organ-confined disease and a much higher disease free survival rate post RP [42-45]. In a very recent study [46] it was found men that younger than 62 with screening PSA < 4 had smaller, lower-grade tumors and lower recurrence rates post RP than those with PSA ≥ 4. This was not true for men over 62. A cut-off of 4 will fail to detect many of these small but highly treatable cancers. In fact, the Johns Hopkins urologist H. Balentine Carter [47] supports the lower cut-off of 2.5 for men under 50 whereas for all others he sees little advantage of lower cut-offs over the traditional value of 4, but this is the subject of debate.

Bosch *et al* [48] have attempted to establish an age dependent set of PSA values that characterize individuals with no prostate cancer. In some cases biopsies were used to exclude candidates for inclusion but this "cancer-free" cohort was probably to some extent contaminated with individuals with undetected cancer, especially since considerable reliance was placed on the DRE. Table 4-2 gives the results. Prostate volumes were also measured and included for comparison. At age 60, the cut-off of 4 given by Walsh would be close to one standard deviation (SD) above the mean, giving support to this age-adjusted cut-off. The linear correlation of prostate volume and PSA is also evident from these data.

Table 4-2. Distribution of PSA values and prostate volumes (in cc) according to age [48].

Age	Mean PSA (SD)*	Mean Prostate Volume (SD)
<55 years	1.1 (1.0)	28.4 (8.0)
55-59 years	1.4 (1.4)	30.5 (9.3)
60-64 years	1.8 (1.8)	34.8 (14.2)
65-69 years	2.3 (2.9)	36.5 (17.1)
70-74 years	2.5 (2.4)	41.9 (19.1)
>75 years	3.1 (3.0)	46.2 (23.2)

* SD—standard deviation

The 2.5 vs 4.0 Cut-Off Debate

Some of the arguments have been presented above. Facts that do not appear debatable include the following. The probability of detecting cancer is a direct function of the PSA level, and therefore the lower cut-off should increase the number of men above threshold who would presumably be counseled to undergo a biopsy, and this would result in finding cancers that otherwise would have escaped detection until the old cut-off was exceeded. A lower cut-off would also result in an increase in the number of benign biopsies, since lowering the cut-off has the inevitable consequence of decreasing the specificity of the screening test [27]. Another argument, as discussed above, is that a lower cut-off will identify more younger men with PC, most of whom are curable, and clearly have a life expectancy that justifies treatment.

Two papers by Catalona and associates [49,50] relate to the objection that a lower cut-off will detect too many insignificant tumors. They conclude that a cut-off of > 2.5 identifies a substantial number of cancers and will indeed find small, organ-confined tumors, but without over-detecting clinically insignificant cancers, but over-detection depends on how it is defined. On the other hand, Carter [47] argues that there is no convincing evidence that with present-day therapy, men treated when their cancers are detected at PSA levels below 4 have any less favorable outcome than men treated when they exceed 4.0 by a small amount. But this argument is confounded by age, as Carter recognizes. He argues that the detection of PC at a younger age should have a greater effect on the probability of being disease-free after treatment than would the detection at a PSA of less than 4.

A recent estimate of the effect of lowering the PSA threshold to 2.5 indicated that whereas approximately 1.5 million American men have a PSA level > 4.0, a threshold of 2.5 would more than double this number adding 1.8 million [51]. The authors also estimate that if all 1.8 million had a biopsy, about 1.35 million would have benign results, i.e. the PSA test gave a false positive. Even with the current threshold of 4.0, the authors estimate, using a 10-year risk of death from prostate cancer as defining clinically important disease, that roughly 10 times the number of men had abnormal PSA as would be expected to die from the disease in the following 10 years. Lowering the threshold would make this comparison even more unfavorable.

There appears no simple answer to the question of the optimum cut-off or the merits of using one lower than the traditional value of 4. The critical need is for new non-invasive tests that have both high sensitivity and higher specificity. Some of these will be discussed below.

FREE AND COMPLEXED PSA, PSA DENSITY AND PSA RATE OF CHANGE

The lack of specificity associated with the total PSA test (tPSA), has prompted considerable interest in refinements and variations that decrease false positives and false negatives. These "second generation" PSA tests include *free* PSA, *complexed* PSA, PSA *density* based either on total prostate volume or transition zone volume, and finally the rate of change of PSA with time expressed as a PSA *velocity* or *doubling time*. Complexed PSA appears to offer no advantage over the other second generation tests and will not be discussed [52]. Of special interest is improving the specificity in the 4-10 PSA range in order to reduce the number of unnecessary biopsies that a cut-off of 4 might provoke for individuals with total PSA levels in this grey area. But the PSA range of 2-4 is also of great interest, given that one in four men with PSA levels between 2.0 and 4.0 have PC at biopsy, more than a fifth of these lesions are judged high grade, and even a cut-off of 2.0 leaves 9% of men below this cut-off with cancer [6]. The need for greater specificity over the whole range from 2 to 10 is generally recognized.

Free PSA

The form of PSA called free PSA is one of the most interesting in this context. While PSA is predominantly complexed with proteins, the form called free PSA (fPSA) is unbound. Early work suggested an enhanced discriminatory power of fPSA over total (tPSA), especially in differentiating PC from BPH. In fact, a crude generalization commonly seen is that free PSA is from BPH and bound PSA is from cancer cells. This has prompted clinical trials of considerable interest. In these studies, free PSA is generally expressed as a percentage of total PSA, so it is

$$\%fPSA = 100 \times fPSA/tPSA$$

The %fPSA has been the subject of a number of studies aimed at evaluating its merits relative to tPSA for indicating the advisability of a biopsy [53]. The incidence of PC in the grey area of tPSA of 4-10 is typically 20-25%, but if everyone with a tPSA above 4 but below 10 is subjected to a biopsy, 75-80% will be benign. The motivation in using %fPSA is to avoid some of these benign biopsies on the basis of a scheme that selects for those with low probability of PC. Thus the interest in determining if a suitable cut-off for %fPSA will accomplish this. The typical study is designed as follows. A group meeting a certain set of criteria (e.g. tPSA between 4 and 10 and a non-suspicious DRE) is recruited who are willing to undergo a biopsy. The %PSA is determined and from the biopsy results of the whole group, the merits of a given cut-off are determined. For example, in a recently reported large study [54], 500 patients underwent biopsy. In 107 PC was found, and thus 393 benign biopsies were generated by the tPSA cut-off of $\geq$ 4.0. If a cut-off for %fPSA of < 23% had been used instead as a biopsy trigger with this particular group, 77 participants were above this cut-off and would have avoided biopsy. Of the 77, 71 were actually benign and 6 had cancer. Thus the percentage of benign biopsies avoided by using this cut-off was 71/393 = 0.18 or 18%. The price for avoiding 77 biopsies was missing 6 cancers, all of which, according to the authors, were significant. The 6 cancers out of a total of 107 represents 5.6%, which allows one to judge the risk of avoiding the biopsy by making use of this %fPSA based cut-off rather than the >4 PSA cut-off. Since any cut-off can be examined from the data in hand, this type of study allows the selection of an optimum cut-off in the trade-off between avoiding unnecessary biopsies and missing cancers. If the desire is not to miss any cancers, then the exercise is pointless since it is necessary to biopsy everybody. In this study, the overall incidence of PC was 107/500 or 21.4%, which is normal. It is important that the incidence be comparable to that found in other cohorts since otherwise there would be a suspicion that the group did not represent the general public in the age range studied. Also, it is typical and perhaps necessary in studies of this sort to ignore the fact that the biopsy itself will miss some cancers. Thus it is possible that not all of the 71 benign biopsies in the above study were in fact benign, but there is no simple solution to this defect since finding participants who will undergo a more extensive biopsy protocol is presumably very difficult.

A second large study reported in 1997 [3] also dealt with the grey PSA area of 4-10 , but a high proportion of cancer cases was found (49%) which may not be representative of a normal patient population [54]. Nevertheless, when a 25% fPSA cut-off was used, 95% of cancers were detected while 20% of unnecessary biopsies were avoided. It is beyond the scope of this review to examine in detail the large number of studies related to the use of %fPSA, but it is frequently but not always found that a cut-off of 20 to 25% results is the avoidance of about 20% of unnecessary biopsies when the population studied has a total PSA in the range of 4-10. Since this grey area represents, for the majority of individuals, the PSA elevating effects of BPH, the use of the %fPSA for this range of tPSA involves an attempt to differentiate PC from BPH. Studies of %fPSA for men in the tPSA range of < 4 range are encouraging but limited [55], and it is too early to draw definite conclusions [55,56].

Along with the problem of the specificity of the PSA test, the other big challenge is to determine with some degree of certainty the presence of a significant tumor or tumors that indicates the advisability of aggressive treatment and at the same time exclude from either a biopsy or treatment those who have insignificant or indolent tumors that are judged to present little current risk and can be merely watched without putting the patient at undue risk. Evaluating a proposed protocol involves either the pathological examination of prostates removed at radical prostatectomy (RP) or an evaluation scheme based on a set of conditions applied to the biopsy core analysis. The information is combined with preoperative or pre-biopsy blood test data required by the proposed test. A number of studies have examined the %fPSA in this context.

In what Dr. Patrick Walsh describes [41] as a landmark study, Epstein *et al* [57] in 1998 reported the results of examining the power of %fPSA in predicting insignificant tumors in a series of radical prostatectomy cases. Insignificant cancers were defined as organ confined with tumor volumes of less than 0.5 mL and Gleason score of < 7. The best model for *preoperatively* predicting insignificant tumors was a %fPSA of ≥ 15% and favorable needle biopsy findings (less than 3 cores involved, none with greater than 50% tumor involvement). This model correctly predicted in the group studied that 17 out of 18 tumors were insignificant when the removed prostates were subjected to pathological examination.

In a study based on radical prostatectomy samples, Southwick *et al* [58] examined a cohort with total PSA between 4 and 10 and a non-suspicious DRE. They also found that a cut-off of 15% fPSA provided the greatest discrimination in predicting a favorable pathological outcome. Aus *et al* [59] examined the use of %fPSA in predicting non-organ-confined PC, which would be classified as aggressive. For a %fPSA of 10.7% (first quartile), the risk of non-organ confined PC was 46.5%, whereas for the fourth quartile (> 20.7 %fPSA) the risk was 13.6%. Grossklaus *et al* [60] used tumor density (tumor volume divided by gland volume as determined in prostates removed during RP) as a measure of "tumor involvement" as estimated by either tPSA or %fPSA. It was found that the %fPSA inversely correlated with tumor volume as well as Gleason score and extra capsular extension (tumor identified outside the prostate capsule). These results further support the notion that %fPSA is inversely related to the aggressive nature of the cancer and that this has clinical significance.

A recent meta-analysis [53] systematically examined a large number of studies related to the use of %fPSA for men in both the 2-4 and 4-10 PSA ranges. The authors found that up to 50% of unnecessary biopsies could be avoided for those in the 4-10 range compared to 35% in the 2-4 range while missing 20% of cancers. From a somewhat different point of view, Dr. Peter Scardino [2] summarizes the results with %fPSA by pointing out that its use improves the ability by 20 to 40% to predict whether the cause of an elevated PSA is due to cancer but reduces by only about 5% the cancers that would otherwise not be detected. He also remarks that at one extreme, a %fPSA value over 25% suggests that elevated PSA is largely caused by BPH and any cancer present is more likely to be small and confined to the gland. At the other extreme, a level %f PSA under 10% suggests that an elevated total PSA is mostly due to cancer and it is more likely than not that the cancer is significant and the patient would benefit from treatment. There is a grey zone between 10 and 25% where the picture is less clear.

Dr. Patrick Walsh in his 2002 book on prostate cancer [41] poses the question "Should you get it?" in reference to the %fPSA test. He introduces two points to consider. First, it is twice as expensive since two blood tests are required. This is an issue only if insurance does not cover the test or if it not on the approved list for public or private health care plans. The second consideration is simply the inevitable consequence of tests that are not 100% specific—5-10% of cancers may be missed. Walsh goes on to mention two situations where this test is, in his view, particularly useful. In the first case, there is the man with an elevated PSA who has had several biopsies that are negative. If the %fPSA is high, the patient can "relax." If the %fPSA is very low, this suggests that more biopsies are in order! The second situation involves an individual with a strong family history of PC but with a low age-adjusted tPSA. If the %fPSA is high, this provides reassurance that cancer is probably absent, whereas if it is low, it is an indication for a biopsy.

PSA Density

The theoretical motivation for using PSA density (PSAD) is partly based on the fact that men with BPH will in general have both higher levels of PSA and enlarged prostates, and that this can be taken into account when trying to distinguish BPH from PC by dividing the tPSA by the measured prostate volume. Since BPH results almost exclusively from transition zone (TZ) hyperplasia, a refinement of the density argument introduced in 1994 leads to a density based on only the TZ volume (PSATZD).

Total PSA can be converted into densities by dividing by the prostate volume. The DRE is notoriously inaccurate in providing a measure of prostate volume, and thus the use of PSA density (PSAD) requires an ultrasound determination, generally with a transrectal probe. Since general practitioners and internists generally do not have such equipment in their offices, this necessitates a visit to the ultrasound facility at a hospital or diagnostic clinic. However, urologists may be able to provide these prostate density tests in the office setting. There is, incidentally, at least one study suggesting that trans-abdominal ultrasound is very much inferior to transrectal ultrasound in this context [61]. Total and TZ volumes can be obtained from ultrasound data available during an ultrasound guided biopsy, but this is irrelevant in the context of the problem of increasing the specificity of the PSA test if the purpose is avoiding unnecessary biopsies.

Most tests of the hypothesis that using a PSA density will improve specificity and avoid unnecessary biopsies involve comparing biopsy results with the levels of PSA density. Some studies also include a comparison with %fPSA. The PSA ranges from 2-10 or 4-10 and ≤ 4.0 are of interest in this context. In a study by Horninger *et al* reported in 1998 [62], 308 individuals underwent ultrasound guided biopsy with 228 showing only BPH and 58 (19%) diagnosed with PC (22 had prostatitis!!). By using a cut-off of > 0.22 ng/mL/cc (the standard unit used) for the PSATZD as a biopsy trigger, 24.4% of negative biopsies could have been avoided. Djavan *et al* published a study [63] in 1998 that involved 559 consecutive men referred for early prostate detection or lower urinary tract symptoms who had tPSA in the range of 4-10 . The diagnosis of PC was based on one or more ultrasound guided biopsies. The PSATZD and the %fPSA were the most powerful and significant predictors of PC, and both were better than PSAD. By tolerating a 5% failure rate in PC detection, a cut-off of >0.25 ng/mL/cc as a biopsy criterion would have resulted in the lowest number of unnecessary biopsies. However, when the total prostate volume was less than 30 mL, the TZ based method was inferior to the %fPSA in sensitivity and specificity. Three much smaller studies published between 1999 and 2005 also examined the utility of PSATZD in diagnosing cancer while avoiding unnecessary biopsies. All involved participants with PSA in the range of 4-10. One study found PSATZD superior to PSAD [64]. Another found PSATZD superior to %fPSA [65] but the third [66] failed to find an advantage over %fPSA. All three found a cut-off of 0.35 ng/mL/cc to give the best compromise between sensitivity and specificity.

Thus it appears that using a PSA density calculated from a measured TZ volume or combining this with %fPSA offers a protocol for decreasing the number of benign biopsy results for men with PSA levels in the grey area of 4-10 who would normally undergo biopsies simply due to exceeding the threshold of 4.0. However, the studies quoted would all have missed some cancers by using either the PSATZD or %fPSA or a combined indicator if their optimum cut-offs were used. By now it should be clear that this is inevitable.

There has been considerable discussion of the question of decreasing the "normal" cut-off from 4.0 to 2.0 or 2.5 for tPSA (see above). Thus tests that have improved specificity as compared to tPSA are of considerable interest for application to men with levels in this range. There have been several studies that address this question [61,67,68]. These studies examined the biopsy results for men with tPSA in the range of either 2.5-4.0 or 2.0-4.0 and relate to using the lower limit of these ranges as a cut-off that would trigger a biopsy. Djavan *et al* [68] studied 273 men with serum PSA between 2.5 and 4.0. The found that patients with a %fPSA > 41% and a PSATZD of less than 0.095 ng/mL/cc could safely have been spared unnecessary biopsies. However, for small prostates (<30 mL), the PSATZD was less effective than in patients with larger prostates, and they suggest in this case the use of %fPSA alone. Koyayashi *et al* [61] found that PSAD and PSATZD were similar in terms of predicting PC in men with tPSA in the range of 2-4 and better than %fPSA.

In a small study, Ohi *et al* [67] found that the diagnostic efficiency of PSATZD showed the highest value for a cut-off of 0.23 and 0.28 for men with tPSA levels of 2.1-3.0 and 3.1-4.0 respectively, and that the use of these cut-offs as biopsy indicators would reduce unnecessary biopsies without missing most PC cases for men with tPSA in the range of 2.1 to 4.0.

The suggestion of lowering the cut-off for triggering biopsies from 4.0 to 2.0 or 2.5 mainly applies to younger men who are less likely to have BPH elevated PSA and who appear most likely to benefit from early detection and treatment of PC. For men who feel lower cut-offs are wise, have serum levels in excess of one or the other of these cut-offs and are referred to a urologist for consultation, a discussion of the possibility of using TZ based PSA density and %fPSA would seem to be in order when considering the pros and cons of a biopsy.

PSA Velocity and Doubling Time (Kinetics)
PSA velocity (PSAV) involves repeated measurements over time to establish the pattern of change or stability in an individual's serum level. It has been known for a number of years that a rapid increase in PSA either in asymptomatic men or in those who have undergone treatment is generally a sign of trouble. As an adjunct to screening, PSA velocity is receiving ever-increasing attention. Some studies also calculate the doubling time. In the context of diagnosis a linear model is generally used, frequently with only two or three measurements. When PSAV is used in the post-treatment setting, it not uncommon to encounter a linear-logarithmic model (i.e. assumed exponential growth) used for calculating doubling times. Several recent studies are of interest.

Berger *et al* [69] recently reported on a large study where men were followed for up to 10 years (average 6 years). In this retrospective study 2,462 men free of PC underwent

PSA testing very two years. Over the total time period 353 patients were diagnosed with PC. In men with cancer mean tPSA increased from 2.28 at baseline 10 years before diagnosis to 6.37 at the time of positive biopsy (PSA velocity 0.409 ng/mL/year). In the benign group, the mean tPSA increased from 1.18 to 1.49 over ten years for a velocity of 0.03 ng/mL/year. For subjects with tPSA levels of 2 or less two years prior to diagnosis, 11.4% had values of more than 4.0 at the time of positive biopsy. The authors concluded that an annual measurement was not required for men with levels below 1.0, but for those above this level annual measurements were suggested on the basis of the observation that a significant percentage of men with initial levels > 1.0 had levels of over 4 two years later. Finally, an interesting observation was that about 24% of men with no evidence of PC had *lower* tPSA values at the end of the study than the value found 10 years earlier. They also comment that the currently used threshold velocity of ≥ 0.75 ng/mL/year may be too high, at least in a Caucasian population. However, two early studies, one in 1992 [70] and one in 1994 [71] found that a cut-off of 0.75 ng/mL/year was optimum for distinguishing men with high risk of progressing to PC or as a biopsy threshold. It was found that when the PSAV was based on a time span of 18 months or more, 95% of men without PC who had a PSA less than 10 had a PSAV less than 0.75 ng/mL/year. Dr. Peter Scardino [2] also takes the position that a PSA velocity of more than 0.75ng/mL/year indicates an increased risk that a biopsy would be positive for PC.

In a small study published in 2002, Fang *et al* [72] studied men with initial PSA levels between 2.0 and 4.0. Men who maintained a PSAV of less than 0.1 ng/mL/year had a 97% probability of remaining disease free for at least 10 years compared to only 37% for those with a PSAV exceeding 0.1 ng/mL/year. Their data indicated that 80% of PC cases could be identified with this cut-off, but the false positive rate would be 50%.

Large annual increases in PSA prior to diagnosis are a strong indication of poor prognosis [73]. Two recent studies strongly suggest that a PSA change of greater than 2 ng/mL in the year preceding diagnosis predicted poor outcome following either RP or RT [74,75], or metastatic disease and progression following hormone therapy.

There have been a few other studies that address the utility of PSAV, but they are difficult to compare due to different designs and populations studied [76-78]. As Dr. Patrick Walsh points out [41], PSAV offers an improvement over the raw PSA score but it is important to realize that 25% of men with prostate cancers that are growing do not have a big increase in their PSA. Like the other variations of the PSA test, perfection is not in sight. Nevertheless, PSAV appears to add a significant piece of information, not only if the PSAV is very low but especially if it is very high. The usefulness of PSAV also provides a rationale for annual or biannual testing in order to acquire the necessary data. Once a man has agreed to have a PSA test, it can be argued that it makes sense to continue the practice for this reason.

Intra-Individual Variations in Measured PSA
A serious problem associated with PSAV, as well as with PSA cut-offs in general, involves the intra-individual variations. In a recent study, Boddy *et al* [79] tested men with biopsy demonstrated absence of PC. Four measurements of PSA levels were made over one month. The average variation was almost 10%, and when stratified by PSA level, 0-4.0 gave, 14.1%, and 4.1-10 gave 10.8% variability. The authors review earlier studies

which showed similar variations, with typical values of about 15%. A 15% variation takes a value of 3.9 to 4.5. Variations of this magnitude are of consequence when either PSAV is being tracked or a patient crosses or is near a cut-off. For example, Eastham *et al* [80] examined 972 men and acquired five consecutive blood samples over a 4-year period. Among men with an abnormal PSA result, a high proportion had a *normal* result at one or more subsequent visits during the follow-up period (44% with an initial PSA result > 4, 40% with an initial level higher than 2.5 and 55% with an initial elevated level above the age specific cut-off). The authors conclude that an elevated PSA (i.e. one that crosses a cut-off) should be confirmed with a repeat test several weeks later before attributing clinical significance to the result. Perhaps even more caution is indicated.

Artificial Lowering or Elevation of PSA

The following factors can raise or lower serum PSA levels to an extent that can be significant in connection with both cut-off crossing and PSA velocity measurements.

- The DRE can artificially raise PSA levels for a day or more. The largest immediate effect is on %fPSA. For example, in one study, the average value from before to 30 minutes after the DRE for total PSA was 3.4 to 4.3 and for %fPSA from 27.9% to 38%, with both changes highly statistically significant [81]. Thus blood for a PSA test should be drawn before a DRE. However, this is controversial due to other studies which indicate an insignificant effect on total PSA.

- Both total and free PSA increase after ejaculation with different rates of return to baseline. PSA testing within 24 hours of ejaculation may lead to an artificial elevation and erroneous clinical conclusions [82].

- Bladder cystoscopy and/or catheterization can elevate PSA levels for at least two weeks.

- Laboratories using different assay procedures (kits from different companies) can experience variations that have significance when the value is near a cut-off or when PSA velocity is an issue. In a recent study of two currently used commercial assays, 19% of patients would have been candidates for a biopsy with one test but not with another used in comparison. The cut-off in this study was 4.0 [83]. This is a serious problem since changing primary care physicians is not uncommon and might result in a different assay being used, and also physicians may change the laboratory they patronize.

- Acute urinary retention can elevate PSA levels for up two weeks.

- Prostate needle biopsy or TURP to treat BPH can elevate PSA values for up to six weeks.

- The two medications used to treat BPH, Proscar and Avodart; both reduce PSA levels by about 50%. Incidentally, Propecia used for treating hair loss is low-dose Proscar. Some physicians correct for this but it is hard to believe that the correction is more than just approximate. For example, in the Prostate Cancer Prevention Trial, the correction factor was increased from 2 at 2 years to 2.5 at 7 years [84]. But these correction factors are based on averaging over a population *believed* free of cancer. The combined uncertainty of the PSA determination itself and the inherent uncertainty in the exact correction factor for any given individual leads to an increased total uncertainty as to what is the real corrected PSA. At this point the magnitude of the uncertainty appears unknown but should be of concern to anyone using Proscar or Avodart who is near a commonly used cut-off or is having their PSA measured periodically for the purposes of using PSA kinetics as a decision making tool. When it was found that the 5α-reductase inhibitors significantly reduced PSA levels, it was clear that considerable diagnostic potential was lost. Attempting to salvage the situation with a correction factor may in fact not be a satisfactory solution.

- Prostatitis can strongly elevate PSA levels which will generally come back down with treatment.

- It has just been reported in a small study that statin treatment for hypercholesterolemia (elevated cholesterol) can lower PSA levels [85]. The study involved 15 airline pilots. Over about 6 years, the average PSA dropped 41.6 % in the statin group and increased by 38% in the comparison group, the latter increase presumably being age related. These are large and statistically significant changes. This observation will no doubt receive additional study in the next few years since the number of men taking statins is very large indeed and there is pressure to increase the number dramatically by lowering LDL cholesterol targets. The mechanism of the interaction is unclear as is the answer to the question; did this reduce the risk of PC? Thus while these results need confirmation, statins appear to significantly interfere with the use of PSA cut-offs for diagnostic purposes. Also, there is actually some evidence that statins do in fact decrease the risk of PC [28,86,87].

- While PSA on average increases with age, across age groups men with greater Body Mass Index (BMI, weight in kg divided by the square of the height in meters—also 704 times the weight in pounds divided by the square of height in inches) have significantly lower total PSA. Obesity (generally BMI > 30) appears to affect the level of PSA mainly in the range of less than 4. This is relevant to the use of adjusted cut-offs and may also impact diagnostic accuracy [88]. Age *and* BMI adjusted tables have been suggested.

The information provided above should be of value to men prior to getting a PSA test and as well, men should be aware of other reasons aside from prostate cancer that might account for an elevated PSA. Most physicians will of course consider these various factors, but men should be informed simply on general principles. Also, an artificially reduced value could mask the presence of cancer, and it is important that men inform urologists if they are taking 5-α-reductase inhibitors such as Proscar, Avodart, or Propecia or statin drugs. The statin effect was reported only recently (2005), and many physicians, especially internists and GPs, may be unaware of it, especially if they do not religiously read the *Journal of Urology*!

THE PROSTATE BIOPSY

The ultrasound guided hollow needle biopsy is the so-called *gold standard* for the diagnosis of PC. In the US, according to 2002 cancer statistics, about 1,300,000 prostate biopsies were performed annually and detected 189,000 new cases of PC (15%) [89]. However, if the gold were "24 carat" for a single biopsy, it would never be necessary to repeat the procedure to "find" a suspected tumor or tumors. Unfortunately, this is not the case. The reason is that the procedure may miss the tumor or tumors because either they are small or in a part of the prostate that is not biopsied. Consider a small blueberry muffin containing only one or two or even a few blueberries and imagine trying to see if there are any at all with a few random thrusts of a hollow needle. However, once a biopsy has revealed the characteristic cells associated with PC, the diagnosis takes on a fairly high level of certainty. In fact, the nature, distribution and quantity of cells recovered that are suggestive or indicative of cancer are the basis of a scoring system, although the resultant scores are frequently changed if a pathological study of the removed prostate is carried out. This is always done after an RP but those who elect radiation therapy do not have the opportunity for this definitive check on the information provided by their biopsy.

The importance of a correct diagnosis, including a correct assessment of the significance or seriousness of the disease if present, cannot be understated. The diagnosis of prostate cancer judged significant will most certainly lead to a discussion of treatment, and the common treatments for localized cancers all have side effects that may profoundly alter an individual's quality of life. To have a radical prostatectomy or radiation therapy when in fact there is only insignificant or indolent cancer present is obviously something to avoid, although there are no doubt some who would debate this point. Likewise, to have a false negative diagnosis when an aggressive cancer is present is also highly undesirable unless the individual has a very short life expectancy attributable to comorbidities or rejects treatment altogether. Thus the imperfections inherent in the standard diagnostic method are disturbing.

The prostate is relatively inaccessible and to acquire tissue samples requires an invasive procedure. Since sampling needles are used, the two most direct routes are through the wall of the rectum or through the perineum, which is the area between the anus and the scrotum. Almost all biopsies employ the former approach. The first reported needle biopsy occurred in 1930 and the first transrectal procedure was reported in 1937. The procedure was revolutionized in the mid 1980s with the advent of both a transrectal ultrasound device of adequate imaging resolution and its combination with a needle device which allowed the operator to direct needles under ultrasound guidance into the targeted sections of the prostate. Shortly thereafter a spring-loaded core biopsy device (a so-called gun) was developed that operated in conjunction with the ultrasound probe. Continued improvements in the resolution of the ultrasound and the design of the needle gun have resulted in the present day instruments which provide both a satisfactory level of visualization coupled with the ability to direct the biopsy needle into a variety of regions of interest. The procedure can be done in an urologist's office or an ultrasound facility, generally requires less than an hour, and is generally accompanied by minimal or at worst tolerable pain, especially if local anesthetic used. However, a small minority of men reports severe pain.

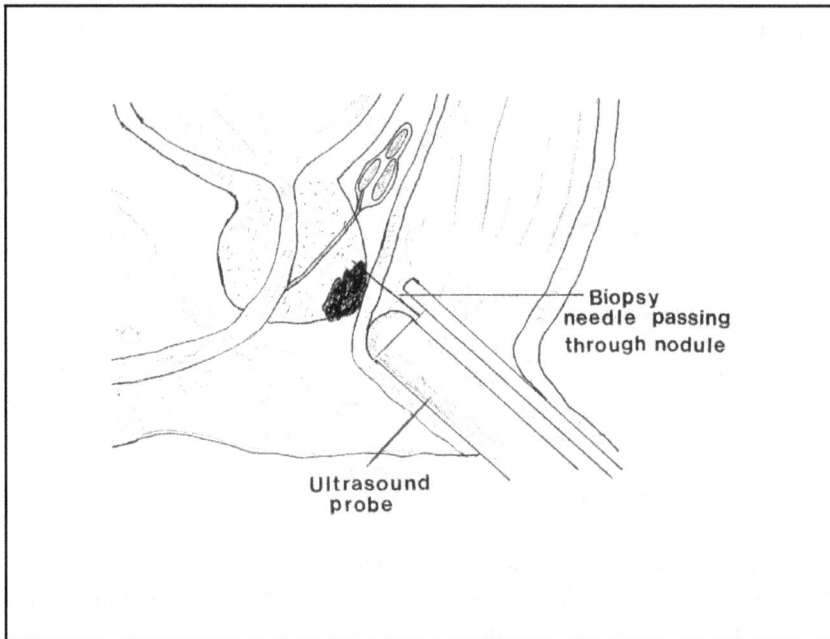

Figure 4-2. Ultrasound Guided Needle Biopsy

Some tumors can be imaged by the ultrasound device used in biopsy, and this can prompt targeting these areas for sampling. However, many tumors, especially early ones, are effectively invisible on the current grey-scale ultrasound [90]. Thus using ultrasound alone is not a solution to the diagnostic problem. While the ability to visualize and study the prostate gland has increased greatly with modern transrectal ultrasound, this has not resulted in substantially improved cancer detection without biopsy confirmation [90].

Since a biopsy is at present the *only* means of PC diagnosis, it is difficult to test its false negative rate since there is no "standard" for comparison. One can obviously not recruit a group of men who agree to radical prostatectomies after a negative biopsy to see if PC was missed! The solution to this dilemma is repeating the biopsy in cases where there is a high risk or a suspicious DRE, since repeating such an invasive procedure can be justified on medical grounds, and if enough biopsies are done, it turns out that a limiting and reasonably accurate estimate is achieved regarding the presence or absence of cancer. Men should be aware that repeat biopsies following a negative result in patients with high risk or suspicious DRE represent normal practice. The repeat procedures are done six to twelve weeks apart in order that the trauma associated with the previous test has resolved.

BIOPSY TECHNIQUE AND THE OPTIMUM NUMBER OF CORES

Men undergoing a prostate biopsy need some knowledge of the technique and the number of cores required in order to understand the rationale for various aspects of the procedure they are about to undergo. As well, they need to be aware of the potential for false negative results and that occasionally the repeat of a positive biopsy comes up negative. When ultrasound guided biopsies became routine, they initially involved taking six samples in the peripheral zone, the so-called sextant biopsy. In a sense this was a random biopsy since no attempt was made to target selected spots. It soon became apparent that the sextant procedure missed a significant number of cancers, the percentage frequently quoted being around 25%. Thus protocols that used a single sextant biopsy to determine the presence or absence of cancer in, for example, studies of the success of screening with PSA, were in fact using a rather imperfect diagnostic tool. That is, in general more subjects below a given PSA cut-off had PC than the biopsy data indicated. Also a single sextant biopsy, when used to define a "cancer free" population for the purposes of a study, in fact left open the possibility of serious misclassification. The situation is even more serious in subjects with large prostates where even a higher percentage of cancers are missed with the sextant protocol. As will be discussed below, acquiring more cores and targeting specific areas has now become much more common, although many studies that still influence practice were based on the sextant biopsy.

A recently study reported in 2005 provides an example of the problem of missed tumors. Djavan *et al* [91] studied 1051 men with risk defined by a PSA between 4 and 10 and compared the results of multiple biopsies with those obtained at the initial biopsy. A random sextant set plus two additional transition zone samples were used in all the biopsies. The first biopsy revealed an incidence of 22% PC. A second biopsy on those who were negative found 10% had PC giving an overall incidence for the two procedures of 30%. The third biopsy on the remaining "negatives" found 5% PC for an overall incidence of 33.3%. The fourth biopsy increased the incidence to only about 34% overall. If one assumes that the fourth biopsy found most of the remaining cancer, the first biopsy missed 123 out of 354 total cancers found, or about 35%. However, two biopsies found about 90% of cancer cases. A subset of patients had an RP. Organ-confined disease was present in 58% of cancer found in the first biopsy, 60.9% in the second, 86.3% in the third and 100% in the fourth. As might have been expected, cancers detected in the fourth biopsy had lower grade, stage and tumor volume as compared to those found in the first or second biopsy, i.e. the smaller the tumor or tumors, the harder they are to find. The third and fourth biopsies were accompanied by slightly higher level of morbidity than the first two. Thus an initial so-called extended biopsy protocol involving 8 cores still had a false negative rate of approximately 35%. The authors recommend that the three or four biopsies be reserved for very selected patients with high suspicion of cancer.

In a large serial biopsy study (2526 subjects), Roehl *et al* [92] found cancer detection rates of 29%, 17%, 14%, 11% 9% and 7% for one to six procedures. In this study the number of cores was variable but frequently the sextant scheme was used. In agreement with Djavan *et al* [91], there was a trend toward more organ confined cancers detected in subsequent biopsies as compared to the initial biopsy. Nearly 25% of the cancers ultimately detected were missed in the initial biopsy. Viewed another way, 77% of cancers were detected on first biopsy, 91% after two, 97% after three and 99% after four. This is similar to the results found by Djavan *et al* as discussed above.

Both of these studies indicate the need for improving the first biopsy. Ochiai *et al* [93] have recently reviewed the current status of this problem. This review of the recent literature makes it clear that both altering and increasing the regions sampled and increasing the number of cores from 6 to 10 or 12 significantly increases the rate of cancer detection on first biopsy. This improvement is in part due to directing sampling to regions of the prostate with high probability of harboring tumors. For example, Presti *et al* [94] found that a more judicious use of even the sextant protocol yielded an 83% detection rate as compared to 78% with the random standard sextant approach, while a 10-core scheme which included high probability regions yielded 97% detection. The reference standard in this study was the 12-core biopsy which was not validated with repeat biopsies. Thus the number of missed cancers, while probably small, was in fact unknown, as it was also in the technique comparison studies reviewed by Ochiai. It in fact appears that the optimum number of cores and the core location strategy remains unknown if the ultimate concern is how many cancers were missed. Studies that compare two or more protocols employed during a single biopsy are relatively easy to accomplish since the protocols are combined in a single procedure, but to test several different protocols where three or four identical repeat biopsies are used to approximate the cancers missed in each protocol represents a much more complex study, both to organize and implement.

In what is called a saturation biopsy, a large number of cores, even over 40, are taken! General anesthetic is generally required and the procedure is frequently accompanied by higher morbidity than observed in normal biopsy procedures. Scardino recommends against this protocol [2]. However, when the goal is to predict insignificant cancer as part of a program of an active surveillance program, Epstein *et al* [18] in a study reported in 2005 found an improvement using saturation techniques over the conventional 12 needle biopsy. They compared an extended 12 core (sextant plus 6 more cores) with 22 and 44 cores, and examined prostates removed during RP. With both the 22 and 44 core biopsies, around an 11% false negative rate was observed (based on significant cancer being present when insignificant cancer was predicted by the protocol being used for watchful waiting). This means that in an active surveillance program, about 90% of the group comprising candidates for active surveillance selected with saturation biopsy as part of the protocol would indeed have insignificant tumors. They would benefit from watchful waiting with active monitoring and temporarily or perhaps even permanently avoid treatment. This topic is discussed in detail in Chapter 6.

Current practice involves taking more cores than in the traditional sextant protocol, typically, 8, 10, 12 or 13. In addition, when a negative first biopsy is obtained with a patient judged at high risk because of a suspicious DRE, a very high PSA, or a family history of PC, one or more additional biopsies are generally recommended. After three or four negative results, the probability is cancer being present is low, typically less than 5%, but still finite and, unless the specific biopsy protocol has been studied locally with repeat biopsies, it is unknown. Coming back to the individual who wants to know for sure whether he has cancer, it appears from what is currently known that not only is a biopsy required, but one would not be enough unless a highly reproducible protocol was used that had been validated locally by repeat biopsies to establish the false negative rate and the initial biopsy was found to give a very low rate. One 12-core protocol yielding 2.3% false negatives on first biopsy has been reported, but the group studied was very small [70]. Thus journal articles can be misleading when a high detection rate is quoted for a particular protocol. For example, Philip *et al* [95] report that their 10-core biopsy technique found 98.6% of cancers in the group studied, but this was based on the reference standard of the number found with a 12 core protocol, not on repeat biopsies until there was a negligible increase in the discovery rate. It is also now fairly clear that men with large prostates require a larger number of cores to achieve the same detection rate as a man with a small prostate [93]. This further complicates studies of the false negative rate of biopsies. Knowledge regarding prostate size should be available to the patient after the first biopsy, and when it is large, the patient should recognize the increased possibility of a false negative and perhaps discuss this with the urologist.

The ultrasound guided needle biopsy can also be used to investigate such questions as whether or not the cancer has spread to the surrounding tissue. Information from such targeted sampling can be of great help in assessing the probable extent of the cancer. Thus a positive biopsy can sometimes prompt a repeat biopsy, the object being to obtain more information about the tumor or the presence of cancer in adjacent areas accessible with the transrectal biopsy. Such information may impact treatment decisions.

BIOPSY PAIN

The pain associated with the biopsy procedure arises mainly from the prostate itself rather than from the needle puncture of the wall of the rectum. In the past it has been generally considered that pain was not an issue. However, discomfort associated with the procedure is indeed experienced with 60-80% of men reporting mild to moderate pain and 6% of patients judging the pain so uncomfortable that they considered general anesthetic indicated [96]. In unusual cases, the pain may be so severe as to limit the number of cores that can be taken [97]. The current practice of taking up to 12 cores aggravates the problem [96]. Several approaches can be used to minimize this pain. One involves "conscious sedation" such as is used in colonoscopy or with surgery done under local anesthetic. Complications from sedation are extremely rare. With sedation, one is semi-awake, feels little pain, and generally does not recall the details of the procedure [41].

Another approach involves a local anesthetic gel (lidocaine gel) used to lubricate the ultrasonic probe, while a more direct approach involves injecting (infiltrating) lidocaine directly into the vicinity of the nerves leading into the prostate, a procedure done under ultrasound guidance. This latter technique is reminiscent of the dental nerve block used for work on the lower jaw. Studies that have either compared the use of lidocaine gel with infiltration or simply evaluated the infiltration method in a randomized fashion find the infiltration protocol superior to the gel and very effective in pain reduction [96-99]. However, lidocaine, even when used as a nerve block, is effective only for a few hours, and patients frequently report rebound pain by the evening of the biopsy. This can be relieved by the use of a long-lasting anti-inflammatory (diclofenac) administered via a suppository about an hour prior to the procedure [100]. The lidocaine nerve block became popular after the study of Soloway and Obek was published in 2000 [101].

If pain can be controlled, what else is there to worry about in connection with having a prostate biopsy? Two things come to mind. The first one is dealing with positive results which require a decision regarding treatment or some form of watchful waiting, a process than can be stressful. Also a positive result may induce psychological stress, perhaps severe, associated simply with the knowledge that cancer is present. Some patients successfully prepare ahead of time for the possibility of bad news, as part of the decision making process for having the biopsy. The second area of concern involves the potential for complications associated with the needle biopsy. The incidence of biopsy related complications have received considerable study. Complications include blood in the urine and semen (hematuria and hematospermia), prostate or urinary infection, a serious or even life-threatening systemic infection, an acute urinary retention episode, temporary erectile dysfunction, and finally rectal bleeding, which if severe can require immediate intervention including surgery. Also, moderate to severe so-called vasovagal responses can occur with drops in systolic blood pressure requiring intravenous fluid administration and in severe cases can be accompanied by neurological events such as seizure or loss of consciousness. The complications of the prostate biopsy merit further discussion.

BIOPSY COMPLICATIONS

Since the rectum is not sterile there is risk of the needle puncture carrying intestinal bacterial into the prostate with the resultant possibility of infection. To guard against this eventuality, it is now standard practice to prescribe antibiotics both before and after the procedure, with the fluoroquinolones class the most popular (e.g. ciprofloxacin, levofloxacin or ofloxacin). However, even with antibiotic prophylaxis, there is still a small risk of post-biopsy infection. In rare instances the fluoroquinolone class of antibiotic can cause very serious and even life-altering side effects [102]. See also Chapter 1.

It is difficult to quote meaningful combined statistics from studies of complications due to a variation in definitions, the failure to distinguish early from delayed morbidity, mild from severe complications and the lack of stratification with regard to antibiotic use. Reviews of large numbers of studies produce huge ranges in percent incidence. For example, Ghani et al [103] give the following ranges: hospitalization 0-4%, hematuria 12.5-80%, hematospermia 1.3-58%, and urinary retention, 0.2-10%. It is perhaps more meaningful to look at a study where early and delayed as well as mild vs. severe complications were distinguished. Djavan et al [104] examined the complication rate associated with 1051 initial biopsies which were all done with fluoroquinolone antibiotic prophylaxis preoperatively and for 4 days thereafter. For early morbidity, between 97.2 and 98.2% of patients had no or mild complications. For moderate to severe early complications, they found rectal bleeding 2.1%, hematuria 62%, vasovagal episodes 2.8%, and urinary retention 1.8%. Delayed morbidity results are given in Table 4-3.

Table 4-3. Incidence of delayed complications after prostate biopsy

COMPLICATION	INCIDENCE
Urinary tract infections	10.9%
Fever	2.9%
Urinary tract infections with fever	2.1%
Urinary retention	0.9%
Hematospermia	9.8%
Recurrent mild hematuria	15.9%
Persistent dysuria (difficulty or pain during urination)	7.2%

The authors also present a review of eleven studies. In all but two cases antibiotic prophylaxis was used. The range of incidence was smaller than reported by Ghani et al [103] but still rather large.

Rectal bleeding can be serious. Scardino [2] gives a rate of 1 in 1000 patients that required hospitalization for transfusion, cauterization or sutures to resolve biopsy induced severe rectal bleeding. He also quotes a rate of about 3% for urinary tract infections or prostatitis if antibiotic prophylaxis is used, with 6-10% otherwise. He makes a very strong point as does Walsh [41] that patients must be very vigilant after a biopsy for symptoms of complications that can quickly become severe. The warning signs are a fever of 101°F (38.3° C) or higher, chills, muscle aches, or urinary problems such as abnormal frequency, urgency or burning. In his opinion, immediate action is indicated, at an emergency room if necessary, in order that the infection apparently present can be cultured and treated. Patients should inform the ER staff or attending physician of the recent transrectal biopsy. Failure to take immediate action (even a 6-12 hour delay is serious) can result in some cases in an overwhelming septic condition with attendant long hospitalization, serious health risks and even death. Scardino gives a risk of 1 in 200 of this scenario. Because of the risk of delayed infection or bleeding, Scardino suggests avoiding long air trips or travel to remote areas where immediate medical attention is unavailable until the risk of these complications has subsided.

Biopsy candidates who have previously undergone total joint replacements are at increased risk of hematogenous prosthetic joint infections. The American Academy of Orthopedic Surgeons (AAOS) and the American Urological Association (AUA) have issued a joint advisory statement regarding this potential problem (http://aaos.org/wordhtml/papers/advistmt/1023.htm). Those at increased risk include all patients during the first two years after joint replacement, patients immuno-compromised or immuno-suppressed, and patients with previous prosthetic joint infections, malnourishment, hemophilia, HIV infections, diabetes and malignancy. Patients corresponding to one or more of these criteria should inform their urologist of the situation prior to a biopsy. The AAOS/AUA recommendations include a special antibiotic prophylaxis regimen.

It is important to realize that most of the complications of the transrectal ultrasound guided biopsy are mild and short lived. The use of anesthetic, especially the prostatic nerve block, should reduce the procedural pain to a minimum, and while severe complications are unpleasant to contemplate and of finite but low probability, it is hard to see that they should be a deterrent to having a medically justified biopsy. However, as has been discussed at length above, what is medically justified is sometimes far from clear, subject to debate and an essential feature of the screening controversy.

THE GLEASON SCORE

The biopsy generates a set of tissue samples (cores) approximately 0.4 mm in diameter and 15 mm in length which are then examined by a pathologist who will look for cells indicative of PC and characterize the type and extent in each core. The number of cores yielding positive results is reported and in most studies is correlated with the risk of non-organ confined disease. Finally, a score, called the *Gleason Score* is calculated and forms part of the basis of clinical judgments as regards treatment and prognosis. While this is the now a widely accepted protocol for the analysis of biopsy cores, it turns out to be somewhat less than perfect in either identifying the seriousness of the cancer or the prognosis. It is, however, all that there is available aside from PSA levels and kinetics and DRE observations to guide the urologist down the path to treatment or watchful waiting unless the patient presents with symptoms of advanced disease or distant metastasis. Pathologists also grade the cancer with the Gleason system when it is found in tissue samples recovered during the TURP surgical procedure for BPH. Gleason Scores can also be calculated from an examination of the prostate after a RP.

The Gleason score is derived from low-power microscopic examination of cells on slides prepared from the core samples. Normal cells, also called *well differentiated*, are characterized by distinct clearly defined boarders and clear centers. Johns Hopkins pathologist Jonathan Epstein describes them as "little round doughnuts" [41]. As differentiation is lost, cell borders become irregular, cells appear to clump together, and highly irregular shapes become more and more common until at the highest grade, the cells have little or no resemblance to normal cells. Gleason divided this transition from normal to poorly differentiated into five patterns which generate the numbers one to five used in the pattern grading system.

Gleason dealt with the problem of more than one malignant pattern in a biopsy sample by having the pathologist characterize what is termed a primary or dominant and a secondary pattern, the latter representing at least 5% of the cancer. The dominant and secondary patterns are graded according to the Gleason 1-5 system, and then the two grades added to give the Gleason Score, with the first number the primary grade and the second the secondary. Thus the score runs from 2 to 10. When there is no secondary pattern, the primary pattern score is simply doubled. Some doctors will give the patient just the sum, whereas the individual numbers are also of interest. A description of each core provides the best information.

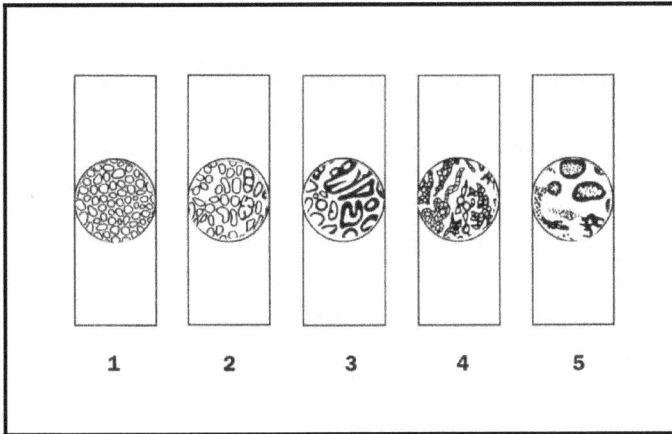

Figure 4-3. Gleason Scores

A Gleason score of 6 could be 4+2 with the predominant finding being poorly differentiated cells, whereas 2+4 indicates that the poorly differentiated cells were present in smaller amounts. Patients with high Gleason scores (7-10) are more likely to have cancer that has penetrated the prostate wall to the point where it perhaps can not be removed surgically, and as well have cancer that is more likely to have spread to the seminal vesicles or lymph nodes, and to other organs. Also, the presence of poorly differentiated cells which yield a high Gleason score suggests a cancer which is aggressive. Thus high Gleason score cancers may be less likely to respond to localized curative treatment such as RT or RP.

At the opposite end of the Gleason scale is the 2 to 4 score. According to Hopkins pathologist Jonathan Epstein [105], most 2-4 scores obtained from needle biopsy are graded 5-6 when reviewed by experts in prostate pathology. In a study at Johns Hopkins Hospital, it was found that their pathologists agreed as to the 2-4 scoring in only 4 of 87 reviews of slides graded initially at other institutions. Sixty-eight were regraded as 5-6, thirteen as 7, and two as 8-10. He also remarks that the few cases actually graded 2-4 at Hopkins showed higher-grade tumor at RP. Epstein points out that in a study involving 10 expert pathologists, no agreement was found on what a 2-4 score looked like in a slide review. This is a serious matter since a true grade of 2-4 from a needle biopsy suggests that there is no need for immediate definitive therapy where in fact, the real score is probably higher and may indicate the need for treatment. In a series of cases with Gleason scores of 2-4 from outside institutions who underwent RPs at Hopkins, 55% of the patients showed extraprostatic extension, including four cases with either lymph node or seminal vesicle invasion. Epstein quotes his experience with 2-4 grades at Hopkins [105]. He assigned a Gleason grade of 2-4 in only 1.1% of 2285 needle biopsies, whereas 24% of 83 pathological examinations of TURP tissue sent to Hopkins for consultation were given grades in this range. The low-grade cancers typically seen in TURP samples reflect the fact that cancers tend to be small when located anteriorly in the prostate within the TZ where tissue is removed during the TURP procedure.

Dr. Peter Scardino expands on the validity of the 2-4 grade in his recent book [2]. He points out that today many pathologists believe that Gleason patterns 1 and 2 may not be cancer at all, and thus it is rare to have a Gleason score of less than 6, i.e. 3 + 3. He suggests for anyone having a score of 5 or lower that a review of the slides by a pathologist considered an expert in prostate cancer is advisable. Another reason why it is wise to get a second opinion in any case is that pathologists in general differ in their interpretation of what they see through the microscope, and there is a variation in expertise as regards the Gleason grading system. He mentions three so-called referee centers where a second opinion can be obtained: the Armed Forcers Institute for Pathology, Memorial Sloan-Kettering, and Johns Hopkins, all of which have pathologists whose principal occupation is examining prostate tissue. If a man has a Gleason 2-4 result confirmed by expert review, he should raise the question of the merits of proceeding with treatment if recommended. The issue is confused by studies in the literature that include the 2-4 score in RP or RT series when in fact, the probability is high that an expert review of the slides would have upgraded these cases into a range where there would be less debate about treatment.

After Gleason score 6, a score of 7 is as the most common found with needle biopsy [106]. There are two ways to get this score, i.e. 3 + 4 or 4 + 3. In the former the lower grade Gleason pattern predominates, whereas in the latter it is the higher grade. Thus the patient should ask to see a breakdown of a score of 7. The score 4 + 3 is generally considered more ominous than 3 + 4, although the evidence is as yet not compelling [107]. Scardino points out that the real issue is the presence or absence of poorly differentiated cancer (patterns 4 and 5), and if so, how much, since poorly differentiated cancer should, in his opinion, be treated promptly [2].

Both the Gleason scores of 2-4 and 8-10 are relatively rare in current needle biopsies. The former have an incidence of about 2%, the latter about 8% [41,107]. *Authentic* scores of 2-4 are generally considered harmless, but as discussed above, they may actually be of higher grade. Many experts feel that scores of 2-4 should not be reported. Grade 5-6 tumors are considered slow-growing, whereas 7 are considerably more dangerous and 8-10 very dangerous. Scores of 7 or greater are more likely to involve extra capsular extensions, seminal vesicle involvement, and lymph node infiltration. The higher the score, the poorer the expected outcome of treatment and the greater the risk of metastasis [107]. But the score is rarely used in isolation, but rather combined in the calculation of prognostic factors using the number of cores containing cancer and how much, tumor stage (see below) and PSA at the time of biopsy. Examples are given below.

An obvious question relates to the correlation in general between the Gleason score derived from needle biopsy and the corresponding score found upon pathological examination of the prostate itself after a RP is performed. Sved *et al* [108] investigated this question for men with a biopsy score of 6. Out of 451 patients, 41% had a score of 7 or greater when the prostate itself was examined, whereas 8% had a lower score and 51% retained the same score. Those who were undergraded at biopsy were more likely to have extraprostatic extension, seminal vesicle invasion and recurrence post-RP.

Lattouf and Saad [109] also found significant undergrading in a study of 390 patients with biopsies who went on to have a RP. Undergrading was found in 38.2%, and overgrading in 32.6%. The discrepancies were somewhat smaller when the patients were grouped into categories (Gleason score 2-4, 5-6, 7 and 8-10) with 48.5% of the patients remaining in the same group after pathologic grading. There was also an improvement when only a subset was considered where a single pathologist examined both the biopsy cores and the RP pathology. Nevertheless, it is clear that the Gleason score is only an approximation to the true state of affairs, if it is assumed that the histological examination of the sectioned prostate is really a gold standard. Perhaps this is not surprising considering that the tissue collected in the needle biopsy represents only 0.04% of the average prostate volume.

A recent study from Johns Hopkins [110] also addresses the matter of upgrading and downgrading when clinical and pathological (post-RP) Gleason scores are compared. The study involved a group of men with Gleason score of 7 and divided them into four groups: (A) biopsy 3 + 4, RP $\leq$ 3+4; (B) biopsy 3 + 4, RP $\geq$ 4 + 3; (C) biopsy, 4 + 3, RP $\leq$ 3 + 4; (D) biopsy 4 + 3, RP $\geq$ 4 + 3. Group B represented 24% of the A and B groups, i.e. 24% upgrade, whereas group C represented 47% of the C and D groups, i.e. 47% downgrade when the Gleason scores was derived from pathological samples. There was a significant and rather dramatic difference in PSA detected RP failure between the four groups, with those ending up in the $\leq$ 3 + 4 post-RP groups faring much better. The 10 year likelihood of survival recurrence free post RP based on PSA was about 85% for Group A and 45% for Group D. This study underlines the uncertainties in the Gleason Score, especially one of 7, when based on clinical biopsy results, and as well suggests that the prognosis of pathological 3 + 4 differs significantly from 4 + 3. In this study nearly half of all patients with a clinical 4 + 3 score were downgraded after RP. The authors point out that the lack of agreement may in part be due to sampling errors since the needle biopsy samples only a small fraction of prostate tissue whereas the pathological Gleason score involves the type and degree of cancer found throughout the gland. Obviously there is need for improvement in the clinical assessment of the nature of the cancer present, and the Gleason score as currently determined is not an entirely satisfactory guide to prognosis or even as a guide in deciding among treatment options.

Finally, there is a problem with both intra-observer and inter-observer variability. For the former, studies find only 43-78% exact agreement on blinded reexamination of slides, whereas the disagreement between observers of plus or minus one score unit has been reported to range from 72-87% [107]. To say the least, some men may find these numbers and the downgrading and upgrading numbers given above to be a bit disconcerting! Perhaps more confidence is placed in the Gleason numbers than is actually deserved. At the very least, men need to realize that when given their Gleason score after a biopsy, it may significantly fail to correspond to reality. It is not clear at this point what they can do about it, aside from seeking second and perhaps even third opinions. If additional opinions disagree, what does one do, calculate an average?

ATYPICAL RESULTS, INTRAEPITHELIAL PROSTATIC NEOPLASIA

Aside from the unfortunate fact that the initial biopsy may fail to detect a cancer present in the prostate, the results of the needle biopsy may not be clear-cut (i.e., benign or PC).

The report may come back with terms such as "inconclusive" or "atypical hyperplasia" or prostatic intraepithelial neoplasia (PIN). PIN is sub-classified as low- or high-grade. The low-grade is generally considered clinically insignificant. High-grade PIN (HGPIN) is thought to be an early stage in prostate carcinogenesis and is regarded as a premalignant lesion that has the potential of progressing to adenocarcinoma [111]. Thus HGPIN is viewed as an early warning sign. The incidence of a HGPIN diagnosis in needle biopsies averages 9% (range 4-16%). Thus somewhat over 100,000 new cases of HGPIN are diagnosed each year in the US. Low-grade PIN is sufficiently hard to distinguish form normal cells that Epstein, for example, suggests it not be included on pathology reports [112].

Studies of PC risk subsequent to or associated with the observation of HGPIN have produced widely variable results. When both PC and PIN are found at the initial biopsy, the classification is PC because for diagnostic purposes the presence of PIN becomes irrelevant. However, until recently the sextant biopsy was the standard protocol and missed approximately 20-25% of cancers in the initial biopsy. Finding HGPIN but not PC generally indicates one or more repeat (immediate) biopsies, and a number of large studies [113] found the repeat biopsy yielded 23 and 35% PC. This range is close enough to that for normally missed cancer in the sextant biopsy that the risk of PC being present in newly diagnosed cases of PIN was not clear. However, Lefkowitz *et al* [114] reported in 2001 that when HGPIN but no cancer was found in an initial 12-core biopsy, the cancer yield of a repeat 12-core biopsy within one year was only 2.3%. However, this result was inconsistent with that of Rosser *et al* [115] who also used an extended biopsy protocol. The reason is not clear. Nevertheless, in a subsequent study, Lefkowitz *et al* [116] used the observation that only 2.3% of patients undergoing repeat 12-core biopsy within 1 year had cancer as validating their particular 12-core protocol and they then examined the incidence of PC after three years in 31 men who had only HGPIN initially and no cancer as determined by this initial 12 core biopsy. They found 25.8 % had developed PC.

Scardino quotes [2] the statistic that 50% of men with high grade PIN will be found to have prostate cancer on a subsequent biopsy over a 5-year period, but it is not clear how effectively undiagnosed cancer at baseline was excluded. Only additional studies will resolve the important question of the real risk of progression of HGPIN to PC if one has HGPIN but no cancer present initially. HGPIN and cancer frequently coexist. For example, 85% of patients diagnosed with PC will also have areas of high grade PIN on examination of the prostate itself [2].

There is no consensus on when a repeat biopsy should be done when HGPIN is found, with some experts recommending six month, others recommending as soon as possible [112]. As regards atypical needle biopsy results in general, Epstein recommends a repeat biopsy within 3 months [112]

STAGING OF PROSTATE CANCER

There are two types of "stage" of prostate cancer, the *clinical* and the *pathological* stage. The first is an estimated stage based on what the physician believes the patient's cancer to represent, which in turn is based on the DRE and needle biopsy. It is to some extent an educated guess. The pathological stage is determined after surgery when reliable information is available regarding the extent, not only of the cancer within or outside the gland, but also whether or not it has spread to the lymph nodes, seminal vesicles or regions adjacent to the prostate. However, the lymph-node status is not investigated in all RPs and the decision to ignore the question is generally based on probabilities determined from tables or nomograms. In cases where advanced disease is suspected, the information available for the clinical staging can be enhanced by bone scans or knowledge of metastasis found in distant sites. Staging information can also be obtained when an operation is performed to examine the lymph nodes. Information gathered from the DRE is of necessity incomplete since only part of the prostate can be explored. Nevertheless, staging based just on the DRE and the biopsy is commonly done and is a very important guide with regard to treatment. It is however important to realize that all the information required may be unavailable when the cancer is not organ confined. The so-called TNM staging system is given in Table 4 (after Walsh [41]).

The TNM stage is central to therapy decisions [41]. T1 and T2 cancers are viewed as favorable for treatment with RP or RT with the intent to cure, whereas T4 cancers have traditionally been considered suitable only for systemic treatment, e.g. hormone therapy, as are the non-zero M and N stages, although the prognosis associated with positive lymph nodes and the merits of surgery in this case are debatable and changing with time [117]. T3 tumors are in the grey area. However, there is growing evidence that for clinically staged T3 tumors, RP offers a number of advantages over other forms of treatment [118,119]. This is discussed in Chapter 6.

As indicated in the table, individuals with a non-suspicious DRE and an elevated PSA who have a positive biopsy are staged as T1c. Approximately 25% of the radical prostatectomies performed for this stage disease reveal potentially insignificant tumors [57]. Epstein *et al* [57] and Walsh [41] provide guidance regarding the prediction of tumor significance in T1c grade disease (adapted from [41]).

Significant stage T1c cancer if *any one* of the following characteristics is present:
- Cancer found in three needle cores or is present in greater than half of any one needle core
- Gleason score ≥ 7
- PSA density > 0.1-0.15 ng/mL/cc (volume should be available from ultrasound directed biopsy)
- %fPSA $< 15\%$

T1c cancer *probably* insignificant if *all* of the following characteristics are present:

- Cancer found only in one or two needle cores and makes up less than half of each needle core.
- Gleason score ≤6
- PSA density < 0.1-0.15 ng/mL/cc
- %fPSA > 15%

Walsh states that the above guidelines are only about 75% predictive [41]. If one is in the low risk group, gambles with watchful waiting (more recently called expectant management—see Chapter 6) and suffers progression, the cancer *may* still have a high probability of being curable [41]. The challenge is acting before it is too late.

Table 4-4. The TNM staging system of 1997 for prostate tumors

---

T1a: Not palpable with DRE. Cancer found incidentally during TURP; 5% or less of removed tissue cancerous.
T1b: Not palpable with DRE. Cancer found incidentally during TURP; more than 5% of tissue cancerous.
T1c: Not palpable with DRE. Cancer found with needle biopsy prompted by elevated PSA. Most common stage presently.

T2a: Palpable with DRE. Involves one lobe.
T2b: Palpable with DRE. Involves both lobes.

In an earlier (1992) scheme still extensively used, the T2 stages are different:-

T2a: Palpable with DRE. Involves less than half of one lobe.
T2b: Palpable with DRE. Involves one lobe.
T2c: Palpable with DRE. Involves both lobes.

Thus T2c is equivalent to the 1997 T2b.

T3: Palpable with DRE and penetrates the wall of the prostate and/or involves seminal vesicles.
T4: Spread to adjacent muscles, bladder neck, external sphincter and/or rectum.
N: Lymph node status. NX – unknown, NO – none, N1 – metastasis to a single node <2 cm, N2 – metastasis to a single node, 2-5 cm or multiple nodes none >5 cm, N3 – metastasis to a node >5 cm.
M: Presence of distant metastasis. MX – unknown, MO – none, M1 – distant metastasis

---

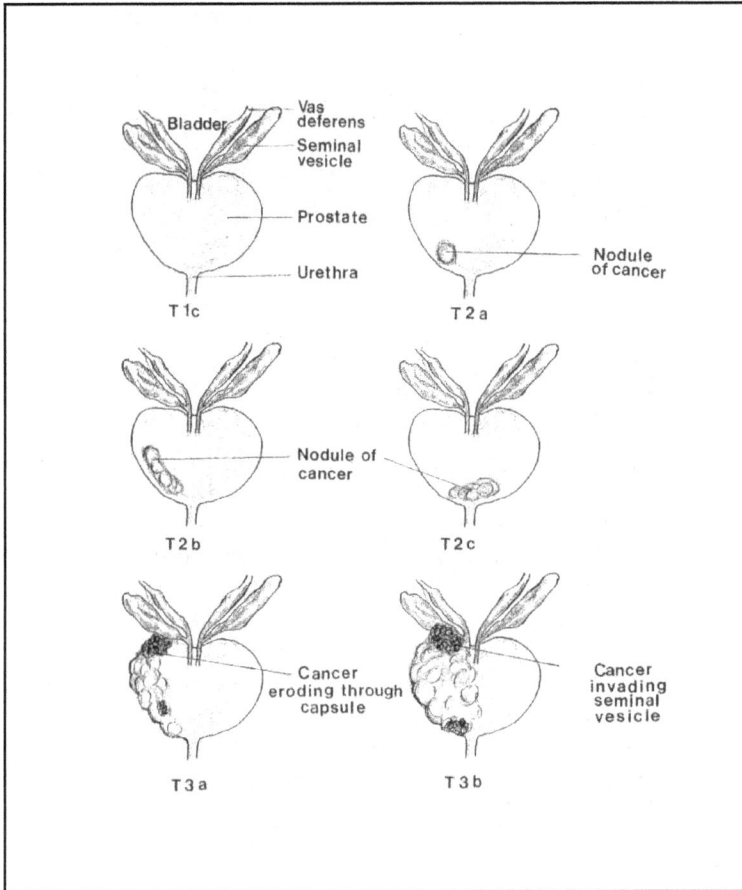

Figure 4-4. Staging of Prostate Cancer

DIAGNOSING ADVANCED PROSTATE CANCER

The needle biopsy can reveal spreading outside the gland, but only into areas accessible during the transrectal procedure. In particular, no information is obtained regarding lymph node or bone metastasis aside from the enhanced probability of advanced disease inferred from a high Gleason score. Pelvic lymph-node metastasis has significant adverse prognostic implications and it presence impacts treatment decisions. While modeling techniques such as nomograms (see below) or probability tables are used to estimate the chances of lymph-node metastasis, surgical removal followed by histological examination has been the only satisfactory way to obtain a dependable answer. Traditionally, one common protocol was for an examination of the question of lymph-node (LN) metastasis to be done at the start of the RP operation. If lymph-node involvement was found upon frozen section analysis, some surgeons would not proceed with the RP but simply close the incision. This approach is now less common, partly because it is evident that surgery can benefit some patients even if there is lymph-node metastasis [41,120]. Nevertheless, it is generally desirable to know the LN status. The performance of a lymphadenectomy to obtain lymph nodes for pathological examination as a stand alone procedure, as would be required if RT was the planned mode of treatment, is only justifiable if the results are going to significantly impact treatment. If hormone therapy is planned anyway as an adjunct to RT, knowledge of the LN status is unnecessary. The removal of the lymph nodes associated with the prostate at present appears to have no therapeutic value, but knowledge of the LN status is important in both judging prognosis and, in some cases, making treatment decisions. If a patient is of very low risk of LN metastasis, as determined from tables or nomograms, some surgeons will omit the removal of these nodes. A recent study [121] justifies this approach for low-risk patients, but the merits of omitting pelvic lymph node dissection have also recently been questioned by Weckermann *et al* [122] who suggest not dispensing with surgical LN staging even in apparently low-risk disease. Some surgeons routinely remove the easily accessible nodes, while some remove all the relevant ones in a so-called extended pelvic node dissection. There is no doubt that patients with LN metastasis are at high risk of not remaining progression free, and the more extensive the LN involvement, the poorer the prognosis [123].

Non-invasive procedures such as CT scans and traditional MRI would be attractive as procedures to acquire information on lymph node status, but at present both lack the sensitivity, especially for clinically occult disease where there has not been as yet an enlargement of the infiltrated nodes. In what appears to be a major diagnostic breakthrough, Harisinghani *et al* [124] have recently reported the results of a study using a special imaging agent which collects in lymph nodes but does not image areas where metastasis has occurred. MRI with superparamagnetic nanoparticles, as these special imaging agents are called, correctly identified all patients with nodal metastases, and had a significantly higher sensitivity than conventional MRI or nomograms. Only in the case of nodes measuring less than 5 mm was there a decrease in sensitivity. This approach has the advantage of being none-invasive, does not require hospitalization for surgery, and is free of side effects. The reference standard for the presence of metastasis was based on surgical lymph-node resection or a biopsy.

Metastasis frequently involves the spread of the cancer to bones, and thus if this is suspected, a bone scan may be offered or recommended prior to treatment decisions. There have been a number of studies that attempt to establish guidelines for when a bone scan is appropriate. The most recent appears to be that of Lee *et al* [125] from Columbia University. They studied 631 patients with bone scans for whom they had a Gleason score, PSA value and clinical staging. From this study they developed a guideline for identifying patients for whom a bone scan would have a low probability of being positive. The guidelines were a Gleason score of 2-7, a PSA of 50 or less, and a clinical stage of T2b or less. For patients with clinical stage $\leq$ T2b and Gleason score 2-7, and PSA $\leq$ 15, zero out of 237 patients had a positive bone scan. Raising the limit to PSA $\leq$ 50 resulted in 3 out of 545 patients with a positive bone scan. Positive bone scans were obtained in 49.5% of patients with PSA > 50. They recommend a bone scan in all patients not meeting the above criteria and especially those with a PSA > 50. The authors review the literature up to 1999-2000 and find similar but not identical results. The studies reviewed looked only at a PSA cut-off. Patients with a PSA of $\leq$ 10 always had negative bone scans, whereas $\leq$ 20 produced a small percentage of positive results. The guidelines presented by the authors are similar to that given by Scardino [2] where he states that a bone scan may provide useful information if the Gleason score is 8-10, PSA > 20 , and the clinical stage is T3 or greater. For those who do not meet these criteria, he suggests that the scan offers little value and has considerable potential to generate unnecessary problems due to false positives and possible recommendation of a bone biopsy, which itself is not necessarily conclusive. These results also provide some insight into the potentially serious indication of a PSA > 20 and certainly for one >50.

CRUNCHING THE NUMBERS EVALUATING THE PRE-TREATMENT PICTURE

At the time of diagnosis the patient usually has a PSA value, a Gleason Score, and a stage based on the TNM system. In the last few years considerable effort has gone into developing mathematical models that allow predictions based on these clinical diagnostic results [126-130]. These models are based on pathological and medical outcomes from large databases, but to some extent contain institutional bias (the institutions specializing in PC may get the best treatment results). The results are presented in the form of tables (Partin Tables, http://urology.jhu.edu) or so-called nomograms (a diagram where numerical "points" can be assigned to the various predictive factors and then summed to yield a total which is used to predict outcome). The pencil and paper analysis using nomograms or tables can now be avoided by using the Internet based nomogram from the Memorial Sloan Kettering Cancer Center (http://www.mskcc.org/mskcc/html/10088.cfm), which does all the calculations. The patient inputs the PSA, Gleason score and tumor stage and the program calculates and displays the *probabilities* of organ confined disease, extra capsular penetration, seminal vesicle involvement, LN involvement, and the 5-year progression-free probability after RP or RT. This provides the patient with an easy to understand analysis of the *probable* significance of the set of parameters that characterize their diagnosis. The probabilities are based on databases that use clinical rather than pathological (post surgical) input. Nomograms such as these are used by some surgeons to decide if looking for LN metastasis can be omitted during surgery because the probability is very low.

As an example of the application of nomograms, the online Memorial Sloan Kettering calculator will be used to examine various outcomes for just exceeding the two commonly suggested PSA thresholds for biopsy, 2.5 and 4.0. In this example, it will be assumed that the cancer stage is T1c, the most common situation today (T2a and T2b are next in incidence [42]). The Gleason scores used were from 3 + 3, 4 + 3 and 5 + 5. The results are given in the Table 5. The second, third and fourth items stratify the non-organ confined disease. Note that on the basis of the databases used to construct this model, Stage T1c and a "low" PSA did not completely rule out non-organ confined disease. The low biochemical failure rate (high % progression free) for these two typical screening scenarios for a Gleason score of 6, a common score with screened patients, is consistent with the view that early detection is highly curative. This table also illustrates that the lower cut-off for triggering a biopsy had a negligible influence on 5-year disease-free outcome as compared to the traditional cut-off. This was one of the principal arguments presented by H. Ballentine Carter from Johns Hopkins in an editorial discussing lowering the cut-off [47]. In fact, in a 1999 study by Carter *et al* [43] it was found that the probability of curable cancer was only slightly different within the range of PSA values from 2.5 to 6.0 for men with clinical T1c cancer. Increasing the PSA to 4.5 for a Gleason score of 6 does not change the figures in the Table 5. From these results it would appear that, for example, a PSA of 4.5 is not a crisis situation. In fact it can be argued that there is merit in repeated measurements at this point to determine the PSA velocity. It is even possible that the value would come back down below 4.0. However, recovery from PSA spiking above a cut-off does not rule out PC [131].

Table 4-5. Sample results from the Memorial Sloan-Kettering Cancer Center online calculator

	PSA = 2.6 ng/mL			PSA = 4.1 ng/mL		
Gleason score	6	7	8-10	6	7	8-10
Organ confined disease (%)	78	63	52	67	49	37
Extra-capsular Penetration (%)	21	31	34	30	40	40
Seminal Vesicle Involvement (%)	1	4	9	2	8	15
Lymph Node Involvement (%)	<1	1	4	1	3	8
5-year % Progression Free (After A Radical Prostatectomy)	93	86	86	92	85	84
5-year % Progression Free (After Radiation Therapy @ 76 Gy)	97	96	95	95	94	92

GENERAL CONCLUSIONS

It should be clear from the information presented in this chapter that diagnosing prostate cancer in asymptomatic men is not a simple matter of doing one or more tests and then saying, yes you do or no you don't have cancer. All that a man can expect is a probability statement, and if he is told the truth, that is given a reasonable accurate number, he may not be very happy or satisfied with the answer. There is a difference, from the point of view of the patient, of between being told that "you probably do not have cancer" and being told that "the probability is one in four that you do have cancer." One in four odds would bother some men. If one wants to eliminate the possibility of having cancer such that the probability of being wrong is less than 10 percent, then as discussed at length in this chapter, it is probably necessary to have at least two biopsies or one so-called saturation biopsy, a solution that is not very appealing to the asymptomatic man simply wanting an answer to what he may have viewed as a simple question. A very low PSA might suffice since as Thompson *et al* found (see above), only about 7% of men with PSA ≤ 0.5 had cancer based on a single biopsy, but then there is the problem of age adjustment.

Definitive testing for prostate cancer becomes an issue, which in fact is downplayed, in studies where it is desired to start with a cohort that is prostate cancer free. It is also an issue when a man is considering testosterone or DHEA replacement therapy or taking growth hormone or its amino acid precursors. These have become rather popular actions in the context of so-called anti-aging therapy. The universally given advice is not to become involved in such interventions if prostate cancer is present or suspected. In fact this cannot be implemented since to be certain of the answer with a high level of confidence, one or more biopsies must be carried out, something that seems a bit extreme in order to decide about taking a supplement. The point is that the general male public, while embracing the PSA test in huge numbers to "see if they have cancer," do not appreciate that in terms of sensitivity and specificity the test does not get very high marks. This is in fact at the root of the great screening controversy and debate regarding PSA. Yet to go beyond this simple test with more sophisticated blood tests, many of which are still being developed, or the biopsy, would involve costs that many would not wish to bear personally and which insurance plans or public financed health care would probably not in general support in the case of asymptomatic men. And presumably, the biopsy would never be considered for screening.

One of the characteristic features of prostate cancer is the uncertainty surrounding practically every important aspect. Screening is a probability game. Both the total PSA test and the modern variations have significant false positive and false negative rates. What is now quite clear is that *while PSA testing can indicate the risk of PC, it cannot be used to rule out the presence of the disease.* Intra-individual PSA variations from day to day and year to year are significant and confuse the issue of decision making with regard to biopsy advice. A number of conditions unrelated to prostate cancer can artificially change PSA levels. Drugs used to treat BPH (5α-reductase inhibitors) and perhaps elevated cholesterol (statins) significantly lower PSA levels, and the accuracy of corrections required before applying diagnostic benchmarks is not well established. As discussed above, there is an indication that the correction for long-term use of finasteride requires a factor larger than 2, the commonly used number. The use of "one-size fits all" correction factors may in retrospect turn out to be unsatisfactory and adjustments for duration of use may simply add more uncertainty to the result. Other drugs that influence PSA levels may turn up any time. To look for them is far from simple since the interaction can develop slowly over time. The transrectal ultrasound guided needle biopsy only *approaches* 100% diagnostic accuracy when biopsies, if negative, are repeated several times. Pathologists reading needle biopsy generated slides when establishing Gleason scores exhibit alarming intra- and inter-observer variations. The DRE is notorious for false positives and false negatives. Imaging techniques still fail to provide definitive diagnosis in most cases. These are all complex issues. It is not for lack of research that these uncertainties exist. At present, nothing better appears available and accepted for general clinical use. A vast amount of careful and thoughtful research has brought us to this point. Clearly there are great challenges ahead. Knowledge of this rather unsatisfactory state of affairs is no doubt limited among the general public unless they have made a considerable effort at self-education.

It will be recalled that avoiding so-called unnecessary biopsies was an important endpoint in a number of studies discussed above, but that while other types of PSA test (i.e. percent free or density) appeared to decrease the frequency of these benign biopsies, the improvement was somewhat marginal at about 20%. Even with the low long-term morbidity associated with the modern biopsy and the availability of effective pain control both during the procedure and for the period after, it is understandable that merit is attached to avoiding this procedure if it is unnecessary. However, it would seem more to the point to concentrate on identifying, with the highest level of certainty possible, individuals who have insignificant tumors. As discussed, there is interest and progress in this area, but characterizing insignificant tumors appears to require *both* biopsy and PSA data. Thus in the sequence of events where PSA exceeds a threshold and a biopsy is done, in general the result will be either no cancer or cancer (or in some cases, no decision) and the composition of the cores examined and various pre-biopsy PSA parameters are both needed in defining the nature of the cancer if found. If criteria can then be applied to differentiate those needing only surveillance from those needing treatment, it would seem that such a protocol successfully addresses the matter of overdiagnosis and overtreatment by restricting treatment to those who would most benefit. This puts the biopsy in a somewhat different perspective and may make it more acceptable to some men. In other words, avoiding unnecessary treatment may be a more important goal than avoiding unnecessary biopsies. It also highlights the necessity of overcoming a serious problem with biopsies, the false negative result. Thus the current interest in a first biopsy procedure that will have a very low percentage of false negatives, as well as in developing protocols that successfully differentiate those who need treatment from those who do not [18,132].

It is clear that PSA screening has revolutionized, albeit indirectly, the diagnosis of PC. Strictly speaking, however, it is not PSA per se that is yielding PC diagnosis, but rather PSA acts as a trigger for diagnosis by biopsy. The disease is being identified and treated at a much earlier stage than was possible before the PSA era. The PSA test, imperfect as it is, offers the *only* approach to early diagnosis in general and routine use today. PSA screening is gaining popularity worldwide and is well established in the practices of urologists, internists and general practitioners, the majority of whom have also had the test. The problems and uncertainties are clearly not compelling enough to discourage this widespread use.

This chapter is concerned mainly with two issues. The first involves the PSA test—what does one need to know to decide whether or not to have the test or if modern variations in the PSA test, especially the %fPSA, and the PSA density, should also be requested if not offered. The second principal issue concerns the basic knowledge deemed desirable prior to agreeing to proceed with the biopsy phase of diagnosis.

The pros and cons of getting the PSA test are those elaborated above in connection with the screening debate. To these must be added age, life expectancy, race and family history (see also Chapter 3). It is not possible to resolve this debate since it depends not so much on disputing the facts as how each argument is weighted. The arguments of those opposed to screening are to some extent weakened by the studies which suggest that the %fPSA and the PSAV enhance the specificity of the tPSA test. There is still no escaping the fact that all three tests have their grey areas. At the extremes the indication of high or low risk has a fairly high probability of being correct, and this supports either feeling good about the low risk of having PC or being forced to consider the merits of a biopsy or even a bone scan if the risk is high. It is the grey area that causes the most anguish, and it unfortunately includes the majority of men. However, being in the grey area or at high risk also brings up the question of the merits of treatment vs. doing nothing (classical watchful-waiting—WW), since there is little point is getting a biopsy or even worrying about screening if the decision has been made to reject conventional treatments, at least until the cancer, if present, causes major problems requiring palliative treatment. Such a rejection might be motivated by what the individual views as unacceptable adverse effects associated with either the radical prostatectomy (RP) or radiation treatment (RT) coupled with what the individual perceives as only marginal benefits of treatment over doing nothing when it comes to prostate cancer specific mortality. As discussed above, such a rejection ignorers or rejects a considerable body of evidence supporting the advocates of screening which suggests a definite shift to favorable probabilities associated with having a PSA test and a DRE and, if indicated, receiving treatment.

A compromise between the extreme options of aggressive treatment such as RP or RT and classical WW followed if necessary by palliation calls for so-called active surveillance in selected low-risk patients until evidence for progression suggest it is now or never for treatment with the intent to cure. This protocol is currently under study [132] and offers an approach which may be attractive to some men. It requires PSA and DRE monitoring and biopsies. For men with diagnosed but possibly indolent cancers, such a compromise may be attractive. It will be a number of years before long-term survival data associated with this protocol are available. This interesting option and the current evidence in its favor are discussed in detail in Chapter 6. It is doubtful if very many men are even aware of this option, the evidence in its favor, or the fact that is being studied and offered at least two major PC centers.

The discussion of the prostate biopsy in this chapter makes it clear that a single biopsy is by no means a gold standard for the presence or absence of PC. Quite the contrary, it misses a substantial percentage of cancers. Men should be aware that once an individual has agreed to a biopsy, one or more repeats may be suggested for good reason. Also men should be aware that the "classical" sextant biopsy is in general inferior to the so-called extended biopsies which utilize more needles, some directed to higher probability zones, with 12 or 13 needles now being common. While the biopsy is far from perfect as a method for finding tissue exhibiting the characteristics of cancer, with all due respect neither are the pathologists who read the slides, and men should be aware of the advisability in some cases of a second opinion, preferably from someone with no potential conflict of interest (e.g. avoid having slides reviewed by an office or department associate). Also, if one elects to have a biopsy, there appears no reason to hesitate in asking for local anesthetic and in particular the nerve block, especially if the extended protocol is used. Being aware of the potential complications associated with the transrectal needle biopsy, their signs and symptoms, and what action is indicated is extremely important. Serious complications associated with the needle biopsy are rare but some can develop very rapidly and can be life-threatening. Also, one probably should not have a biopsy unless the decision has been made beforehand as to what the next step will be if the result is positive. However, some men who have no intention of being treated may still want to know in detail the nature of what they have decided not to treat, just for future reference or in case they change their mind.

Finally, one of the cornerstones of the pro-screening position is that prostate cancer detected early with PSA is likely to be organ-confined and amenable to successful treatment with intent to cure. The results obtained with both RP and RT seem to support the likelihood of a favorable outcome if the Gleason score is 6 or less and even those opposed to screening do not appear to have confronted the alternative of returning the pre-PSA era where most of the cancer diagnosed was already advanced.

Chapter 5

Prevention of Prostate Cancer

Hans R. Larsen MSc ChE

INTRODUCTION

Despite impressive advances in medical, surgical and radiation technology, the treatment of prostate cancer is, by no means, a simple matter and the potential side effects can be devastating. Radical prostatectomy (RP) is the "gold standard" of treatment and involves removal of the entire prostate gland and seminal vesicles. It is usually quite effective as long as the cancer is contained within the prostate, but of little value if it is not. Among the more common side effects are impotence, incontinence, leaking of urine during sexual intercourse, shrinking of the penis, dry orgasms, and, no doubt, other less publicized effects[1]. It is estimated that about 8% of men undergoing RP become permanently incontinent and 42% have problems with sexual functioning[2]. Radiation therapy is used when RP is not desirable. It also has serious potential side effects including fecal and urinary incontinence and an impotence rate exceeding 60%[2]. Androgen deprivation therapy basically amounts to chemical castration and thus carries with it its own set of problems. For more on success rates and side effects of conventional treatments see Chapter 6.

If ever there was a place for the old adage "an ounce of prevention is worth a pound of cure", it certainly applies to prostate cancer. Fortunately, because prostate cancer, in the vast majority of cases, is very slow-growing there is usually time to take preventive measures before resorting to drastic ones.

The need for prevention cannot be overstated and the earlier it is begun the better. Nearly half of all men in their sixties have a latent (dormant) form of prostate cancer, and for men in their seventies the prevalence rises to 70%. Even 25% of men in their thirties have latent prostate cancer[3]. The goal of prevention is to ensure that any latent cancer remains dormant for the life of the individual man, that the initiation of new cancer is prevented, and that progression of cancer to a full-blown, detectable tumor is halted or, at least, delayed for a long time, preferably a life-time. The first and foremost step in any prevention plan is clearly to avoid known risk factors as outlined in Chapter 3.

Apart from risk avoidance, there are four major approaches to prostate cancer prevention:

- Prevention with pharmaceutical drugs
- Prevention with diet and lifestyle changes
- Prevention with vitamins and minerals
- Prevention with botanical medicines

PREVENTION WITH PHARMACEUTICAL DRUGS

FINASTERIDE

Androgens (male sex hormones) are believed to fuel the growth of both BPH and androgen-dependent prostate cancer. There is evidence that dihydrotestosterone (DHT) rather than testosterone itself is the major culprit in this regard. DHT is formed by conversion of testosterone through the action of the enzyme 5-alpha-reductase. Drugs and herbs that inhibit 5-alpha-reductase have been found effective in the treatment of BPH and it is therefore not surprising that the 5-alpha-reductase inhibitor finasteride (PROSCAR) has been evaluated for its possible role in the prevention of prostate cancer.

In 1998 researchers at the University of California presented a study which showed that finasteride does not reduce the risk of prostate cancer in high-risk men, but may in fact increase it. The study involved 52 men with PSA (prostate-specific antigen) levels over 4.0 nanogram/ml and negative biopsies for prostate cancer. The men were randomized to receive either 5 mg/day of finasteride (27 patients) or no medication (25 patients) for a 12-month period. At the end of the trial period prostate biopsies were again performed. Eight patients (30%) of the men in the finasteride group were found to have developed prostate cancer (adenocarcinoma) as compared to one patient (4%) in the control group. The researchers conclude that their study "raises serious questions about the probable efficacy of finasteride in preventing prostate cancer".[1]

A more recent study involved 18,882 men 55 years of age or older with a PSA level of 3.0 ng/mL or less and a normal digital rectal examination (DRE). The men were assigned to receive either 5 mg/day of finasteride or a placebo for the 7-year duration of the trial. The men were examined annually and underwent biopsy if their DRE was abnormal or their PSA level exceeded 4.0 ng/mL. They also underwent biopsy at the end of the trial.

A total of 9,060 men were included in the final analysis. The number of cases of prostate cancer detected in the finasteride group was 803 or 18.4% (2.6% per year) as compared to 1147 cases or 24.4% (3.5% per year) in the placebo group. The cancers detected in the finasteride group were, however, more advanced than those detected in the placebo group. A Gleason score of 6 or less is usually associated with a less serious cancer that can be managed successfully with watchful waiting. A Gleason score of 7 or higher, on the other hand, indicates a more aggressive cancer demanding swift attention. Considering only cancers of grade 7 or higher, it is clear that the participants on finasteride fared worse than those on the placebo. Of the men diagnosed with cancer in the finasteride group, 74% had a Gleason score of 7 or higher as compared to only 44% in the placebo group.[2]

Several prominent cancer researchers have raised serious concerns about the study.[3-6] One important difference between the finasteride group and the placebo group was that significantly more biopsies were performed among men in the placebo group (56.5%) than among men in the finasteride group (48.4%) because of elevated PSA levels. As one researcher put it, "Fewer biopsies in the finasteride group resulted in fewer cancers detected."[5]   Dr. Peter Scardino points out that the cancer rates detected in the 7-year study (24.4% in placebo group and 18.4% in the finasteride group) are substantially higher than the estimated lifetime risk of 16.7% for a 50-year-old man.   This would indicate massive over-diagnosis and Dr. Scardino questions whether all the cancers really were clinically relevant.   He concludes, "On balance, finasteride does not seem to be an attractive agent for the chemoprevention of prostate cancer".   Dr. Scardino also recommends that men taking finasteride for BPH be carefully monitored for the development of cancer.[4]

Researchers at the University of Southern California state, "The routine use of finasteride for the chemoprevention of prostate cancer cannot be advocated and may be contraindicated".   They suggest that altering the testosterone/DHT ratio through the use of finasteride may result in more aggressive cancers fuelled by testosterone rather than by DHT.[6]

Side effects were common in both the finasteride and placebo groups with effects on sexual functioning being more common in the finasteride group and urinary problems being more common in the placebo group.[2]

Should finasteride be part of a program to reduce the risk of prostate cancer? In my opinion, no – there are too many unanswered questions remaining and there are equally effective and less dangerous alternative options for reducing prostate cancer risk.

DUTASTERIDE

The enzyme, 5-alpha-reductase, which converts testosterone to DHT comes in two types. Type 2 is the predominant form in normal prostate tissue and in tissue affected by BPH. However, there is some evidence that type 1 may be predominant in prostate cancer cell lines. Finasteride inhibits only type 2, while the drug dutasteride (Avodart) inhibits both types. Like finasteride, dutasteride is approved for the treatment of BPH and trials are underway to test it in prostate cancer prevention.

In a recent trial 46 men with stage T1 and T2 prostate cancer scheduled for radical prostatectomy were randomized to receive a placebo or 5 mg/day of dutasteride for 6 to 10 weeks prior to the surgery. Treatment with dutasteride resulted in a 97% decrease in DHT level in prostate tissue (accompanied by a 95% increase in intraprostatic testosterone concentration).   The treatment also caused a substantial increase in apoptosis (cell death) in cancerous tissue and a reduction in angiogenesis (creation of new blood vessels to supply the tumors). The authors of the study conclude that short-term treatment with dutasteride can result in the regression of some prostate cancers.[7] Other researchers have found that dutasteride therapy shrinks prostate tumors.[8]

In follow-up of these promising findings a large clinical trial (REDUCE or Reduction by Dutasteride of Prostate Cancer Events) has now been launched. The study will involve 8,000 men who will be randomized to receive placebo or 0.5 mg/day of dutasteride for 4 years. The men selected will be between 50 and 75 years old, have a PSA value between 2.5 and 10 ng/mL and must have had a negative biopsy within 6 months prior to enrollment. Repeat biopsies will be required after 2 and 4 years. The purpose of the study will be to determine the relative cancer rates in the treatment and placebo groups, and to evaluate the effect of dutasteride treatment on BPH, prostatitis and PSA levels (total and free). Side effects will also be carefully monitored.[9]

ASPIRIN AND NSAIDS

Canadian researchers observed an 18% relative decrease in the risk of prostate cancer among participants taking aspirin in an 8-year study involving 13,326 participants. At the end of the 8 years a total of 2221 (17%) had developed prostate cancer (2.1% per year). The researchers found that men who had taken 80 mg/day or more of aspirin for at least 8 years had an 18% lower incidence of prostate cancer than did men who had not taken aspirin. More recent aspirin users only had a risk reduction of 7% and one year after stopping the drug there was no discernable risk reduction. The researchers found no connection between the use of other nonsteroidal antiinflammatory drugs (NSAIDs) and the risk of prostate cancer.[10]

Spanish researchers investigated the use of aspirin, other NSAIDs, and acetaminophen (Tylenol, Paracetamol) on the incidence of prostate cancer among 12,000 men between the ages of 50 and 79 years. They found that men who took aspirin on a regular basis reduced their risk of prostate cancer by 30% after correcting for other known variables affecting the risk. The protective effect was independent of dose (75 mg/day to 300 mg/day). The researchers also noted that the regular use of acetaminophen for longer than a year was associated with a 35% risk reduction, while use for less than a year was associated with a slightly higher risk. The use of NSAIDs other than aspirin (diclofenac, ibuprofen, indomethacin, naproxen, piroxicam, etc) was associated with a 11% decreased risk if used for more than a year, but a 14% increased risk during the first year of use.[11]

Researchers at the Johns Hopkins School of Public Health found a trend (statistically non-significant) for aspirin and ibuprofen to be protective among 1244 men enrolled in the Baltimore Longitudinal Study of Aging. There was no association between PSA levels and aspirin usage.[12]

Researchers at the American Cancer Society examined the association between NSAID use and prostate cancer risk among 70,000 men enrolled in the Society's Cancer Prevention Study II Nutrition Cohort. The men were followed for almost 10 years during which time 4,853 cases of prostate cancer were diagnosed. The incidence was 1.01% a year for men who had never reported NSAID use and 0.85% a year for those who had used NSAIDs regularly for 5 or more years. They conclude that long-term, regular NSAID users have an 18% lower risk of prostate cancer after adjustment for the effect of known risk factors. Long-term aspirin users had a 15% reduced risk.[13]

The preponderance of evidence would thus indicate that long-term, regular use of aspirin, other NSAIDs, and acetaminophen is associated with a modest reduction in prostate cancer risk. However, weighing in against regular use of aspirin and other NSAIDs is the fact that these drugs have several serious side effects, chiefly, internal bleeding and hemorrhagic stroke.   Long-term acetaminophen use could also be problematical as it can cause liver problems, especially if combined with alcohol abuse.

NO-NSAIDS

There is substantial evidence that the cyclooxygenase (COX) pathway is involved in prostate cancer. Research has shown that the COX-2 enzyme is more prevalent in prostate cancer tissue than in normal tissue. There is also evidence that medications such as aspirin and selective COX-2 inhibitors (Vioxx and Celebrex) can reduce the risk of prostate cancer. Both aspirin and the COX-2 inhibitors do, unfortunately, have some bad side effects and Vioxx was recently withdrawn from the market because it was found to double the risk of heart attack.

French researchers have developed a new drug called NO-ASA. NO-ASA or nitric oxide donating aspirin (nitroxy-butyl-acetylsalicylate) combines the proven anti-inflammatory properties of aspirin with the anti-bleeding properties of nitric oxide. Nitric oxide (NO) helps the immune system destroy tumour cells, bacteria, viruses, and other invading micro-organisms and also plays a role in planned cell death (apoptosis). NO is widely distributed in the body and is found in especially high concentrations in prostate tissue.

Sarah Royle and colleagues at the University of Edinburgh have found that NO-ASA and its cousin, NO-ibuprofen, may have important roles in preventing and halting prostate cancer. Although human trials are no doubt a long way off initial results are promising. The researchers studied the effect of NO-ASA and NO-ibuprofen on hormone-sensitive and hormone-insensitive prostate cancer cell lines as well as on primary cultures of prostatic stroma (the cells forming the overall structure of the gland). They found that both NO-NSAIDs (NO-aspirin and NO-ibuprofen) were potent inhibitors of cell proliferation and strongly induced apoptosis (planned cell death) in all three cultures. The researchers conclude that these new drugs show great promise for prostate cancer prevention and treatment and may also prove useful in the treatment of BPH.[14]

STATIN DRUGS

Early cell culture experiments hinted at the possibility that statin drugs such as lovastatin (Mevacor), atorvastatin (Lipitor) and simvastatin (Zocor) might suppress the growth of breast and prostate cancer cells. However, in May 2002 Patricia Coogan and her team at the Boston University School of Medicine reported that female users of statin drugs experienced a slightly higher incidence of breast cancer (predominantly carcinoma *in situ*) than did non-users and that male users had a higher incidence of prostate cancer. The study involved over 1000 women and 1000 men with breast and prostate cancer and a similar number of controls.[15]

In June 2005, Mfon Cyrus-David and associates at Baylor College of Medicine reported that statin therapy significantly reduced PSA levels in a group of airline pilots being treated for high cholesterol levels over a 10-year period. The study involved 100 pilots of whom 15 had high cholesterol levels and received statin therapy, while the remaining 85 had normal levels and did not receive statins. The PSA level dropped from an average of 1.15 ng/mL to an average of 0.8 ng/mL in the statin group, while it rose from 1.41 ng/mL to 1.68 ng/mL in the untreated group. The researchers speculate that statin drugs may have a role in preventing prostate cancer, but call for larger trials to confirm this.[16]

The 10-year Scandinavian Simvastatin Survival Study observed no statistically significant differences in cancer incidence or cancer mortality between statin users and non-users in a population of heart disease patients.[17] Similarly, the General Practice Research Database study of about 20,000 statin users and non-users concluded that statin use was not associated with a significantly altered risk of cancer, including prostate cancer.[18]

In contrast, Dutch researchers reported in 2004 that statin use was associated with a 20% reduction in the risk of cancer (mainly renal cancer) when used for 4 years or more. The observed reduction in prostate cancer incidence was statistically non-significant.[19]

The most recently reported study on statin use versus prostate cancer risk was carried out by Jackilen Shannon and colleagues at the Oregon Health and Sciences University. The study involved 100 men with prostate cancer and 202 cancer-free controls. Thirty-six per cent of cancer cases had a record of statin use as compared to 49% among controls. The researchers conclude that statin use may reduce the risk of prostate cancer or, more specifically, the risk of aggressive prostate cancer (Gleason score equal to or above 7).[20]

As in so much research concerning prostate cancer, there is no clear-cut answer to the question, "Do statin drugs reduce the risk of prostate cancer?" Thus, taking statin drugs in the hope of reducing prostate cancer risk is probably premature at this point. However, if statin drugs are already "on the menu", then it is possible that prostate cancer prevention may be one of their more desirable side effects.

PREVENTION WITH DIET AND LIFESTYLE CHANGES

FRUITS AND VEGETABLES

Edward Giovannucci and his team at the Harvard Medical School have found that fructose protects against prostate cancer. Men who consumed more than 70 grams/day had half the risk of developing advanced prostate cancer than did men who consumed only 40 grams/day or less. The main sources of fructose in the study were fruits, carbonated beverages, and sweet bakery products. A high fruit intake as such was also found to be protective with men consuming five servings a day having a 37% lower risk of advanced prostate cancer than men who only consumed one serving a day or less.[1]

A major study carried out at the University of Massachusetts Medical School found that the consumption of members of the *Brassica* family of vegetables (kale, cauliflower, brussel sprouts, kohlrabi, and broccoli) was highly protective.[2]

British researchers have observed a protective effect of peas and baked beans. Men who consumed beans or peas more than once a week were found to have a 37% reduction in prostate cancer risk compared to those who ate these foods less often.[3]

Several other studies provide abundant evidence that a high intake of vegetables affords significant protection against prostate cancer. Researchers at the Fred Hutchinson Cancer Research Center have found that the intake of vegetables, but not fruits, is significantly associated with prostate cancer risk. Their study involved 628 men from the Seattle area between the ages of 40 and 64 years who had been diagnosed with prostate cancer between January 1 and December 31, 1996. An age-matched sample of 602 men without prostate cancer served as the control group. All participants were interviewed and completed a 99-item food frequency questionnaire which included 12 fruit items and 21 vegetable items. The participants were asked to estimate their intake of the foods (ranging from "never or less than once per month" to "2+ per day") over the 3-5 years preceding the date of diagnosis or date of interview (for controls). The intake of fruit did not significantly affect prostate cancer risk. However, men who consumed 28 or more servings of vegetables per week were found to have a 35 per cent lower risk than men who consumed fewer than 14 servings per week. When limiting the analysis to cruciferous vegetables only, the protective effect was found to be even more pronounced. Men who ate three or more servings of cruciferous vegetables (broccoli, cauliflower, brussel sprouts, cabbage) per week had a 41% lower risk of developing prostate cancer than did men who ate less than one serving a week.[4]

The Giovannucci team at Harvard Medical School have followed up on this study and found a more modest benefit of a high intake of cruciferous vegetables. They found that men under the age of 65 years who consumed these vegetables 5 or more times per week had a 19% reduced incidence of prostate cancer as compared to men who ate cruciferous vegetables once a week or less. They conclude that an increased consumption of cruciferous vegetables may be highly beneficial for younger men as it may prevent initiation of the cancer. However, cruciferous vegetable intake may be less beneficial among older men with advanced cancer.[5]

The main protective components in cruciferous vegetables are sulforaphane (SFN), an isothiocyanate and indole-3-carbinol (I3C). Researchers at the Mount Sinai Medical Center in New York have isolated SFN and found it to be highly effective in preventing both initiation and progression of prostate cancer in cell cultures.[6] Other researchers have found that SFN works by generating reactive oxygen species (free radicals) which induces apoptosis in cancer cells.[7]

James Brooks and colleagues at Stanford University have found that sulforaphane and an extract from broccoli sprouts both increase the production of phase 2 enzymes (potent cancer fighters) and the intracellular level of glutathione. They believe these findings help explain the observed inverse correlation between the consumption of cruciferous vegetables and prostate cancer risk.[8]

Researchers at the University of California have studied I3C and found it to be highly effective in controlling the growth of human prostate cancer cells.[9,10] Researchers at Wayne State University have also studied I3C extensively and conclude that it and its dimer (DIM) inhibit prostate cancer through the regulation of the cell cycle, cell proliferation, apoptosis, and cell-signal transduction. They suggest that I3C and DIM may be effective as anti-cancer agents in their own right and may also be useful in sensitizing cancer cells to chemotherapy.[11]

Both sulforaphane and indole-3-carbinol are now available in supplement form. However, it is likely that broccoli remains a superior source of these and other cancer-protective compounds.

Jed Fahey and his team at the Johns Hopkins University School of Medicine report that sprouted broccoli seeds may be much more effective than mature plants. The researchers sprouted pesticide-free commercial broccoli seeds. After three days of sprouting at 25° C the sprouts were harvested, boiled in water for three minutes and cooled, filtered, and freeze-dried to provide a dry powder. The powder was extracted with a solvent system designed to capture the glucosinolates which were then enzymatically converted to the active isothiocyanate form. The researchers measured the potency (Inducer Activity) of the extracts in terms of their ability to activate the body's cancer defense mechanism and found that broccoli sprouts had an Inducer Activity 10 to 100 times higher than the mature plants. They also tested the activity of other crucifer sprouts and found broccoli and cauliflower to be the most potent ones. Fresh, mature heads of broccoli were found to be, on the average, three times as active as frozen broccoli, but no difference was found between organically and commercially grown samples of fresh broccoli. The researchers finally tested the broccoli sprout extracts on laboratory rats with induced breast cancer. They found that rats who received as little as 100 mg of dried sprout extract in their 15-gram daily food intake had a significantly lower incidence of tumours and a much slower growth of the tumours they did have. The researchers note that 0.54 - 2.83% of sprout extract in the daily diet of the rats provided the same protection as 5 – 40% of mature broccoli. They are now evaluating the implications of their findings in the prevention and regression of human cancers.[12]

Researchers at the University of Ulster have found that a mixture of broccoli, radish, alfalfa and clover sprouts is highly effective in preventing peroxide-induced DNA damage involved in the initiation of cancer. They tested an extract (juice) of the sprouts on the HT29 colon cancer cell line. It was found that cells incubated with the juice were about 50% more resistant to DNA damage caused by exposure to hydrogen peroxide than were non-incubated cells. The researchers also tested the effect of the sprouts on 10 male and 10 female healthy volunteers. Half the volunteers were randomized to consume their usual diet as well as 113 grams/day of the sprouts for a 2-week period. The other half of the group consumed their regular diet. Blood samples were drawn from all participants at baseline and at the end of the 2-week period. Lymphocytes were isolated from the blood and checked for DNA damage before and after exposure to hydrogen peroxide. The researchers found that the DNA in lymphocytes from the sprout-eating group was substantially less likely to be damaged by peroxide at the end of the 2-week sprout consumption period than was DNA in lymphocytes taken at baseline or from the control group. The researchers conclude that young sprouts may be a potent source of cancer-protecting compounds.[13]

It is clear that broccoli sprouts are the most potent source of beneficial sulphoraphanes and other phase 2 detoxification enzymes. However, most people probably consume their cruciferous vegetables cooked. Steaming is by far the best way of preserving the essential nutrients of vegetables. A team of Spanish researchers have found that microwaving broccoli virtually eliminates its vital antioxidant nutrients. The researchers cooked broccoli in 4 different ways – steaming, pressure-cooking, boiling, and microwaving. They found that steaming preserved about 90% of the bioflavonoid antioxidant content, pressure-cooking preserved about 45% (the rest being lost in the water), boiling preserved about 35%, and microwaving only about 2%. In other words, 98% of perhaps the most important components of broccoli as far as health protection and cancer prevention are concerned were lost in microwaving. The same group of researchers has also found that broccoli heads lose 50-80% of their vital nutrient content between harvest and actual sale at the retail level.[14] Although the Spanish researchers did not specifically evaluate the sulphoraphane content of the broccoli after preparation, it is likely that light steaming would be the best way of preserving this compound as well.

A very recent study involving almost 1000 men (433 prostate cancer patients and 538 controls) from New York State confirmed that a high intake of vegetables (more than 500 grams a day) is associated with a 50% decrease in the risk of prostate cancer.[15]

Not all studies, however, have found that a high vegetable intake is protective. A 1994 study involving 20,000 Hawaiian men of various ethnic backgrounds found no association between vegetable intake and prostate cancer risk.[16] A 1998 study of 58,000 Dutch men also found no statistically significant effect of overall vegetable intake, although the researchers do suggest that a protective effect may be associated with certain specific vegetables.[17]

More recently a group of researchers at Oxford University in the UK reported on a very large nutritional study involving 130,544 men from 7 countries who were followed for 5 years. They found no association between prostate cancer risk and the intake of fruits, vegetables or cruciferous vegetables specifically.[18] It is possible that, at least, part of the reason for this finding is that the highest intakes of fruits (410 grams a day) and vegetables (242 grams a day) observed in the sample population are actually fairly low. As a matter of fact, the highest vegetable intake in the European study was lower than the lowest intake reported in the study of New York State men.[15] It is also possible that the glycemic load of the North American and European diets were quite different. A high glycemic load would be associated with increased insulin production and concomitant increase in IGF-1, a known promoter of prostate cancer. Thus, it would likely be desirable to emphasize low glycemic index fruits and vegetables in a prostate-healthy diet (see Appendix C).

Thus, overall, it would seem that a high intake of vegetables, especially cruciferous ones is associated with a reduced prostate cancer risk. A high intake of vegetables is also recommended as a protective measure against numerous other disease conditions including heart disease and most other cancers. Although sprouts seem to be particularly effective in cancer prevention, it is important to ensure that only organic, pesticide-free seeds are used in their preparation.

TOMATO PRODUCTS

In 1995 Edward Giovannucci and his Harvard team reported that frequent consumption of tomato sauce and tomatoes provides significant protection against the development of prostate cancer. Their study involved over 47,000 male health professionals 812 of whom developed prostate cancer in the period between 1986 and 1992. All participants in the study completed validated food-frequency questionnaires in 1986, 1988, 1990 and 1992. Analysis of the collected data clearly showed that men with a high consumption of tomato sauce, tomatoes, and pizza have a significantly lower risk of developing prostate cancer. The protective effect of tomato sauce (ripe tomatoes cooked in oil) was particularly noteworthy; men who consumed tomato sauce two to four times per week had a 35 per cent lower risk of developing prostate cancer than did men who never ate tomato sauce. The researchers believe that it is the high content of lycopene which gives tomato products their protective effect. They also speculate that oil or fat is necessary for proper absorption of the lycopene from the tomatoes. Tomato juice on its own has no protective effect and its lycopene is poorly absorbed. However, if tomato juice is cooked in oil and then ingested the blood level of lycopene rises very significantly within 24 hours. The researchers believe that lycopene protects against prostate cancer because it is a very powerful antioxidant, more than twice as effective as beta-carotene, and because it is the most abundant carotenoid in the prostate gland. No protective effect was found for vitamin A, beta-carotene, alpha-carotene, lutein or beta-cryptoxanthin. The researchers also found that a high intake of fruit and vegetables other than tomatoes had no significant protective effect.[1]

A follow-up on the original Harvard study confirmed the initial findings. By 1998 a total of 2481 men had developed prostate cancer. The researchers found that a high intake (2 or more servings a week) of tomato sauce was associated with a 23% reduction in the risk of prostate cancer when compared to an intake of less than one serving a month. A high intake of lycopene (19 mg a day) was associated with a cancer incidence of 0.42% a year, while an intake of only 3 mg a day was associated with an incidence of 0.51% a year – a 16% reduction in risk.[2]

A nested case-control study based on the data from the Male Health Professionals Study found that a high lycopene intake reduced prostate cancer risk by 34%. However, detailed examination of the data for the 450 prostate cancer patients involved revealed that the protective effect was limited to men with no family history of prostate cancer who were 65 years or older when the blood sample measuring serum lycopene was drawn. For these men, the reduction in risk was 57%.[3]

Greek researchers have confirmed that lycopene and other micronutrients may have age-dependent effects on prostate cancer risk. They investigated the effect of cooked tomatoes (lycopene), polyunsaturated fatty acids (PUFAs), and vitamin E in a sample of 320 prostate cancer patients and 246 controls. They found that a high PUFA intake increased risk among men under the age of 70 years, but had little effect among older men. Cooked tomatoes had a strong protective effect among older men, but no effect on men under 70 years of age. Conversely, vitamin E was found to be highly protective for younger men, but not for those over the age of 70 years.[4] The same group of researchers also observed a strong inverse correlation between the intake of cooked tomatoes and blood level of IGF-1, a known promoter of prostate cancer.[5]

Another Harvard study involved over 22,000 male American physicians aged 40 to 84 years at the start of the study in 1982. The original purpose of the study was to investigate the effects of beta-carotene supplementation (50 mg every other day). However, the availability of stored blood samples made it possible to investigate the effects of other carotenoids as well. By 1995, 578 men had developed prostate cancer. These were matched with 1294 cancer-free controls according to age and smoking status. Analysis of the blood levels of carotenoids and vitamin E showed that men with the highest lycopene levels and no beta-carotene supplementation had a 41% lower risk of prostate cancer than did men with the lowest levels. No risk reduction associated with lycopene levels was observed in physicians who received beta-carotene supplementation. However, beta-carotene in itself also appeared to be protective with men assigned to supplementation having a 37.3 per cent lower risk than men with low lycopene levels assigned to placebos. Men with high vitamin E (alpha-tocopherol) levels were found to have a lower incidence of aggressive prostate cancer. The researchers conclude that increased consumption of tomato products might reduce prostate cancer risk.[6]

A recent meta-analysis of 11 case-control studies and 10 cohort studies confirmed the protective effect of tomato products, but found a more modest association with men with the highest intake of cooked tomatoes having a 19% lower risk.[7]

Canadian researchers have provided an excellent overview of the role of lycopene in the human body. Lycopene is a powerful antioxidant with a singlet-oxygen quenching capacity 10 times greater than that of vitamin E. It is the most abundant carotenoid in human plasma and is highly concentrated in the adrenal glands, testes, prostate, and breast tissue. Several studies have found an inverse correlation between serum and tissue levels of lycopene and the risk of breast and prostate cancers. Other studies have linked a high intake of tomatoes to a 50% reduction in cancer mortality among elderly Americans. A recent study found that supplementation with a tomato extract significantly lowered the level of prostate-specific antigen (PSA) in patients with prostate cancer. High tissue (adipose) levels of lycopene have also been found to be protective against heart attacks. No published studies have shown any adverse effects of high lycopene levels or a high intake of tomato products. It has been hypothesized that lycopene prevents cancer and heart disease by protecting lipids, lipoproteins (especially low-density lipoprotein), proteins, and DNA. There is also evidence that lycopene counteracts the proliferation of cancer cells induced by insulin-like growth factors.[8]

There is evidence that lycopene and its metabolites increase direct gap junction communication between cells by increasing the level of connexion 43. Proper gap formation is important in the regulation of uncontrolled, rapid cell growth.[9]

Several studies have confirmed that an increased intake of processed tomato products results in a substantial increase in lycopene in both blood and prostate tissue and a commensurate decrease in blood levels of prostate specific antigen (PSA).[10,11]

Indian researchers recently reported that supplementation with 4 mg of lycopene twice a day for a year is highly effective in preventing high-grade prostate intraepithelial neoplasia (HGPIN) from developing into prostate cancer.[12]   However, American researchers have expressed concern about using lycopene to treat potentially advanced and metastatic prostate cancer. Cell culture experiments have shown that lycopene may actually accelerate these forms of prostate cancer.[13]

A small study carried out at the University of Illinois concluded that tomato sauce may suppress the progression of prostate cancer by increasing apoptosis (planned cell death).[14]

Christine Gartner and colleagues at the Heinrich Heine University in Germany have discovered that lycopene in tomato paste has a far greater bioavailability (absorption) than does lycopene in fresh tomatoes. Their experiment involved five healthy volunteers who consumed either 400 g fresh tomatoes or 40 g tomato paste together with 15 g corn oil and 100 g bread. The meals each contained 23 mg of lycopene (of which 46% was *all-trans*-lycopene). Five hours after the ingestion of the tomato meal the concentration of lycopene in the chylomicrons (microscopic fat particles) of the tomato paste group was 2.5 times higher than in the fresh tomato group. All told the tomato paste group absorbed almost four times more lycopene than did the fresh tomato group. Previous research has shown that the bioavailability of lycopene from tomato juice is extremely low.[15]

It is clear that the best sources of bioavailable lycopene are processed (cooked with oil) tomato products such as tomato paste, tomato sauce, and tomato-based spaghetti sauce. Raw tomatoes and tomato juice are not very good sources. German researchers have found that heating tomato juice converts *trans*-isomers of lycopene to the *cis*-isomers and that only the *cis*-isomers are absorbed.[16]

In addition to its protective effect against prostate cancer, lycopene may also be beneficial in the prevention of stroke and heart attack. Finnish researchers have discovered that middle-aged men with low blood serum levels of lycopene (less than 0.07 micromol/L) have a 3.3-fold greater risk of suffering a stroke or heart attack than do men with higher levels.[17]

German researchers have found that a low lycopene level is associated with a substantially increased risk of adenomatous polyps (adenomas) in the colon. Adenomas are believed to be precursors for colon cancer. They point out that low lycopene levels have been associated with an increased risk of lung and stomach cancers as well.[18]

Research has also shown that supplementation with synthetic beta-carotene reduces blood levels of lycopene – an effect not seen with beta-carotene from natural sources.[19,20] Since most multivitamin supplements contain synthetic beta-carotene, which suppresses lycopene absorption, it is quite possible that a significant proportion of the population is deficient in lycopene.

There is indeed overwhelming evidence that an adequate lycopene status is crucial to health. A daily intake of 15 mg is likely needed for ongoing protection against the development of prostate cancer, but double this (30 mg/day) is required to actually help reverse the cancer. Three-quarter cup of tomato sauce provides about 30 mg of lycopene.

Although most of the evidence concerning the benefits of lycopene has come from epidemiologic studies of tomato product consumption and small clinical trials involving tomato sauce, there is some evidence that properly formulated lycopene supplements may also be beneficial. The best-researched supplement is probably *Lyc-O-Mato* which is produced from a specially bred and cultivated lycopene-rich tomato variety developed in Israel. These tomatoes contain approximately three times more lycopene than do regular tomatoes. *Lyc-O-Mato*, in addition to concentrated *trans-* and *cis*-lycopene, also contains small amounts of other carotenoids (gamma-carotene, beta-carotene, phytofluene and phytoene) found in the special tomatoes. An early clinical trial carried out by the US Department of Agriculture found that lycopene supplementation (75 mg/day) increased the blood level of lycopene by about 40% after 4 weeks.[21]

A later trial by Israeli researchers found that supplementation with 30 mg/day of tomato lycopene oleoresin doubled serum lycopene concentration and also increased the concentration of lycopene in skin and adipose tissue (obtained during haemorrhoidectomy or peri-anal fistulotomy) by about 50%.[22]

Although tomato-based sauce or paste is probably still the safest bet when it comes to preventing or treating prostate cancer, it is unlikely that consuming relatively large amounts of tomato or spaghetti sauce every day will catch on in a big way. If consuming processed tomato products on a regular basis is not an option then certainly supplementation with a proven product like *Lyc-O-Mato* would seem to be an acceptable alternative.

FISH AND FISH OILS

There is convincing evidence that fish and fish oils can help prevent prostate and other cancers. There is also evidence that the ratio of omega-6 fatty acids (linoleic acid, arachidonic acid) to omega-3 fatty acids (linolenic acid and fish oils) has a marked influence on prostate health.

Researchers at the Korea Institute of Science and Technology have discovered that men with prostate cancer and benign prostatic hyperplasia (BPH) have markedly different ratios of omega-3 to omega-6 as compared to men with healthy prostates. Their study involved 24 men with BPH, 19 men with prostate cancer in various stages, and 21 age-matched men with normal prostates. All participants provided blood samples that were analyzed for a total of 21 different fatty acids. The researchers found no significant differences in the overall levels of saturated, monounsaturated, and polyunsaturated fatty acids. However, there was a very marked decline in the levels of EPA (eicosapentaenoic acid) and DHA (docosahexaenoic acid) from the normal men to the men with BPH to the men with prostate cancer. The serum ratios of omega-3 to omega-6 polyunsaturated acids were also quite different for the three groups ranging from 0.89

for normal subjects to 0.71 for men with BPH to 0.50 for men with prostate cancer. The men with prostate cancer also had significantly higher levels of omega-6 acids than did the normal men and the men with BPH. The researchers conclude that their work supports the contention that omega-6 polyunsaturated fatty acids have a tumor-promoting effect while omega-3 acids have a protective effect.[1]

Norrish, *et al.* in New Zealand provide convincing evidence that an increased consumption of fish oils helps reduce the risk of developing prostate cancer. Their study involved 317 men who had been diagnosed with prostate cancer during 1996-97 and 480 age-matched controls. Blood samples were obtained from all participants and the erythrocyte (red blood cell) phosphatidylcholine fraction of the plasma was analyzed for EPA (eicosapentaenoic acid) and DHA (docosahexaenoic acid), the two main components of fish oils. Evaluation of the collected data showed a clear correlation between blood level of EPA and DHA and the presence of prostate cancer. Study participants with levels in the highest quartile were found to have a 40 per cent lower incidence than participants with levels in the lowest quartile. This relationship held true even when adjusted for age, height, use of NSAIDs (non-steroidal anti-inflammatory drugs), socio-economic status, and estimated intake of lycopene and polyunsaturated fats. The researchers also found that men with low socio-economic status, a low intake of lycopene, and non-regular use of NSAIDs were more likely to develop prostate cancer. They speculate that fish oils may prevent the progression of prostate cancer by inhibiting the biosynthesis of eicosanoids from arachidonic acid.[2]

Swedish researchers studied 3136 pairs of male twins born between 1886 and 1925. The participants completed food frequency questionnaires in 1961 and 1967 and were then followed up for 30 years. By December 31, 1997 the researchers had recorded 466 diagnoses of prostate cancer (340 fatal ones). The average age of diagnosis was 76.7 years. After adjusting for other known risk factors the researchers conclude that men who never eat fish have a two- to three-fold higher risk of prostate cancer than do men who eat moderate to high amounts. The researchers emphasize that only fatty fish such as salmon, herring and mackerel, which contain high amounts of omega-3 fatty acids (EPA and DHA), would be expected to be beneficial.[3]

A team of researchers from the National Cancer Institute, the Harvard Medical School, the Harvard School of Public Health, and the Karolinska Institutet in Stockholm have found a protective effect against prostate cancer associated with a high intake of fish oils - eicosapentaenoic acid (EPA) and docosahexaenoic acid (DHA). The study involved 47,866 male American Health professionals who were followed over a 14-year period beginning in 1986. The participants completed detailed food frequency questionnaires in 1986, 1990 and 1994. By the year 2000, 2965 new cases of prostate cancer had been reported with 448 of these being advanced (metastasized) or fatal. The overall incidence of new prostate cancer detected over the 14-year period was 0.5% per year. Men with a daily intake of more than 0.214% of daily energy (about 470 mg/day) of EPA + DHA were 11% less likely to develop prostate cancer than were men with an intake less than 0.057% of energy (about 125 mg/day). The beneficial effect of EPA plus DHA was particularly pronounced in regard to the incidence of advanced prostate cancer. Fish oil supplements were slightly less effective than fish oils from fatty fish perhaps indicating that vitamin D and vitamin A may be necessary to obtain the maximum benefit.[4]

A high intake of fish or fish oils has many benefits besides a protective effect in regard to prostate cancer. An enormous amount of medical literature testifies to the fact that fish oils prevent and may help to ameliorate or reverse atherosclerosis, angina, heart attack, congestive heart failure, arrhythmias, stroke, and peripheral vascular disease. Fish oils help maintain the elasticity of artery walls, prevent blood clotting, reduce blood pressure, and stabilize heart rhythm.[5-12] Fish oil supplementation has also been found helpful in alleviating depression, Alzheimer's disease, ulcerative colitis, arthritis, and high blood pressure.[12-36]

There is now also evidence that fish oil consumption can delay or reduce tumor development in breast cancer. Studies have shown that a high blood level of omega-3 fatty acids combined with a low level of omega-6 acids reduces the risk of developing breast cancer. Daily supplementation with as little as 2.5 grams of fish oils has been found effective in preventing the progression from benign polyps to colon cancer and Korean researchers have reported that prostate cancer patients have low blood levels of omega-3 fatty acids.[1,2,37-40]

It is estimated that 85% or more of people in the Western world are deficient in omega-3 fatty acids and most get far too much of the omega-6 fatty acids. Vegetarian diets, for example, tend to be very high in omega-6. The recommended daily intake of EPA plus DHA is about 650 mg rising to 1000 mg/day during pregnancy and lactation. Clinical trials have used anywhere from 1 g/day to 10 g/day, but little additional benefit has been observed at levels above 5 g/day of EPA and DHA combined. The benefits of therapeutic supplementation may become evident in a few weeks when blood parameters (triglycerides, fibrinogen) are involved, but may take 3 months or longer to materialize in degenerative diseases like atherosclerosis and rheumatoid arthritis. [41,42]

The processing and packaging of the fish oil are crucial in determining its quality. Low quality oils may be quite unstable and contain significant amounts of mercury, pesticides, and undesirable oxidation products. High quality oils are highly purified through molecular distillation, are stabilized with adequate amounts of vitamin E, and are packaged in individual foil pouches or other packaging impervious to light and oxygen.

Supplementing with fish oils has been found to be entirely safe even for periods as long as 7 years and no significant adverse effects have been reported in hundreds of clinical trials using as much as 18 grams/day. Fish oil supplementation does, however, lower blood concentrations of vitamin E so it is a good idea to take extra vitamin E when adding fish oils to the diet. A clinical trial carried out by the US Department of Agriculture found that taking 200 mg/day of synthetic vitamin E (equivalent to about 100 IU of natural alpha-tocopherol) is sufficient to completely counteract this effect of fish oil supplementation. [41,44]

SOY PRODUCTS

Both the incidence and mortality associated with cancer are substantially lower in Asian countries than in western ones. The mortality from prostate cancer in Japan, for example, is 4 per 100,00 men as compared to 24 per 100,000 among white Americans and 55 per 100,000 among African Americans.[1,2] The incidence of the cancer in some parts of China is 1.9 per 100,000 as compared to 182 per 100,000 in the US for white men and 247 per 100,000 for African Americans.[1,3] It is likely that genetic, environmental and dietary factors are involved in the explanation of these differences. It has, for example, been observed that Asian men who move to the US eventually reach an incidence of prostate cancer somewhere between that observed in their homeland and that observed in the US.[1]

There seems to be fairly general agreement that isoflavones (phytoestrogens) abundant in soy products are, at least partly, behind the relative immunity against prostate cancer enjoyed by many Asian populations.[2,3] A small study found that isoflavonoid content in the blood of Japanese men (average age of 55 years) was 110 times higher than that found in Finnish men of the same age. The researchers doing the study (from the University of Helsinki and the Japanese National Cancer Research Institute) concluded that dietary isoflavonoids inhibit the growth of prostate cancer cells.[4] Other studies have determined that the average Asian diet contains 10 times the amount of soy products as does the typical American diet, and that the Asian intake of isoflavones is approximately 50 mg/day as compared to the average American intake of 2-3 mg/day.[5]

The main soy-based food products are tofu, miso, tempeh, tamari, soy milk, soy yogurt, soy cheese, and soy ice cream. Soybeans can also be sprouted and used in salads and oriental dishes. One-half cup of tofu contains 20 grams of protein, 11 grams of unsaturated essential fatty acids, and provides 183 calories.

Sonoda, *et al.* recently reported the results of a study aimed at determining the association between fish and soy consumption and prostate cancer risk. Their study involved 140 men with prostate cancer and 140 matched controls from various regions in Japan. Food frequency questionnaires were used to estimate the intake of fish and soy products 5 years prior to diagnosis. The researchers found that men with the highest intake of fish (more than 130 grams/day) had a 55% lower risk of prostate cancer than those with the lowest intake. Similarly with tofu and natto (a fermented soy product). High consumers of tofu (more than 187 grams/day) reduced their risk by 53% and high consumers of natto (40 grams/day) reduced their risk by 75%. Consumption of even moderate amounts of meat, however, was found to double prostate cancer risk. The researchers conclude that the traditional Japanese diet, which is rich in soybean products and fish, might be protective against prostate cancer.[6]

A small study of Seventh Day Adventists found that men who consumed soy milk regularly had a 70% lower incidence of prostate cancer than those who did not.[7]

Researchers at the Harvard Medical School have found that a combination of tea (green or black) and soy extract is highly effective in inhibiting progression of prostate cancer, shrinks tumours, prevents metastasis, and reduces serum levels of testosterone and dihydrotestosterone in laboratory mice. They conclude that, "further research is warranted to study the role of soy and tea combination as effective nutritional regimens in [human] prostate cancer prevention."[8]

Soy products have also been found to decrease hot flashes in menopausal women. Japanese women whose consumption of soy products amounted to about 115 grams/day had half the risk of experiencing hot flashes of moderate to severe intensity than did women with a median intake of 45 grams/day.[9] Nagata, *et al.* have also observed that regular soy consumption tends to reduce total cholesterol levels.[10]

Genistein and daidzein are the most abundant isoflavonoids (isoflavones) in soy products. Isoflavonoids, like other phytoestrogens, have weak estrogenic properties, but it is now believed that they exert their anti-cancer effects through their role as antioxidants and their ability to induce apoptosis and to inhibit tumor cell proliferation, angiogenesis (creation of new blood vessels to supply the tumor), and metastatic invasion.[2,5] Japanese researchers compared blood serum levels of genistein and daidzein for 40 prostate cancer patients and 101 controls and found that men with the highest levels of genistein had a 62% lower risk of prostate cancer, while men with the highest levels of daidzein had a 59% lower risk, and men with the highest levels of equol a 66% reduction in risk. They conclude that men with high serum levels of genistein, daidzein, and equol have a reduced risk of prostate cancer.[11]

American researchers have found that genistein inhibits the growth of both BPH, androgen-dependent, and androgen-independent prostate cancer tissue in histoculture and Austrian researchers have reported that genistein levels are reduced in prostatic tissue from men with prostate cancer and large-volume BPH.[12,13]

So, should soy products be consumed daily by both men and women? In moderation perhaps, but not in excessive quantities. Soy products are a rich source of phytic acid which is known to seriously inhibit the absorption of many important minerals such as calcium, magnesium, iron, copper, and zinc. Thus, mineral supplements should not be taken in conjunction with a soy-containing meal.

Ishizuki, *et al.* have observed that soybean consumption suppresses thyroid function and that elderly people may develop hypothyroidism (goiter) after consuming as little as 30 grams/day of soybeans for 3 months. They also noted that soybean consumption decreased body stores of inorganic iodine and resulted in an increase in the level of TSH (thyroid stimulating hormone). The hypothyroidism symptoms disappeared 1 month after stopping the trial.[14]

Researchers at the US National Center for Toxicological Research warn that soy products may cause harm in humans because of their estrogenic effects and their effects on the human thyroid gland. They point out that an iodine deficiency may potentiate soy's detrimental effect on the thyroid.[15]

The Honolulu Heart Program has been following the health of 8000 Japanese-American men since 1965. In the year 2000 the researchers involved in the program reported the startling finding that a high consumption of tofu (2 or more servings per week) in midlife was associated with poor cognitive test performance, brain atrophy, and heart (ventricle) enlargement in later life. The researchers also noted a higher incidence of stroke among the high tofu consumers.[16,17] Although these findings are preliminary and certainly need confirmation, they are nevertheless disturbing.

So, although there is substantial evidence that soy products can help prevent and retard prostate cancer, there is also evidence that an excessive soy consumption can have adverse effects. So what is excessive? There seems to be no clear-cut answer to this. The Ishizuki study found that 30 grams/day of soybeans increased the risk of goiter, particularly in elderly people.[14] The Nagata study on the effects of soy consumption on cholesterol levels found that soy intakes varied between 25 and 100 grams/day.[9] The study by Sonoda, *et al.* found that the maximum protection against prostate cancer was obtained with a daily intake of 40 grams or more of natto, or more than 187 grams/day of tofu.[6] It is likely that the maximum safe soy intake depends on the other components of the diet. If the diet is rich in seafood and seaweed then a higher intake would likely be tolerable.

In 2000 the American Heart Association concluded that, "it is prudent to recommend including soy protein foods in a diet low in saturated fat and cholesterol." Just recently (January 2006) the Association reversed this recommendation in new guidelines that conclude that isolated soy protein with isoflavones have little or no effect on cholesterol levels and is not effective in preventing breast and colon cancer. The guidelines emphasize that the negative stand on isolated soy protein and isoflavones does not include whole soy products such as tofu, soy butter, soy nuts, and soy burgers. Quite the contrary, natural whole soy products are believed to be beneficial both for cardiovascular and overall health.

In conclusion, a high daily intake of whole soy products has been found to reduce the risk of prostate cancer, but may introduce hypothyroidism, especially in older or iodine-deficient people. Soy products should not be consumed at the same time as a mineral supplement is taken since it will inhibit its absorption. In view of the synergy between soy products and tea, it may be desirable to settle on a low to moderate soy intake combined with 2 cups of green or black tea a day. In this way benefits would be realized, but adverse effects avoided.

GARLIC

British researchers studied the diets of 328 men with prostate cancer (diagnosed before age 75 years) and 328 age-matched controls. They found that men who consumed garlic at least twice a week had a 44% reduced risk of prostate cancer as compared to men who never consumed garlic. The estimate of reduced risk did not change when the use of supplements was factored in.[1] Other studies have noted a distinct association between garlic consumption (raw or cooked) and a reduced risk of stomach and colon cancer.[2]

Researchers at the National Cancer Institute in Bethesda, Maryland have reported that a high consumption of allium vegetables, garlic and scallions in particular, is associated with a reduced risk of prostate cancer. Their study, carried out in Shanghai, China, involved 238 patients with confirmed prostate cancer and 472 controls. Men with an intake of more than 10 grams/day of allium vegetables (garlic, scallions, onions, Chinese chives, and leeks) were found to have half the risk of prostate cancer compared to men with an intake of less than 2 grams/day. The protective effect was more pronounced in patients with localized disease than in patients with advanced disease. Garlic and scallions (green onions, *Allium cepa*) were found to be particularly protective. Men with a garlic intake above 2.14 grams/day (one clove) were found to have a 53% lower risk of prostate cancer than were men who did not consume any garlic. Men with a scallion intake above 2.14 grams/day were found to have a 70% lower risk of prostate cancer than did men who never consumed scallions. The risk reduction was particularly impressive for localized disease where it amounted to 83% (59% for advanced disease). A small scallion (about 3 inches in length) weighs about 5 grams, so consuming just one small scallion a day would, according to this study, provide very meaningful protection against prostate cancer. The Cancer Institute researchers are not entirely sure why allium vegetables are protective, but point out that they block metabolism of polycyclic hydrocarbons and nitrosamines, inhibit microbial activity, enhance immune function, suppress cell division and proliferation, modulate phase I and II enzymes and DNA repair, and induce apoptosis (planned cell death).[3]

Two Dutch studies examined the effect of garlic supplements on the risk of breast and lung cancer and found no protective effect.[2] However, a study carried out at the Memorial Sloan-Kettering Cancer Center and Cornell University reports that certain extracts from aged garlic is highly effective in halting the growth and proliferation of human prostate cancer cells *in vitro*. Human prostate cancer cells (LNCaP cells) were cultured for 24 hours and then exposed to a saline solution containing 50 ppm of either S-allylcysteine or S-allylmercaptocysteine. Both of these water-soluble garlic components are found in crushed garlic that has been aged for at least a year; they are not present in fresh garlic. The researchers incubated the cancer cells for an additional 1, 4, 6 and 8 days and then measured the number of active cells. They found that S-allylmercaptocysteine reduced the number of cancer cells by more than 50% after 6 and 8 days. Incubation was then continued for another 4 days after rinsing and removal of the S-allylmercaptocysteine. A new cell count showed that the inhibitory effect of S-allylmercaptocysteine continued even after its removal. S-allylcysteine also inhibited cancer cell growth, but to a much lesser extent than S-allylmercaptocysteine. Both compounds were also effective in regenerating the important antioxidant glutathione and in reducing the amount of certain proteins necessary for the proliferation of cancer cells. The researchers conclude that aged garlic components or derivatives may be useful in controlling the proliferation of prostate cancer cells.[4,5]

GREEN TEA

The interest in the cancer-preventive properties of green tea began 11 years ago when a team of American and Chinese researchers reported that green tea was highly effective in preventing the development of esophageal cancer. Their study involved about 1000 Shanghai residents who developed esophageal cancer between October 1990 and January 1993. The researchers concluded that women who drank green tea regularly had a 50% lower risk of developing esophageal cancer than did women who did not consume green tea. This risk estimate took into account the known cancer-promoting effects of cigarette smoking and alcohol consumption. When the scientists looked at the data for a subgroup of men and women who neither smoked nor drank alcohol they found that women who drank green tea reduced their risk of developing esophageal cancer by 60%; the corresponding reduction for men in this subgroup was 57%. The study also revealed that drinking burning-hot liquids increases the risk of developing esophageal cancer two- to four-fold. No added risk was found due to consumption of herbal teas at normal temperatures.[6]

In 2004 Chinese researchers reported on a case-control study involving 130 patients with confirmed prostate cancer and 274 age-matched healthy controls. After adjusting for age, education, income, body mass index, physical activity, alcohol consumption, tobacco smoking, total fat intake, marital status, age at marriage, number of children, history of vasectomy, and family history of prostate cancer, the researchers concluded that tea drinkers had a significantly lower risk of prostate cancer. About 80% of controls were regular tea drinkers as compared to only 55.4% among prostate cancer cases. The researchers found the prostate cancer risk declined with increasing frequency, duration and quantity of green tea consumption. Compared to non-tea drinkers, regular green tea consumers had a 72% lower (adjusted) risk of developing prostate cancer. Those drinking 3 cups or more per day had a 73% lower risk, those having consumed green tea regularly for 40 years or more reduced their risk by 88%, and the real heavy consumers, those consuming more than 1.5 kg of tea leaves yearly, reduced their risk by 91%. The researchers conclude that green tea may be protective against prostate cancer.[7]

More recently Italian researchers reported the results of a clinical trial involving 62 men between the ages of 45 and 75 years who were at high risk for developing prostate cancer because they had been diagnosed with high-grade PIN (precursor to prostate cancer). The men were randomized to receive either placebo or three 200-mg tablets a day of green tea catechins (50% of which were in the form of EGCG). Follow-up biopsies were performed after 6 months and again at 12 months after the start of the study. At the latest follow-up 9 men in the placebo group had been diagnosed with prostate cancer compared to only 1 man in the catechin-supplemented group. The study will continue for 5 years, but the researchers suggest that consideration should be given to using green tea catechins to prevent prostate cancer in groups at high risk, such as the elderly, African-Americans and those with a family history of prostate cancer.[8]

In 1998 researchers at the Mayo Clinic reported that epigallocatechin-3-gallate (EGCG) is the active component in green tea and that it kills human prostate cancer cells *in vitro*.[9]

Hussain, *et al.* at the University of Wisconsin point out that cyclooxygenase (COX)-2 has been implicated in prostate cancer development and that inhibiting COX-2 could serve as a promising target for prevention or therapy of cancer. In a recent study they showed that EGCG (the active component in green tea) inhibits COX-2 without affecting COX-1 at both the mRNA and protein levels in both androgen-sensitive and androgen-insensitive human prostate cancer cells. They conclude that, "it is tempting to suggest that a combination of EGCG with chemotherapeutic drugs could be an improved strategy for prevention and treatment of prostate cancer."[10] The Wisconsin group of researchers has also shown that green tea reduces the level of IGF-1 and increases the level of

IGFBP-3, the protein that binds IGF-1 and prevents it from initiating and promoting cancer.[11]

University of Chicago researchers have found that EGCG inhibits type 1 5-alpha-reductase, the enzyme responsible for the conversion of testosterone to the more powerful dihydrotestosterone (DHT)[12] and Japanese researchers report that ECGC also inhibits the formation of cancer-causing heterocyclic amines formed during grilling or barbecuing of foods.[13]

Although prostate specific antigen (PSA) is primarily known for its property as a marker for prostate cancer, it is also involved in actively promoting cancer progression through its effect on cell migration and metastasis and through degradation of type IV collagen. A team of Italian researchers reported that EGCG inhibits all the negative actions of PSA in a dose-dependent manner with even the ingestion of one cup of green tea having a significant effect. The researchers conclude that green tea (EGCG) may serve as a natural inhibitor of prostate cancer progression.[14]

British researchers recently reviewed the evidence supporting an association between green tea consumption and prostate cancer risk and concluded that, "Based on all the evidence, green tea clearly has a marked effect in reducing the development of prostate cancer."[15] Although, there is thus ample and growing evidence that green tea and ECGC help prevent prostate cancer, there is much less evidence that they are effective in treating existing cancer. As a matter of fact, one recent study found that green tea extract capsules had no effect on the progression of advanced (androgen-independent) prostate cancer.[16]

Drs. Siro Trevisanato and Young-In Kim of the University of Toronto have published a fascinating report detailing the history, biochemistry, and health benefits of tea. It is the richest source of flavonoid antioxidants in the northern European diet and contributes about 63% of all flavonoids in the diet. Tea drinkers have been found to have substantially lower risks of stroke (73% lower) and heart attack (44% lower) than non-tea drinkers. Tea has also been found to lower cholesterol and blood pressure. A Norwegian study found that men who drink one or more cups of tea every day have a 40% lower risk of dying from coronary heart disease than do men who drink less than one cup per day. An American study of 35,000 women found that women who drank two or more cups of tea a day had a 60% lower incidence of cancers involving the digestive tract (mouth, esophagus, stomach, pancreas, colon and rectum) and a 32% lower incidence of urinary tract cancers than did women who did not drink tea. A Canadian study found that men who drink two or more cups of tea a day reduce their risk of prostate cancer by 70% compared to non-tea drinkers.

Tea is safe; it contains only 25 to 34 mg of caffeine so one would need to drink 10-12 cups a day to approach the caffeine limit given in the Canada Food Guide. It inhibits the absorption of non-heme iron, but only if drunk with meals. Therefore vegetarians who get their iron from non-heme sources should refrain from drinking tea with their meals or should drink it with milk or lemon juice added. Tea leaves contain a relatively high level of aluminum and concern has arisen that a high consumption of tea may increase the risk of developing Alzheimer's disease. Fortunately, the aluminum in the leaves is not very soluble in hot water and there is no scientific evidence that heavy tea drinkers have higher blood levels of aluminum than do non-tea drinkers. The Canadian researchers conclude that tea has many health benefits, is pleasant to drink, and is entirely safe.[17]

Nevertheless, concern has recently been raised about the levels of pesticides contained in teas imported from certain Asian countries. To be safe, organic teas or teas from a reputable supplier should be sought out or, for those who cannot tolerate caffeine at all, a standardized ECGC extract in decaffeinated green tea may be a good option. ECGC/green tea capsules are available from reputable supplement suppliers such as the Life Extension Foundation.

FLAXSEED

Wendy Demark-Wahnefried, *et al.* at Duke University concluded that a low-fat diet (daily fat intake of less than 20% of total energy intake in kilocalories) supplemented with ground flaxseed (30 grams) is effective in reducing cholesterol levels, testosterone levels, and free androgen levels. Their clinical trial involved 25 prostate cancer patients scheduled for prostatectomy. After following the diet for an average of 34 days (21 to 77) the average total cholesterol level had dropped from 201 mg/dL to 174 mg/dL, the total testosterone level from 422 to 360 ng/dL, and the free androgen index from 36.3% to 29.3%. Among men with Gleason sums of 6 or less, the average PSA level decreased from 7.1 ng/dL to 6.4 ng/dL and the mean proliferation index declined to 5.0 from the 7.4 measured in historic controls. The researchers conclude that a flaxseed-supplemented, fat-restricted diet may favourably affect prostate cancer biology and associated biomarkers.[18]

More recently the same group of researchers investigated the effect of the flaxseed-supplemented, low-fat diet on prostate growth and PSA in 15 men who were scheduled for a repeat biopsy 6 months after having been diagnosed with high-grade PIN and/or atypical small glands. After the patients had followed the diet for 6 months, the researchers made the following observations. Average PSA level decreased significantly from 8.47 to 5.72 ng/mL and total cholesterol declined from 241 mg/dL to 213 mg/dL. No statistically significant changes were seen in testosterone level, but the rate of growth of normal prostatic tissue (benign proliferation rate) decreased significantly. Two of the 15 men who were originally scheduled for repeat biopsy had their procedure cancelled because their PSA level had stabilized. A review of biopsy slides by a reference pathologist revealed that only 7 of the 15 men had atypia or high-grade PIN at the start of the trial. At the end of the trial only one of the 13 men undergoing repeat biopsy was found to have atypia or high-grade PIN, but three (23%) were diagnosed with prostate cancer. This percentage of cancer incidence is in line with published reports on the discovery of carcinoma in men who undergo repeat biopsy 6 months after diagnosis of atypia or high-grade PIN. The researchers conclude that the flaxseed-enriched, low-fat diet is effective in reducing PSA and cholesterol, and may be useful in controlling prostate growth, especially the proliferation involved in BPH. They plan further work to determine the relative contribution of fat restriction and flaxseed to their intriguing findings.[19]

Although there is some indication that certain alpha-linolenic acid containing foodstuffs may increase the risk of prostate cancer, there is no evidence that flaxseed supplementation is, in any way, harmful, so adding a tablespoon of freshly ground flaxseed to the diet every day is likely to be an excellent way of not only reducing cholesterol and improving heart health, but would also be expected to significantly reduce PSA level and perhaps prevent or at least ameliorate BPH.

LIFESTYLE FACTORS

Although diet is clearly very important in prostate cancer prevention, it may be equally important to get sufficient exercise and exposure to sunlight. Researchers at the Harvard School of Public Health and the Cooper Institute for Aerobics Research report that physically active men are much less likely to develop prostate cancer than are less active men. Their study involved almost 13,000 men aged 20 to 80 years who had a medical examination at the Cooper Clinic between 1970 and 1989. The men were questioned as to their participation in sports and other physical activities and underwent a maximal exercise treadmill test to determine their cardiorespiratory fitness. The researchers conclude that men with the highest cardiorespiratory fitness level (>21 minutes) are four times less likely to develop prostate cancer than are men with a low cardiorespiratory fitness level (<13.7 minutes). The protective effect was only found in men below 60 years of age. The researchers also found that men who are physically active (energy expenditure >1000 kcal/week) have about a three times lower risk of developing prostate cancer than do men who are less active (energy expenditure <1000 kcal/week). The researchers believe that high testosterone levels are involved in the development of prostate cancer and that physical activity and cardiorespiratory fitness tend to lower these levels.[1]

Edward Giovannucci and his team at the Harvard Medical School did not find any correlation between overall prostate cancer risk and the level of physical activity among 48,000 participants in the Health Professionals Study; however, they did find a lower risk of metastatic prostate cancer in men engaging in high levels of vigorous activities.[2] Researchers at the American Cancer Institute also found no correlation between the level of recreational physical activity and overall prostate cancer risk; however, they did find a reduced risk of aggressive prostate cancer among men who reported a high level of vigorous physical activity.[3] Dutch researchers found no association between prostate cancer risk and physical activity level in a group of 58,000 men aged 55 to 69 years followed for 9 years.[4] Italian researchers also found no association between leisure time physical activity or sports participation and prostate cancer risk, but did note a significant decrease in risk among men in the age groups 30-39 years and 50-59 years who experienced a high level of physical activity in their daily work.[5] Canadian researchers also found that a high degree of work-related physical activity reduced the risk of prostate cancer very significantly, whereas sedentary work was associated with an increased risk.[6] Researchers at Stanford University reviewed 13 cohort studies and 11 case-control studies conducted between 1988 and 2002 in order to determine the relationship between physical activity and prostate cancer. They concluded that 9 out of 16 studies showed a statistically significant reduction in prostate cancer risk (10-30%) with an increased level of physical activity.[7]

So, although there is no definite consensus as to the effect of physical exercise, there is no indication whatsoever that a high level of physical activity increases the risk of prostate cancer. Overall, it would seem that a regular, moderate to vigorous exercise program is likely to reduce prostate cancer risk, especially the risk of advanced and metastatic cancer.

British researchers have found that exposure to sunlight helps prevent prostate cancer. Their study involved 210 men diagnosed with prostate cancer and 155 men with an enlarged prostate (BPH), but no prostate cancer (controls). The men were interviewed in order to estimate their lifetime sun exposure. Men with the lowest exposure were found to have a three times greater incidence of prostate cancer than did men with a high lifetime exposure. Sunburns in childhood were found to be particularly protective with men having had one or more childhood sunburns being six times less likely to develop prostate cancer than men who had not experienced childhood sunburns. A history of regular foreign holidays, presumably in sunnier climes, also had a protective effect with men having had such holidays having a 60% lower risk of prostate cancer. Regular sun bathing was also found to be protective. The risk of prostate cancer was not associated with skin type, hair colour or eye colour, and the associations with sun exposure were not affected by including occupation, vasectomy or dietary factors in the analysis. The researchers are not sure why sun exposure is protective, but speculate that vitamin D and parathyroid hormone may somehow be involved. Excessive sun exposure has been linked to an increased risk of certain non-melanoma skin cancers. These cancers, however, are rarely fatal whereas prostate cancer often is. So on balance, cultivating a healthy suntan is still a good idea.[8]

The British researchers later reported on a study involving 453 prostate cancer patients and 312 BPH patients. They found that regular sunbathing was highly protective. Patients who rarely engaged in sunbathing were much more likely to have been diagnosed with prostate cancer than were patients with a high sunbathing score. The researchers also confirmed that holidays in sunny climates and sunburns in childhood are associated with a significantly lower risk of prostate cancer.[9]

Researchers at the Northern California Cancer Center recently confirmed the British findings. Their study involved 3414 men of which 153 had been diagnosed with prostate cancer. Men who lived in the southern US had a 30-40% lower risk of prostate cancer and men born in a southern state had half the risk of developing prostate cancer than did men born in a northern state.[10]

PREVENTION WITH VITAMINS AND MINERALS

VITAMIN A

Vitamin A (retinol) is a fat-soluble vitamin required by the body to ensure proper function of the immune system and to counteract the development of night blindness and weak eyesight. There is also some indication that it may help prevent the development of breast cancer and adenomatous polyps (a precursor to colon cancer).[1,2]

Evidence of a preventive role against prostate cancer is not convincing. Researchers at the Baylor College of Medicine reported in 1996 that vitamin A might play a role in the prevention and treatment of prostate cancer. They analyzed prostate tissue from patients with prostate cancer, tissue from patients with benign prostatic hyperplasia (BPH), and normal tissue. They made several interesting observations:

- All tissues tested contained retinol and retinoic acid in various concentrations. The retinol concentration in tissue from enlarged prostates was 2.5 times higher than in normal tissue or tissue from cancer patients. Tissue from cancer patients contained near normal levels of retinol, but only barely detectable levels of retinoic acid.
- The prostate contains enzymes which enables it to convert retinol supplied in the diet to the biologically active retinoic acid.

The researchers speculate that enlarged prostate tissue contains more retinol than normal and cancerous tissue either because it is less efficient in converting it to retinoic acid or because enlarged prostate tissue is more efficient in absorbing retinol from the blood. They also suggest that the low level of retinoic acid in cancer patients could be due to a more rapid degradation of retinoic acid in cancer tissue. The researchers conclude that retinol (vitamin A) and carotenoids may be useful both in the prevention and treatment of prostate cancer.[3]

Other researchers have failed, however, to find a protective role for vitamin A. The authors reporting on the Health Professionals Study involving almost 48,000 male health professionals found no consistent association between vitamin A intake and the risk of prostate cancer.[4] Swedish researchers, in a study of 526 prostate cancer patients, found no association between the risk of prostate cancer and the intake of protein, vitamin A or zinc.[5] Researchers at the Fred Hutchinson Cancer Center in Seattle recently concluded that there is no evidence that vitamin A is effective in preventing prostate cancer.[6]

Italian researchers compared the diet of 1294 prostate cancer patients and 1451 controls and observed no statistically significant protective effects associated with vitamin A, but did observe a weak protective effect of carotenes, especially beta-carotene.[7]

So, until more convincing results become available indicating a protective effect of vitamin A, it should probably not be high on the list of supplements to take in a prostate cancer prevention program. This, of course, does not mean that vitamin A is unimportant and supplements unnecessary. The current Recommended Daily Allowance (RDA) in North America is 5000 IU or, more correctly, 1000 RE equivalents for men and 4000 IU or 800 RE for women. Children need between 400 and 700 RE daily depending on age. Any intake above the daily requirement is stored in the liver. This fact has led to cautions about taking too much vitamin A as it can be toxic in large quantities. Vitamin A toxicity may occur in adults who take more than 10,000 RE daily for several years. Pregnant women should keep their daily intake below 1000 RE/day.

Vitamin A is obtained from the diet in two forms either as retinol (from animal products) or in the form of carotenes (from fruits and vegetables), which the body converts to retinol. In 1967 the World Health Organization reported that it took six micrograms of beta-carotene to produce one microgram (1 RE) of pure vitamin A. This conversion factor has been used ever since to determine the average daily vitamin A intake throughout the world. Using the WHO factor it was estimated that the average daily vitamin A intake varied from about 600 RE in South America and Asia to about 1000 RE in Europe and North America. In other words, it's adequate in Europe and North America, but deficient in Asia and South America.

Dutch and Indonesian researchers have found that the 1967 WHO conversion factor is seriously wrong. Using up-to-date analysis techniques and new information about bioavailability and bioconversion of vitamin A and carotenes they conclude that it takes not six micrograms of beta-carotene from fruits and vegetables to yield one microgram of vitamin A, but rather 21 micrograms. This finding puts a completely different complexion on things. Essentially, the entire world is likely to be vitamin A deficient. The revised estimated daily intake of vitamin A is now only 780 RE in Europe, 581 RE in North America, 372 RE in South America, and a mere 258 RE in Asia where blindness among children is becoming endemic.[8]

The most convenient way of obtaining the daily recommended intake of vitamin A is through supplementation with cod or halibut liver oil. These oils also provide vitamin D and the beneficial fish oils eicosapentaenoic acid (EPA) and docosahexaenoic acid (DHA). However, there are some indications that overdosing on fish liver oils is not a good idea. A Swedish study concluded that women with a daily intake of more than 7500 IU of vitamin A increase their risk of osteoporosis and hip fracture.[9]

BETA-CAROTENE

Numerous studies have shown that people who consume a diet rich in dark yellow-orange vegetables (eg. carrots) and dark green vegetables (eg. kale and broccoli) are much less likely to develop cancer and heart disease.[10-17] It has also been established that people with low levels of beta-carotene in their blood have a higher incidence of heart disease and cancer, particularly lung cancer.[10,12,18-23]

In 1981 it was suggested that beta-carotene is the "active component" in the protective vegetables and that supplementing with beta-carotene might prevent certain cancers.[10] The idea was based on the fact that beta-carotene is an antioxidant and the most abundant carotenoid in vegetables. Antioxidants counteract the free radical-induced damage to DNA which initiates cancer.[10,12,24-31] At the time there was also some evidence to the effect that vitamin A prevents or retards certain cancers, so the fact that beta-carotene is readily converted to vitamin A in the liver and intestine was seen as an added bonus.[10,32] More recent research suggests that beta-carotene's preventive effect is due to its antioxidant property rather than to its ability to form vitamin A.[11,12,14,18,19,33]

Beta-carotene is a member of the carotenoid family and has over 500 relatives. Carotenoids are yellow-to-red pigments found in all green plant tissues and in some species of algae. So far 21 different carotenoids have been found in human blood.[34] The most abundant ones are alpha-carotene, beta-carotene, lutein, lycopene, cryptoxanthin and zeaxanthin. A molecule of alpha-carotene, beta-carotene or cryptoxanthin can be split into two molecules of vitamin A in the body, but the conversion of beta-carotene is by far the most effective. The six carotenoids are all antioxidants. They are very effective in neutralizing (quenching) a highly reactive form of oxygen called singlet oxygen but also, to some extent, act to break up the chain reactions involved in lipid peroxidation (a precursor of atherosclerosis).[25,27,35-37] Lycopene is the most abundant carotene in the human body and is by far the most effective quencher of singlet oxygen - more than twice as effective as beta-carotene.[4,12,19,31,35,38]

Beta-carotene exists in several different configurations (isomers). Synthetic beta-carotene is almost 100% *trans*-beta-carotene; beta-carotene found in fruits and vegetables contains about 10% of *cis*-isomers and beta-carotene derived from algae contains about 50% of the 9-*cis* isomer.[37,39]

The 1981 suggestion that beta-carotene might act as a cancer prevention agent led to several trials of controlled supplementation.

In 1994 Finnish researchers reported that male smokers supplementing with 20 mg/day of synthetic beta-carotene had a higher incidence of prostate cancer than those who did not supplement.[40] In January 1996 investigators at the Fred Hutchinson Cancer Research Center cut short a trial involving 18,000 smokers because they observed a higher mortality among the participants supplementing with beta-carotene and vitamin A.[41,42]

In May 1996 Charles Hennekens and colleagues at the Harvard Medical School and cooperating research centers reported on a study of beta-carotene supplementation involving over 22,000 male physicians 11% of whom were smokers. Half of the physicians were given 50 mg of beta-carotene every second day, while the other half was given a placebo. At the end of the 12-year study period there was no significant difference in the incidence of lung cancer or prostate cancer, cardiovascular disease or death from all causes between the supplement and placebo groups.[43] A recent re-evaluation of the Health Professionals Follow-up Study concluded that a diet rich in beta-carotene is protective against prostate cancer in men younger than 65 years of age, but not among older men. The protective effect of lycopene, on the other hand, was found only among men older then 65 years.[44] Italian researchers, after studying 1294 confirmed prostate cancer cases, concluded that beta-carotene may have a weak protective effect against prostate cancer, but that vitamin A and lycopene have no effect.[7]

All told, a very mixed picture with no conclusive evidence that beta-carotene helps prevent prostate cancer and some indication that it may actually promote it in smokers. So, is beta-carotene a friend or foe? The answer is fairly straightforward. Supplementing with excessive amounts of synthetic beta-carotene in isolation is of no benefit and may be harmful, especially for smokers. This conclusion in no way detracts from the epidemiologic evidence that dark green and yellow-orange vegetables protect against the development of cancer. Research shows that people with a relatively high intake of beta-carotene (6-8 mg/day) from natural sources have about half the risk of developing lung or colon cancer as do people with a low intake.[14,17] Unfortunately, a recent survey carried out in the United States also shows that less than 20% of men and less than 30% of women consume the recommended five servings a day of fruits and vegetables - so there is lots of room for improvement without resorting to supplementation.[45]

It is possible that a beta-carotene supplement derived from natural sources and formulated so as to preserve the normal carotene ratio in the blood may be of benefit for people at high risk for cancer and cardiovascular disease. This, however, remains to be proven.[46]

So, until the remaining riddles in the carotene puzzle are solved, the prudent course of action is to avoid smoking and exposure to second-hand smoke and to increase the intake of protective vegetables and fruits while avoiding large intakes of beta-carotene in isolation.

B-VITAMINS

Only folic acid (vitamin B9) and cobalamin (vitamin B12) have been investigated for a possible association with prostate cancer.

Folic acid (folinic acid, folacin, pteroylglutamic acid) is essential for the synthesis of adenine and thymine, two of the four nucleic acids that make up our genes, DNA and chromosomes. It is also required for the proper metabolism of the essential amino acid methionine that is found primarily in animal proteins. Folic acid deficiency has been implicated in a wide variety of disorders from Alzheimer's disease to atherosclerosis, heart attack, stroke, osteoporosis, cervical, breast, pancreatic and colon cancers, depression, dementia, cleft lip and palate, hearing loss, and neural tube defects. It is estimated that many North Americans suffer from a folic acid deficiency clearly indicating that the standard diet does not provide enough. This has led to the fortification of grains and cereals, and recommendations for supplementation to achieve a minimum daily intake of 400 micrograms (600 mcg for pregnant women).

Vitamin B12 (cobalamin) is an important water-soluble vitamin. In contrast to other water-soluble vitamins it is not excreted quickly in the urine, but rather accumulates and is stored in the liver, kidney and other body tissues. As a result, a vitamin B12 deficiency may not manifest itself until after 5 or 6 years of a diet supplying inadequate amounts. Vitamin B12 functions as a methyl donor and works with folic acid in the synthesis of DNA and red blood cells and is vitally important in maintaining the health of the insulation sheath (myelin sheath) that surrounds nerve cells. The classical vitamin B12 deficiency disease is pernicious anaemia, a serious disease characterized by large, immature red blood cells. It is now clear though, that a vitamin B12 deficiency can have serious consequences long before anaemia is evident. The normal blood level of vitamin B12 ranges between 200 and 600 picogram/mL (148-443 picomol/L).

A vitamin B12 deficiency often manifests itself first in the development of neurological dysfunction that is almost indistinguishable from senile dementia and Alzheimer's disease. There is little question that many patients exhibiting symptoms of Alzheimer's actually suffer from a vitamin B12 deficiency. Their symptoms are totally reversible through effective supplementation. A low level of vitamin B12 has also been associated with asthma, depression, AIDS, multiple sclerosis, tinnitus, diabetic neuropathy and low sperm counts. Clearly, it is very important to maintain adequate body stores of this crucial vitamin. The amount of vitamin B12 actually needed by the body is very small, probably only about 2 micrograms or 2 millionth of a gram/day. Unfortunately, vitamin B12 is not absorbed very well so much larger amounts need to be supplied through the diet or supplementation.

Both folic acid and vitamin B12 are crucial in ensuring DNA replication through their action as efficient methyl donors. While DNA replication and associated cell renewal are clearly highly desirable in healthy tissue, it can be detrimental in cancerous tissue. It is therefore not too surprising that two recent studies come to different conclusions regarding the role of folic acid and vitamin B12 in prostate cancer. Italian researchers observed that men with a high dietary intake of folic acid had a 34% lower risk of prostate cancer than did men with a low intake.[1] However, results of a Swedish study contradicts these findings.

The Swedish study, part of the Northern Sweden Health and Disease Cohort, involves over 37,000 men who underwent medical examination and extensive blood work at ages 40, 50 and 60 years. By 2001 254 cases of prostate cancer had been diagnosed and these were matched with 512 healthy controls. The average age at diagnosis was 64 years and the prostate cancer patients had been under observation an average of 4.9 years (2.9-7.0 years) prior to diagnosis. Average PSA level at diagnosis was 11 ng/mL (range of 6.8-26.0). The researchers found that prostate cancer patients had significantly higher plasma levels of folate and vitamin B12 than did the controls. After adjusting for body mass index and smoking the researchers conclude that high vitamin B12 levels are associated with a 3-fold increased risk of prostate cancer. High folate levels were associated with a 1.6-fold increase in risk, but this increase became statistically insignificant when adjusting for other relevant variables. The researchers conclude that high levels of folic acid and vitamin B12 are not protective against prostate cancer, but may actually promote its development. They suggest that hypermethylation may be behind the risk increase and point out that several genes, including the one for glutathione-S-transferase (the main antioxidant in prostate tissue), have been observed to be hypermethylated and inactivated in prostate cancer.[2]

Canadian researchers have also warned that excess folic acid may accelerate cancer growth. Dr. Young-In Kim of the University of Toronto points out that, while folic acid is effective in preventing the initiation of many forms of cancer, it may actually accelerate the growth of already existing cancers. Folate plays a very important role in DNA synthesis and replication, which is great when it comes to healthy cells, but not when it comes to cancerous cells. Rapid replication and proliferation is the last thing you want in the case of cancer cells. As a matter of fact, experiments have shown that inducing a folate deficiency inhibits tumor growth and at least two chemotherapy agents (methotrexate and 5-fluorouracil) owe at least part of their effect to the fact that they counteract the cell proliferation effect of folic acid.[3]

As in so much of the research involving cancer in general and prostate cancer in particular, there is no clear consensus as to the role of folic acid and vitamin B12. However, based on current knowledge it would seem prudent to limit daily intake to 400-600 micrograms/day of folic acid and 500-1000 micrograms/day of vitamin B12, and to have regular blood tests to ensure that plasma levels are within the normal range. If cancer is suspected or diagnosed, maintaining blood levels in the lower part of the range may be desirable.

VITAMIN C

Vitamin C (ascorbic acid) is the primary water-soluble dietary antioxidant in the human body. It is particularly effective in deactivating hydroxyl radicals before they can damage DNA. Vitamin C plays an important role as a component of enzymes involved in the synthesis of collagen and carnitine and helps regenerate vitamin E, the body's main fat-soluble dietary antioxidant.

Numerous studies have shown that an adequate intake of vitamin C is effective in reducing the risk of a variety of cancers, including cancers of the lungs, stomach, esophagus, oral cavity, pancreas, colon and cervix.[4-19]   An analysis of 12 studies concerning breast cancer and vitamin C concluded that a high vitamin C intake is associated with a reduced risk of breast cancer in women.[6]   The cancer preventive effects of vitamin C are quite significant. Researchers at the National Heart, Lung and Blood Institute in the US have found that men with a blood level of vitamin C below 28.4 micromol/L have a 62% higher risk of dying from cancer than do men with serum levels above 73.8 micromol/L.   The researchers also found that the use of vitamin supplements was vastly more prevalent among men with high vitamin C status and lower mortality.   Nineteen per cent of the men in the high survival rate group used vitamin C supplements versus 0.2% in the low survival rate group (low vitamin C status).[20]

Researchers at Cambridge University have reported that men with a blood serum level of vitamin C of 72.6 micromol/L or higher have a 24% lower risk of dying from cancer than do men with a serum level of 20.8 micromol/L or lower. The researchers also found that a 20-micromol/L rise in plasma ascorbic acid level can reduce all-cause mortality rate by 20 per cent independent of age and other risk factors. A 20-micromol/L increase can be obtained by increasing fruit and vegetable intake by 50 grams per day. The researchers also noted that higher vitamin-C levels were associated with lower systolic blood pressure and body mass index as well as with a higher level of "good" (HDL) cholesterol.[21]

There is conflicting evidence regarding the role of vitamin C in prostate cancer prevention. The large Western Electric Study involving 1899 middle-aged men found no correlation between high vitamin C intakes and a reduced risk of prostate cancer.[22] Researchers at the Johns Hopkins School of Public Health also found no association between prostate cancer risk and serum level of vitamin C.[23]

A study comparing vitamin supplementation in 697 prostate cancer patients and 666 controls found that those taking a daily zinc supplement had a 45% lower incidence of prostate cancer than did men not using supplements. The daily use of vitamin A, vitamin C, and vitamin E was associated with a 41%, 23%, and 24% statistically non-significant decrease in risk.[24] Johns Hopkins researchers recently reported that there was no indication that a high plasma level of vitamin C is associated with a reduced risk of prostate cancer.[25] However, researchers at the National Cancer Institute in Montevideo, Uruguay believe otherwise. Their study involved 175 patients with prostate cancer and 233 controls. Both patients and controls had face-to-face interviews with researchers and also filled out detailed questionnaires, which covered family history of cancer, sociodemographic variables, height and weight, alcohol and tobacco consumption, and usual diet. A high intake of vegetables, fruits, and vitamin C and vitamin-E was found to significantly decrease the risk of prostate cancer. After adjusting for other risk factors the researchers concluded that men with a high intake of vitamin-C (greater than 162 mg/day) reduce their risk of prostate cancer by 60 per cent as compared to men with a low intake (less than 86 mg/day).[26]

The results of this study need to be confirmed by other researchers before it can be concluded that vitamin C, in the amounts available through diet or supplementation, is helpful in preventing prostate cancer. However, there is evidence that very high serum levels of vitamin C, achievable only through intravenous administration, can be effective in the treatment of prostate cancer.[27] There is also some evidence that a combination of vitamin C and vitamin K-3 (menadione) may be effective in the treatment of prostate cancer, either on its own or in combination with radiation or chemotherapy.[28]

Nevertheless, an adequate vitamin C level is associated with so many benefits that everyone should ensure an ample daily intake. A team of medical researchers at the National Institutes of Health in the USA recently completed a study designed to determine the vitamin C requirements of healthy, young men. They found that a minimum intake of 1000 mg/day was required to completely saturate the blood plasma with vitamin C. They also found that vitamin C should be taken in divided doses throughout the day as urinary excretion increases rapidly when individual doses exceed 500 mg. The researchers conclude that the RDA should be raised to 200 mg/day. This amount of vitamin C can be obtained from a diet containing five daily servings of fresh fruit and vegetables; unfortunately, less than 15 per cent of children and adults in the USA actually consume such a diet.[29,30]

Daily supplementation with 500 mg of vitamin C for 10 years or more has been found to cut the risk of developing bladder cancer by 60 per cent.[31] The spread of breast cancer (metastasis) is now believed to be predominantly due to free radical damage which can be controlled through intake of increased amounts of vitamin C. [32] Supplementation with 3 g/day of vitamin C has been found to effectively prevent further polyp growth in colon cancer and a vitamin C intake of more than 157 mg/day has been found to reduce the risk of developing colon cancer by 50 per cent.[18,33]

Dr. Linus Pauling believed that vitamin C combats cancer by promoting collagen synthesis and thereby preventing growing tumors from invading adjacent tissue.[27]

Many researchers now believe that vitamin C prevents cancer by deactivating free radicals before they can damage DNA and initiate tumor growth while others believe that vitamin C may sometimes act as a prooxidant helping the body's own free radical defense mechanism destroy tumors in their early stages.[10-13,34]

The current RDA of 60 mg/day is clearly far too low and the proposed new RDA of 200 mg/day, while perhaps adequate for healthy, young males, would seem to be quite inadequate for older people and certainly way too low for sick people. As a matter of fact, a scientific advisory panel to the U.S. Government sponsored Alliance for Aging Research has recommended that all healthy adults increase their vitamin C intake to 250-1000 mg/day.[35]

Vitamin C is best taken in divided doses throughout the day as it is fairly rapidly used up. The Institute of Medicine (National Academy of Sciences) has established a tolerable upper intake level of 2000 mg/day. People with hemochromatosis (iron overload) should not take large amounts of vitamin C as this would increase iron absorption.[29,36-38]

VITAMIN D

There is ample evidence that men with low sunshine exposure and low blood levels of vitamin D (cholecalciferol) are at increased risk for prostate cancer. Several studies have elucidated the mechanism whereby vitamin D and its metabolites (25-hydroxyvitamin D3 [25D] and 1alpha,25-dihydroxyvitamin D3 [1,25 D or calcitriol]) exert their protective effect. It is believed that it is not vitamin D as such, but rather its metabolite, calcitriol, which is the active component. Studies have shown that prostate cancer cells lack 1alpha-hydroxylase, the enzyme responsible for converting 25 D to calcitriol.[1]

Studies have also shown that calcitriol induces cell cycle arrest, apoptosis, and increases the level of IGFBP-3, the protein that binds IGF-1, so as to prevent it from promoting cancer.[1] Other studies have shown prostate cancer cells respond to vitamin D3 with increases in differentiation and apoptosis, and decreases in proliferation, invasiveness and metastasis.[2]

Synthetic calcitriol has also been used in trials aimed at preventing or halting progression of prostate cancer, but its use is likely to be limited as it is toxic in high doses and can lead to hypercalcemia.[3,4] However, it is possible, but not proven, that a combination of lower calcitriol doses with NSAIDs (ibuprofen) or dexamethasone may be beneficial.[5,6]

It is to be hoped that large-scale trials of vitamin D supplementation in prostate cancer prevention will eventually be undertaken. However, in the meantime, it would seem prudent to ensure adequate daily sunlight exposure and/or vitamin D supplementation.

A prominent vitamin D researcher, Dr. Reinhold Vieth of the University of Toronto, is convinced that vitamin D deficiency is widespread and that the current RDA

(Recommended Daily Allowance) for vitamin D is totally inadequate. He points out that total-body sun exposure easily provides the equivalent of 10,000 IU of vitamin D a day and that this amount is what the human race originating in Africa was originally accustomed to. With our current, officially sanctioned phobia about sun exposure most people expose only their face and hands to the sun on a regular basis and as a result become woefully deficient. The use of sunscreens prevents the formation of any vitamin D at all and makes matters even worse. Dr. Vieth recommends a minimum vitamin D intake from supplements of 800-1000 IU/day and feels that a more optimum intake from sunlight and diet would be 4000 IU/day. He also states that numerous studies have shown that daily intakes as high as 10,000 IU are safe (in the absence of sunshine). Dr. Vieth also points out that the RDA for vitamin D (400 IU/day) used until 1997 was based on the amount of vitamin D found in a teaspoon of cod liver oil. The rationale being that one teaspoon of cod liver oil a day had been found over the years to protect children from rickets![7,8]

VITAMIN E

Naturally occurring vitamin E is a mixture of 4 tocopherols and 4 tocotrienols. Vitamin E is not merely a vitamin, but is also the most powerful antioxidant in the lipid (fat) phase of human cells. Very small amounts of the vitamin are required to fulfill the role as a vitamin (catalyst for enzymatic reactions), but very large amounts may be needed to effectively combat oxidative stress. Vitamin E cannot be synthesized by the body and must therefore be supplied in the diet or through supplementation. It is only stored in the body for a relatively short time and must be replenished on a regular basis. Unlike the other fat-soluble vitamins, A, D and K, which are stored in the liver, vitamin E is stored throughout the body in the lipid phase. This fact is of crucial importance in the utilization of the vitamin to modify metabolic reactions.

The two most researched vitamin E compounds, when it comes to cancer prevention, are alpha-tocopherol and gamma-tocopherol. There is also some indication that alpha-tocopheryl succinate, a reaction product between alpha-tocopherol and succinic acid, may be useful in the prevention of prostate cancer.

In 1996, Swiss researchers reported that male smokers with low serum levels of vitamin E had an increased risk of developing prostate cancer.[1] These findings were confirmed in the Finnish Alpha-Tocopherol, Beta-Carotene (ATBC) Cancer Prevention Study. This large clinical trial involved 29,133 male smokers who were randomized to receive a placebo or 50 mg/day of alpha-tocopherol (vitamin E) for an average of 6 years. During the follow-up period, 246 new cases of prostate cancer were diagnosed and 62 deaths resulted from the disease. The researchers found that the incidence of clinically-evident prostate cancer was 32% lower in the vitamin E group than in the placebo group and mortality 41% lower.[2] June Chan and colleagues at the Harvard School of Public Health confirmed that vitamin E supplementation (100 IU/day or more) protects smokers against metastatic and fatal prostate cancer, but found no protective effect among non-smokers.[3] Scientists at the Fred Hutchinson Cancer Research Center found that men who supplemented with vitamin E daily had a 24% lower risk of developing prostate cancer than did men who did not supplement. This study did not distinguish between smokers and non-smokers.[4]

A large comprehensive study carried out by Johns Hopkins researchers found that both alpha-tocopherol (common supplement form of vitamin E) and gamma-tocopherol (most common form of vitamin E in dietary sources) provide significant protection against prostate cancer. Men with a serum level of 1.74 mg/dL of alpha-tocopherol had a 35% lower risk than did men with a serum level of 1.05 mg/dL. The protective effect of gamma-tocopherol was even more impressive with a serum level of 0.41 mg/dL conferring a 75% lower risk than that observed for men with a level of 0.17 mg/dL or less. Combining the two vitamin E forms with selenium further improved the level of protection. The researchers conclude that a mixture of alpha- and gamma-tocopherol should be used in future trials of vitamin E supplementation in the prevention of prostate cancer.[5]

At least two cell culture studies have found gamma-tocopherol to be significantly more effective than alpha-tocopherol in inhibiting proliferation of human prostate cancer cells.[6,7] Until quite recently gamma-tocopherol was thought to be of little importance. Laboratory experiments using rats had shown that gamma concentrations in blood and tissues were insignificant compared to the levels of alpha. This lead to the conclusion that the active form of vitamin E was alpha-tocopherol and future research therefore concentrated on this compound. It is worth noting that alpha-tocopherol is usually the sole component in vitamin E supplements. In 1998 researchers at the Canadian National Research Council concluded that when it comes to gamma-tocopherol people are not rats. They found that blood and tissue levels of gamma in humans are far higher than the rat experiments had indicated. Particularly noteworthy is the finding that gamma-tocopherol constitutes as much as 30 to 50% of the total vitamin E content of human skin, muscles, veins and fat (adipose) tissue.[8,9] There is also evidence that gamma is exceptionally important in protecting lung tissue.[10-12]

Research has shown that gamma-tocopherol is superior to alpha when it comes to trapping reactive nitrogen dioxide specimens and preventing lipid peroxidation under oxidative stress.[9,11-13] The gamma form of vitamin E is also less likely to act as a prooxidant than is alpha-tocopherol.[9] As if this was not enough, gamma-tocopherol also helps prevent cardiovascular disease, prostate cancer, lung inflammation, and perhaps type 1 diabetes and has potent anti-inflammatory properties.[9,11,14]

As mentioned above, gamma-tocopherol is the main form of vitamin E in the diet and accounts for about 70% of the total dietary vitamin E intake with the main sources being nuts, seeds, and vegetable oils.[12] Unfortunately, studies have shown that between 25 and 40% of all Americans are deficient in vitamin E.[15] The realization that the daily diet cannot provide an adequate intake of vitamin E has lead many people to supplement with vitamin E or rather, alpha-tocopherol. Unfortunately, ingesting large amounts of alpha-tocopherol has a disastrous effect on gamma levels.[9,16] Researchers at the University of California found that supplementing for one year with 800 mg/day of synthetic alpha-tocopherol resulted in a dramatic drop in gamma levels in both blood plasma and adipose tissue. The plasma concentration of alpha more than doubled within 2 weeks of starting supplementation and remained elevated for the remainder of the supplementation period. Gamma-tocopherol levels in adipose tissue, however, declined by more than 70% by the end of the supplementation period and the gamma/alpha ratio in adipose tissue decreased by almost 200%. Of equal concern is the finding that it took as long as 5 years for gamma levels to return to normal after the alpha-tocopherol supplementation was stopped.[16] Thus, people who supplement solely with alpha-tocopherol may deprive themselves of the benefits of gamma-tocopherol. In contrast, supplementation with gamma-tocopherol increases blood and tissue concentrations of both alpha- and gamma-tocopherol.[9]

Gamma-tocopherol is usually derived from natural sources, but alpha-tocopherol may be from natural sources or synthesized as a petrochemical. Natural vitamin E comes in two main forms: d-alpha-tocopherol (100 mg=149 IU) and d-alpha-tocopheryl acetate (100 mg=136 IU). The "d" designation in front of the "alpha" indicates that the products are derived from natural sources such as vegetable oils or wheat germ. A prefix of "dl", such as in dl-alpha-tocopherol, shows that the vitamin has been synthesized from a petroleum base. Recent research has shown d-alpha-tocopherol and d-alpha-tocopheryl acetate to be equally effective on an International Unit basis.[17] Synthetic alpha-tocopherol acetate however, has been found to be considerably less effective than its natural equivalent in raising the blood plasma level of vitamin E and in preventing peroxide hemolysis even when ingested at equivalent IU levels.[18]

Vitamin E is quite clearly a prime example of a vitamin/antioxidant that is present in the diet in an amount insufficient to sustain health. To obtain a daily dosage of vitamin E equivalent to 400 IU it would be necessary to consume 200 cups of brown rice, 10 cups of almonds, 80 cups of cooked spinach, or 12 tablespoonfuls of unrefined, fresh wheat germ oil - clearly not a viable alternative. Vitamin E should be taken as a mixture of natural alpha-tocopherol and gamma-tocopherol. If the supplement also contains other tocopherols and tocotrienols, so much the better.

There is evidence that alpha-tocopheryl succinate may be even more effective than plain alpha-tocopherol or alpha-tocopheryl acetate when it comes to preventing prostate cancer. Researchers at the University of Rochester have found that alpha-tocopheryl succinate suppress androgen receptor expression and the formation of PSA and inhibits the growth of prostate cancer cells (LNCaP line).[19] The same group has also reported that succinate inhibits prostate cancer cell invasiveness by inhibiting the activity of matrix metalloproteinase-9. This means that alpha-tocopheryl succinate could play an important role in preventing existing prostate cancer from metastasizing.[20] There is also evidence (from cell culture experiments) that alpha-tocopheryl succinate inhibits the growth of androgen-independent (hormone-refractory) prostate cancer.[21] It is likely that alpha-tocopheryl succinate needs to be given intravenously in order to be effective as it is easily hydrolyzed in the gastrointestinal tract.[22]

Based on the substantial evidence that vitamin E (and selenium) may be protective against prostate cancer, the National Cancer Institute has embarked upon a major trial, the Selenium and Vitamin E Cancer Prevention Trial (SELECT). The trial, opened for recruitment in July 2001, now has a total enrollment of 35,534 men with a median age of 62 years (range of 50-93 years) who were free of prostate cancer at enrollment. The expected follow-up time is 7-12 years. After much deliberation and a thorough review of the literature, the SELECT Steering Committee decided that the supplements to be evaluated would be 200 micrograms/day of elemental selenium in the form of L-selenomethionine and 400 IU/day of synthetic alpha-tocopheryl acetate. The trial design will involve 5 pair-wise comparisons of prostate cancer incidence, in association with – vitamin E vs placebo, selenium vs placebo, vitamin E plus selenium (combination) vs placebo, combination vs vitamin E, and combination vs selenium. The Steering Committee points out that there is strong evidence that 200 micrograms/day of elemental selenium is entirely safe, as is up to 1000 mg/day of vitamin E. They acknowledge that natural alpha-tocopherol is significantly more effective than synthetic alpha-tocopheryl acetate and that gamma-tocopherol may be even more effective than either as far as prostate cancer prevention is concerned. However, due to the fact that more clinical trial data is available on synthetic alpha-tocopheryl acetate they decided to go ahead with this form. All study participants will also receive a daily multivitamin devoid of selenium and vitamin E, but including 400 IU of vitamin-D3.[23]

So the question is, should you wait for the results of SELECT or be proactive and begin supplementing with vitamin E and selenium? In view of the fact that the ULs (upper tolerable limits) for vitamin E and selenium are 1000 mg and 400 micrograms respectively[24], it would seem to be safe and prudent to supplement with 400 IU/day of vitamin E (a 50:50 mixture of natural alpha- and gamma-tocopherol) and 200 micrograms/day of selenium from selenomethionine.

COENZYME Q10

Coenzyme Q10 (ubiquinone/ubiquinol) is a fat-soluble quinone with a structure similar to that of vitamin K. It is a powerful antioxidant both on its own and in combination with vitamin E and is vital in powering the body's energy production (ATP) cycle. CoQ10 is found throughout the body in cell membranes, especially in the mitochondrial membranes and is particularly abundant in the heart, lungs, liver, kidneys, spleen, pancreas and adrenal glands. The total body content of CoQ10 is only about 500-1500 mg and decreases with age.[1]

Research carried out in Denmark has provided some tantalizing evidence that CoQ10 may be effective in the fight against breast cancer. A trial involving the treatment of 32 breast cancer patients with mega doses of vitamins, minerals, essential fatty acids and coenzyme Q10 (90 mg/day) in addition to conventional therapy showed a highly beneficial effect of the supplementation. Two of the patients in the trial whose tumours had not regressed had their CoQ10 dosages increased to 390 mg/day and 300 mg/day respectively with the result that their tumours disappeared completely within three months.[2-4]   CoQ10 supplementation is also very important for cancer patients undergoing chemotherapy with heart toxic drugs such as adriamycin and athralines.[5]

Turkish researchers have found that the concentration of coenzyme Q10 is much lower in breast cancer tissue than in surrounding healthy tissue. They speculate that the level of reactive oxygen species (free radicals) in cancer tissue is elevated and that coenzyme Q10 is consumed in an attempt to keep oxidative stress under control. They conclude that, "administration of coenzyme by nutrition may induce the protective effect of coenzyme Q10 on breast tissue."[6]

The effect of coenzyme Q10 on prostate cancer initiation and progression has been much less researched. However, Spanish researchers have confirmed that prostate cancer tissue, like breast cancer tissue, produces more reactive oxygen species than does surrounding normal tissue. They have also found that coenzyme Q10 significantly reduces the growth of prostate cancer cells without affecting nearby healthy cells. They conclude that coenzyme Q10 may be useful in cancer therapy.[7]

Coenzyme Q10 has also been found beneficial in the prevention or treatment of atherosclerosis, angina, congestive heart failure, mitral valve prolapse, irregular heart beat, high blood pressure, muscular dystrophy, gingivitis (gum disease), and AIDS. Truly a wonder nutrient![8]

The body can synthesize coenzyme Q10 and it is also found in several dietary sources, notably organ meats. The level of CoQ10 in humans peaks around the age of 20 years and then declines fairly rapidly. The decrease in CoQ10 concentration in the heart is particularly significant with a 77-year-old person having 57 per cent less CoQ10 in the heart muscle than a 20-year- old.[9] Some experts involved in CoQ10 research believe that many people, especially older people and people engaging in vigorous exercise may be deficient in CoQ10 and may benefit from supplementation. The recommended daily dosage for health maintenance varies from 30 mg to 300 mg[10-12]; however, considerably higher amounts may be used in the treatment of the various diseases for which supplementation has been found beneficial. CoQ10 should be taken with a meal containing some fat or even better, in combination with soy or vegetable oil which enhances its absorption quite substantially. Coenzyme Q10 supplements vary considerably in regard to efficacy and bioavailability, and effective ones are generally quite expensive. No toxic effects from CoQ10 supplementation have been reported for daily dosages as high as 300 mg.[1,10]

ALPHA-LIPOIC ACID

Alpha-lipoic acid (ALA), also known as thioctic acid, was first isolated in 1953 and was quickly discovered to be a very important cofactor in the Krebs cycle (citric acid cycle), the body's main process for converting carbohydrates into energy. ALA is a medium length (8 carbon atoms) fatty acid containing two sulfur atoms. It is readily synthesized in the body and is well absorbed from the diet through the stomach and intestines. Liver and yeast are especially good dietary sources of ALA. ALA is the oxidized form of dihydrolipoic acid (DHLA), is water-soluble, and is found in varying concentrations in all muscles and internal organs.[13,14]

In 1959 it was discovered that both ALA and DHLA are powerful antioxidants. ALA scavenges hydroxyl radicals, singlet oxygen and hypochlorous acid, can remove heavy metals by chelation and regenerates other antioxidants like glutathione, vitamin C, ubiquinol (coenzyme Q10) and indirectly, vitamin E. DHLA has similar properties.[13]

Glutathione is the body's most important internal antioxidant and is in the frontline in the battle against cancer. Experimental studies have shown that alpha-lipoic acid is highly effective in regenerating glutathione and that glutathione inhibits the progression of prostate cancer.[15,16] The findings of these studies are of a preliminary nature and need to be confirmed in clinical trials.

Alpha-lipoic acid and its cousin DHLA are active in both cell fluids and membranes and have no serious side effects. There is substantial experimental and clinical evidence to the effect that ALA may be useful in the prevention and treatment of such diverse conditions as diabetes, heart attack, stroke, HIV infection, AIDS, neurodegenerative diseases, heavy metal poisoning and radiation exposure. The recommended daily maintenance dose is 20 to 100 milligrams, but much higher doses are needed in the treatment of diseases such as diabetes and AIDS.[17]

BORON

Boron is a trace mineral found in nuts, fruits, and vegetables. As is the case with selenium, the actual content in specific fruits and vegetables is entirely dependent on the soil's boron content. Nuts, leafy vegetables, apples, raisins, prunes, and grapes are considered good dietary sources of boron.

Boron plays a major role in the metabolism of calcium and magnesium and a deficiency has been associated with osteoporosis and osteoarthritis. Studies have shown that daily supplementation with 6-9 milligrams can provide significant relief in arthritis patients.[1,2] It is estimated that the average boron intake in the US is between 1.7 and 7 mg/day. There is no RDA for boron, but the upper safe intake level (UL) has been set at 20 mg/day.

Researchers at the UCLA School of Public Health in Los Angeles have evaluated the effect of boron intake on prostate cancer risk. They compared boron intake for 95 prostate cancer cases with that of 8720 male controls without cancer as part of the NHANES III Survey. After controlling for age, race, education, smoking, alcohol consumption, body mass index, and caloric intake, they concluded that men with a high boron intake had a 54% lower risk of prostate cancer than did men with a low intake.[3] Other researchers have, in animal studies, found that boron supplementation is associated with a significant decrease in PSA level, a decrease in tumour size, and a reduction of the IGF-1 (a cancer promoter) concentration in the tumour.[4]

Prostate-specific antigen (PSA) is intimately involved in the initiation, progression, and metastasis of prostate cancer. Researchers at the National Institute of Environmental Health Sciences have confirmed that boric acid (in cell cultures) inhibits PSA's ability to release IGF-1 and also helps prevent PSA's degradation of extracellular matrix glycoproteins – an important step in metastasis.[5]

The recommended daily intake of boron is 3-9 mg/day with the best forms being sodium borate or chelated boron.[6]

MAGNESIUM

Researchers in Taiwan have discovered that men with a high intake of magnesium from drinking water have a 27% lower risk of dying from prostate cancer than do men with a lower intake. The researchers conclude that, "there might be a significant protective effect of magnesium intake from drinking water and other dietary sources against the risk of prostate cancer development."[7] I have not come across any follow-up to this finding; however, an adequate magnesium status is important for a number of other reasons.

Magnesium is of key importance to human health. It participates in over 300 enzymatic reactions in the body. A deficiency has been linked to such varied conditions as irregular heart beat, asthma, emphysema, cardiovascular disease, high blood pressure, mitral valve prolapse, stroke and heart attack, diabetes, fibromyalgia, glaucoma, migraine, kidney stones, osteoporosis, and probably many more.

The RDA is 420 mg for men. Unfortunately, recent surveys have shown that many Americans have a dietary intake of 200 mg/day or less.[8] Almonds, nuts, blackstrap molasses, wheat bran and wheat germ are good sources of magnesium; however, many people will, no doubt, prefer to take a magnesium supplement as an easy and reliable way of assuring an adequate daily intake. Up to 800 mg/day of elemental magnesium is probably safe; however, people with kidney disease or severe heart disease should not supplement with magnesium without their doctor's approval.

Some magnesium supplements, when taken in excess, cause a looser stool and even diarrhea. Taking too much magnesium is not a good idea since diarrhea is likely to cause the loss of most, if not all, of the supplemented amount.

The most common magnesium supplements are magnesium oxide, magnesium carbonate, chelated magnesium (magnesium glycinate), magnesium orotate, magnesium citrate, magnesium maleate and magnesium gluconate. These supplements provide different amounts of elemental magnesium (the constituent that matters) and also vary significantly in their bioavailability (absorption).

Magnesium oxide is the most dense magnesium compound and the one most often used in mineral supplements and multivitamins. It contains 300 mg of elemental magnesium per 500 mg tablet, but is extremely poorly absorbed. Only about 4% of its elemental magnesium is absorbed or about 12 mg out of a 500 mg tablet.[9]

Magnesium carbonate contains 125 mg of elemental magnesium per 500 mg tablet, but is poorly absorbed.

Chelated magnesium (magnesium glycinate) is magnesium bound in a complex of glycine and lysine. It is easily absorbed and highly bioavailable. The magnesium (elemental) content per tablet or capsule is usually 100 mg.

Magnesium orotate contains only 31 mg of elemental magnesium per 500 mg tablet. However, it is well absorbed and has been found highly effective in daily intakes of 3000 mg (186 mg elemental).[10-12]

Magnesium citrate contains 80 mg of elemental magnesium per 500 mg tablet. It is far better absorbed than is magnesium oxide.[13] The water soluble form (Natural Calm) contains 205 mg of elemental magnesium per teaspoon, is totally soluble in hot water and is highly bioavailable.

Magnesium maleate contains 56 mg of elemental magnesium per 500 mg tablet.

Magnesium gluconate contains 27 mg of elemental magnesium per 500 mg tablet. It is easily absorbed and quick acting.

All forms of oral magnesium supplements are better absorbed when taken with a meal.[14,15]

SELENIUM

There is ample evidence that a selenium deficiency is associated with a significantly increased risk of prostate cancer[1-10]. It is generally accepted that selenium's most important role is that of a vital component of the body's most powerful antioxidant enzyme and DNA protector, glutathione peroxidase. Research has shown that a daily selenium intake of 40-50 micrograms is sufficient to maximize the glutathione level, but meaningful cancer protection has only been achieved at intakes exceeding 200 micrograms/day.[11,12] It is thus clear that selenium must be a component of other enzymes and proteins involved in disease prevention. Indeed, German researchers have, so far, identified at least 13 selenium-containing proteins that are likely to have beneficial effects.[13]. It is not clear what the role of these selenoproteins is, but there is no doubt that some of them may be even more important than glutathione peroxidase.[13] American researchers have concluded that selenium compounds prevent and combat cancer by inhibiting cell proliferation and promoting apoptosis (planned cell death). The processes involved in these ultimate results are complex and wide-ranging and include altering the synthesis and/or activities of signalling molecules, proteases, cell cycle regulatory proteins, transcriptional factors, tumour suppressor genes, and various factors associated with mitochondrial activity.[14]

In December 1996 came the first evidence that selenium supplementation could be effective in cancer prevention. The Nutritional Prevention of Cancer Study Group found that cancer mortality was cut in half in a group of patients who supplemented with selenium. The double-blind, randomized, placebo-controlled cancer prevention trial involved 1312 patients aged 18 to 80 years (75% males) who had previously been diagnosed with basal or squamous cell carcinomas of the skin. The purpose of the trial, started in 1983, was to test the hypothesis that selenium supplementation helps prevent skin cancer. Half the patients were randomized to receive 200 micrograms/day of selenium supplied as a 0.5 gram high-selenium brewer's yeast tablet; the other half received a placebo. Patients were treated for a mean of 4.5 years and had a mean total follow-up period of 6.4 years. At the end of the study, the researchers concluded that selenium supplementation does not prevent skin cancer. They did, however, find strong evidence that selenium supplementation is very effective in preventing other types of cancer. The overall mortality rate from cancer in the supplemented group was found to be only half of that in the placebo group. The reduction in mortality and incidence was particularly impressive in the case of cancers of the lung, prostate, colon, and rectum. The incidence and mortality rate from lung cancer was twice as high in the placebo group as in the selenium group. Supplement users developed only one third the number of prostate cancers as did the members of the placebo group and the incidence of colon and rectal cancer was similarly reduced in the supplement group. Unfortunately, there was not enough data to statistically evaluate the effect of selenium supplementation on the incidence of breast and ovarian cancers. The researchers were so impressed with the results of the trial that they decided to stop it early so that all patients could benefit from selenium supplementation. They believe selenium combats cancer by inhibiting the late stage promotion and progression of tumors. No toxic effects of selenium supplementation were observed.[15,16]

A meta-analysis covering 16 studies of the association between selenium intake and prostate cancer risk concluded that a moderate selenium intake is associated with a 25% reduction in risk.[17] Other researchers have found that high selenium levels are associated with improved immune function; this could be another avenue by which selenium prevents cancer.[18,19] If selenium proves to be cancer preventive it is clearly important to know whether selenium levels as measured in a blood sample correlates with actual selenium levels in prostate tissue.

Researchers at the University of Queensland in Australia have now answered this question. Their clinical trial involved 51 men who had been scheduled for transurethral resection for prostate enlargement. The men were randomly assigned to serve as controls or to receive selenium yeast tablets daily for one month prior to surgery. The tablets provided a total of 200 micrograms/day of selenium. Blood samples were taken at the beginning of the 30-day trial and on the day of surgery and the selenium content of red blood cells was compared to the selenium content of prostate tissue removed during surgery. The researchers found that the red blood cell level of selenium had increased from 173 ng/mL to 209 ng/mL in the supplemented group with no significant change among controls. The selenium level in prostate tissue from supplemented men was significantly higher than among controls (241 ng/g versus 196 ng/g). The researchers conclude that selenium supplementation is effective in raising selenium levels in both prostate tissue and red blood cells, but that selenium values from blood testing do not correlate with values obtained from testing of prostate tissue.[20]

The current RDA (Recommended Daily Allowance) for adult men is 60 micrograms and the tolerable upper intake (safe) level is 400 micrograms.[21] It is likely that most men in North America meet the RDA, but men in many other countries, notably Australia, New Zealand, Finland and France may not.[13] It is almost certain that the selenium intake among men in any part of the world is well below the 200-300 micrograms/day found beneficial in cancer prevention, thus making supplementation mandatory in any prostate cancer prevention program.

Selenium supplements come in two forms, inorganic and organic. The inorganic compounds, selenium selenite and selenium selenate, are both effective in increasing blood levels of glutathione. The organic form, selenomethionine (from yeast), also effectively increases glutathione levels, but is far more effective in raising blood and erythrocyte (red blood cell) levels of selenium than are the inorganic forms. Thus, for long-term supplementation, selenomethionine or high selenium content yeast are the preferred forms.[22,23] Assuming a daily intake from the diet of about 60-80 micrograms, a daily supplement of 200 mcg should be adequate and sufficient to obtain meaningful protection from prostate cancer. Supplementation with more than 300 mcg/day is not recommended since selenium can be toxic in excessive amounts. It is, of course, also possible to obtain additional selenium from food sources. Brazil nuts and wheat germ are both excellent sources of selenium provided they are grown in selenium-rich soils. As this cannot always be guaranteed, it is more reliable to supplement with a known amount of selenomethionine or selenium in the form of selenium-rich yeast.

A large trial (SELECT) was recently undertaken by the National Cancer Institute in the US to evaluate the effect on prostate cancer risk of supplementation with selenium and vitamin E. The supplementation protocol used in the trial consists of 200 micrograms/day of selenomethionine and 400 IU of alpha-tocopheryl acetate (vitamin E) along with a standard multivitamin pill containing 400 IU of vitamin D, but no vitamin E or selenium.[24]

ZINC

Zinc is a component of over 200 enzymes and, like selenium, is vital to human health. Zinc is necessary for the proper functioning of insulin, growth hormone and sex hormones. Zinc is highly concentrated in red and white blood cells and is also found in high concentrations in the prostate, pancreas, retina, liver and kidneys. The most abundant source of zinc is oysters, but appreciable amounts are also found in other shellfish, fish and red meat. Pumpkin seed and ginger root are also good sources, as are many grains. Zinc is, however, not well absorbed from grains as it binds to phytic acid found in fiber and produces an insoluble complex that is not absorbed. The human body contains about 2 grams of zinc and the RDA for men is 11 mg/day with an upper safe limit (UL) of 40 mg/day. Several studies have shown that much of the population, in particular older men and women, are deficient in zinc.[1,2]

Zinc is very important for proper immune system functioning and for the maintenance of vision, taste and smell, and it also plays a vital role in pregnancy outcome. Zinc concentrations are especially high in prostate tissue reflecting its crucial role in male reproductive health. It is a vital component in prostatic antibacterial factor, which protects the seminal fluid and also serves to protect citrate from oxidation. Citrate is found in very high concentrations in prostate peripheral cells and is critical for the proper functioning of the prostate and reproductive system.[3,4]

Several studies have shown that zinc levels are substantially lower in cancerous prostatic tissue than in normal prostatic tissue. Zinc levels in tissue affected by benign prostatic hyperplasia, on the other hand, are substantially higher than in normal tissue. Researchers at the University of Maryland have found that zinc levels in normal peripheral prostate tissue is about 3000 mmols/g as compared to 4000 mmols/g in BPH-affected tissue and only 500-900 mmols/g in cancerous tissue.[4] Indian researchers have found that blood serum levels of zinc increase by about 78% in the case of BPH and decrease by about 37% in the case of prostate cancer as compared to normal levels.[5] The finding that zinc serum levels are substantially elevated in BPH and substantially depressed in cancer has led to the idea of combining the PSA test with a serum zinc level determination in order to better distinguish between BPH and cancer.[6,7]

The fact that zinc levels are lower in prostate cancer has, not surprisingly, spawned the idea that zinc supplementation may be beneficial. Several cell culture and animal experiments have indeed shown that zinc is effective in inhibiting the growth of prostate cancer cells.[8-11] A British study found a 27% reduced risk of prostate cancer in men with an adequate zinc intake as compared to men with a sub-optimal intake.[12] Researchers at the Fred Hutchinson Cancer Research Center found that daily supplementation with zinc reduced the risk of prostate cancer by about 45%. Their study involved 697 prostate cancer patients and 666 healthy controls between the ages of 40 and 64 years.[13]

Unfortunately, zinc supplementation has also been found to increase plasma levels of testosterone and dihydrotestosterone in zinc-deficient men and increase the level of DHT in men with normal zinc levels.[14] This is obviously of concern since testosterone and, especially, DHT have been associated with the promotion of prostate cancer. One large study involving 47,000 male health professionals found a 2-fold greater risk of being diagnosed with advanced prostate cancer among men who had supplemented with over 100 mg/day of zinc or who had used zinc supplements for 10 years or more. No risk increase was observed in the risk of localized (confined to the prostate gland itself) prostate cancer.[15] It is worth noting that the overall risk of developing prostate cancer during the 14-year follow-up period was 0.49% per year. The probability of being diagnosed with advanced prostate cancer was 0.07% per year. It is also interesting that there was a trend for zinc supplementation up to 25 mg/day to be protective against both localized and advanced cancer and that this protection was not diminished in the case of localized cancer if supplementation was continued for longer than 10 years.[15]

Dr. Leslie Costello and colleagues at the University of Maryland point out that the increase in prostate cancer risk observed in the Health Professionals Study was limited to a group of men who had supplemented with more than 100 mg/day of zinc for more than 10 years. They also point out that the men were all diagnosed with androgen-independent (advanced) cancer rather than with localized cancer. The Maryland researchers conclude that, "the use of supplemental zinc at levels less than about 75 mg/day does not exhibit any increased risk factor for prostate cancer." They also state that, "compelling clinical and experimental evidence supports the expectation that an appropriate regimen of zinc supplement that would increase the uptake of zinc by malignant prostate cells could be efficacious against the development and progression of prostate cancer."[4]

So, at this point, it would appear that moderate zinc supplementation (probably up to the UL of 40 mg/day) is safe and may be beneficial in prostate cancer prevention. Larger amounts, however, should be discouraged until more information is available.[16]

The most effective and well-absorbed zinc supplements are zinc citrate, zinc picolinate, and zinc monomethionate. Chelated zinc compounds may be contaminated with lead, so should be used with caution.[4] Zinc supplements should not be taken in isolation. Zinc competes with copper for absorption, so increasing zinc intake can lead to a copper deficiency, which presents a whole different set of problems. Zinc and copper intake should be balanced in a ratio of approximately 10:1.[17] This means that an extra 25 mg/day of zinc should be accompanied by an extra 2.5 mg of copper.

PREVENTION WITH BOTANICAL MEDICINES

When it comes to degenerative diseases such as cancer it is often difficult to distinguish between a prevention and a treatment effect. This is especially true for prostate cancer. Most men harbour dormant (latent) cancer cells by the age of 65 years. However, in most cases, the cells do not become active and, by far, the majority of men die with prostate cancer rather than from it. Is this caused by a preventive effect that prevents the cancer from "blossoming" in the first place, or is it caused by a treatment effect that kills cancer cells as they become more aggressive?

Whatever the case may be, it would seem reasonable to assume that medicines that destroy cancer cells as they appear should be classified as preventive as well as curative.

Many botanical medicines exhibit both preventive and treatment effects. For example, the polyphenol resveratrol is a powerful antioxidant that prevents free radicals from interfering with DNA repair mechanisms and thereby helps to prevent the initiation of cancer. Resveratrol has also been found to inhibit the proliferation of existing prostate cancer cells – clearly a treatment effect.[1]

Botanical medicines that have been found effective in preventing (or treating) prostate cancer can conveniently be discussed under two headings – plant extracts and polyphenols.

PLANT EXTRACTS

The most "famous" plant in the treatment of prostate problems is **saw palmetto** (*Serenoa repens*). Extracts from the saw palmetto plant have been used for hundreds of years to treat BPH and Veterans Affairs (US) medical researchers have confirmed its potent effects in controlled trials involving almost 3000 men.[7] Saw palmetto inhibits the enzyme 5-alpha-reductase responsible for converting testosterone to dihydrotestosterone. Saw palmetto also has strong anti-inflammatory properties in the prostate and has been found effective in inhibiting the growth of prostate cancer cells in culture experiments.[8,9]   At least one progressive medical doctor recommends supplementing with 320 mg/day of extract as a preventive measure.[11] Scottish researchers recently confirmed that *Serenoa repens* is effective in inhibiting 5-alpha reductase and that it does so without affecting PSA values.[10] See Chapter 2 for more details.

Another extract famous for its beneficial effect on BPH is **Pygeum africanum**, an extract from the bark of the pygeum tree native to Central and Southern Africa. Spanish researchers have reported that *Pygeum* is highly effective in not only inhibiting prostatic cancer cell proliferation in cultures, but also inhibits the growth of the benign hyperplasia epithelial cells involved in BPH.[12] So far, there have been no clinical trials evaluating the effectiveness of *pygeum africanum* in human prostate cancer prevention. See Chapter 2 for more details.

Curcumin, the yellow pigment in the spice turmeric, has received a lot of attention recently as a potent remedy against cancer. Researchers at Columbia University in New York have reported that curcumin is effective in inducing cell death in both androgen-dependent and androgen-independent prostate cancer cell lines. They conclude that, "curcumin could be a potentially therapeutic anti-cancer agent, as it significantly inhibits prostate cancer growth and has the potential to prevent the progression of this cancer to its hormone refractory state."[13-15]

Brazilian researchers have confirmed that extracts of turmeric produced via supercritical fluid (CO_2) extraction are effective in inhibiting the growth of prostate cancer cells.[16] So far, curcumin has not been clinically evaluated for cancer prevention or treatment. However, as curcumin is inexpensive, safe and widely available a small daily intake of this plant extract may to be a tasteful addition to a prostate cancer prevention program.

Ginger has a long history of use in Malaysian traditional medicine. It is widely used in the treatment of stomach problems, nausea, vomiting, epilepsy, sore throat, cough, bruises, wounds, childbirth, sore eyes, liver complaints, rheumatism, asthma, and many other disorders. Researchers at the Forest Research Institute of Malaysia now report that several members of the Zingiberaceae family effectively block the promotion of cancerous tumors. They tested 11 different species and found that seven of them had strong anti-tumor properties. Their test involved a short-term assay of the inhibitory effect of extracts of the rhizomes (roots) on human cancer cells. They found that turmeric (*Curcuma domestica*) extracts (turmeric root extracted with petroleum ether, chloroform or ethanol) completely inhibited further growth of the cancer cells. Ginger (*Zingiber officinale*) extracts, especially the chloroform extract, also inhibited further growth, but the concentration of extract was more critical than for the turmeric extracts. The researchers conclude that turmeric, ginger and other Zingiberaceae rhizomes may be useful in preventing the promotion of cancer and that populations with high risks of cancer should be encouraged to include them in their diet.[17]

Brazilian researchers have confirmed that extracts of ginger produced via supercritical fluid (CO_2) extraction are effective in inhibiting the growth of prostate cancer cells. The ginger extracts were also found to be effective in killing leukemia cells.[18]   So far, there have been no clinical trials that have evaluated ginger for cancer prevention or treatment. However, increasing the use of ginger in the daily diet can do no harm and may have considerable benefits.

Beta-sitosterol is a phytosterol found in many plants. It is similar to cholesterol in structure. Several clinical trials have found beta-sitosterol highly effective in alleviating urinary symptoms caused by prostate enlargement.[18-21]. In 1995 German researchers treated 100 men with BPH with beta-sitosterol (20 mg 3 times a day). After 6 months the men experienced significantly improved urine flow and less retention.[1] These benefits were maintained for at least another 18 months with continued supplementation.[19] In 1997 another group of German researchers performed a similar randomized, double-blind, and placebo-controlled clinical trial involving 177 patients with BPH. The patients treated with beta-sitosterol (130 mg/day for 6 months) experienced significant improvement in urine flow as well as less urine retention.[20] A meta-analysis of clinical trials employing beta-sitosterol to treat BPH confirmed its beneficial effects.[21]

Laboratory experiments have shown that beta-sitosterol is highly effective in inhibiting the growth of both androgen-dependent (LNCaP cells) and androgen-independent (PC3 cells) prostate cancer.[22,23] More recently American researchers reported that both beta-sitosterol and resveratrol are effective in inhibiting the growth of PC3 prostate cancer cells. Beta-sitosterol was the most effective agent, but the combination with resveratrol was more effective than either agent alone.[24] No clinical trials, so far, have investigated the possible prostate cancer preventing effects of beta-sitosterol in humans. However, beta-sitosterol is entirely safe and readily available. Peanuts are an excellent source of phytosterol, particularly beta-sitosterol. Peanut butter contains about 150 mg per 100 grams.[25] See Chapter 2 for further details.

Extracts from **milk thistle** (*Silybum marianum*) have been used in herbal medicine for 2000 years. Pliney The Elder (AD 23-79) reported that a mixture of the plant's juice and honey was excellent for "carrying off bile". Since then many scientists have lauded milk thistle's ability to treat liver disease. Since 1969 milk thistle extracts have become very popular and now account for sales of $160 million a year in Germany alone. Researchers at the Oregon Health Sciences University recently released a major report reviewing the scientific papers dealing with silymarin, the active ingredient in milk thistle extracts. A standard silymarin extract contains 70 per cent silymarin, which in itself is a mixture of flavonolignans, silydianin, silychristine, silybin (silibinin), and isosilybin. Silybin is believed to be the most biologically active component and is rapidly absorbed into the blood stream and bile after an oral dose. Silybin acts as an antioxidant, decreases the activity of tumor promoters, and acts as a mild chelator of iron. Studies have shown that silymarin is beneficial in the treatment of acute viral hepatitis and some toxin and drug-induced forms of hepatitis. There are also reports that silymarin is effective in the treatment of alcoholic liver disease and chronic hepatitis. Therapeutic dosages range from 140 mg twice a day to 560 mg/day for periods from six months to six years. No adverse side effects of silymarin have been documented and the researchers conclude that well-designed, double-blind, placebo-controlled studies should be carried out to further investigate silymarin's benefits in the treatment of a variety of diseases.[26]

In 1999 researchers at the University of Colorado found that silibinin inhibits the growth of human prostate cancer cells (LNCaP cells) and decreases both intracellular and secreted PSA. They conclude that, "silibinin could be a useful agent for the intervention of hormone-refractory human prostate cancer."[27] In 2004 the same researchers confirmed that silibinin is strongly protective against prostate cancer progression and announced the start of a phase I clinical trail in prostate cancer patients.[28,29] Further research elicited the finding that two components of silymarin, isosilybin A and isosilybin B are more effective than silibinin in suppressing both cell growth and PSA secretion. The researchers conclude that, "extracts enriched for isosilybin B, or isosilybin B alone, might posses improved potency for cancer prevention and treatment."[30] In their latest report the University of Colorado researchers conclude that silymarin and silibinin are also effective in halting the growth of androgen-independent (advanced) cancers (PC3 cells).[31]

It is clear that silymarin, silibinin, and isosilybin B hold great promise for both prostate cancer prevention and treatment. Silymarin and its components are safe and a supplement containing silymarin and isosilybin B (4.5%) is now commercially available.[32]

POLYPHENOLS

Polyphenols constitute a very large group of phytochemicals responsible, among other things, for the brightly coloured pigments of many fruits and vegetables. Polyphenols also help protect plants from diseases. Flavonoids are an important subclass of polyphenols and include such popular supplements as quercetin, flavones, isoflavones, anthocyanins, and proanthocyanins. All polyphenols are powerful antioxidants and thus help protect against the initiation of cancer through their ability to inactivate free radicals before they can interfere with the body's normal DNA repair mechanisms. Some flavonoids have also been found to slow down the progression of existing cancers.

Quercetin is abundant in many fruits and vegetables. Studies have shown that it has important anti-tumour, anti-inflammatory, anti-allergic, and antiviral activities. Researchers at the State University of New York recently reported that quercetin is effective in inhibiting the growth of the most aggressive prostate cancer cells. It does this by increasing (up-regulating) tumour suppressor genes and inhibiting (down-regulating) oncogenes and cell cycle genes.[1] Appreciable amounts of quercetin can be obtained from a diet rich in parsley, onions, oranges and tomatoes. Quercetin can also be taken as a supplement (preferably in combination with bromelain). The recommended daily dose is 200-400 mg taken 3 times a day 20 minutes before meals.[2]

Resveratrol is found in grapes and red wine and is increasingly being touted as an important cancer fighter. Researchers at the University of Illinois have reported that resveratrol is a strong antioxidant, has powerful anti-inflammatory effects, is a COX-2 inhibitor, and prevents the initiation of some cancers in laboratory mice.[3,4]

In 2001 Italian researchers reported that resveratrol inhibits the growth of prostate cancer cells and prevents oxidative damage to DNA.[5]

In 2003 Korean researchers confirmed that resveratrol inhibits the growth of prostate cancer cells and induces apoptotic cell death. They conclude that, "our study suggests that resveratrol has a strong potential as an agent for the prevention of human prostate cancer."[6]

Just recently, researchers at the Fred Hutchinson Cancer Research Center in Seattle reported that men who drank a glass of red wine daily had a 50% lower risk of developing prostate cancer than did men who did not imbibe. Their study included 753 patients with newly-diagnosed prostate cancer and 703 cancer-free controls. The researchers found no association between prostate cancer risk and the consumption of beer or liquor and only a weak association with white wine consumption. They conclude that resveratrol is likely behind the protective effect of red wine. Resveratrol is a major component of the skins of grape varieties used to produce red wine, but is much less abundant in grapes used for white wines. Peanuts and raspberries are also good sources.[7]

Having a glass of red wine a day has long been advocated for its benefits in preventing cardiovascular disease. The finding that it also helps prevent prostate cancer only adds to the value of this preventive measure – and women do not need to feel left out – Greek researchers have reported that red wine polyphenols also inhibit the growth of breast cancer cells.[8] Of course, for those who prefer not to imbibe, red wine extracts and resveratrol are also available as supplements.

Grape seed extract has been found to kill human prostate cancer cells, but clinical trials are, undoubtedly, some way off.[9,10]

Pycnogenol, an extract from the French maritime pine, has been found to induce apoptosis in certain lines of breast cancer cells, but no research would appear to have been done on its possible use in preventing prostate cancer.[11]

CONCLUSION

It is clear that there is an astonishingly large variety of foods, vitamins, minerals, herbs and plant extracts that have been found effective in preventing and inhibiting the growth of prostate cancer. Some have undergone clinical trials and some have not, but all are likely to be safe and well-tolerated. It is estimated that about two-thirds of all cancers are preventable through diet and lifestyle modifications.[1] As far as prostate cancer is concerned, the most important preventive measures, apart from avoiding the risk factors outlined in Chapter 3, are:

- Ensure an adequate daily intake of vegetables, especially cruciferous ones (broccoli, cauliflower, etc).
- Consume tomato sauce or other processed tomato products frequently, or supplement with lycopene capsules.
- Ensure an adequate daily intake of fish oils. A minimum of 650 mg/day of EPA (eicosapentaenoic acid) plus DHA (docosahexaenoic acid) is recommended.

- Consider including tofu, natto or other whole soy products in the daily diet.
- Ensure daily consumption of garlic, scallions (green onions) or other allium vegetables.
- Drink green tea regularly or supplement with standardized green tea extract containing EGCG.
- Engage in moderate to vigorous exercise on a regular basis.
- Ensure 15-30 minutes of unprotected sun exposure daily, or supplement with vitamin D (1000 IU/day).
- Maintain blood levels of folic acid and vitamin B12 within the normal range.
- Supplement with 200 mcg/day of selenomethionine and 400 IU/day of vitamin E while awaiting the results of the SELECT trial.
- Have a glass of red wine daily, or supplement with resveratrol (more speculative).

Other potential candidates for prostate cancer prevention are listed below, but please bear in mind that the evidence supporting their effect is considerably weaker than the evidence for the above-mentioned measures.

- Ensure an adequate daily intake of vitamin C (250-1000 mg/day) and coenzyme Q10 (30 mg/daily).
- Ensure an adequate daily intake of boron (3-9 mg/day) and magnesium (420 mg/day).
- If supplementing with zinc ensure a zinc:copper ratio of around 10:1.

The following herbal compounds have shown some protective effect in cell cultures and could be considered in a prostate cancer prevention program:

- Saw palmetto
- *Pygeum africanum*
- Curcumin
- Ginger
- Beta-sitosterol
- Milk thistle
- Quercetin
- Resveratrol
- Grape seed extract

There are no pharmaceutical drugs specifically approved for the prevention of prostate cancer. However, the following drugs have undergone preliminary evaluation and shown some promise of effectiveness:

- Finasteride (Proscar)
- Dutasteride (Avodart)
- Aspirin and NSAIDs
- NO-ASA and NO-ibuprofen
- Statin drugs

Chapter 6

Treatment of Localized Prostate Cancer

William R. Ware PhD

INTRODUCTION

"Is cure necessary in those in whom it is possible, and is cure possible in those in whom it is necessary?" W. F. Whitmore, Jr., 1990 [1]

The diagnosis of prostate cancer (PC) can be psychologically devastating and leave a man unprepared to deal with his options. Nevertheless, there are options which need to be weighed, and considerable research has been reported that provides guidance. A critical and essential component in this decision making process is the clinical picture presented by the patient which in turn is based on the PSA history and level at diagnosis, the Gleason score and the details of the pathology report generated by the biopsy, the tumor grade, evidence of metastasis or advanced disease, age, and comorbidities. Another important component of the decision making process involves what is called *the natural history* of the disease, and this relates to the rate and nature of progression of untreated disease after diagnosis, and this in turn relates to the strategic question—to treat or not to treat or to wait and then perhaps treat. Current practice involves the patient taking an active role in the decision making process and selecting the most appropriate treatment. Men with localized prostate cancer on average have rather long disease-free intervals regardless of the treatment selected. Thus the post-treatment quality of life and satisfaction with the treatment are very important.

Treatment is generally described with the terms primary, adjuvant, neoadjuvant, secondary or salvage. Primary is the initial treatment given, whereas neoadjuvant treatment comes before a given protocol, adjuvant generally immediately after, and the term salvage is generally restricted to the secondary treatment of a failed primary protocol. Palliative refers to treatment carried out to alleviate pain or complications, in this case of advanced cancer.

In this chapter it is assumed that the reader is familiar with the contents of Chapter 4, in particular TNM tumor staging, the Gleason score, and the measurement and use of PSA levels. The various aspects of the treatment of prostate cancer cannot be adequately discussed without frequent reference to these common indicators of the seriousness of the disease. With regard to the tumor staging, i.e. T1, T2 etc., and the Gleason score, it is also important to keep in mind the distinction between information gained prior to treatment vs. that obtained from the pathology report on the prostate and other tissue after surgical removal. These are generally differentiated by the terms *clinical* and *pathological* with the former referring to the pre-treatment presentation, including information gained through biopsy.

TO TREAT OR NOT TO TREAT, OR TO COMPROMISE

Subsequent to the diagnosis of prostate cancer, not all patients receive treatment. Some patients are judged to have cancer that has advanced to the point where palliation is the only option offered. For others, it may be recommended that the course of their disease be followed closely and treatment initiated when progression is observed but before it is too late for the treatment to be potentially curative (active surveillance). Some men reject treatment even when advised that it would be beneficial if not in fact strongly indicated. Some of these men may change their minds later on while others will hold out until palliative measures are forced on them by end-stage disease or they die of some unrelated cause. It is of interest to first examine some of the reasons why treatment might be rejected.

- Belief that treatment will not influence overall survival, and thus there is no point in undergoing procedures which may impact the present quality of life. Some men may feel that their chances of dying of PC are less than from some other health problem, and they are willing to take the risk of a decrease in quality of life associated with palliative treatment if necessary, or perhaps they just choose to ignore this possibility.

- Fear of surgery and the belief that the side effects and complications associated with surgery or any form of radiation therapy or cryotherapy are unacceptable.

- Some men who have examined the matter carefully may have concluded that the decision making process is merely a probability game where the probabilities are uncertain, and unlike other games, the game of life is played through only once which prevents taking advantage of probabilities through repeated trials, as would for example happen in a casino or in the game of baseball.

- Some men will fail to understand or appreciate the significance of the physician's arguments for the desirability of treatment; others will simply give different weights to the factors being discussed.

- The decision not to accept treatment may be merely based on an irrational gut reaction to the prospect of treatment options, may be based on very limited data such as the bad experiences related by the fellow who lives down the street, or may even be the perceived result of seeking divine direction.

Many of these reasons obviously can not be addressed through evidence-based arguments, but it is of interest to examine what is known about the impact of treatment on overall survival, and in addition, the impact on PC-specific survival, the risk of metastasis and local progression.

Of greatest interest in the context of treatment and overall survival is a study from Scandinavia given landmark status that was first reported by Holmberg *et al* in 2002 [2] with a sequel reported by Bill-Axelson *et al* extending data analysis period from 8 to 10 years [3]. This study is very important because the designers randomized 695 men to either surgery (RP) or watchful waiting (WW). Men in the watchful waiting group received no initial treatment other than the transurethral resection (TURP, see Chapter 2) some had already undergone. For both the surgery and WW groups, hormone therapy was recommended for all men with disseminated disease, and as well, for RP patients with local progression. Table 1 summarizes the results.

Table 6-1. Causes of death for the radical prostatectomy (RP) and watchful-waiting (WW) groups during 8.2 years (median) follow-up after diagnosis

Cause of death	RP Group (N = 347)	WW Group (N = 348)
	Number of Patients	
Prostate Cancer	30	50
Other Causes	53	56
Any Cause	83	106

In the WW group, close to 50% of the deaths during follow-up were from PC. Treatment with surgery reduced mortality from prostate cancer by 40%. Radical prostatectomy resulted in an estimated 26% relative reduction in overall mortality. This appears to be the only long-term randomized study to indicate improved overall survival attributable to treatment (in this case radical prostatectomy) as compared to watchful waiting. However, as the table indicates, the number of patients in each mortality category was rather small, and as the authors point out, the absolute reduction in mortality due to treatment was moderate and "clinical decision making and patient counseling will remain difficult." The study also found a 40% reduction in the risk of distant metastasis and a 67% reduction in local progression. Taken together, these results indicate positive benefits from surgical treatment and the authors predict the benefits will increase during longer follow-up. However, the reduction in PC-specific mortality as a result of surgery was limited to patients younger than 65 years of age, although the study lacked power to fully investigate this aspect. Interestingly enough, the earlier report from this same study covering a shorter follow-up showed no significant effect on overall survival.

In the follow-up period, the Scandinavian study found substantial absolute differences between the two groups in terms of local progression, which can cause problems with urination, pain and anxiety. The WW group had a greater need for hormone treatment and palliative radiation for pain relief. Both these interventions are accompanied by side effects that influence the quality of life. The authors point out that the more immediate but stable side effects associated with surgery must be weighed against the increasing incidence of symptoms and use of treatments after progression in the WW group. The point is that there are more factors to consider than overall or PC-specific survival and that the decision making process is multifactorial and complex.

However, the results of the Scandinavian study are not that clear-cut. As Chodak and Warren point out in a recent review [4], the mean PSA at randomization was 12.9 ng/mL. Today, that average would be closer to 6 ng/mL. This could reduce the overall relative survival benefit of RP and illustrates one of the problems with studies of this type being currently reported, i.e. to have the long follow-up, the cohort will generally include a higher percentage of men with more advanced disease than would be the case if the study had been initiated recently and the effect of PSA screening on lead-time well established in the study population [5]. Thus it is not clear how applicable these results are to men diagnosed with PC today.

The issue is further confused by a recent study from Columbia University which revealed a significant dependence of the outcome for radical prostatectomy on the year of surgery [6]. Three periods were identified, 1988-1993, 1994-1998, and 1999-2003. The rate of biochemical failure after surgery (median follow-up 54 months), expressed as a percentage of patients in each group, was 40.0%, 17.8% and 8.1% for these three periods, respectively. The authors were unable to account for this dramatic improvement in outcome even after correcting for all obvious confounders. The Scandinavian study started in 1989 and follow-up lasted through 2003. If the phenomenon found in the Columbia University study was also present in the Scandinavian study, this complicates the application of these results to today's population of PC patients, and in fact might make the benefits of surgery greater than reported by Bill-Axelson *et al*.

When overall survival is the issue, there is a race, so to speak, between the prostate cancer and other causes of death, and what becomes significant is which cause crosses the finish line first. Making the decision to have surgery only on the basis of the results of Bill-Axelson *et al* ignores a number of factors including the individual's age and other diseases competing in the race to death. Also, since the time frame can be 15-20 years from today, there are bound to be changes in the prevention, diagnosis and treatment of not only PC, but also the competing major causes of death. No one can predict the net result of this continuously changing picture on the overall survival question. The point is that of necessity, trying to use overall survival as the critical factor in the decision to treat or not to treat is simply a probability game, but the data one has to work with is uncertain, changing with time, and the game is played only once!

A man may elect RP over WW merely because of studies suggest a large decrease in the probability of metastasis and local progression. Also, RP does indeed offer the chance of a permanent cure, while classical WW does not. As will be discussed below, if the cancer is organ confined and not aggressive, the probability of recurrence 10 years after RP can be less than 10%, i.e. a high probability of a "permanent" cure. Also, recurrence is not the end of the game since so-called salvage RT can also be highly curative. In addition, the RP, because it involves the removal of the gland, eliminates most cancer related causes of urinary obstruction which in the WW case, would require treatment. The RP also provides much more prognostic information than was available prior to surgery, which can be an advantage in planning additional treatment if indicated. In rejecting surgical treatment, a man elects to forgo these potential advantages.

However, a man over 65 may point to the Scandinavian study and conclude that there is no benefit from surgery if the criterion is PC-specific survival. This ignores the low power of the subgroup analysis, but more importantly, he is taking an average result and applying it to himself. This in fact is at the root of the problem of decision-making based on studies or probabilities, and why, ideally, as many factors as possible need to be considered by both the patient and his physician.

In the end, however, it seems inevitable that attempts at rational analysis will fail to provide a really clear-cut answer to the treatment dilemma. The pessimist would simply argue that there are too many variables, too many uncertainties, and besides, an integral part of the process of decision making involves predicting the future which at best is a tricky business.

It is widely recognized that a small but significant percentage of patients receiving a RP will be found to have tumors deemed insignificant or indolent. The surgery may well have been unnecessary. While these tumors may never have posed a threat during the lifetime of the patient, the word *may* is important. Again, no one really knows, especially if the time frame is 15 or 20 years. One solution is active surveillance, which represents a compromise between immediate treatment and the classical WW described above. This will be discussed in detail below, but the essential features are as follows. If the probability is high that the cancer is not aggressive and may never present a problem during a man's lifetime, then the option is to closely follow the case with periodic PSA tests, DREs, and biopsies. If no progression is seen, nothing is done. Treatment may never be necessary. If progression suggesting a threat to the patient's life expectancy is observed, he is offered treatment. Patients are initially selected so that if the decision to treat is made, the chances of a cure are high and have not been significantly influenced by the waiting period.

Active surveillance reduces the uncertainties associated with the initial assessment because the repeated follow-ups provide more reliable information on the nature of the cancer than was available from the initial clinical assessment based on PSA, Gleason score and Tumor grade. It can be argued that this is a much more intelligent approach to the question of to treat or not to treat than simply accepting or rejecting treatment on the basis a number of considerations, many of which were elaborated above. Active surveillance allows the decision not to treat to be reconsidered periodically, which makes more sense than the black and white options, to treat or not to treat. In particular, it reduces considerably the uncertainty in the educated guess made after the initial biopsy as to the true nature of the cancer present in what is really somewhat of a black box.

Active surveillance may also be elected by individuals at higher risk of post-treatment failure than those currently considered ideal for this option (see below). These men may want confirmation of the clinical assessment by experiencing progression before taking action, or they may simply hope to buy some time before undergoing treatment by taking advantage of what they hope is a slowly developing disease.

The reader will probably have observed that the only treatment modality discussed so far has been surgery. This is because there is no equivalent long-term overall survival data from randomized studies for radiation therapy or cryotherapy vs. WW.

Following untreated patients reveals the so-called natural history of PC, which can be an important component in the process of selecting among the treatment options. Two factors combine to confuse this natural history. These are the advent of PSA testing in the late 1980s and the fact that PC is in many cases a very slowly developing disease. For example, estimates of the chances of dying of untreated PC are based mostly on the study of individuals diagnosed in the pre-PSA era and would be expected to be considerably higher than the probabilities for individuals diagnosed with PSA screening [7] because in the pre-PSA era most PC was diagnosed at an advanced stage. However, due to the slow progression of this disease in many individuals, there are insufficient data for the required analysis at present, mainly because the clinical characteristics of the present-day population with newly-diagnosed PC have only more or less stabilized recently. However, there have been attempts to model this problem based on existing data. The work of Nicholson and Harland [7] is of particular interest. They calculate the 10-year probabilities of death from prostate cancer in a PSA-era population assuming no treatment after diagnosis. Involved is an estimated lead-time of 9 years due to the early detection feature of PSA screening. After this lead-time, the older mortality data was applied. For men with Gleason Scores of 6, they obtain the results given in Table 2.

Table 6-2. A model of the natural history of untreated prostate cancer. Probability (%) of untreated PC-specific death 10 and 15 years after diagnosis by PSA screening and biopsy for men with a Gleason score of 6 compared with the probability of death from other causes [7]

Age at screen diagnosis	Alive	Death from PC	Death—other causes
	PROBABILITY OF DEATH (%) (no definitive treatment)		
	Ten-year results		
50	85.0	6.3	8.7
60	74.0	5.8	19.6
70	55.6	6.3	38.1
80	11.7	3.4	84.9
	Fifteen-year results		
50	72.1	12.2	15.7
60	56.3	11.1	32.6
70	31.4	10.5	58.1
80	2.2	4.0	93.8

These numbers can be compared, for example, to pre-PSA results where, for untreated men between 65 and 75 years of age with Gleason Scores of 6, 20% were expected to die of PC over the following 15 years [8]. Comparison with the data of Bill-Axelson *et al* is also interesting. Nicholson and Harland also give data for age 65 (not shown) which is the average age of the Bill-Axelson cohort, which also had about 50% of participants with Gleason 5-6. Ten-year numbers from Nicholson and Harland were 66.3%, 6.0% and 27.7% for being alive, death from PC or death from other causes, respectively. Comparable numbers from Bill-Axelson *et al* (Table1) were 69.5%, 14.4% and 16.1%

respectively. Thus if the Scandinavian survival study had involved a more modern cohort, the death rate from untreated PC might have been substantially lower. However, survival after RP might have been higher and the overall survival advantage between the treated and untreated groups might have disappeared. This underscores the problems caused by the changing characteristics of the modern-day recently diagnosed population as compared to a less recent cohort.

Parker [9] points out that even the numbers for PC-specific death of Nicholson and Harland may in fact be too large since the mortality data they used may be too high given recent decline in PC-specific mortality. Thus it is important for men to recognize that older, much less favorable survival figures, which still influence clinical decisions, should be questioned. When confronted with this argument, they should inquire as to whether or not the PSA-era lead-time has been integrated into the survival data.

Other aspects of the natural history of PC that relate to the question of treatment are as follows [10].

- The lifetime risk of PC is 16% in the US but the risk of PC-specific death is only about 3%.
- The median time from diagnosis to death for men with biopsy detected PC prompted by elevated PSA is about 17 years, where at age 65, the life expectancy is 16 years. This raises the question of the extent to which treatment will add years to a man's lifespan, which of course depends on age.
- Up to 1/3 of men in PSA screened populations undergoing radical prostatectomies (RPs) have small (< 0.5 cc), low-grade (≤ 6 Gleason scorer) tumors. Such small tumors may not impact the lifespan in older men. Walsh [11] gives a slightly lower estimate.
- Approximately 30% of men older than 50 have PC at autopsy after dying of non-PC related causes, but the diagnosis rate for this age group is only about 11% [12].
- Average age at diagnosis in the pre-PSA era was approximately 70. Now it is 60 [13].
- If the lead-time due to PSA screening is 5-7 years; this is equivalent to 10-12 years to the symptomatic stage of untreated PC. A lead-time of 9 years gives 14 years.
- At present in the US, 75% of men diagnosed with PC have non-palpable disease (negative DRE) and have a biopsy because of elevated PSA (stage T1c).

Two recent studies concerning the natural history of localized PC merit mention. Albertsen *et al* [8] presented the results of a 20-year follow-up of patients treated only with either observation or immediate or delayed hormone treatment. Their results, which received considerable media coverage, did not support the aggressive treatment of localized low-grade PC. However, editorial comment [14] pointed out that the authors failed to emphasize that the cohort studied had a preponderance of very low-grade (Gleason 2-4) tumors which are rarely if ever seen today. And as well, the work was criticized for not really describing the natural history of untreated PC since 42% of the patients received hormone therapy within 6 months of diagnosis [15].

In the second study, the opposite conclusion was reached by Johansson *et al* [16]. They found that for early, localized cancer an indolent course for 15 years can be followed by significant local progression and metastatic disease over the next 5 years. Given that a number of patients have a 20-year or greater life expectancy, this result impacts treatment decisions. However, as Neugut and Grann point out in an accompanying editorial [17], these results may have been influenced by better detection of progressing disease near the end of the study, resulting in a false impression of more aggressive disease late in the natural history of untreated PC. However, the chance that these results are valid raises questions as to the relevance of shorter-term studies including those discussed above and strengthens the commonly held view that young men with PC should be encouraged to have definitive treatment even if the cancer appears organ confined and non-aggressive. The results presented by Johansson *et al* may never be confirmed since it is probably true that 20-year follow-up studies involving a large number of untreated men with prostate cancer, all recently diagnosed, are now for the most part impossible to organize and implement. Thus major questions persist and will probably continue to persist.

What can be concluded? The above discussion should indicate the complexity of the treatment question, its many aspects, and the impact of PSA screening on the clinical characteristics of present-day populations. Just-diagnosed patients can be thought of in terms of several groups. There are those who reject treatment out of hand and as well, those who say, "doctor, just tell me what to do," i.e. they have no opinion or preferences or wish to follow what they perceive as expert advice. There are those who are comfortable with treatment but do not want unnecessary therapy, and those who regard the cancer as a definitely unwanted foreign invader and emphatically want it eradicated no matter what, even given the risk of an unnecessary operation or the risk of complications and side effects that may diminish their quality of life. They may even elect or demand definitive treatment knowing that the chances of durable disease-free period are poor. This group is unable to live with the untreated disease, the stress of which would also pose a health problem. Evidence based arguments will have little or no impact on the decision making process for most of these men.

Another group may have extensively researched the question of risk vs. benefit associated with definitive treatment for their clinical presentation. This group would then divide into those rejecting treatment and those embracing it, with some electing active surveillance. While they would probably maintain that the decision was rational and evidence-based, this was perhaps imaginary since the weight given to various probability arguments may in part have been both emotional and irrational. The bottom line is that there appears to be no simple or satisfying answer to the treat or not to treat question. Unfortunately, the decision to accept or reject treatment for prostate cancer is not like deciding whether or not to have an appendectomy! However, there is growing evidence to support the merits of a middle ground, active surveillance for carefully selected patients. The quotation given at the beginning of this chapter neatly summarizes the situation.

THE TREATMENT OPTIONS AND GUIDELINES

There are four general post-diagnosis options, and within each there are additional options. Which of the general options selected will depend greatly on the nature of the disease, but the patient generally has the power to force the decision to take a particular route, a decision that that may go against the advice of the attending physician and may not correspond to the most appropriate mode of treatment given the clinical picture. An extreme example is the rejection of treatment with intent to cure at a stage where the treatment should be initiated soon to have the greatest probability of a favorable outcome and instead to elect to do nothing until the end stage is reached and pain control is required, or death occurs from an unrelated cause. At the opposite extreme, if the estimated life expectancy is short compared to the estimated time to prostate cancer related death; this can strongly impact the choice of treatment. There are many other scenarios, including unnecessary treatment of indolent tumors. The probability of successful treatment must also be weighed against the probability of adverse treatment effects influencing the quality of life, and different treatment options each have their set of adverse side effects. Like using the clinical picture to predict treatment success, the risk-reward considerations for treatment reduce to probabilities. Life is rarely simple in our modern high-tech world.

Positive and unequivocal diagnosis (see Chapter 4) of prostate cancer (PC) leads to four currently favored primary treatment options, active surveillance, radical prostatectomy, radiation treatment with or without the implantation of radioactive needles (brachytherapy) and androgen ablation (hormone treatment or castration). As briefly described above, the term *active surveillance* implies monitoring with the intent to intervene with treatment intended to cure if warranted by changes in the clinical picture. Treatment guidelines in the literature [18-20] related to the four options can be summarized with respect to risk factors for post-treatment recurrence based on the clinical presentation after diagnosis (see www.nccn.org). Not everyone agrees with all of the aspects of these guidelines, but they probably represent the majority viewpoint. See Chapter 4 for a detailed discussion of the TNM staging, the significance of PSA levels, and the meaning of the Gleason score.

GUIDELINES FOR TREATMENT

I. **LOW RECURRENCE RISK**—StageT1-T2a, Gleason score 2-6, and PSA < 10 ng/mL
* *Life expectancy* < **10 y:** Active surveillance (AS) or radiation therapy (RT).
* *Life expectancy* ≥ **10 y:** AS or radiation therapy (RT) or brachytherapy or radical prostatectomy (RP) with or without lymph node dissection.

II. **INTERMEDIATE RECURRENCE RISK**—StageT2b-T2c *or* Gleason Score 7 *or* PSA 10-20 ng/mL
* *Life expectancy* < **10 y:** AS or RT (with or without brachytherapy) or RP with pelvic lymph node (LN) dissection unless probability of LN metastasis is < 3% (from nomograms or tables).
* *Life expectancy* ≥ **10 y:** RT (with or without brachytherapy) or RP with pelvic LN dissection unless probability of LN metastasis is < 3%.

III. **HIGH RECURRENCE RISK**—StageT3a *or* Gleason score 8-10 *or* PSA >20 ng/mL
* RT plus hormone treatment (HT, i.e. androgen ablation)
* *Or* RT with or without short-term HT if only single adverse risk factor is present.
* *Or* RP with pelvic node dissection in selected patients.

IV. **VERY HIGH RECURRENCE RISK**—LOCALLY ADVANCED—T3b-T4
* HT
* *Or* RT plus HT.

V. **METASTATIC**
* Any T Stage, N1 (positive lymph nodes): HT or RT plus HT
* Any T Stage, any N, M1 (evidence of metastasis): HT.

These guidelines exhibit a number of interesting aspects. The risk of recurrence after definitive treatment clearly depends on other factors than the three clinical parameters, PSA, TNM stage and Gleason score that are used. Aspects of the patient's real disease status which would make the prediction of recurrence much more reliable are of necessity unknown since the treatment decisions are made either before surgery or before an exploratory operation (e.g. examining lymph node status). Also, it is impossible to take into account the possibility of substandard therapy. The higher the recurrence risk status as defined by the three clinical parameters, the higher the probability that the disease is not organ confined and thus less amenable to therapy directed at the gland itself, such as RP or RT. Likewise, the more unfavorable the recurrence risk factors, the higher the probability that the disease has spread to the lymph nodes or beyond. However, the clinical parameters on which this risk assessment is based, as used in the guidelines and discussed in detail in Chapter 4, are subject to significant error, especially the TNM stage and Gleason score. Because of the uncertainty concerning the true disease status due to the inherent inadequacy of the clinical assessment, using treatment guidelines leading to recommendations and patient decisions represents in fact simply an educated guess.

Estimates of the relevant probabilities are available from on-line calculators as discussed in Chapter 4. For example, what is the probability range associated with the low recurrence risk status? If someone is at the high end of the low-risk category (T2a, PSA 9.9 and Gleason score 6) the recurrence probability, i.e. the five-year disease free survival for RP or RT is approximately 80%, i.e. a 20% failure rate. Thus the low-risk category presumably encompasses a failure probability of near 0% to 20%. These are considered favorable odds. The intermediate risk category yields a rather wide range of recurrence probabilities depending on the selected clinical picture, but fall in the range of 30-70%. It will be noted that this does not alter treatment options significantly except that AS is not recommended if the life expectancy (LE) is ≥ 10 years and RP is now a recommended option even if the LE is < 10 years. The RP allows LN dissection which provides additional information. If the LNs turn out to be positive, the probability is much higher that the cancer has spread and that systemic therapy (HT) is indicated. It appears that these guidelines take the position that even if the probability of treatment failure is, say 50%, the chance that the disease severity has been overestimated, the potential for delay of progression, the avoidance of acute urinary problems and the opportunity of gaining therapeutic guidance (in the case of the RP), make it worthwhile to still consider definitive therapy with intent to cure. The alternative is to assume disseminated disease and treat accordingly, thus abandoning all hope of a cure. For the high-risk category, the probability of definitive treatment failure is very high, but the guidelines still suggest RT or RP for selected patients. Nevertheless, now hormone therapy figures prominently among the options, as it does for locally advanced and metastatic disease.

Consider as an example, a patient in the intermediate-risk category with a PSA of 15, Gleason score of 7 (4 + 3) and TNM stage of T2b. The probability of five-year disease-free survival after RP is 30%. If after surgery the pathological Gleason is also 7 and there is no capsular invasion and both the seminal vesicles and lymph nodes are negative, then, based on this new information, which would otherwise not have been available, the five-year recurrence-free probability jumps to 95% and if there is seminal vesicle involvement, it is still 87%. The patient has obviously benefited from this option even when the pre-treatment risk was unfavorable and might have prompted some to consider only systemic therapy. The point is that the three clinical parameters are providing only probabilities of the true extent of the disease, and these probabilities have significant uncertainties themselves. The decision-making process with regard to therapy involves just how much weight the physician and patient are willing to give to probabilities that are unfavorable but do not reflect a hopeless situation. This is in fact much more complex than it might seem from the simple process of placing the patient in one of the three categories.

For low, intermediate or high recurrence risk, there are two treatment outcomes that warrant consideration of immediate additional (adjuvant therapy). If RP results in positive surgical margins, the guidelines recommend that adjuvant RT should be considered. If RP reveals LN metastasis, HT should be considered. In either case, observation until recurrence is an alternative. These guidelines indicate the complexity of the options offered and the need for men diagnosed with PC to educate themselves as to the pros and cons of the options that apply to their clinical picture (risk status). These issues and those raised in the above discussion will receive further discussion in the remainder of this chapter.

The application of these guidelines requires, at least for those in the low and intermediate risk groups, an estimate of life expectancy (LE). This estimate must take into account the presence of health problems known to significantly decrease life expectancy such as congestive heart failure, end-stage renal disease, oxygen-dependent chronic obstructive lung disease and severe functional dependencies in the activities of daily living. Table 3, which applies to the general US male population, illustrates the range of life expectancies for three different age groups [21]. The large range in life expectancy at any age is of course due to the large variation in the state of health.

Table 6-3. The range of life expectancy for three age groups [21]

	LIFE EXPECTANCY (years)		
AGE	70	75	80
Top quartile	18.0	14.0	10.8
50th percentile	12.4	9.3	6.7
Lowest quartile	6.7	4.9	3.3

Thus the 70-year-old, even if not in perfect health (e.g. 50th percentile), can have a LE of 10 years, and an 80-year-old in excellent health also has a LE of about 10 years. The lowest quartile in general reflects poor health. Obviously, there are serious judgment calls to be made when the physician attempts to estimate the LE of a cancer patient since the above numbers, based on so called life tables, are not broken down according to the presence or stage of prostate cancer or comorbidities. If a man is diagnosed with localized low or intermediate recurrence risk PC, then given that the average time to disease specific death from diagnosis is in excess of 10 years, the comorbidities (other than PC) that influence the range of LE in the Table 3 for a given age become a primary factor in placing the individual in the > 10 years or < 10 years category. This in turn can influence treatment decisions based on these guidelines. The urologist or oncologist assisting a man having both heart disease and diabetes in making treatment decisions may not be in a position to make the best evaluation of this particular individual's LE. Even the individual's internist or GP might have a problem with this type of assessment. Predicting the future is never easy.

If a man wishes to take an active and informed role in the decision making process, it is highly desirable that he equip himself with the appropriate knowledge as to what evidence based medicine has to say about this subject. For example, post-treatment recurrence or side effects should not be a total surprise, and the patient should know ahead of time approximately what the probabilities are for such eventualities, and how these probabilities may unfortunately depend on the medical center or hospital where the treatment is done. Obvious questions include the comparison of surgery with radiation treatment when judged by side effects and the probability of disease-free survival for, say, five, ten or even more years. There are many other issues, some of which are quite complex.

The rate of progression of prostate cancer is such that, for example, if a man takes a few months after diagnosis to educate himself on the subject of treatments and seeks a second opinion, this delay should have minimal or negligible impact on the outcome [22,23]. Prostate cancer is not like a serious infection that must be treated immediately or a life-threatening situation may rapidly develop. As Gwede *et al* [24] point out in a recent study of the decision-making process, "Patients with localized prostate carcinoma need to be afforded ample time and resources to facilitate what is sometimes a lengthy, difficult and distressful decision-making process." This chapter will discuss the subject of conventional treatments of localized PC and attempt to provide useful resources. Treatment of patients with recurrent and advanced cancer and as well alternative treatments will be discussed in subsequent chapters.

WATCHFUL WAITING AND ACTIVE SURVEILLANCE

Modern usage distinguishes traditional watchful waiting from active surveillance, which is also called expectant management, expectant management with curative intent, delayed therapy with curative intent, active monitoring or temporarily deferred therapy. While some use these terms interchangeably, watchful waiting historically applied to the option where no treatment with intent to cure was attempted but palliative treatment was provided when required. This was a frequently encountered situation in the pre-PSA era when it was common for PC to be diagnosed at a stage where neither radiation treatment nor surgery offered significant benefit, the possibility of a "cure" or a significant delay in progression. Active surveillance (AS), on the other hand, is based on identifying, among those diagnosed with PC, individuals for whom there is an interest and a high probability of treatment producing a cure or at least very long-term freedom from recurrence. At the same time if AS is contemplated the clinical picture presented by these individuals must be such that treatment can be delayed without significant risk that waiting will adversely impact the chances of success if treatment is eventually initiated. Also, the protocol must include clinical parameters to identify men progressing to the point where treatment becomes advisable.

AS is intended to address the problem of men diagnosed with low-grade PC or indolent disease who may never experience progression to the point where the disease influences their life expectancy or causes bothersome symptoms. Thus treatment of insignificant cancers, which is one of the major concerns associated with PSA screening, is theoretically avoided. The fact that both RP and RT are accompanied by side effects that can impact the quality of life (e.g. impotence, incontinence, and bowel problems) adds to the attractiveness of the AS option since, as pointed out above, a significant fraction of RPs reveal cancers that would probably not have influenced the life expectancy or quality of life of older men, and yet many of these men must endure the side effects of an operation that was perhaps unnecessary. Another objective of AS is to take advantage of the lead-time generated by PSA screening and add as many treatment-free years (i.e. side effect-free years) as possible before radical intervention is indicated or death from some unrelated cause intervenes.

TRADITIONAL WATCHFUL WAITING AND ITS MODERN VERSION

Traditional watchful waiting was equivalent to doing nothing. To quote Dr. Patrick Walsh [11], "There have always been, and always will be, many men who are best served by watchful waiting." A common characterization of those who are most appropriate for this approach includes men who are too old or too sick to survive more than ten years. When symptoms became bothersome, palliative treatment is indicated. Doing nothing until pain relief or the treatment of urinary obstruction is necessary is much less common today than it was a 10 or 15 years ago. Thus it is important to dig beneath the terminology "watchful waiting" to see the modern variations. For men with incurable cancer, watchful waiting can involve treatment, perhaps delayed, to slow progression even when there is no intent to cure. Such treatments have their unpleasant side effects, and thus there is incentive to delay as long as possible without losing the opportunity to extend the time-course of the disease. Age enters into the treatment decision process, since in some cases traditional watchful waiting is indicated simply because the individual is too old and has too many comorbidities, with the result that, for example, surgical treatment would offer little benefit, a high risk of side effects that would adversely impact the quality of life, and an enhanced risk of treatment associated mortality.

An interesting group of patients in this context are those diagnosed before the PSA era who had palpable evidence from a DRE prompting a biopsy or TURP specimen evidence (see Chapter 2) which revealed PC. This is a different patient population than is encountered today because of the lead-time associated with PSA screening and thus this pre-PSA era population had a higher percentage of more advanced disease at diagnosis than seen today. As discussed above in connection with the question of treating or not treating PC, a recently reported [2] and then updated [3] study from Sweden, which has been hailed by many experts as a landmark study, examined in a randomized fashion the difference in outcome for a large cohort receiving either surgery or traditional watchful waiting for localized PC, mostly diagnosed by DRE. In this latter arm of the study, only disseminated disease was treated. The results discussed above indicated that there were benefits associated with the radical prostatectomy as compared to traditional watchful waiting, which included reduced risk of death from prostate cancer, reduced risk of metastasis, and in addition, at 10 years, there was a significant benefit in terms of overall survival. This was the first study to provide clear evidence that surgical treatment of localized cancer not only reduces death from prostate cancer but also increases survival. However, 75% of the patients had palpable disease and only 11% had T1c stage cancer (biopsy prompted by elevated PSA). Thus the watchful waiting group was not typical of patients seen today, at least in the US, and the extrapolation of this data to modern watchful waiting (which is really or should be active surveillance) in present-day populations presents difficulties.

MODERN WATCHFUL WAITING–ACTIVE SURVEILLANCE

Successfully implementing active surveillance (AS) requires determining criteria for the selection of suitable patients, setting the clinical parameters that trigger treatment, and establishing the frequency of reassessment. The success of a given protocol is then determined by long-term studies of a large cohort meeting the selection criteria where

AS is compared with immediate treatment, ideally in a randomized fashion. Endpoints might include the number under AS ultimately treated, and the 10- or 15-year recurrence-free survival and the PC-specific mortality for those under AS compared to those given immediate treatment. Unfortunately, AS has only recently been used with significant frequency and there are no long-term studies as yet completed, nor will there be any completed for quite some time. Only short-term follow up has so far been possible. However, as will be discussed, the initial experience with this option as indicated by recently published results has been very interesting. Studies currently available look at the number on AS that progress to treatment, and the nature of the progression as seen on examination of the prostate and other tissue removed at RP. The protocols differ mainly in the triggers for treatment. It is convenient to consider separately the Johns Hopkins and Memorial Sloan-Kettering protocols and then other studies

Active Surveillance Program at Johns Hopkins Hospital [10,25]
At Hopkins this is called the "Expectant Management with Curative Intent Program." The admission criteria are: stage T1c (non-palpable, discovered by biopsy prompted by elevated PSA), PSA density ≤ 0.15 ng/mL/cc, *absence of all* of the following results from a biopsy involving at least 12 cores: Gleason score of 7 or more, any Gleason pattern of 4 or 5, three or more cores involved or more than 50% involvement found in any one core. Strict follow-up includes a DRE and a PSA measurement every 6 months and a biopsy every year. Disease progression was defined as a Gleason score of 7 or more, any Gleason pattern of 4, more than 2 cores involved with cancer or more than 50% involvement of any core with cancer. Thus the biopsy provides the only trigger for recommending treatment. For the purpose of evaluating results, "curable cancer" was defined as greater than an estimated value of 70% for the disease free progression *probability* for 10 years after surgery, which in turn was based on the pathological Gleason score and individual core patterns, whether or not the cancer was organ confined, and as well as seminal vesicle and lymph node status.

Thus far results have been reported for only 81 men involved in the Hopkins program, but a number of interesting observations have already been forthcoming. The median follow-up period was about 2 years (range 12 to 58 months). Some patients exhibited progression after only one or two years, but the authors suggest that this was not real progression since the time interval is too short as judged by the natural history of this disease. Thus men who experienced treatment triggers during the first two years were viewed as under-diagnosed at the first biopsy. Of the 81 participants, 25 showed progression, but only 7 may have experienced true progression. It can thus be argued that 18 may not in retrospect have really met the admission criteria, but this was missed in the first biopsy. Of the 63 who apparently actually met the admission criteria, the observed number that progressed to trigger a treatment recommendation was thus 7 (11.1%), or about 89% of this smaller group remained on AS during the follow-up period. Of the 25 men with progression, 13 underwent RP, and 92% had cancers judged curable according to the above criteria. Unfortunately, the follow-up time was short, and additional results over a longer period will be of great interest. The authors conclude that expectant management with curative intent may be a reasonable alternative for carefully selected men who are older and thought to have small volume cancers. This study [10] also looked at other potential ways to predict progression. An important result was that neither the percent free PSA nor the PSA density (see Chapter 4) was satisfactory because of extensive overlap in both measures for men with and without progression. This result has a bearing on the interpretation of other studies of AS which used only various PSA measurements as triggers.

The Hopkins study also highlights the biopsy problem discussed in Chapter 4. A recent study from this same institution [26] addresses this issue. A total of 103 men were studied who were predicted to have insignificant cancer. However, at RP 71% were classified as insignificant whereas 29% were misclassified, i.e. the cancer was not insignificant. The study showed that by using so-called saturation biopsy techniques, the misclassification rate could be reduced to about 11%. This approach used on average 44 cores (range 24-54) but a modified protocol using half the number of cores produced similar results. The authors conclude that saturation biopsy provides an accurate prediction of tumor volume and grade for the selection of candidates for AS therapy. While 44 cores may not be very appealing to some men, the merits of avoiding or delaying radical treatment should be weighed against the potential added discomfort and potential increased morbidity of the saturation biopsy. However, these appear to be minor issues.

Memorial Sloan-Kettering Approach To Active Surveillance
The criteria given by Scardino [27] will be taken as representative of the current Memorial Sloan-Kettering (MSK) approach to what they term *deferred therapy* or *active monitoring*. To be a candidate, the patient must have a PSA < 10, tumor stage no greater than T1c, i.e. no palpable tumor on DRE, only one or two biopsy cores positive with a Gleason ≤ 6 (3+3 only), and no poorly differentiated Gleason pattern 4 or 5 cancer. Those selecting the AS option are required to have a post diagnosis biopsy with preferably 10-14 cores. There are three possible outcomes of this second biopsy: (a) no cancer (40 to 50% of second biopsies had this result!); (b) more extensive cancer such that the patient no longer meets the criteria for AS; (c) agreement with the first biopsy. Studies done at MSK found that 85% of patients found cancer-free on second biopsy exhibited no signs of disease progression over the next 10 years [28]. The follow-up protocol involves a DRE, PSA and %fPSA every three months during the first year. At one year, imaging with ultrasound or MRI is also suggested and as well a biopsy is necessary. If the biopsy yields a Gleason sum of 3 + 3 or less and there is no change in the DRE or adverse indication from the PSA behavior, then the protocol is continued with another biopsy at the end of the second or third year, as well as continued PSA and %fPSA monitoring. The DRE and PSA are done every 6 months, and biopsies are continued every two to three years until life expectancy is less than 5 years. While PSA is followed, the definitive trigger for advising treatment is the biopsy. This protocol is quite similar to that used by Hopkins.

MSK was involved in a long-term study (1984-2001, median follow-up 44 months, range 1-172 months) of AS with a cohort that was similar to the Swedish study described above. They found that about half the patients remained progression-free at 10 years and definitive treatment appeared effective in those with progression. The MSK criteria given above for their current AS program would have excluded a number of the participants included in this long-term study [28].

Other Studies

Khatami *et al* [29] recently reported on the results of a study which addressed the question "Does initial surveillance in early prostate cancer reduce the chance of cure by radical prostatectomy?" A total of 26 patients with PC (T1c-T2, Gleason score < 7, PSA 3-13) were managed by initial surveillance (mean 23.4 months, range 8-55 months) followed by a RP. Each case was matched for PSA, Gleason score and TNM stage with two controls who had received immediate surgery. They found that tumor volume did not differ significantly between cases and controls and as well, extra-capsular growth, pathological Gleason score and time to recurrence after RP over a follow-up period of 2 years were also similar between the two groups. They conclude that AS followed by treatment when signs of progression appear is a low-risk option. This group of patients also contained some individuals who would have been ineligible (tumor stage > T1c) if the protocols described above of either Hopkins or MSK were applied.

As was pointed out above the Hopkins group found that PSA changes do not appear to be a reliable indicator of progression in men with low grade disease electing watchful waiting. Nevertheless, studies indicate that men electing watchful waiting in the PSA era and their urologists are strongly influenced by PSA changes as a trigger for initiating therapy [12,25,30].

Finally, Harlan *et al* [31,32] examined the temporal trends in watchful waiting from 1989 to 2000. Since the early 90s the use of watchful waiting as the initial management protocol has been decreasing. What is interesting is that this decrease is seen particularly in low-risk patients. By the year 2000, the percentage of patients electing watchful waiting was less than 10% and at least half reversed their initial choice within 4 years [32]. It has been suggested that physicians who treat prostate cancer contribute to a climate that strongly favors immediate treatment [33]. This trend may be reversed by the favorable early results from Johns Hopkins, the positive comments regarding this option for appropriately selected men on the Hopkins prostate website (Johns Hopkins Prostate Bulletin) and in the recent review by Allaf and Carter [25], and favorable commentary in Peter Scardino's recent book [27]. Nevertheless, widespread acceptance of this option may have to wait until there are large, long-term, randomized studies. But some men may find the AS option attractive, even at this stage in its development. It is important to realize that while studies of men with T1c cancer selecting the AS option are limited, the Hopkins criteria are based on research over more than a decade where the question of clinically detecting low-grade, more or less indolent cancer has been greatly clarified [25]. Also, the use of repeat biopsies as the only trigger for abandoning AS and starting treatment removes some of uncertainties associated with determining the nature of the prostate cancer at any given point in time.

While many prostate cancers are slow-growing and if caught in the initial stages, may be effectively managed with active surveillance, for young men the issues are more complex. A healthy man aged 50 will have 30-40 years life expectancy, and even a slowly developing cancer may well become dangerous well before this period is up. Thus there is understandable reluctance among urologists to suggest AS for young men with low-grade PC which can be immediately treated with very high probability of a resultant long disease-free period. The wisdom of this stance must await long-term studies where young men who qualify for and elect AS are compared with those who present with the same clinical picture who receive immediate definitive treatment. It may be years before the answer is known, and even longer before the results influence every-day clinical practice.

In summary, the advantage of AS is the potential for avoiding unnecessary treatment or delaying treatment to maximize the years without side effects which may adversely influence the quality of life. In addition, the delay in treatment associated with carefully orchestrated AS does not appear to adversely impact the success of subsequent treatment if required. It is important to keep in mind that AS is not watchful waiting in the traditional sense. Examination of the NCCN guidelines given above reveals less stringent selection criteria for AS than currently employed at Hopkins or Memorial Sloan-Kettering. AS addresses one of the key objections to screening, offering a middle ground according to its proponents where those with a high probability of indolent cancers are identified and treatment delayed, and when this assessment is wrong or changes in an unfavorable direction, the warning signs used are timely and definitive action can be taken when it is quite probably not too late. The disadvantage is that there is as yet no long-term evidence-based information much less randomized studies available concerning the long-term merits of this approach. Modern AS has not been in use for a sufficient period of time. Unfortunately, this will continue to be the case for a number of years. Thus men need to consider AS on the basis of current research results. AS also seems to offer a strong counter argument to those who are against screening. If screening leads to a positive biopsy it need not inevitably result in a recommendation for definitive treatment but rather, the decision to treat or wait can be based on the probability that treatment at that point in time may be unnecessary, and this decision can be reviewed periodically.

DEFINITIVE PRIMARY THERAPY

"Diseases that harm require treatments that harm less." Sir William Osler, M.D.

Definitive primary therapy consists of either surgery or radiation therapy, although there is growing interest in hormone treatment and cryoablation (cryosurgery) as a primary treatment in some situations. The need for definitive therapy is presumably dictated by the clinical picture which indicates that active surveillance is not a wise or attractive approach either to initiate or continue. The patient can compare his clinical parameters with those discussed in the above section to examine the consistency between the current suggested practice in two of the best prostate centers in the US and what is being used by the attending physician as a threshold for recommending definitive treatment. The trend is for the physician to present the patient with his options along with the pros and cons of each. The patient may then go away to think about these options, perhaps acquire detailed knowledge, and finally reach a decision, perhaps after additional discussions. Unfortunately, as discussed in Chapter 4, the data the patient has available after his last PSA test and DRE and his subsequent biopsy may or may not accurately reflect his true clinical picture, but aside from one or more additional biopsies, the measurement of other PSA indicators and perhaps imaging if thought appropriate, there is little a man can do in the quest for the elusive absolute certainty. But it may be realistic for him to request these additional tests to increase the certainty of his staging, tumor grade, and detailed PSA profile. In addition, evidence has accumulated and is getting increased attention which suggests that surgery is appropriate in situations where a decade ago it would not be considered. Thus it is important that a man diagnosed with advanced cancer thought to still be localized should become aware of the current thinking and clinical results related to the relative merits of surgery, radiation and hormone therapy.

The question of which therapy is most appropriate has recently been made more complex by the increased use and promotion of hormone therapy either prior (neoadjuvant) to or immediately after (adjuvant) either RP or RT and in addition the use of RT immediately after RP when the surgical or pathological picture suggests benefit. Also, changes and improvements in RT in the past decade confuse the issue when long-term freedom from recurrence vs. side effects is an issue. While the general term *External Beam Radiation Therapy* (EBRT) is widely used, some authors fail to distinguish the more traditional method from the modern 3-dimensional confocal protocol (3D-CRT) which has a somewhat lower incidence of side effects and can employ higher, more effective doses of radiation.

In the following two sections, the essential aspects of the surgical and radiation approach to primary therapy will be discussed in order to provide the reader with an information base for the decision making process. This will be followed later by a head-to-head comparison of surgery and radiation which will attempt to put these two sections in perspective for the individual who has been told that either therapeutic approach would be prudent. The use of adjuvant or neoadjuvant therapies in conjunction with radiation therapy or surgery will be discussed in Chapter 7.

THE RADICAL PROSTATECTOMY

...as surgical procedures go, radical prostatectomy remains one of the most delicate, intricate, and flat-out difficult to perform correctly. Dr. Patrick Walsh [34].

The radical prostatectomy (RP) normally involves the complete removal of the prostate, the seminal vesicles, and frequently the easily assessable pelvic lymph nodes. The operation was first done through an incision in the perineum (the area between the scrotum and the anus), and later (1947) with an abdominal incision. This latter approach, termed the *retropubic radical prostatectomy,* gained popularity because it offered a wider surgical field which allowed flexibility in adapting the operation to the individual's anatomy, easier control of bleeding, and complete resection of the cancer in most patients. In addition, the abdominal incision facilitated the dissection of the pelvic lymph nodes without additional morbidity. Recently a laprascopic technique has been gaining popularity and the RP is also now being performed robotically. Today, the route to the prostate via an abdominal incision is by far the most common. Historically, the first published report of surgery for prostate cancer in the US was on 40 patients at Johns Hopkins and appeared in 1905.

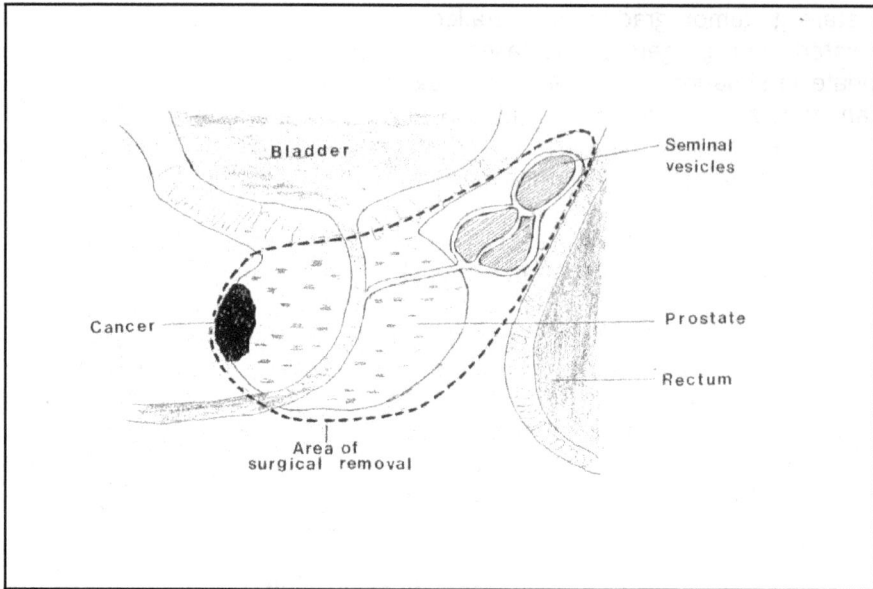

Figure 6-1. Radical Prostatectomy

When the RP first came into used for the treatment of PC, it was accompanied by a very high level of morbidity and mortality and most of the patients were at an incurable stage. Also, into the 1960s, less than 10% of prostate cancer patients were deemed candidates for a RP and these were generally men with small tumors [35]. Heavy bleeding was common, blood transfusions almost always required, impotence a universal outcome and incontinence and serious infections very common. For good reason, the operation developed a very bad reputation and both hormonal intervention and radiation were more frequently used for a number of years due to their somewhat lower mortality and morbidity. One reason for the poor results accompanying the early RP experience was related in part to an abysmal knowledge at that time of the anatomy of the prostate, the nerves involved in erectile function, and the delicate and fragile nature of the lower urinary sphincter. Also, decades passed before surgical procedures were developed that avoided the very heavy bleeding that led some surgeons to describe the operation as working almost blind in a pool of blood.

The modern RP *as carried out by an experienced and skilled surgeon* bears little resemblance to the older operation and because the critical problems have been essentially solved, it has now become a very common procedure and for many men, the preferred option for the treatment of cancer deemed either curable or likely to respond favorably to the complete removal of the prostate. Much of the credit for the rebirth of the RP must be given to the Johns Hopkins urologist Dr. Patrick Walsh. In the 1970s he pioneered techniques that resulted in a bloodless field and later developed the surgical protocol associated with minimizing the long-term side effect of impotence. The initial incentive for investigating the problem of impotence came from an interaction with a retired Dutch urologist Pieter Donker who was investigating the anatomy of the nerve system associated with the prostate and the erectile process. In 1982 Walsh performed the first so-called "nerve-sparing" RP. Walsh devised surgical procedures that allowed, in many cases, the preservation of both nerve bundles that contained the nerves responsible for erections by painstakingly dissecting the nerve bundles away from the prostate prior to its removal. This nerve-sparing approach, techniques to control bleeding and avoiding injury to the critical lower sphincter resulted in a dramatic decrease in the rate of impotence, incontinence and the need for transfusions. In the years to follow, he systematically perfected all aspects of this operation. The current status is described in a recent review by Herbert Lepor [36]—"In the modern era, radical prostatectomy is a procedure that should be performed with negligible mortality, minimal morbidity, a short hospital stay, a quick return to normal activities, a very high probability of continence, a good chance for preserving potency, and a high probability for a cure. An important caveat is that outcomes following radical prostatectomy are intimately related to the experience of the surgeon performing the procedure."

In his quest for what is now recognized as a level of perfection that others strive to emulate, Walsh actually video-taped hundreds of his operations and studied his technique down to the minutest detail as it related to the outcome of each operation. Recently a CD containing a video of his RP techniques was provided free for all subscribers to major urology journals, presumably in the hope that this would result in a higher standard of perfection for this operation. Nevertheless, studies of the rate of adverse outcomes from RPs that span many institutions and surgeons reveal a very large variation in achieving the level of perfection found not only at Hopkins but also reported by some other US centers. Inferior results are not only found for individual surgeons but also found even in hospitals where a high volume of RPs is performed. This state of affairs strongly impacts the determination of the rate of adverse effects and the comparison between the RP and the RT since the results, as measured by the incidence of such adverse results as impotence, incontinence and rectal damage, depend on where the surgery was done and by whom. A man may get very good results when the operation is done at his local hospital, but then he may not, and he frequently has no way of obtaining relevant information ahead of time. This is a more or less insoluble problem that is inherent to the RP because, as the quote at the beginning of this section indicates, the operation involves great technical difficulties.

The RP has several merits. First, if the cancer is indeed totally confined to the gland, then the complete removal of the prostate also removes all the cancer cells and theoretically constitutes a permanent cure. The second major advantage is that with the prostate gone, there is no possibility of cancer related urinary obstruction, at least from the prostate itself, which can present serious problems if the prostrate remains in place and the cancer progresses. In contrast, radiation therapy leaves the prostate in place, and if unsuccessful, the continued growth of the cancer may eventually obstruct the urinary pathway and require major intervention. In addition, if RT does not kill all the cancer cells, then those remaining are free to grow and eventually cause problems including metastasis, whereas if the cancer is indeed organ confined, the removal of the prostate eliminates this eventuality. Finally, the complete removal of the prostate simplifies the use of PSA levels when monitoring for recurrence during follow-up, permits the early detection of recurrence (failure) and also allows for the complete pathological examination of both the prostate and other tissues removed during surgery. A grey area involves the situation where the cancer has penetrated the prostate capsule. In some cases the surgeon can successfully excise this cancerous tissue and produce what amounts to a cure. In less favorable cases or because of a lack of surgical skill, some cancer tissue is left behind—a result described as leaving *positive margins*. If these cancer cells proliferate, which is generally termed *local recurrence*; this will frequently be indicated by an increase in PSA. Radiation directed at the prostate bed can kill these cells and potentially yield a permanent cure. If the cancer has spread beyond the prostate to the seminal vesicles, the lymph nodes, or even more extensively to other organs or bone, then the removal of the prostate obviously does not result in a cure. The whole idea behind active surveillance discussed above is to estimate the probability that the cancer is indeed organ confined and of a relatively non-aggressive nature. When this probability is very high, then active surveillance becomes a viable and for some a very attractive option, but this is also the ideal situation for a successful outcome for a RP. The true state of affairs is only more or less clear when the patient is opened, the prostate, seminal vesicles and lymph nodes removed and pathological examination completed.

WHEN IS A RADICAL PROSTATECTOMY A GOOD THERAPEUTIC CHOICE?

This in fact is a complicated question with a complicated set of answers. Examination of the treatment guidelines given above reveals the use of life expectancy (LE) and thus age is an important parameter. For example, individuals with low recurrence risk but with a life expectancy of less than 10 years are directed to AS or RT rather than RP. But as discussed above, life expectancy is not something that can be determined with certainty. Not only is it slowly but constantly increasing, but sudden progress in dealing with heart disease or diabetes could significantly impact such estimates. Nevertheless, using current guidelines (e.g. www.nccn.org), a RP is considered appropriate for tumor grades up to T3a, or a Gleason score up to and including 8-10, or a PSA of greater than 20 ng/mL. The difference between stage T3a and T3b is that for latter there is seminal vesicle invasion, whereas for T3a the tumor is judged to have only gone beyond the prostate capsule itself, either on one or both sides, as revealed in a DRE. That is, aside from the individual with low risk and a LE < 10 years, the low, intermediate and high risk patients are all considered eligible for a RP, and in addition, for the intermediate and high risk categories, there are no life expectancy considerations for deciding between RP and other options, although if patients in the high risk group have multiple adverse factors it is suggested they be shifted to the very high risk group where only hormone therapy or radiation or both are considered appropriate [20]. The patient with a low risk of recurrence but with a life expectancy of less than 10 years is steered away from surgery because of quality of life considerations associated with RP related morbidity which is considered in general greater than that associated with modern external beam radiotherapy or brachytherapy, and as well, the observation that the probability is less than 20% that a low-risk patient will die of PC within 10 years of diagnosis [20]. Some men may feel that this relegates more importance to the LE estimate than it deserves, given that is at best an informed guess. Some may elect an RP anyway simply because they consider this a way of increasing the chances of completely eradicating the cancer and avoiding obstructive urinary problems down the road.

The conventional wisdom holds that age is an important determinant in the recommendation of a RP and over 50% of North American urologists believe that 70 should be an upper limit for this procedure. This view appears based in part on studies that revealed increased risk of short-term complications in older men, but the problem is that these studies were not adjusted for existing comorbidity [37]. In a study published in the *Journal of the National Cancer Institute*, Alibhai *et al* [37] examined mortality and complications occurring within 30 days of RP surgery. The information was culled from medical records of over 11,000 men who underwent this surgery between 1990 and 1999. Over 200 separate potentially coexisting medical conditions were included which ranged over cardiac, respiratory, vascular, wound/bleeding, and genitourinary conditions to which they added a large number of miscellaneous medical and surgical factors. Trends for 30-day complications with age were statistically significant only with preexisting cardiac and respiratory problems. Increasing comorbidity was found to be a much stronger predictor of early complications than age in most groups of comorbid conditions. Also, the authors conclude that the risk of postoperative mortality after surgery was relatively low for otherwise healthy men up to age 79 and while the risk increased with age after adjusting for comorbidity, the absolute mortality risk remained fairly small (0.66% for men between 70 and 79 as compared to the overall mortality for the whole study cohort of 0.48%). Nevertheless, for some men comorbidities exclude surgery or render it unacceptably dangerous.

The guidelines presented above do not recommend RP for patients with locally advanced disease which includes T3b *or* a Gleason score of 8-10, although this remains controversial [38]. In fact Dr. Patrick Walsh in his book on prostate cancer for lay audiences [34] published in 2002 states that "Men with T3a disease are usually not good candidates for a radical prostatectomy." But he qualifies this position by stating that some patients with minimal spread of cancer, and Gleason scores lower than 8 may benefit from surgery, especially if they are in their fifties or younger. If one uses T3b as a stage in the Memorial Sloan-Kettering online nomogram calculator (see Chapter 4), it refuses to calculate predictions unless radiation therapy is selected as the treatment of choice. Also, the preoperative nomogram published in 2004 by Ohori et al [39] from this same institution does not include T3b as a stage option in calculating predicted 5-year recurrence free probabilities after RP.

Recently published studies from the Mayo Clinic [38,40,41] suggests that surgery may be more appropriate for patients clinically staged T3 including T3b and Gleason 8-10 than is generally recognized. In fact, they have been treating some T3 cancers with RP for over 20 years. Their experience was summarized in the journal *Urological Oncology* in 2005 [38]. Over the period from 1987 to 1997 they studied 5621 men of which 841 had clinical T3 disease with the remainder clinically staged T2. The issues studied were slightly confused by the fact that some patients received hormone treatment prior to or after surgery. Freedom from local recurrence or systemic disease for men with clinically staged T3 cancer was 85%, 73%, and 67% for 5, 10 and 15 years after surgery respectively. Cancer specific survival for this group for the same periods was 95%, 90% and 79% respectively. This can be compared to the 5-year survival rate for patients with clinically assigned stage T3 if left untreated which is only 60-70%. It is of interest that 27% of men clinically staged T3 in this study were in fact T2 upon pathological staging. Walsh [34] also mentions over-staging in this context. Walsh points out that over-staging has denied the RP option to some patients, especially when anyone with T3 disease was considered as an unfavorable candidate for surgery. The current guidelines (e.g. www.nccn.org) partly solve this problem by admitting T3a or Gleason 8-10 cases for consideration as RP candidates but fail to recognize the merits described by the Mayo Clinic urologists of also treating T3b patients with surgery.

Comparisons of the RP with other treatment options will be provided later in this chapter. However, in connection with the merits of treating patients clinically staged T3b with RP, additional results reported from the Mayo Clinic by Barry et al [42] are of particular interest. They found that there was no statistically significant difference in cancer-specific survival over 15 years in 1063 men treated for prostate cancer with RP as the primary therapy when the results were stratified by the findings of pre-operative DRE (T1c to T3b) whereas there were large and significant differences when the same outcome from radiotherapy was subjected to similar analysis by also stratifying with respects to stage.

Radiation therapy is an alternative that always accompanies the RP option in the current guidelines for patients with localized PC with low, intermediate or high risk of recurrence [20]. In a study published in 2001, Meitzer *et al* [43] found that US surgery rates were only 30% for patients with newly diagnosed T1-T2 cancer and only 6% for those with T3 stage. For men with a long life expectancy the RP rates were approximately 67% for the youngest with T1-T2 cancer but only 19% for those staged T3. In many discussions of the treatment of T3 disease, there is no distinction made in general between T3a and T3b. Overall, approximately 45% of men currently diagnosed with PC will be treated with RP [44].

In summary, the results of recent studies have modified the traditional view that RP should be restricted to cases where there was a low risk of recurrence. If fact, proponents of the RP as the ideal therapy for many men even with advanced localized prostate cancer are now presenting what appear to be strong arguments in favor of this position.

INTRAOPERATIVE AND EARLY POSTOPERATIVE COMPLICATIONS OF THE RADICAL PROSTATECTOMY

Short-term complications associated with prostate cancer surgery are rare. Based on a series of 1000 consecutive cases performed by a single surgeon at New York University Medical Center between 1994 and 2001 reported by Lepor *et al* [36], the following incidence figures are of interest: mortality rate—zero; any technical intraoperative complication, all with no long-term sequelae 0.8%; heart attack—0.5%; deep vein thrombosis—0.1%; and pulmonary embolism—0.3% (during the first 30 days post-op). Approximately 10% of the patients required blood transfusion. The mean hospital stay was 2.3 days. In his review [36], Lelpor quotes similar results from another high-profile institution. Lepor encourages his patients to return to normal activities within three weeks. Walsh quotes a 2% rate for the combined incidence of deep vein thrombosis and pulmonary embolism with a zero mortality rate for blood clots in a recent series of 1500 operations [34]. Walsh points out that blood loss is the most common complication during RP surgery and that it is very important that the surgeon masters the techniques for controlling bleeding and achieving a "bloodless field."

Studies of complication rates associated with the RP that are not institution specific have been obtained by the study of U.S. Medicare-Medicaid billing data. The study by Yao and Lu-Yao [45] is particularly interesting because they provide detailed data on a large number of complications related to the surgery or anesthetic which occurred during or soon after the operation. They examined claims associated with over 100,000 RPs from 1991 to 1994. The rates of complications considered serious are given in Table 4

Table 6-4. Serious immediate or early complications associated with the RP procedure from a multi-center study [45]

Complications	% of Patients
Cardiac	3.49
Respiratory	6.08
Vascular	1.53
Wound or bleeding related	0.65
Miscellaneous medical problems	0.48
Miscellaneous surgical problems	0.80

Included under respiratory complications were pulmonary embolism, 0.44% and deep vein thrombosis at 0.05%. If however, one adds up all of the complication rates, typical results obtained in a number of studies range from 20-30% [46], but it seems more meaningful to look at the rates for individual problems or small groups of problems. One patient will not have all of the complications, and in fact probably only one or two at most, if any.

Mortality rates typically range from about 0.2 to 0.5% when large numbers of procedures are considered [46]. There appears to be a connection between the mortality rate and the hospital's surgical volume. Yao and Lu-Yao [45], as part of the study described above, found the mortality for low vs. high volume hospitals increased from 0.39 to 0.63. This appears to be a general phenomenon for cancer surgery [47].

The influence the surgical volume of individual surgeons has on the outcomes they achieve is not clear. In a recent editorial, Begg and Scardino [48] comment with regard to picking a surgeon that the busier ones will probably get better outcomes but volume is an insufficient guide. They conclude "We are left with little more than word of mouth from family and friends and the subjective recommendations of personal contacts within the medical community." The point is well taken. In many jurisdictions information on hospital or specific surgeon volume and outcomes is impossible to obtain, neither surgeons nor hospitals in many places are rated, and some of the information is carefully guarded because of possible legal implications. It is unfortunately not as simple as consulting Consumer *Reports* to pick out a toaster.

Thus while the RP is not a totally risk-free surgical procedure, mortality is very low and the immediate and short-term complications are minimal, at least when the procedure is performed by a skilled surgeon with competent support and the patient has no comorbidities that put him at significant risk for some particular complication.

LONG-TERM SIDE EFFECTS OF THE RADICAL PROSTATECTOMY

Incontinence

The two major long-term side effects of the radical prostatectomy are incontinence and impotence. An additional adverse result is the leaving of so-called positive margins, i.e. all the cancerous tissue is not removed. This latter situation, while not really a side effect, nevertheless, may lead to recurrence and advanced stage cancer at some time after the surgery. Other side effects such as rectal damage are rare but can be serious and also influence the quality of life. Incontinence and impotence also obviously impact the patient's quality of life and the specter of one or both are uppermost in the minds of many men as they consider their treatment options. The perceived possibility of urinary incontinence in fact limits the widespread acceptance by both urologists and patients of radical prostatectomy as a treatment of prostate cancer [49]. As will be discussed below, the actual rate of incontinence observed in first-rate institutions is in fact very low.

In men there are two major "valves" that control urinary flow: the urethral sphincter (so-called striated urethral sphincter or distal sphincter) below the prostate and the pre-prostatic sphincter-bladder neck. The radical prostatectomy generally removes the latter sphincter leaving only the former. Thus incontinence results in general from insufficient control arising from the proper functioning of this sphincter, either due to surgical injury or aging. Thus one of the critical issues in prostatectomy related incontinence is the avoidance of surgical injury to the striated sphincter. However, there has been some interest in so-called bladder neck preservation [50,51] where the circular fibers of the bladder neck and the sphincter located within are preserved. The bladder neck runs into and is more or less indistinguishable from the prostate. The aim is to improve continence, but a major potential pitfall of this technique is a positive surgical margin, i.e. the surgical procedure may fail to remove all the cancer. However, while positive margins exist in the region of the bladder neck, the anatomical preservation of the neck was not found to increase the percentage of positive margins at this location [52]. Bladder neck preservation does not appear to be a common variation of the RP operation.

Carlson and Nitti [53] have recently reviewed continence rates following prostate surgery ascertained by self-administered questionnaires. Tremendous variability was observed. Between 7 and 47% of men utilized protective pads (diapers) and 13-69% experienced at least some leakage. As Herbert Lepor points out in his recent review [36] of the RP, there is no way to predict prior to the surgery those men at risk of developing severe incontinence, although men over 65 have greater difficulty regaining urinary control [27]. He also comments that this tremendous variability is likely due not only to the variations in the skill of the surgeon and the age of the patient, but variations in defining and quantifying incontinence probably play a role as well. Some surgeons obtain outstanding results. For example, the well known surgeon William J. Catalona recently reported on 2737 men followed for more than 18 months after RP [54]. Overall, 93% of these patients recovered urinary continence, defined as not requiring pads or other protection to keep outer garments dry. Walsh reports an identical percentage but the study was much smaller [55]. Lepor *et al* report continence rates of between 94 and 97%, depending on the definition of incontinence, after 24 months post RP. In this study over 600 men operated on by a single surgeon (H. Lepor,

Department of Urology, New York University School of Medicine) during a period between 2000 and 2004 were followed up with a questionnaire.

Patients should realize that continence improves progressively over the first two years after surgery and that in addition, there is considerable variation in how long is required before continence is restored [27,56].   Early problems should not be viewed too pessimistically. Patients should also realize that unless they have very good information regarding the incontinency rates for the surgeon doing their operation, they may be gambling that their results will compare favorably with those obtained at the top centers in the US.

Impotence and Infertility
The radical prostatectomy eliminates the possibility of ejaculation. Men who wish to consider the possibility of parenthood after surgery should bank a number of sperm samples. Failing this, it is sometimes possible to harvest sperm from the testicles using a biopsy type needle under local anesthetic. When small numbers of sperm are recovered, intracytoplasmic sperm injection is generally required to successfully fertilize an ovum and the success rate in achieving pregnancy is about 50%.

Historically, impotence was a universal side effect of the RP since both nerve bundles were excised. These nerve bundles pass along either side of the prostate like string on a package. The nerves are exceedingly fragile and in the nerve sparing operation, the process of separating the nerve bundles from the prostate surface can result in permanent damage or temporary trauma, and in addition, post surgical inflammation can cause nerve dysfunction. Patrick Walsh of Johns Hopkins University Medical School pioneered the modern-day so-called nerve-sparing operation, which when done by a surgeon skilled in this procedure generally results in a very favorable outcome. Since the primary goal of the RP is to remove all cancerous tissue, if the cancer has spread from the gland to the region of the nerve bundles, it may not be possible to preserve either one or both while still removing all the target tissue. The excellent in results preserving potency obtained by top-notch surgeons suggest that nerve bundle removal because of cancerous infiltration is somewhat rare. However as will be discussed below, when this is necessary, nerve grafting is now a possibility for restoring potency.

A recently published study by Blanco, Scardino and Eastham [57] provides an indication of impotency rates. The study involved men with localized prostate cancer having RPs between 1983 and 2003 at either Baylor College of Medicine or at Sloan-Kettering Memorial Cancer Center by one surgeon (P.T. Scardino). Only 5% of patients had a clinical stage > T2b and 4% had a Gleason Score > 7. It is interesting that less than 1% of these men required resection of both neurovascular bundles and the majority had bilateral nerve-sparing prostatectomies. Data on the recovery of erectile function was available for 785 men. Estimates of recovery of potency were 63% by 18 months and 70% by 24 months. In another study co-authored by Scardino, it was found that the probability of recovering full potency (full erections) post-RP was 37% at 1 year and 62% at 2 years [58].

In a recent review, Lepor [36] quotes studies where the percentage regaining potency after a RP ranged from 18.5% to 86%, but gives a more representative value for men less than 60 years of age with good preoperative erectile function is 70%, i.e. a 30%

rate of impotency. Thus men have in general a higher risk of impotency than incontinence after prostate cancer surgery and potency, if it improves with time, exhibits a slow and not necessarily complete recovery. There is current interest in the question of the benefit of early stimulation or assisting erections after surgery and the early use of sildenafil (Viagra) is being tested [36].

There seems little disagreement that the potency outcome is a strong and critical function of the skill of the surgeon, but as well depends on the preoperative potency. General risk factors for erectile dysfunction include advanced age, diabetes, high cholesterol, and coronary artery disease, all of which potentially are associated with lower the blood flow the penis and may adversely impact the recovery of potency [27,36].

Restoring Potency With Nerve Grafting
In the case of extraprostatic extension of tumor in the vicinity of the neurovascular bundles carrying the nerves involved in the erection process, some surgeons elect to remove one or both bundles and offer nerve grafting while others will if at all possible dissect the bundle from the tumor to preserve potency. Opinions differ as to which is prudent, given that the goal is to avoid positive margins. The nerve used in the graft is the genitofemoral nerve from within the pelvis or the sural nerve taken from the ankle. Removal of the sural nerve can leave some residual numbness which may resolve in time, whereas loosing using the genitofemoral nerve can result in numbness in the scrotum and inner thigh. The nerve grafting procedure also adds to the duration of the surgery. The availability of the nerve graft option no doubt encourages those skilled in its use to elect a more conservative approach to the problem of tumor involvement in one or both nerve bundles, and when there is any doubt, remove one or both. However, Walsh claims that in his experience, the need for a nerve graft is very rare. In his book on prostate cancer for lay audiences [34] as well as in a recent editorial [59], Walsh claims that in his experience it is almost never necessary to remove both neurovascular bundles. In a series of 2700 RPs he performed between 1986 and 1999, only seven men potent pre-op had both bundles removed. Four were not cured anyway because they had disseminated disease, and for the other three it turned out to be unnecessary. He takes the position that if a man has reached the point where it is necessary to remove both bundles because of bilateral capsular penetration, then this man is probably not curable with surgery because the disease has already spread.

Scardino and Kim [60] appear to disagree. They point out that even in the presence of disseminated disease, the slow progression frequently seen justifies the attempt to improve the quality of life by restoring potency. Scardino and Kim [60] also argue that in their experience resecting either one or both nerve bundles impacts the occurrence of positive margins in cases where there is extraprostatic extension in the nerve bundle region, and the existence and effectiveness of nerve grafts offers both patients and surgeons a solution to the dilemma of nerve-sparing to retain potency vs. wide resection of the nerve bundle to avoid positive margins. Also, in many cases the conservative approach involves unilateral resection i.e. just one nerve bundle. Scardino and Kim report [60] modestly improved erectile function with the unilateral graft since loosing even one nerve bundle impacts potency. However, they indicate that prospective, controlled trials are needed to prove the value of unilateral grafts.

Patients requiring neurovascular bundle resection, especially bilateral, may also be candidates for adjuvant hormonal or radiation therapy, and the strong adverse effect of either of these two secondary treatments on erectile function makes one wonder at the merits of the nerve graft in some if not many cases. However, aside from prolonging the surgery, there appears to be very limited morbidity associated with this procedure.

SUCCESS OF THE RADICAL PROSTATECTOMY IN LONG-TERM CANCER CONTROL

Since the number-one goal of the radical prostatectomy is the total eradication of the cancer, the success of the surgery in accomplishing this result becomes the major outcome concern. A more severe evaluation combines cancer control and recovery of urinary and sexual function. The term *trifecta* has recently been used to denote these three combined outcomes [57]. First the question of how successful the RP is in long-term cancer control will be examined.

A patient might ask his doctor, will a radical prostatectomy really cure my cancer? Does it really work? There is no yes or no answer to this question and the necessity of providing an answer based on probabilities may seem unsatisfactory to the patient. As has been discussed above, the probability of being cured or termed cancer free or having such and such a cancer free survival period depends strongly on a man's cancer stage, Gleason score, PSA at diagnosis, and the findings of the surgeon and pathologist during and after the surgery. Put simply, patients presenting with a very low risk of recurrence can have probabilities of 10 or 15-year postsurgical cancer-free survival above 90%, whereas if the clinical and pathological factors indicate intermediate or high risk, this probability can drop significantly with high risk patients having numbers below 50%.

The classification according to low, intermediate and high risk of recurrence has real significance, and is reflected in the observed risk of recurrence found in studies. Studies from a single center with a reputation for very good outcomes provide the information as to the best possible scenario. Nomograms such as the online version from Memorial Sloan-Kettering also provide excellent guidance since the database used was developed from data acquired from several centers. An example is given Table 5 of the variation of recurrence risk with pre-operative stage, Gleason Score, and PSA.

Table 6-5. Five-year probability of being recurrence free after radical prostatectomy based on the pre-operative presentation***

Clinical Stage	Clinical Gleason Score	PSA*	Rec. Risk**	5-yr Probability
T1c	3 + 3	4.1	Low	92%
T1c	4 + 3	4.1	Low	84%
T2a	3 + 3	9	Low	83%
T2b	4 + 3	20	Intermediate	31%
T3a	4 + 3	25	High	6%

* PSA prior to surgery
** From Guidelines, www.nccn.org
*** www.mskcc.org/mskcc/html/10038.ctm Memorial Sloan-Kettering Cancer Center online nomogram

The tumor stage and Gleason score can change after surgery when more information is available about the tumor extent and differentiation, size, and extra-capsular extension and the extent, if any, of spreading to the seminal vesicles, and lymph nodes. Also, the pathologist will provide information regarding the presence of positive or negative surgical margins. This then provides the data for a revised prognosis. There are obviously a large number of permutations of the various factors. The best case scenario is of course totally organ-confined disease with negative margins and no evidence of spreading to seminal vesicles or lymph nodes. The Memorial Sloan-Kettering website also has an online nomogram for predicting the post-RP probability of being recurrence free based in part on post-surgical pathological observations

The results obtained over the years at Johns Hopkins are also of interest. The results reported by Han *et al* [61] given in Table 6 based on the follow-up of 1050 men with organ confined disease as observed at surgery are instructive. The probability of being recurrence free (PSA < 0.2 ng/mL) for 10 years is presented stratified by the surgical (pathological) Gleason score and the preoperative PSA. Note that the tumor staging is replaced by the actual observed stage, in this case organ confined, which is accompanied by the best prognosis. Note that both a high pre-operative PSA and a high Gleason score dramatically reduce the chances of remaining cancer free after surgery.

Table 6-6. Ten-year recurrence free survival probabilities (%) for organ confined (≤ T2b) prostate cancer*

Surgical Gleason Score	Pre-operative PSA (ng/mL)			
	0-4.0	4.1-10.0	10.1-20	>20
5	99	97	95	90
6	97	94	91	84
3+4	92	84	83	75
4+3	82	77	70	62
8-10	63	57	52	46

*adapted from Han et al [61]

It is also informative to look at overall survival figures rather than those stratified by tumor grade etc. In the study by Han *et al* [61] from which Table 6 was derived, the authors also calculated overall recurrence free survival rates of 84%, 72% and 61% for 5, 10 and 15 years. Overall cancer specific survival rates were 99%, 96% and 89% for 5, 10 and 15 years respectively. No patient had a clinical stage greater than T2b, 4% had PSA > 20, and 6% had a clinical Gleason score of 8-10.

In the study by Bianco et al [57] discussed above in the context of side effects, the authors also examined the overall success of the RP in 1746 patients. At 5, 10 and 15 years cancer-specific survival was 99%, 95% and 89% respectively. Over the same three time intervals, 82%, 77% and 75% were free from recurrence (disease progression). The 15-year probabilities of death from prostate cancer vs. other causes were similar at 32% and 33%, respectively. In terms of clinical stage, only 5% of the patients were >T2b. In terms of the clinical Gleason score, only 4% were in the 8-10 range. There was significant Gleason score upgrading from postoperative pathological findings. The percentage with Gleason 7 went from 26% to 45%.

It is well known that the advent of PSA testing has been responsible for significant stage migration. As many as 75% of men now present with only an elevated PSA and a normal DRE, i.e. stage T1c disease. A recent study from Johns Hopkins focuses on this group with respect to the question of recurrence [62]. 1149 patients staged T1c who underwent a RP between 1998 and 2000 were stratified into two groups, T1cI and T1cII. The former had a preoperative PSA of < 10 *and* a clinical Gleason score of < 7, whereas the T1cII group had a PSA > 10 *or* a clinical Gleason of ≥ 7. The 5, 10 and 15 year rates of freedom from recurrence (PSA > 0.2 ng/mL) were 98%, 96% and 96% for the T1cI group and 86%, 83% and 73% for the T1cII group, respectively. In addition, the recurrence- free probabilities for the T1cII group were virtually identical to a T2a group for whom data was also available from Hopkins. These results emphasize the importance of treatment before the PSA level exceeds 10 and the poorer outcomes when the clinical Gleason score is 7 or greater. The excellent results in group T1cI also indicate the success of surgery in achieving what amounts to a cure in all but 4% of the patients with these clinical characteristics. They also found that patients with less than 50% of any single biopsy core positive for cancer gave a much more favorable prognosis than if the percentage was greater than 50% maximal core involvement.

The range of results presented above indicates that there is no simple answer to the question, has surgery cured my cancer? Reference to the Memorial Sloan-Kettering online nomogram for post-surgical predictions will only reinforce this point. The reader is encouraged to experiment with this nomogram and examine the effect of organ confined vs. non-organ confined disease, positive margins etc., and observe the dramatic decline in the probability of remaining recurrence free as the number of adverse items is increased. It should also be clear from the above tables that the prognosis after a RP is significantly improved for low pre-operative PSA, Gleason score less that 7, and tumor stage T1c or less. This reinforces the argument that PSA screening and early detection have real merit. Also, the Han *et al* study [61] found 5, 10, and 15 year metastasis-free survival rates of 96%, 89% and 81%. The average time from observing metastasis to PC related death is typically 5 years, so being metastasis free at 15 years post RP means that one can expect, on average, at least not dying from PC before a total of 20 years have elapsed.

POSITIVE SURGICAL MARGINS

Of the various factors influencing recurrence of prostate cancer after RP, only the surgical margin status can in general be influenced by the surgeon's skill and judgment. In establishing the presence of positive surgical margins, the pathologist looks at the edges of the tissue that has been cut out during surgery. The external surface of the prostate is generally painted with indelible ink with different colors denoting the right and left sides. Any tumor cells in the inked area are considered margin positive. If no cancer appears on these areas, the margin is negative and this implies that the cancerous tissue is totally contained in the tissue removed. If a margin is positive, there exists the possibility that cancer tissue was left on the other side, i.e. it is still present in the patient at the end of the operation, and may be contribute to recurrence. While one might think that this is obviously an unsatisfactory situation, the actual prognostic importance of positive margins is unclear and the subject of debate [63]. Swindle *et al* have recently studied this question with data collected from about 1400 patients undergoing RPs at Baylor College of Medicine [63]. As they discuss in their paper, an important factor in the inconsistent results obtained when an attempt is made to connect positive margins with outcome is the problem of accounting for the influence of adjuvant therapy prompted at least in part by the presence of positive margins. Swindle *et al* attempted to account for this factor in their statistical analysis and were able to confirm that positive surgical margins had a significant adverse impact on recurrence. Overall, patients with positive surgical margins had a 10-year progression free probability (PSA $\leq$ 0.4 ng/mL confirmed by one subsequent measurement) of 58% whereas those with negative margins had 81%. The difference was statistically highly significant. The difference in progression probability was apparent already in the early months after surgery and virtually the full effect was seen after 5 years (See Fig.1, [63]). The incidence of positive surgical margins has decreased over recent years. Han *et al* [64] associate this with the downward stage migration in the PSA era and the accompanying increase in the percentage of patients presenting with organ confined disease rather than an improvement in surgical technique. They point to the stable percentage of positive margins among men with pathologically staged T3 disease.

Surgical techniques associated with minimizing positive margins interact with the problem of preserving potency in the case where extraprostatic extension occurs in the region of the neurovascular bundle. As might be expected, the more conservative approach can result in a higher level of impotency [40,65]. Researchers from Johns Hopkins have reported a study of this problem which emphasizes the importance of visual and tactile assessment during open surgery which provides valuable information on when and where it is safe to preserve the neurovascular bundle in patients with extraprostatic extension of their tumor. This raises serious questions regarding techniques where the tactile information is absent such as laprascopic surgery [65].

It is interesting that the postoperative margin status has assumed a central position along with short-term PSA elevation in evaluating laprascopic and robotic assisted laprascopic prostatectomies and the associated quality of tumor excision. These procedures are so new that long-term oncological results are not generally available.

SUMMARY—CONVENTIONAL RP

The retropubic radical prostatectomy meets the definition of an effective treatment if it is defined on the basis of the complete removal of the prostate, excision of the lymph nodes, and acceptable margin rates. The following quotation from an editorial [66] by the urologist Gerald Andriole from Washington University School of Medicine in St. Louis (a center of excellence in prostate cancer treatment) nicely sums up as this section on the RP: "Indeed, the urologic community at large should be applauded for its diligence in learning and continually refining open radical perineal and retropubic prostatectomy for the past 20 years. Our collective success in performing an effective radical prostatectomy is evident by the high cancer control rates and by the steadily decreasing morbidity and mortality rates as reported in numerous series."

LAPRASCOPIC AND ROBOTIC PROSTATE SURGERY

LAPRASCOPIC RP

The first laprascopic radical prostatectomy (LRP) was reported in 1997. The technique attracted interest and recently several large series have been reported from France and Germany. These studies demonstrated that LRP offers reasonable operative outcomes and an alternative to open surgery that can result in reduced patient morbidity, shorter hospital stays and more rapid resumption of everyday activities. However, these promising results were obtained by groups with considerable skill in the art of laprascopic prostate surgery developed by doing 600-700 procedures.

In the laprascopic procedure, instruments for viewing, cutting and suturing, manipulation and suction are introduced through small abdominal incisions. The working area is inflated with carbon dioxide to generate space in which to operate. The required skills are generally learned first with a "dry lab" box, then in some institutions by operations on animals, and finally mentored learning during real operations. This last learning phase is considered to be critical [67]. Some countries have organized structured courses including animal surgery to prepare surgeons for the mentored phase. An interesting paradox has arisen in centers where almost all procedures are now done laprascopically—residents and fellows are gaining only limited skill and experience in open surgery. This is a problem because anyone doing a LRP must be ready with the skills and surgical tools at hand to switch (called conversion) to the open procedure if problems arise which cannot be handled laprascopically. For example, in a multi-center study of conversion to open RP, 13 out of 670 operations required this change in procedure [68].

Judging the cancer related success of LRP is difficult because of the short history of the technique. Insufficient follow-up time has elapsed to permit the collection of meaningful recurrence data. In the absence of such data, the percent positive surgical margins has been used as an early surrogate marker for success in cancer eradication. Trabulsi and Guillonneau from Memorial Sloan-Kettering [69] have recently published a review on the LRP in which they discuss this aspect. The percent positive margins found in 9 studies ranged from 11.4 to 26%. The positive margin rate depends on the distribution of tumor stage in the cohort as well as the skill and judgment of the surgeon. In general, it is concluded LRP and open RP are achieving approximately the same results as measured by this yardstick. Also, comparison stratified by pathological tumor stage yielded similar positive margin rates for open RP and LRP. It has been recently suggested [70] that the use of frozen sections during surgery should be considered to attempt to improve the negative margin rate in LRP but at present this is not commonly done.

The two other important outcomes, potency and urinary continence, appear roughly the same when LRP is compared with open RP, although the comparison for potency is complicated by differing definitions and follow-up time [70].

There is a considerable variation in complication rates associated with LRP. Trabulsi and Guillonneau [70] in their review of 13 reports find a range from 3.6 to 34%. They comment that unclear and non-standardized reporting of complication rates makes interpretation difficult, and the learning curve associated with this new technique "skews the results strongly." There are two different laprascopic approaches used, one via the peritoneal cavity and the other extraperitoneal. The former is accompanied by a risk of inadvertent bowel injury and if the connection between the bladder and the urethra leaks after the connection is made, urine leaking into the peritoneal cavity can cause problems. An inexperienced surgeon can do serious damage merely while inserting the laprascopic tools or can encounter problems or a crisis situation that can only be rectified by switching to open surgery. Some surgeons doing mostly or entirely LRPs may not be highly skilled in the conventional operation which they may be forced to undertake. A recent multicenter study of forced conversion to conventional open surgery at seven institutions found a rate of about 2%, and that the need for conversion was more likely to occur during a surgeon's early experience with the laprascopic technique [68]. Forced conversion may thus result in higher morbidity.

Thus in general LRP compares favorably with open RP, especially in centers where laprascopic techniques have been perfected and a high standard maintained. Its growing popularity is also related to the quicker recovery and shorter hospital stay (and perhaps because it is currently very fashionable). There is however, a learning curve, and some surgeons claim several hundred procedures are necessary to achieve a high level of competence [67,69]. It is not uncommon that surgeons already have extensive laprascopic experience from, for example, kidney surgery, prior to learning the LRP, and of course this leads to a much more rapid development of proficiency. Initially, learning is mentored in many centers and men must realize that their laprascopic operation may be done in part by inexperienced hands by an individual just learning the technique. While no doubt the effectiveness of the mentoring is strongly related to the risk of a bad outcome or a disaster, some men would probably prefer not to take such an active part in a training program but rather have their operation done entirely by an experienced surgeon. However, it should be recognized that some surgeons learned the modern nerve-sparing open RP techniques as residents and fellows and honed their skills actually doing the procedure, either in part or entirely on numerous patients. That is the way surgeons are trained! The best institutions in general will also be those with large and active resident and fellowship programs, which complicates the problem for one seeking one of the best laprascopic surgeon to do the whole operation. Also, attempting to determine where a given surgeon is on the laprascopic learning curve may be impossible. The problem of selecting an institution and a surgeon for any highly complex and challenging surgery will always be difficult unless the patient has a really reliable and trustworthy inside track to critical and frequently carefully guarded information. It is also worth remembering that July 1 is an especially significant day in medicine. It is when some of the residents leave and are replaced by the incoming group who, by comparison, are obviously lacking in experience.

ROBOTIC LAPRASCOPIC RP

The evolution of the laprascopic concept has resulted in radical prostatectomies done almost entirely by a robot. The surgeon sits at a computer console and controls the robotic tools that have been inserted in the patient. Using robotics deals with certain limitations of conventional laparoscopy. These limitations include counterintuitive movements associated with the required manipulations, rigid instruments, two-dimensional images and limited ergonomics. A surgeon experienced in the open RP generally finds the robotic operation more akin to the classical surgery and the stereoscopic 3-dimensional view with considerable available magnification an advantage.

As with the conventional LRP, there is a learning curve. In a recent paper in the journal *Urology*, the Vanderbilt urologist J. A. Smith, Jr. discusses his experience in learning the robotic approach. He brought to this undertaking experience with over 2500 open RPs, and as well was working with a fellowship-trained laprascopic surgeon as table-side assistant (the co-author of the report). He was not able to routinely obtain results comparable to the open RP until after more than 150 robotic procedures. While it is impossible to generalize the experience of one surgeon, nevertheless this report emphasizes what others have repeatedly pointed out, i.e. there is a significant learning curve to laprascopic surgery in general (of which the robotic approach is a variation), and early results will probably not be optimal, either for the patient or for the satisfaction of the surgeon. On the other hand, a report from the Urology Centers of Alabama reports a short learning curve of approximately 20-25 cases, and this center reports very favorable functional and oncological results and minimal perioperative complications [71].

In the US, the development of the robotic LRP has taken place principally at the Vattikuti Urology Institute of the Henry Ford Hospital in Detroit using the da Vinci master-slave robot. The surgeon, seated comfortably at the console, manipulates the instruments with his fingers and the camera with his foot. The camera provides a 3-dimensional stereoscopic view with capability for 10- to 15-fold magnification. Finger movements can be scaled to yield high precision in delicate dissection. A disadvantage is a high initial investment (currently over one million US) and high maintenance costs.

In a recent report from the Vattikuti Institute, Menon et al [72] report on a comparison between 100 open RPs, 50 conventional LRPs, and 565 robotic RPs, the latter done over the period from 2001 to 2005. Their current robotic protocol is in fact called the *Vattikuti Institute Prostatectomy* [73]. Currently over 95% of patients admitted to the Vattikuti Institute choose robotic over open surgery. In the comparative study, odds ratios for operative times, blood loss, postoperative pain, complications, and median times to urinary continence and resumption of sexual activity were all lower (i.e. more favorable) for robotic than for open or laprascopic surgery. Positive margins averaged 6%. In a comparison of positive margin results between the open RP, LRP and the robotic LRP, the robotic approach resulted in about one-third the positive margin rates of the other procedures. However, overall positive margin rates are deceptive since they may depend on the distribution of cases within the various tumor stages. Menon *et al* do not provide the required data and other centers using robotic LRP do not in general achieve this low a positive margin rate and in fact obtain results similar to RP and LRP [74].

Only a limited number of centers worldwide have published results with the robotic LRP [74]. According to the review by Perrotti and Moran [74], more than 200 da Vinci robotic surgical systems have been installed worldwide. It is estimated that 9000 robotic RPs were performed in 2004. The authors conclude that the robotic RP has an advantage of less blood loss and shorter hospital stay than open RP. However, Herrell and Smith point out that how significant these and other differences really are is debatable [75]. There is considerable commercial promotion that describes the conventional RP in terms that only apply to somewhat inferior centers and surgeons [75] which of course makes either LRP or the robotic RP look very good. In fact, with variable results from all three approaches depending on the medical center quality and surgeon skill and a wide range of definitions whereby outcome are judged, truly meaningful comparisons are difficult in general and impossible for a patient to extrapolate to his local hospital and urological surgeons. There is also the problem that early experiences are rarely included in the robotic data published. Herrel and Smith make the following points [75]:

- As regards blood loss, in their institution (Vanderbilt University Medical School) only 1% of men having an open RP need blood products, which leaves little room for improvement.
- They also find that their patients undergoing open RP with an 8-9 cm incision have little postsurgical pain and thus there is again little room for improvement.

- When blood loss, pain, time to discharge or time to catheter removal are considered, the Vanderbilt experience is that the results with open RP and the robotic RP are very similar. They emphasize that their robotic results match any of the reported robotic series.
- They have not found that the robotic RP is any less invasive than open RP in "any clinically meaningful manner."
- The morbidity accompanying surgery (perioperative) with the open RP has been diminished to the point where the laprascopic techniques have little opportunity for improvement.

Herrel and Smith go on to argue that the aspects of the procedural outcome discussed above are in fact less important than tumor control, continence and potency, the three outcomes which should be of primary concern to both the surgeon and the patient. Small differences is discharge time, clinically irrelevant differences in blood markers at time of discharge, or minor differences is postoperative pain are really of little consequence compared to whether or not, for example, the patient goes home with positive surgical margins! However, for the three really important outcomes the authors suggest that in the final analysis the robotic procedure may well be better than the open surgery. Part of the reason for this opinion is the exceptional visualization, minimal traction on the neurovascular bundle, and the precision with which tissue can be dissected, incised and sutured. They express "cautious enthusiasm" for the robotic approach. Herrel and Smith make a strong point of the fact that the open RP in the hands of an expert surgeon is already very good indeed with respect to any measure one wishes to apply, and that care must be taken not to overemphasize the significance of marginal improvements.

For men in need of a RP who live in the in an area where the robotic RP has been perfected, is being used on a routine basis with good results from a significant number of cases, perhaps even reported in the literature, this option would appear worth considering. There are very few such places (some of which are Nashville TN, Detroit MI, Birmingham AL, Irvine CA, Paris France). Some men may want to make sure that they are not among the first patients to undergo robotic surgery with a newly acquired robot. Also, there may be financial impediments to selecting this option.

RADIATION THERAPY (RADIOTHERAPY)

Radiation therapy (RT) is administered either by an external beam of radiation or radiation emitted from pellets or other radioactive sources actually inserted surgically into the prostate. The latter is called *brachytherapy*. The first radiation therapy for prostate cancer was apparently performed in the early 20th century at Hopkins. Radium or radon containing pellets were implanted but this was long before the dangers of radiation exposure were appreciated and both patients and practitioners suffered injury. It was not until after the World War II that the dangers of radiation became apparent. This early brachytherapy was not particularly successful because of the highly uneven distribution of radiation due to less than optimal pellet placement. The first external beam therapy employed gamma rays from colbalt-60, a byproduct (fission product) of the operation of nuclear reactors. Since the source radiates uniformly in all directions, shielding was necessary to obtain a collimated beam, i.e. to generate with shielding a beam the radiation will fall on the desired area and then penetrate to and irradiate the prostate, *and incidentally anything else in the beam path before or after the prostate.* Control of dosage and collimation proved difficult and there were severe side effect including damage to both the bladder and rectum, and because of limitations regarding on dose, recurrence was common.

The field of external beam RT was revolutionized by the development of the linear accelerator in the late 1950s. Electrons accelerated to very high energies strike a heavy metal target (e.g. gold plated tantalum). The changes in kinetic energy that result when these high speed electrons are deflected by the nuclei of the target atoms generate high energy electromagnetic radiation (x-rays or more properly gamma-rays) called bremssthralung which in modern machines can reach energies of 20 or more million electron volts (MEV). For comparison, the Co-60 gamma ray energy is 1.66 MEV. For comparison, diagnostic x-rays are in the kilo-electron volt range. RT using a linear accelerator is now called traditional RT. These very high external beam energies are actually enough to cause both electron and gamma induced nuclear reactions with the resultant development of low-level radioactive contamination of the machine and the air in the treatment suite. When adapted to deliver a collimated beam of electromagnetic radiation, therapy could be accomplished with higher dose as well as greater targeting precision and safety than with the Co-60 source. The overall results were nevertheless considerably inferior to those obtained today with what might be termed third generation external beam therapy.

The first big advance came in the late 1980s when highly sophisticated beam definition was combined with accurate information gained from a CT scan or MRI as to the location of the prostate relative to the bladder, rectum and surrounding structures. The use of computer programs allowed much more precise targeting of the prostate and allowed the operator to minimize the dose to surrounding areas, and especially the rectum, where the most serious side effects of traditional RT occurred. If an advantage was to be gained from this advance in technique, exact reproducible positioning of the patient for each treatment became essential. This approach is called *Three-Dimensional Conformal Radiation Therapy* (3D-CRT), conformal because the beam conforms closely to the shape of the target (i.e. the prostate). The 3D-CRT approach (some call it the hypothesis) predominantly aims to reduce surrounding tissue side effects at a given dose compared to conventional EBRT, and by doing this allows for an escalation of dose with the hope of increasing tumor control rates. In the last few years 3D-CRT has been significantly improved by technology which allows modulation of the intensity over the target field and thus permits even more precise control of the dose-area problem. This technique is called *Intensity Modulated Radiation Therapy* (IMRT). If radiation oncology departments using one of these three external beam RT protocols were rated with the famous system used to rank French restaurants, IMRT would get two stars, 3D-CRT one, and traditional RT would probably now be absent altogether from the guide book! The awarding of three stars would await long-term results with IMRT. IMRT is not available at all centers where 3D-CRT radiation therapy is provided, but there seems little disagreement that men electing RT should at least seek out clinics that routinely do 3D-CRT [19].

Even with the state-of-the-art technology represented by 3D-CRT and IMRT, the best results are only obtained if the prostate is located exactly relative to the radiation beam on each treatment (generally daily, 5 times a week). While considerable effort goes into determining prior to the first treatment just where the patient is placed under the machine and attempts to reproduce this day after day are made, the prostate can move in response to the bladder and rectal filling and there is an inherent variation in the daily optimal positioning. This results in the use of a slightly larger beam than is theoretically necessary or desirable in order to "play it safe" and this results in increased exposure of surrounding tissue and the probability of radiation-induced morbidity and as well reduces the dose that can be safely given [76]. Typical beam enlargement to correct for these problems is 10-15 mm [76]. A recent solution is to implant several inert markers into the prostate which are then used daily to refine the patient positioning relative to the radiation beam. The ability to deliver radiation to within 2 mm of the desired location is claimed [76]. This also allows margins of the radiation field to be accurately adjusted according to the clinical presentation of the patient, and in particular the suspected extraprostatic extensions.

The fact that these refinements of the traditional RT are fairly recent makes it difficult to assess the efficacy of 3D-CRT in preventing recurrence over the long-term (>10 years). This is especially true when the variables of dose protocol, tumor staging, etc. also have to be taken into account. Some short term studies of efficacy and safety of 3D-CRT are now beginning to appear which should give a good indication of side effects to be expected both short and long term. All the long term data apply to traditional RT, the longest covering over 20 years [35], but this data is mostly of interest to those studying the improvements obtained by modern RT. If we have reached a plateau of technology (some openly ridicule this notion) with modern RT (3D-CRT and IMRT) which will allow the collection of meaningful recurrence data over 10-15 years with a fixed protocol, then it will be possible to compare modern RT with the modern radical prostatectomy, for which there is data collected over a 10-15 years with only minor changes in technique, changes that probably do not significantly impact recurrence-free survival. For a man weighing his options as regards treatment, using older data that pertains to traditional RT would appear to have little merit except to set a lower limit which modern treatment would be expected to exceed. RT also has the same inherent problem as RP, namely that the results vary with the skill of those involved. With RP it is mainly the surgeon's skill, but with RT there is a team involved in treatment planning, imaging, positioning the patient reproducibly, adjusting the beam dimensions, angles, intensity distribution, and dose protocol. Some of the personnel involved may even change over the course of the treatment schedule. The patient selecting the external beam RT option is obviously well advised to seek out an institution has a reputation for first-class modern RT. Reliable information is not always readily available!

With regard to any therapy for PC, there is always the question of how well the approach works. How is treatment failure identified in order to acquire data on success or failure? The prostate is still there, and thus both biopsies and the DRE can reveal recurrence. In addition, PSA measurements are informative. After RT, the PSA should fall over a fairly extended period to some low value (the so-called nadir). If after this, the PSA level starts to increase, this is generally an indication of treatment failure, although there are several competing definitions as to what constitutes significant failure. Since PSA is the easiest parameter to follow, many studies use this as an indicator. This will be discussed at length in a subsequent chapter. For the present purposes, the observation of recurrence in the context of treatment success or failure will be used without detailed analysis of the criteria used.

Radiation oncologists started using 3D-CRT in the late 1980s and by 1994 there were already very positive and encouraging results being published. Eng *et al* [77] have provided a recent review of the efficacy of 3D-CRT. The principal issue associated with outcomes related to recurrence involves dose escalation since this was one of the main motivations for the evolution of this modern protocol. By the late 80s it had become apparent that the doses being used (60-70 Gy—*Gray Scale*, a unit for measuring radiation intensity) were in many cases too low to produce good disease free survival results and the 3D-CRT approach allowed significant dose escalation without an accompanying increase in serious side effects such as impotence, incontinence and rectal damage. Eng *et al* review a number of studies published between 1994 and 2004 and found that considerable improvements in disease-free survival accompany increases in dose above 70 Gy and that the total dose that is indicated today is at least 76 Gy for patients with favorable prognosis and a higher dose (e.g. 80 Gy) for men with unfavorable prognosis. Favorable prognosis in this context was stage T1-T2, pretreatment PSA < 10, Gleason score < 6 whereas intermediate prognosis was T2b-T3, or PSA > 10 or Gleason >6. Presence of *any two* of these intermediate measures indicated unfavorable prognosis. For example, Zelefsky *et al* [78,79] found for a median follow-up of 5 years, that patients in every risk group had better PSA related disease-free survival when the dose was greater than 75.6 Gy as compared to lower doses and that patients with an unfavorable prognosis appeared to benefit from doses of 81 Gy or higher. In this later case, the 5-year survival rates were 69% for the use of 81.6 Gy compared to 43% and 24% for those who received 75.6Gy or a lower dose, respectively—obviously a strong dose dependence. Eng *et al* also discuss other studies that support these observations. However, one study found no dose effect for patients with pretreatment PSA greater than 20 mg/dL, but it is not clear if the dose this group received reached 81Gy. Clearly, some patients in the unfavorable category will already have undetected disseminated disease which will evolve no matter how much the prostate is irradiated, simply because the problem in part lies elsewhere. Long-term, or even 5-year PSA related disease-free survival rates for the IMRT protocol are not available at this writing. However, Zelefsky *et al* [80] have reported preliminary results for 3 years of follow-up for 772 patients treated with IMRT at 81 Gy. The rates were 93%, 84% and 81% for patients with favorable, intermediate and unfavorable features, respectively. These results are comparable to those with obtained with ordinary 3D-CRT and suggest that the variable intensity within the beam associated with IMRT does not compromise the oncological results. *The authors comment that IMRT has become the standard mode of 3D-CRT for localized PC at their institution (Memorial Sloan-Kettering Cancer Center, New York, NY).*

SIDE EFFECTS OF CURRENT EXTERNAL BEAM RT

During RT some men complain of decreased energy, weight loss, altered appetite and fatigue but according to Scardino, about 85% of patients have no such problems [27]. In his experience and presumably that of his colleagues at Memorial Sloan-Kettering,

10% will have gastrointestinal or rectal bleeding during or soon after treatment. Urgency, frequency and other urinary symptoms are experienced by about half of RT patients. These side effects generally clear up about two months after treatment.

Long-term side effects are of course a major issue with all treatments for PC. Morris and eleven other radiation oncologists have prepared a review of the outcomes of 3D-CRT vs. traditional external beam RT [81]. From an analysis of the literature up to 2002, this task force concluded:

- A reduction in acute toxicity occurred when 3D-CRT was used. Higher doses were possible with the conformal protocol with the same acute toxicity as with lower doses used in traditional RT. Thirty studies were reviewed.
- As regards late toxicity, the task force concluded from the data available from 9 studies that late morbidity, particularly late gastrointestinal morbidity was lower with 3D-CRT compared to traditional RT provided the dose to the rectum was limited. On the other hand, they found no added benefit in terms of urinary symptoms or sexual function.

At Memorial Sloan-Kettering, Zelefsky *et al* [27,79] found that the incidence radiation induced bowel injury was greatly reduced with 3D-CRT as compared to conventional RT. They found a rate of 17% with modern 3D-CRT and a dramatic reduction to 2-3% when IMRT was used. As regards erectile dysfunction, Scardino quotes a rate of 40-50% of patients experiencing this side effect with the risk higher for older men and those with erectile difficulties prior to treatment. However, about three-fourths of men with post-treatment impotence found medications such as sildenafil (Viagra) helpful [27].

BRACHYTHERAPY

CONVENTIONAL BRACHYTHERAPY

Brachytherapy involves permanent radioactive seed or pellet implantation directly into the prostate. Historically this was the first used radiation therapy for prostate cancer. A number of different techniques have been used but until the early 1980s, the oncological results were poor compared to traditional RT or RP. The radioactive seeds were implanted via the retropubic route which turned out to be very imprecise with non-uniformity of radiation common and with excessive radiation on occasion damaging the rectum, bladder or urethra. Brachytherapy was saved in the early 80s from falling into disuse by the use of CT imaging and ultrasound-guided perineal implantation. The initial approach involved pre-planning the optimal location of the seeds and the real-time visualization of the implantation process. Also, implantation through the perineum rather than through the abdomen turned out to be a significant advance. This is called pre-planned implantation and requires the collaboration of the radiation oncologist and a medical physicist, and as well computer software for optimization.

The next significant advance came when pre-planning was replaced by intra-operative planning. This avoided the technical problems associated with variation of the exact configurations of the prostate, rectum, bladder and urethra of the pre-plan obtained on the anaesthetized patient as compared with the actual anatomy during the operation. This avoided intraoperative adjustments and the failure of the final configuration of seeds to match the optimum pattern. Under-dosing was in fact a serious problem if prostate changes were not compensated for in real time. Overdosing of the intraprostatic urethra, bladder and rectum is also avoided. With this so-called intraoperative conformal optimization and planning approach, computer assisted optimization occurs during the operation. This protocol has in fact been used since 1996 at Memorial Sloan-Kettering Cancer Center and as of 2003, 700 patients have been treated with this version of brachytherapy [82]. The time required for the entire planning process requires only about 10-20 minutes which was not considered a significant increase in operating time.

Fundamental to brachytherapy is the concept of the range (distance or depth of penetration) of radiation from a source. With the radioactive isotopes used in seed implants, the energy of the radiation is such that most is absorbed in a very short distance from the seed. This not only allows control over the irradiation of tissue outside the prostate, but also means that the patient is not putting family and associates at risk by in fact being a dangerous radiation source. Two artificially radioactive isotopes are commonly used, Iodine-125 (I-125) and Palladium-103. They have different half-lives (time for the radiation intensity to decrease by ½) of 17 days palladium and 60 days for iodine. The tumor killing ability of these two isotopes appears to be similar but the longer-lived I-125 produces a slower PSA decline. The integrated dose (summed) is much higher with brachytherapy than with external beam RT, but it is of course delivered over a much longer period.

How does brachytherapy compare with IMRT or 3D-CRT as judged by recurrence rates? This is obviously a key question. In a recent review, Zelefsky [82] reports a study comparing intraoperative planned brachytherapy with high-dose IMRT (81 Gy) as regards PSA detected recurrence. The median follow-up was 4 years and the PSA related disease-free survival results were 96% and 90% for the Brachytherapy vs. the IMRT patients, respectively. The patients were all in the favorable risk category. Zelefsky et al [83] found in a comparison of acute urinary symptoms during pre-planned vs. intraoperative planned brachytherapy that the latter resulted in improved urinary tolerance and reduced urethral irradiation. Resolution of urinary symptoms was also more rapid with the intraoperative planning group.

SIDE EFFECTS OF 3D-CRT AND BRACHYTHERAPY

The recovery of sexual function after external radiation or brachytherapy has been reviewed by Hollenbeck *et al* [84]. The comparison of external beam RT and brachytherapy reveals similar results for the two treatment modalities as regards a variety of measures of sexual function. For example, for men over 60 years old, the percentage reporting small or no sexual problems was in the range of 50-58% independent of which mode of RT was used. Miller and Theodorescu [85] have also reviewed the impact of brachytherapy on sexual function. Problems with potency develop over several years after implantation. Miller and Theodorescu quote 5- or 6-year potency rates at 53% and 59% in two studies and 76 in a third. Addition of either external beam RT or hormone therapy to brachytherapy negatively impacts potency rates.

More detailed comparison of side effects associated with 3D-CRT and intraoperative planned brachytherapy does not seem warranted. Comparisons are confounded by pretreatment factors such as pretreatment potency, age, prior treatment for BPH, and urinary function status. Brachytherapy protocol is far from standardized. 3D-CRT protocol is also variable depending on risk status which can control dose and extent of the radiation beam margins. Recent switch to IMRT further complicates comparisons, especially if IMRT and 3D-CRT results are pooled. Nevertheless, it is difficult to ignore the apparent superiority of both IMRT and intraoperative planned brachytherapy as state of the art approaches to the use of radiation in the treatment of localized prostate cancer. They also appear to produce similar oncological outcomes and appeal to many men because they are less invasive than surgery.

It may strike some readers as curious that on the one hand, radiation is used to "cure" cancer, and on the other it is universally recognized and feared as a cause of cancer. The study of the incidence of cancer in the Japanese atomic bomb survivors has in fact provided one of the most informative sources of data concerning the long-term effects of ionizing radiation (alpha, beta, gamma and x-radiation) in the etiology of cancer. Those who feel strongly about the dangers recommend keeping even diagnostic x-rays to an absolute minimum, point out that the effects are probably cumulative, and that one should minimize exposure over and above what is uncontrollable, namely radiation from cosmic rays and from the materials that surround us, including building materials and radon gas seeping into some basements, although this latter source can be more or less eliminated with proper ventilation if its presence is recognized. Also, compared to a chest x-ray, the radiation exposure from a CT scan is many times greater, something that may not be pointed out to asymptomatic individuals eagerly seeking whole body scans in the hope of early detection of some disease or disorder. Clearly this is another of the seemingly endless risk-reward problems confronting those subject to ministrations of modern medicine, which includes most of us.

One of the major concerns in RT technology is to minimize the radiation delivered to the rectum which is just behind the back surface of the prostate. Side effects involving the damage to the rectum are very common. But there is another obvious concern—does RT for PC increase rate or risk of rectal cancer? In a recent retrospective cohort study comparing the incidence of rectal cancer in 30,552 men receiving RT vs. 55,263 undergoing surgery only, Baxter *et al* found a hazard ratio of 1.7 (i.e. nearly twice the risk) for the incidence of rectal cancer among those having RT vs. those treated surgery [86]. Case control studies discussed for comparison by the authors provide weaker evidenced but the large retrospective study of Baxter *et al* was better powered to detect this effect [86,87]. In an accompanying editorial, Grady and Russell [87] point out that because of the shift to younger men selecting RT as a treatment, individuals having RT should be followed up with the same guidelines as those with a family history of colorectal cancer, i.e. an endoscopic exam every 5 years. This recommendation is based on the hypothesis that rectal cancer induced by therapeutic radiation may take a number of years to become clinically evident. This is obviously another example of the risk-reward dilemma, but also highlights the merits of those radiation therapy techniques that minimize the exposure of the rectum, even though the primary motivation is not rectal cancer prevention but rectal damage minimization, especially as the dose is escalated.

HIGH DOSE RATE BRACHYTHERAPY WITH OR WITHOUT EBRT [88]

A variation of conventional brachytherapy involves using high intensity radioactive seeds (actually small pieces of iridium wire containing the radioactive isotope iridium 192 (Ir-192) which are left in place only a short period. This is called *high dose radiation (HDR) brachytherapy* or *temporary interstitial prostate brachytherapy*. Some also call it the Andy Grove (of Intel Inc. fame) treatment. He elected this treatment and later wrote a cover story for Fortune magazine describing his agonizing and research regarding cancer treatments. The HDR-brachytherapy process of inserting and removing the radiation sources is repeated several times over a period days or weeks. It is common practice to introduce the HDR therapy during a pause in the EBRT, but it is also done before or after the EBRT. The sources are placed in hollow needles (also termed catheters) which have been inserted into the prostate through the perineum and generally left in place between treatments. Trans-rectal ultrasound imaging is generally used to position the catheters and computer software is then employed to plan the positioning of the radioactive implants which are actually moved to different dwell places within each catheter during the treatment to implement the dose plan. Recent studies illustrate the importance of minimizing the exposure of both the urethra and the rectum by careful placement of the catheters and radioactive sources [89-92]. Otherwise, acute genitourinary toxicity can result. HDR-brachytherapy is almost always combined with external beam radiation therapy and sometimes with neoadjuvant or adjuvant hormone therapy. The brachytherapy is viewed as *boosting* the EBRT. Using the HDR-brachytherapy in conjunction with EBRT allows for high, carefully targeted doses plus lower EBRT doses. According to Galalae *et al* [93], neoadjuvant/concurrent androgen deprivation therapy (hormone therapy) did not improve outcomes when used in conjunction with HDR-brachytherapy plus EBRT. As will be discussed below, there is also interest and limited studies regarding the use of HDR-brachytherapy as primary monotherapy.

A rationale for HDR-brachytherapy involves the hypothesis that prostate cancer tissue is more sensitive to a short exposure to a high dose as compared to long exposure to a lower dose, and in addition, the reverse holds for normal tissue. Thus the hope that HDR brachytherapy will result in better tumor control along with a lower rate of adverse effects associated with the damage of normal tissue. In addition, being able to vary the dwell time of the radioactive source along each catheter allows coverage of the target tissue without exceeding the radiation tolerance of the urethra, bladder or rectum [88].

Most of the data concerning recurrence rates and short and long-term side effects are based on combined HDR-brachytherapy and EBRT. Two large studies that used approximately the same risk stratification definitions were reported in 2005. Galalae *et al* [93] report the combined results from three institutions, one in Germany and two in the US, and together these involved 593 patients with a 5-10 year follow-up. The other study was from Sweden. Åström *et al* [94] reported on the results of treating 214 patients with a follow-up of 5 years. In both cases both HDR-brachytherapy and EBRT were used. The results are summarized in Table 7.

Table 6-7. Five-year probabilities of no evidence of disease (biochemical, i.e. PSA), both overall and stratified by risk categories, resulting from combined EBRT and HDR-brachytherapy

	Probability (%) of No Biochemical Evidence of Disease			
	Overall	Low Risk	Intermediate Risk	High Risk
Reference [94]	82	92	87	56
Reference [93]	77	96	88	69

When the results of the three-institution study were stratified by institution, the results were similar, which the authors point out gives credence to the reproducibility of this approach to RT. Also, in this study, the 10-year freedom from biochemical recurrence was 73% and 10 year cancer specific survival was 92%. In a third study published in 2005, Deger *et a* [95] found somewhat lower probabilities, but used somewhat different definitions for risk categories.

In 2005 Sathya *et al* [96] reported a randomized trial with approximately 100 participants comparing just EBRT with HDR-brachytherapy plus EBRT. This study was unusual in that all the patients submitted to a lymphadenectomy to pathologically stage their lymph node status, and only those with negative results were included. This eliminated a confounding factor in the analysis of progression. This study also used only one session of brachytherapy that lasted 48 hours and was given prior to the EBRT. At a median follow-up of 8.2 years, 29% (71% recurrence free survival) of those on combined therapy experienced biochemical failure vs. 61% (39% recurrence free survival) of those receiving only EBRT. The patient population had either T2 or T3 disease and both groups had a similar distribution of intermediate (≈ 40%) vs. high risk (≈ 60%) cases. For example, in the intermediate risk group on combined therapy, approximately 81% had recurrence free survival vs. 47% in the EBRT only group.

There is growing evidence that the HDR-brachytherapy "fractionation" (how many times the procedure is repeated) may have a significant impact on outcomes. Brenner *et al* [97] examined the effect of 2 vs 3 sessions with approximately the same total dose in a study that combined HDR-brachytherapy and EBRT. The brachytherapy was given during the pauses in the EBRT. After 3 years follow-up the freedom from biochemical recurrence ranged from 64 to 75% for the three-dose group and 87 to 95% for the two-dose group, the variations being due to different total dose.

Two reviews published in 2003 [98,99] review earlier studies. Detailed comparisons are beyond the scope of this discussion, but in general the results compared favorably with those given below in Table 6-8.

Complications associated with HDR-brachytherapy plus EBRT are minimal, according to the review by Vicini *et al* [98]. Furthermore, this combined treatment modality offers the advantage of reduced treatment times, less acute toxicity, and no additional requirements to account for and correct for organ motion, edema, and set-up uncertainties [98]. However, to achieve the best results requires careful and knowledgeable planning and execution of both the placement of the catheters, the positioning of the sources and the duration of exposure as the sources are manipulated within the catheters to produced the desired dose to the various regions of the prostate [89,90,92].

HDR-brachytherapy has also been employed as a monotherapy, i.e. without EBRT, but at present this approach is considered experimental [88]. Published results are very limited. Martin *et al* [92] in a pilot study published in 2004 found minimal acute toxicity, but the follow-up period was too short to even reveal late toxicity much less biochemical control. Grills *et al* [100] compared HDR-brachytherapy with permanent implantation brachytherapy and examined both adverse side effects and oncological outcomes. The majority of patients were staged T1c or T2a, had a Gleason score of 6 or less and a pretreatment PSA of less than 10 ng/mL. Out of a total of 149 patients 65 received HDR treatment and 84 where given conventional brachytherapy. The median follow-up was 35 months. They found that HDR therapy was associated with a lower rate of urinary and rectal problems and there was a dramatic decrease (66%) in treatment related impotency with HDR. Recurrence as measured by PSA was similar and very low for the two groups (3% vs. 2% for convention vs. HDR therapy) which when taken together with observed lower rate of side effects provides evidence in favor of using HDR-brachytherapy rather than conventional permanent seed implants as a primary monotherapy in low-risk patients. However, more and larger studies are needed.

It is probably safe to conclude that this approach shows considerable merit and promise. At the end of the HDR-brachytherapy the radioactive sources and hollow needles are removed which eliminates the occasional problem of seed migration. It can be expected that over the next few years this technique will continue to be optimized with regard to the number of fractions used and the dose, and in addition, long-term results regarding both adverse effects and oncological outcomes will no doubt appear that exclusively used either 3D-CRT or IMRT for the EBRT. More studies on the use of HDR-brachytherapy as a primary monotherapy can also be anticipated. Since 3D-CRT has allowed dose increases over conventional EBRT, the comparison between HDR-brachytherapy and the current escalated dose 3D-CRT will be especially relevant and interesting.

COMPARISON OF THE THREE MAJOR PRIMARY TREATMENT MODALITIES

Finally, it is of interest to compare outcomes as regards recurrence for the definitive treatment modalities. There are many ways of accomplishing this. Table 8 provides results that take advantage of the database that is the basis of the Memorial Sloan-Kettering nomogram which is available online. Three recurrence risk clinical profiles are selected, low, the top of low and the top of intermediate, as defined by the guidelines given at the beginning of this chapter.

Table 6-8. Five-year progression free probabilities (%) according to treatment selected

Tumor Stage	T1c	T2a	T2b (T2b)
Pre-treatment PSA	7	9.9	20
Gleason Score	3 + 3	3 + 3	4 + 3
Radical Prostatectomy	90%	81%	56%
3D-conformal RT (86.4 Gy)	92%	80%	48%
Brachytherapy	86%	82%	78%

www.mskcc.org/mskcc/html/10088/ctm Memorial Sloan-Kettering Cancer Center online nomogram

The results given in Table 8 when compared to those in Table 7 suggest that HDR-brachytherapy plus EBRT compares favorably with RP, RT and conventional brachytherapy as regards outcomes.

These probabilities indicate rather small differences in oncological outcome for the three major definitive therapies provided the clinical picture indicates low recurrence risk localized cancer. Once the PSA is high and the Gleason score 7 or more, the prognosis is not particularly encouraging. Whether the difference is significant for the intermediate case between brachytherapy and the other two treatment modalities is not clear. Also, as has been emphasized repeatedly in the above discussion, individual outcomes will depend on the skill and abilities of the professionals involved in the any given procedure. In the situation where the predicted oncological outcome is similar for RP and RT it is natural that a consideration of side effects and interference of the treatment with daily activities become important and can influence an individual's ultimate decision regarding his options. In terms of combined oncological, urological and sexual outcomes, results from the best centers would appear to give RP the edge over other definitive treatments modalities because of the low rates of incontinence and impotence.

ANDROGEN DEPRIVATION (HORMONE THERAPY) AS A MONOTHERAPY FOR LOW-RISK LOCALIZED CANCER

The current US guidelines (www.nccn.org) for hormone monotherapy (including castration) restrict its use to advanced cancer with a very high risk of recurrence (T3b-T4). However, in the period 1999-2001, 12% of low-risk patients (PSA at diagnosis ≤ 10 ng/mL, Gleason <7 with no Gleason pattern 4 or 5 and clinical stage T1 or T2a) were treated only with hormone therapy in the US [101]. In Japan, hormone monotherapy which includes low-risk patients is also prevalent [102]. There appear to be no adequate studies that support this practice, but it appears that candidates are considered poor risks for either RP or RT, or simply refuse either and agree to hormone therapy, or elect an inexpensive option compared with RP or RT—an issue in the absence of insurance coverage. Whether or not this primary monotherapy is justified is unknown. Large studies are needed that are stratified by pretreatment clinical parameters, age and comorbidities and by the use of antiandrogen treatments combined with androgen deprivation [101,103,104]. The mechanism of action and use of androgen deprivation and antiandrogen drugs in conjunction with RT after RP or in treating advanced disease will be discussed in detail in Chapter 6. It is this approach that is included in present-day guidelines.

CRYOTHERAPY (CRYOABLATION OR CRYOSURGERY)

In simple terms, cryotherapy kills prostate cells, both normal and cancerous, by freezing the gland. A number of hollow needles are inserted into the prostate and cold gas is circulated to bring down the temperature of the prostate to about -40°C to create what is commonly called an "ice ball." Cryotherapy is used both for primary and salvage treatments, although current US guidelines (www.nccn.org) do not recognize cryosurgery as a recommended primary treatment. This is also true for the latest European Association of Urology guidelines (see www.uroweb.org) on prostate cancer [105]. However, there have been a few of studies examining the effectiveness of this technique in the primary treatment setting, although in some cases cryoablation was preceded by hormone treatment (androgen deprivation therapy) to reduce the size of the prostate.

Attempts to use cryotherapy in the 1960s for BPH-related urinary obstruction were accompanied by a high rate of morbidity and similar problems arose when liquid nitrogen probes were used to treat prostate cancer, mainly because the cooling probe placement was not ultrasound guided and urethral warmers were not used. Resurgence of interest in cryotherapy occurred when ultrasound guided probe placement and continuous temperature monitoring with thermal sensor probes were introduced. The ultrasound image approximately defines the frozen volume but does not give temperature information. Also, the use of a warming catheter reduced the damage to the urethra and concomitant incontinence. This is called second generation cryotherapy. In 1996 an improved probe cooling system using high-pressure argon/helium became available which responded rapidly to user input and resulted in more rapid creation of the ice ball than was possible with the older liquid nitrogen systems. This third generation cryotherapy has subsequently been improved by more sophisticated real-time computer assisted planning and execution of the freeze-thaw cycle, which is frequently repeated once. Some call this the fourth generation cryotherapy.

Cell destruction depends on rapid freezing, slow thawing and the effectiveness is improved by repeating the cycle. To kill malignant cells it is necessary to maintain a temperature of -40°C for at least three minutes. Thus the ideal scenario involves freezing the gland and a few mm of margin without damaging either the urethra, the rectum or the lower sphincter. In practice it is not that simple. In a recent review, Merrkck, Wallner and Butler [106] describe a number of unresolved problems with cryotherapy that include the following.

- A significant number of cancer foci are near the urethra and some actually abut it. Thus heating the urethra and tissue in its immediate vicinity can leave significant tumor tissue at temperatures too high for cryotoxicity, and this will be responsible for some cases of recurrence. This problem has received little study and in fact may be difficult or impossible to solve.

- Biopsies after cryotherapy reveal residual prostate cancer in a significant number of patients. There is no data supporting the contention that repeated cryotherapy addresses this problem.

- During cryoablation, the ice ball normally extends only 2-3 mm beyond the prostate capsule and there is a sharp thermal gradient. Studies are required to establish if cryosurgery can be safely administered with 5 mm margins which would be more effective in, for example, T3 cancers.

- Studies are needed to establish more accurately the temperature distributions within the ice ball and assure that all regions are treated adequately.

Judging the effectiveness of cryosurgery requires one to consider the recurrence risk status of the patients and as well, the criteria whereby treatment success or failure are measured. There is no consensus agreement on what constitutes treatment failure, a situation similar to that encountered in radiotherapy. After cryotherapy the PSA level drops over a period of several weeks or even months, to a nadir and then it either fluctuates about this nadir or increases. Definitions such as the ASTRO criteria for failure in radiotherapy (see Chapter 7), or simply remaining below or exceeding a PSA of 0.5 or 1.0 ng/mL are frequently used to define and identify treatment success or failure. Most studies have involved limited numbers of participants and short follow-up [107-109]. However, two studies of the use of cryotherapy for primary treatment have follow-ups of 5 or more years and involved 80 or more subjects.

The largest study was by Bahn [110] which used either 2nd or 3rd generation cryoablation and involved 590 patients with localized or advanced localized cancer (T2-T3). 91.5% had hormone treatment of 3 months to one-year duration prior to cryotherapy. Two freeze-thaw cycles were employed with a target temperature of -40°C. Follow-up involved periodic PSA measurements and biopsies. No hormone therapy was given post-cryotherapy.

Donnelly *et al* [111] treated 87 patients with clinically localized cancer, PSA < 30 ng/mL and negative bone scans. If the probability of lymph node involvement was grater than 5%, laprascopic pelvic node dissection was done before inclusion in the study. The first 30 patients received no neoadjuvant hormone therapy, but for the remainder, neoadjuvant hormone therapy was used if the ultrasonic estimate of prostate size exceeded 45g. No post-cryotherapy hormone treatment was used. Cryoablation involved the 2nd generation procedure with all but the first 10 patients undergoing the two-cycle process. Follow-up involved repeated PSA measurements and a biopsy 6 months after treatment. Cryotherapy was repeated if the biopsy was positive and the patient agreed.

The results of these two studies are summarized in Table 6-9. The pre-treatment clinical risk categories used for stratification were defined in the same manner by both groups and were as follows: low risk—T2a stage, PSA < 10, Gleason score ≤ 6. Intermediate (moderate) risk—*any one* of the following, T2b or greater stage, PSA ≥ 10 or Gleason score ≥ 7. High risk—two or more of the risk factors for intermediate risk.

Three PSA cut-off criteria were used to judge disease-free survival were <0.3, < 0.5 and < 1.0 ng/mL.

Table 6-9. Long-term (5-7 years) disease-free outcomes after cryosurgery [110,111]

Study	PSA cut-off	Low-risk	Intermediate-risk	High-risk
Bahn et al [110]*	<1.0	87%	79%	71%
	<0.5	61%	68%	61%
Donnelly et al [111]**	<1.0	75%	89%	76%
	<0.3	60%	77%	48%

* 7-year biochemical (PSA) disease free survival
** 5-year biochemical disease free survival

While precisely parallel comparisons with the standard primary with intent to cure treatment modalities are difficult, in part because of the neoadjuvant hormone therapy used in a number of the cryotherapy patients, the success rates given in Table 9 are roughly similar to those obtained by the recommended protocols (see Table 8) and suggest that cryotherapy will become more popular as longer-term studies with larger numbers of patients that employ 3rd and 4th generation techniques are reported. However, the problem of defining failure makes detailed and meaningful comparisons difficult. Salvage cryotherapy will be discussed in Chapter 7.

Biopsies conducted after cryotherapy on occasion find both viable cancer and non-cancer cells, suggesting that cryotherapy results in incomplete and inadequate ablation of the prostate tissue. When cancer cells are identified at post-treatment biopsy, this carries negative implications regarding the probability of recurrence [112]. However, finding viable non-cancer cells has not been found predictive of increased risk or relapse [112,113].

Modern cryoablation is associated with much lower rates of complications than historically observed with this procedure. In a recent review, Vestal [109] gives incontinence rates of 1%-5%, and urethral sloughing 4%-7%. However, the incidence of erectile dysfunction was found to be 80%-100%. Thus the freezing of the gland in general includes damage due to freezing of the neurovascular bundles. However, recovery of some erectile function is seen over time presumably due to nerve regeneration. Nevertheless, some men would probably prefer RP over cryoablation for this reason alone.

CONCLUSIONS

This chapter began with a discussion of the option of rejecting treatment until palliation was required. The decision to treat or not to treat turned out to be complex and while studies provided a number of indications of significant benefit associated with treatment by radical prostatectomy vs. watchful waiting, extrapolating to the present-day man with newly diagnosed prostate cancer was not possible with any degree of certainty, especially if overall survival was the issue. Thus for this question, an evidence-based answer appears to still be elusive.

However, it should be clear from the above discussion that the standard primary definitive treatments for prostate cancer have evolved to the point where very favorable outcomes occur for low-risk patients. In the hands of Patrick Walsh, the techniques for the RP he has championed have become the standard worldwide and most urological surgeons now have a DVD providing all the details. The improvements in the traditional external beam RT which allow precise targeting and amazing control of margins, intensity distribution and control of the irradiation of adjacent structures has, in the hands of skilled technical personnel, reached the point which again starts to approach a level of near perfection and has allowed dose escalation that has improved outcomes substantially. In brachytherapy, intraoperative CT computer assisted planning and precise positioning of the radioactive seeds has elevated this technique to a remarkable level of technological success. For this continued effort and success, the urologic surgery and radiation oncology communities deserve the gratitude of all prostate cancer patients. A corollary is that the outcome a man can expect is strongly dependent on the skill and judgment with which his treatment is provided and in addition how well the whole team involved functions. It is this aspect than may be difficult to research or impossible to even consider if only one treatment facility is either available or financially feasible.

Successful treatments for localized cancer depend on the absence of cancer outside the treatable region. When radiation fails to target all the cancer cells or surgery leaves behind cancer cells or the cancer has spread to surrounding tissue, the lymph nodes or beyond, then RT or RP may well fail to eradicate all of the cancer and recurrence may take place. The clinical parameters such as PSA, Gleason score and tumor stage help predict the probability that the treatment will in fact get at the cancer in its entirety, but these measures of the state of the disease are not fool proof and the disease staging and Gleason score can change upon pathological examination of the removed prostate and associated tissue. Patients electing RT as the primary treatment will never know if the clinical assessment is accurate since the prostate is obviously not examined by a pathologist. Even an individual with T1c stage cancer with a Gleason of 6 and a PSA of 5 still has a small chance of the treatment failing to "get" all the cancer, as indicated by the probability for recurrence-free survival is not 100%. Also, when recurrence occurs, men who have had a RP have a much better picture of the nature of their cancer than do the men who elected to have RT, and this better picture can make the selection of secondary (salvage) treatment more "evidence-based." It is also clear that the generally used clinical and pathological parameters such as pretreatment PSA, clinical or pathological stage and Gleason score, and seminal vesicle and lymph node status are strongly correlated in many studies with the probability of success for the treatment of localized cancer, and men with a low risk profile can look forward to a high probability of being "cured" by either RT or surgery. This knowledge is important since it impacts the psychological aspects of the diagnosis and treatment of this disease.

There are three principal long-term side effects with RP and RT, namely incontinence, impotence and bowel injury. Bowel injury is generally restricted to RT. As regards incontinence, the rate observed at highly-rated institutions for this side effect is very low for RP, and while initially high after RT, it generally resolves over time. The rate of long-term impotence after either RT or RP is similar, with perhaps RP having an edge of ten or so percentage points with 60-70% of all patients recovering potency eventually. For both treatment modalities, patient age and pre-operative potency confuse the potency issue. Impotency after RP, as discussed above, depends on the necessity of removing one or more of the neurovascular bundles in order to completely eradicate the tumor. When this is unnecessary, the skill of the surgeon in preserving these bundles and their functionality is critical to preserving potency. Also, nerve grafting can restore potency. The lowest rate of bowel injury appears to result when IMRT is used, with 3D-CRT offering an improvement over traditional external bean radiation therapy. Also, bowel injury resolves in most patients over time. Thus the side-effect picture evolves with time after treatment and is critically dependent on the skill with which the treatment is executed. Thus generalizations and comparisons are more difficult with regard to side effects as compared to, for example, disease-free survival.

It seems appropriate to return to the quotation that headed this chapter. Is a cure necessary in those in whom it is possible? In 1990 when Whitmore made this comment it was long before the recent progress and interest in active surveillance, but this new form of watchful waiting relates directly to the provocative question he advanced. The understanding of prostate cancer appears to have advanced to the point where it is possible to identify cases where delayed treatment is probably appropriate and carries little risk. Treatment with the intent to cure can be initiated after a delay with little risk of increasing the probability of failure. This makes Whitmore's question particularly relevant at present. It would appear prudent for men to be persistent in pursuing the issue of active surveillance with their oncologists or urologist to ascertain if they qualify according to the Hopkins or Memorial Sloan-Kettering criteria for active surveillance, and if so, perhaps should give this option serious consideration in spite of the fact that the evidence does not as yet satisfy the those who demand trials that may not be completed for a decade. It seems clear that a certain percentage of men who elect to follow this route, if they really qualify according to the criteria being used today, may avoid both treatment and side effects for an indefinite period, perhaps for their remaining lifetime, and apparently with little risk that they have given up the possibility of a cure if they progress. The availability of this option also should encourage men to accept the suggestion of PSA screening and even a biopsy, since the option of active surveillance allows for the possibility of identifying indolent cancer and of avoiding unnecessary treatment that might result from positive screening results. However, if a man elects this option, he must be willing to submit to periodic biopsies if he follows the protocol being promoted for active surveillance. The modern biopsy, carried out with local anesthetic, should not be feared and may be the more attractive option, if the alternative is one of the standard primary treatments for prostate cancer.

At the opposite extreme, men with a highly unfavorable prognosis must recognize that the data on which the assessment is based is extensive, that their prognosis is probably indeed poor, and they should act accordingly and either accept what conventional medicine has to offer by way of delaying tactics, or seek alternative approaches which might help but which have minimal evidence that would satisfy mainstream medicine. It is for these individuals that psychiatric help, support from their partners and prostate cancer support groups may be helpful. Unfortunately, while great progress has been made in primary treatment, mainstream medicine has considerably less to offer those with advanced or metastatic cancer. Nevertheless, this is an active area of research and there is always hope that new advances will provide treatments that will successfully prolong the life expectancy of advanced or metastatic cancer cases. Men should also realize that even advanced cancer can progress slowly. The treatment of advanced cancer is the topic of the following chapter.

Finally, men should never underestimate the value of a second opinion or the repeat of a test. As pointed out in Chapter 4, some experts strongly recommend, incidentally for very good reasons, having biopsy slides read at a center specializing in prostate pathology in order to obtain a second opinion. Repeat biopsies sometimes do not agree, and in some cases the second result is much more favorable than the first, and this can impact treatment decisions. Laboratories make mistakes and even mix up samples or x-rays. Incorrect names can be attached to diagnostic results. The author of this chapter has seen this happen to a friend whose urologist commented on his artificial hip joint as seen on a bone scan, when in fact both his hip joints were his own! The scan also showed extensive bone metastasis, and if this patient had not detected the identification error, the mistake would have had a profound impact on his treatment. He did not in fact have metastatic disease and ended up having a successful RP. Thus men need to be on guard to protect themselves from the inevitable consequences of the fact that the system that has a hold on them is not perfect and is run by human beings who are not immune from error. In fact, no reasonable person would expect the system to be perfect, although some professionals may act as if they believe this to be true. In fact, requesting a second opinion or the repeat of a test may generate hostility and even be considered a personal attack or insult. But the patient has to look out for his own best interests. One of the best ways of doing this is to make sure the information on which treatment decisions are made is as reliable as possible and has had the best available interpretation.

Chapter 7

Treatment of Residual, Recurrent and Advanced Prostate Cancer

William R. Ware PhD

INTRODUCTION

After the primary treatment of prostate cancer with intent to cure, there follows a period of uncertainty concerning the outcome, especially long-term. Prognosis is determined to some extent by the clinical pictured presented prior to treatment and, in the case of the radical prostatectomy (RP), the pathological findings upon examination of the prostate and other tissue recovered during surgery. Many patients worry, some excessively, about such questions as (a) did the radiation kill all the cancer cells or (b) did the surgeon remove all of the cancerous tissue and (c) will my next test show that the cancer is back. In other words, the patient worries that he may not really be cured. This concern is justified—some patients are in fact not cured! The physician involved can advise the patient as to the *probability* of not being cured, i.e. of having a so called recurrence, or put the other way, the probability of being recurrence-free for some period, typically 5-10 years. The best one can hope for in the case of this latter probability is about 95%, and when the clinical or post surgical picture is unfavorable, this percentage can drop to 40-60% or even less. Thus while a rosy picture may have been painted prior to primary treatment, a less than very favorable probability of recurrence can cause profound stress and agonizing worry prior to each new test to determine if the attempted cure has been successful. It is important to realize that recurrence is not a death sentence, that progression can be very slow and that there are secondary treatments available that are frequently effective. Also, the natural history of prostate cancer is such that all pronouncements of "cure" are of necessity tentative, and recurrence or even a new local tumor can occur even after 10-15 years of apparent recurrence-free survival.

After either a radical prostatectomy or radiation therapy (RT) the probability for recurrence averaged over large groups of patients typically ranges from 25-50%. These large groups will include patients with intermediate or high risk of recurrence based on pretreatment clinical data (see Chapter 6). The potential for recurrence exists when the surgeon leaves cancerous tissue at the site of the surgery or when radiation fails to ultimately kill all the cancer cells in the irradiated area or fails to target all of the cancer cells. Also, in the case of RT as the primary treatment, it is possible that while all the cancer cells were killed, a new primary cancer will form and be responsible for the observed recurrence. Finally, disseminated disease may have been present in which case the primary treatment designed to deal with localized cancer would obviously not be totally effective. Prior to primary definitive treatment, the risk of recurrence can be estimated from the PSA at that time, the clinical tumor stage and the Gleason score and detailed characteristics of the cores recovered at biopsy. This was discussed in Chapter 6 and reference made to an online calculator available for making such estimates. If surgery is the selected treatment option, then after the operation additional prognostic information becomes available from both the surgeon's observations about whether or not the cancer was organ confined and from the pathologist's report concerning the actual stage, pathological Gleason score, and the state of the surgical margins, seminal vesicles and, if removed and examined, the lymph nodes. This picture is obviously more accurate than that obtained prior to surgery, and illustrates the difference in prognostic information available after a RP compared to RT, where the latter provides no additional information gained from the treatment procedure.

On the basis of postoperative evaluation, it may be recommended that the patient receive additional treatment without waiting for possible recurrence. This is termed *adjuvant therapy*, and is prompted by the observation of significant risk of recurrence such as positive surgical margins or lymph node metastasis. According to the guidelines in current use, positive margins might prompt adjuvant RT because there is evidence of cancer still present but localized. Lymph node metastasis can prompt androgen ablation (hormone treatment). Hormone treatment will be discussed in detail later in this chapter. Another form of adjuvant treatment is called *neoadjuvant* and is carried out prior to the primary or secondary therapy. One indication for its use is the finding of a large prostate when RT is planned. Neoadjuvant hormone therapy can shrink the prostate and allow for a potentially more successful treatment.

If the prostate has been removed, the detection of recurrence is generally based on PSA measurements although if there has been tumor growth over time in the so-called prostate bed it is sometimes large enough to be detected with a DRE or imaging. As discussed in Chapter 4, if the PSA is very high (e.g. > 30-50) a bone scan is indicated to determine if bone metastasis has occurred, although this is generally done prior to treatment. After RP, the PSA level should fall to the "undetectable" range. With the commonly used assays of normal sensitivity this is between 0.1 and 0.4 ng/mL although 0.1 ng/mL is probably the more common threshold. The point is that if all the tumor and all the prostate tissue were removed there should be negligible PSA in circulation once the residual has been eliminated, which generally takes only a few weeks. If a man is actually cured, this state of affairs should persist for the remainder of his life. If PSA elevation (biochemical recurrence or failure) is being used as a means of identifying recurrence, various aspects of its increase can be use to indicate the seriousness of the failure and predict the success of treatment of recurrence, which has the quaint designation *salvage therapy*. The term "biochemical" is used because when recurrence is detected with PSA elevation the patient generally presents with no clinical (palpable) or radiographic evidence of recurrence.

The situation after RT is far more complex. Months are necessary before the PSA reaches a minimum or plateau, called the *nadir,* and then the characteristics of an increase if it occurs are used to detect the presence of recurrence and judge the prognosis of salvage treatment and as well judge what salvage treatment is appropriate. The various schemes and views for this will be discussed below. However, with RT the prostate is still *in situ* and both the DRE and biopsies are available to aid in detecting and accessing recurrence.

The possibility of recurrence after primary definitive treatment causes some men great anxiety and emotional stress. It is important that men realize that recurrence does not necessarily mean a death sentence or that they have only a few years to live, although in some cases this may unfortunately be the case. In a landmark study, the natural history of PC after surgery was been examined for almost two thousand patients who were operated on by one surgeon at Johns Hopkins. No additional treatment was used before surgery or prior to the appearance of symptoms or clinical evidence of metastasis [1]. The overall metastasis-free survival was 82% at 15 years after surgery and only 15% experienced PSA elevation. Of the 304 men who developed PSA elevation (PSA ≥ 0.2 ng/mL) and did not undergo early hormone treatment, 103 (34%) developed metastatic disease during the study period. The mean time to diagnosing metastasis was 8 years from the time of PSA elevation, and the mean time to death was 5 years from the time metastatic disease was identified. Thus on average, 13 years elapsed between the recurrence identified by a rising PSA and disease specific death in patients receiving no post-RP treatment prior to clinically evident metastatic disease. These are averages and thus obviously, many survived longer. This is then the worst-case scenario since no attempt was made to slow the progression to clinically evident metastatic disease with hormone therapy or salvage radiation treatments. The study also highlights the long time span between the first evidence of biochemical recurrence and the development of metastatic cancer. The probability and time to the development of metastatic disease depended on the time interval between surgery and recurrence, the Gleason score and the PSA doubling time after recurrence. In fact, the clinical experience of patients with biochemical recurrence (BCR) is highly variable; some will die from the disease in a few years whereas other will survive 5-10 years with no evidence of cancer other than a detectable and perhaps slowly increasing PSA level. Because of the impact on the selection of appropriate treatment, the problem of distinguishing at the time of recurrence between local recurrence, indolent disease and metastatic disease represents one of the major dilemmas facing clinicians working in this area [2].

The intent of this chapter is to provide detailed information regarding recurrence and its treatment for men who wish to understand current practice and the pros and cons of the options available. In addition, the current treatments available for advanced prostate cancer will be discussed.

BIOCHEMICAL RECURRENCE (FAILURE) AFTER PRIMARY TREATMENT

BIOCHEMICAL RECURRENCE AFTER RADICAL PROSTATECTOMY

After the removal of the prostate, PSA should become undetectable after about 30 days, which is the time required for the elimination of residual PSA. However, what constitutes undetectable depends on the assay used. Commonly used assays have a detection threshold of 0.1 ng/mL but other assays have both higher and lower limits. High-sensitivity assays are capable of detecting levels below 0.01 ng/mL. When the limit of detectability is 0.1 ng/mL, then a result just above this limit is frequently used as a signal for recurrence. Urologists at Johns Hopkins are still (2005) using a single postoperative PSA of at least 0.2 ng/mL as defining biochemical recurrence (BCR) after RP [3]. The use of this value is supported by a recent study by Freeland *et al* [4] and other earlier studies. On the other hand, researchers at the Mayo Clinic recommend the adoption of 0.4 ng/mL as the threshold for defining BCR on the basis of their study indicating this cut-off to be most strongly associated with continued significant clinical progression. Following RP, BCR occurs in approximately 35% of patients within 10 years of surgery [3]. Men who have had a RP should obviously continue to periodically have PSA tests, probably the rest of their lives, although the frequency is generally depends on what, if any changes are found and, if the level is increasing, what is the rate of increase or doubling time.

There has been only a limited number of studies on the use and merits of ultrasensitive assays for detecting recurrence [5-8]. However, a recent study form New York University may stimulate interest in this approach [5]. The researchers employed an assay that had a lower limit of detection of less than 0.01 ng/mL and defined BCR as 2 consecutive increases in post-nadir PSA of 0.1 ng/mL and used this definition to examine the predictive properties of the nadir itself in patients having had a RP. The ultrasensitive assay allows the observation of the nadir whereas the conventional assay generally does not since the nadir may be less than 0.1 ng/mL. The results they obtained are shown in Table 1.

Table 7-1. Ultrasensitive PSA Nadir after radical prostatectomy and the recurrence rate (BCR) [5]

PSA Nadir (ng/mL)	Recurrence Rate (%)
<0.01	4%
0.01	12%
0.02	16%
≥0.04	89%

Clearly, even if the starting point is < 0.01, two increases of 0.1 yield over 0.2, the most common recurrence signal. However, the authors consider the 89% relapse rate associated with a nadir greater than 0.04 ng/mL sufficiently significant to warrant its being considered as a threshold for additional therapy prior to recurrence in the postoperative follow-up. It is this earlier opportunity to intervene that constitutes a major factor in favor of using the high-sensitivity assay, but some would want the merits of this early intervention examined in randomized trials which would of necessity be very long-term, given the natural history of this disease. An alternative use of these results would be to incorporate ultrasensitive PSA results in postoperative nomograms used to select candidates for adjuvant therapy. A study published in 2000 supports this viewpoint [8] that the ultrasensitive PSA approach allows the early identification of early-relapsing patients and enables clinicians to initiate treatment in a timely fashion. But it has not been demonstrated that immediate treatment of early-relapsing patients is accompanied by cancer-specific or metastatic disease-free survival advantage. It may be some time before ultrasensitive PSA measurements become popular. The threshold of > 0.1 ng/mL appears to have served the urology community very well, at least when used with RP patients.

Once BCR after RP has occurred, the central question concerns the site and extent of the recurrent disease because this impacts directly on decisions as to treatment. There is also the possibility that the rising PSA is due to the presence of small amounts of benign prostate tissue. The challenge presented relates to the common occurrence of BCR as an isolated event without any objective clinical findings that might provide guidance. If the recurrence is local, i.e. in the vicinity of the prostate bed, then localized treatment is indicated, but if the recurrence reflects metastasis, then systemic treatment is appropriate and local treatment would not only be ineffective but cause unnecessary side effects [2]. In a recent review, Ward and Moul [9] discuss this diagnostic problem and make the following observations:

- For men with early PSA-only progression (early BCR), the commonly used CT imaging of the abdomen and pelvis along with a radionuclide bone scan generally yield very little information.

- In the studies they reviewed, the use of a radioactive isotope-labeled monoclonal antibody (the ProstaScint scan) was found to provide little useful information and this type of scan did not predict response to salvage RT. There are however, conflicting results regarding the ProstaScint approach, which the authors ascribe to a high degree of operator dependency and the difficulty of interpreting the scans.

These observations are echoed in a review by Djavan *et al* [10]. In a comprehensive review published in 2003 of markers and the meaning of primary treatment failure, Swindle *et al* [2] evaluate transrectal ultrasound and biopsy of the prostate bed, CT scans, the bone scan, MRI, ProstaScint and positron emission tomography (PET scan). For the identification of local recurrence, all of these approaches were considered to play a minimal post-recurrence diagnostic role, have minimal utility, or require further validation.

Thus there remain the so-called clinicopathologic factors that can be used to predict if the recurrence is local or due to distant metastasis. Swindle *et al* [2] give the following criteria for when the probabilities favor local failure: PSA doubling time of > 6 months; time to PSA recurrence after surgery of > 2 years, and a PSA velocity at 1 year of < 0.75 ng/mL per year. Distant metastasis is favored by a PSA doubling time of less than 6-10 months, a time to PSA recurrence of < 2 years, a PSA velocity at 1 year of > 0.75 ng/mL per year, a Gleason score of 8-10, positive lymph nodes or invasion of the seminal vesicles by cancer cells. Studies which would lead to validated treatment recommendations are not as yet available and a perhaps uncharitable view of the present state of affairs is that deciding on local vs. systemic treatment after BCR is more or less based on an educated guess. The use of PSA dependent parameters also underscores the importance of frequent measurement especially during the first 2 years after surgery.

A recent study [3] from Johns Hopkins and the University of Southern California examined clinicopathologic factors outlined above to attempt to differentiate local from distant recurrence. They used PSA doubling time, Gleason score and time from surgery to BCR and were able to stratify a cohort of patients into groups with varying risk of prostate cancer-specific survival ranging from 100% to < 1%, depending on the risk category, at 5, 10, and 15 years after BCR. The PSA doubling time was found to be one of the strongest risk factors for cancer-specific mortality. Patients with long doubling times ($\geq$ 15 months) were at low risk. For example, patients with recurrence time of > 3 years, Gleason score < 8, and a PSA doubling time of $\geq$ 15 months had 5, 10 and 15 year PC cancer-specific survival probabilities of 100%, 98% and 94%. At the opposite extreme, a recurrence time of $\leq$ 3 years, a Gleason score $\geq$ 8 and a PSA doubling time of < 3 months gave 5, 10 and 15 year cancer-specific survival probabilities of 51%, 1% (range <1-55) and < 1% (range <1-2). The reader is referred to their Table 3 for a complete picture. The authors take the position that low-risk patients can potentially be spared the effects of secondary treatment since it is unlikely to prolong life. They also suggest that these findings, while preliminary, may serve also as a useful guide to patients and their physicians when an attempt is made to identify high-risk situations where enrollment in aggressive treatment trials is appropriate or where the offer of multimodal treatment using hormonal therapy and cytotoxic chemotherapy is indicated. However, the range from low risk to very high risk is a continuum and for the majority in the middle, the approach to treatment of necessity is poorly defined and strongly dependent on the individual clinician's judgment and experience as well as patient preferences.

When the level of PSA increases after surgery, the growth is generally exponential (linear on a semi-log plot) or even super-exponential with an increasing doubling time. The Memorial Sloan-Kettering online calculator mentioned above and in other chapters has a calculator for doubling times where the patient can input a series of times and values and get the desired result. Men familiar with the mathematics of exponential growth can calculate the doubling time from the appropriate equation or from a semi-log plot.

With regard to the possibility that the rise in PSA is due to benign prostate tissue left behind during surgery, Scardino [11] points out that when this is the case the PSA rises slowly and peaks at a low level of about 1 ng/mL, whereas when it is due to residual cancer the rise is more rapid or goes above 1 ng/mL and will continue to rise if untreated. Thus some patients experiencing BCR who are in the low-risk category for recurrence may not have residual cancer at all, but merely benign residual prostate tissue, and treatment would clearly be inappropriate. However, before the PSA level has reached 1 ng/mL, some patients will have been advised to consider salvage therapy.

There is a wide variation in reports in the literature regarding the incidence of local recurrence after a RP (4%-53% [2]). This wide variation is due to problems inherent with the definition and the difficulty of diagnosis. Since local recurrence has been poorly defined, Swindle *et al* [2] suggest that any data on local recurrence must be interpreted with caution.

BIOCHEMICAL RECURRENCE AFTER EXTERNAL BEAM RADIATION THERAPY

The detection of recurrence after RT is complicated by a number of factors. The radiation does not result in instant cancer cell death, but rather the process extends over a number of months. This is in part due to the fact that the effect of radiation on a cancer cell may not be experienced until cell division occurs. Thus it is necessary to follow the decline in PSA and attempt to observe when the value becomes constant or exhibits a minimum—the nadir. The median time to nadir is reported to be typically 18 months or more, and may be longer after brachytherapy [9]. Likewise, a biopsy would not be informative until the same waiting period had elapsed. Experts generally recommend waiting two and a half years to see the full effect of radiation treatment [11]. Thus the early detection of recurrence possible in the case of RP is in many cases not possible with patients treated with radiation. However, failure of RT to halt an aggressive cancer may be evident fairly soon after treatment. Recurrence is identified when the nadir is followed by a rise, but there are a remarkable number of definitions described in the literature for this biochemical recurrence (over 100!).

There are several causes of either real or false biochemical recurrence. Benign tissue can generate a PSA increase as seen in benign prostatic hyperplasia (BPH—see Chapter 2). Also, the RT may not have reached all the cancer cells if it was focused entirely on just the gland or if distant disease was already present at the time of treatment. Finally, the dose used may not have been sufficient to eradicate all the cancer cells even if they were completely within the radiation field.

The fact that the criteria for or definition of biochemical recurrence after RT is controversial, still being debated in the literature, and still the subject of clinical studies does not increase a man's confidence that after RT the presence of recurrence can be established with a high level of certainty or that a definition will be used that guarantees him a low probability of unnecessary salvage treatment. This problem becomes much more serious if androgen ablation (hormone therapy—HT) was used after the course of radiation treatments, since HT has a strong influence on PSA levels which persists for a time after HT is terminated and further confuses the picture when PSA is used as a marker for recurrence. All of this coupled with the above mentioned waiting period due to the slow cancer cell death after RT causes a potentially stressful post-treatment period where the patient has no idea where he stands. Unfortunately, it may be some time before this problem is resolved, and patients must make do with the present state of the art.

Men having RT thus should expect to be followed to see if the treatment was successful, and if the treatment was unsuccessful, to be offered options as what to do next. Thus the challenge of the post-RT follow-up is to correctly identify failure, judge its implications and as well avoid the recommendation of additional treatment when no failure has actually occurred, or the risk of PC-specific death is very low. This becomes a very important matter for any patient concerned with the quality of care and advice he is receiving. For this reason a more detailed discussion of the so-called definitions of failure after RT will be provided.

In 1997 the American Society for Therapeutic Radiology and Oncology (ASTRO) attempted to standardize via a panel consensus the detection of BCR after RT (including brachytherapy) with a set of definitions and qualifications. The panel guidelines as they relate to individuals rather than trials were as follows:

- BF is defined as three consecutive increases in PSA after RT (typically at 6-month intervals.
- Biochemical failure (BF i.e. BCR) is not clinical failure and is does not provide justification per se for initiating additional treatment.

- The nadir PSA is a strong prognostic factor but no absolute level provides a valid cut point for identifying successful treatment. The nadir has similar prognostic value to the standard pretreatment prognostic parameters.

These guidelines were the subject of considerable criticism and prompted comparison with other definitions. One of the largest studies involved 4839 stage T1-T2 cancer patients from several institutions combined into one data base [12]. The follow-up was at least 5 years with a median of 6.3. The object was to test the ability of a number of definitions of BF to predict clinical failure (CF) which was defined as clinically evident local disease recurrence, distant metastasis, PSA > 25 ng/mL or the indication for the administration of hormone therapy. The following definitions were used to calculate the sensitivity, specificity, and the positive and negative predictive values (PV+ and PV-):

- True negative (TN)—no BF and no CF later.
- True positive (TP)—BF followed by CF later.
- False negative (FN)—no BF but CF later.
- False positive (FP)—BF but no CF later.

Sensitivity, specificity, positive and negative predictive values are defined as follows.

$$\text{Sensitivity (\%)} = 100 \times TP/(TP + FN) \qquad \text{Specificity (\%)} = 100 \times TN/(FP + TN)$$

$$PV+(\%) = 100 \times TP/(TP + FP) \qquad PV-(\%) = 100 \times TN/(FN + TN)$$

Thus the sensitivity is the % who will have CF who also have BF, and the specificity is the % of those who will not progress to CF who also do not have BF. The quantities (100 - sensitivity) and (100- specificity) represent the % of those who will progress to CF but exhibit no BF and those who will not progress to CF but exhibit BF, i.e. the failures of the diagnosis. The positive predictive value represents the % of those with BF who will actually progress to CF whereas the negative predictive value represents the % of those with no BF who will not actually progress to CF. Thus these measures reflect the predictive merit or failure of the BF definition designed to detect recurrence, i.e. the definitions that generate the "positive" and "negative" results.

Thames *et al* [12] identified four definitions out of over 100 (!) that were superior in terms of sensitivity and specificity as compared to the ASTRO definition. These are given in Table 2. The improvement over the ASTRO definition provided by these four definitions of failure is not that great, and the sensitivity figures indicate that these definitions including ASTRO miss a significant number of patients who have in fact will develop clinical failure without exhibiting BF—i.e. 26-39% as judged from 100-sensitivity!

Table 7-2. The sensitivity and specificity of various definitions of biochemical failure (recurrence) after approximately 5 years [12]

Definition of BF	Sensitivity	Specificity
ASTRO	61%	80%
1. Two consecutive rises, each > 0.5 ng/mL	68%	87%
2. PSA ≥ absolute nadir PSA + 2 ng/mL	67%	84%
3. PSA ≥ most recent PSA nadir + 2 ng/mL	74%	82%
4. PSA ≥ most recent nadir PSA + 3 ng/mL	66%	86%

Using the most recent nadir (also called current) takes into account the possibility of fluctuations which can produce several minima. Thames *et al* also looked at positive and negative predictive values stratified by pretreatment risk. Low risk was pretreatment PSA < 10 ng/mL, and Gleason ≤ 6 and a tumor stage of T1b-T2a. High risk was defined as PSA ≥ 20 ng/mL or Gleason score ≥ 8. Intermediate was defined as all those falling between these limits. Typical predictive values are illustrated in Table 3 where two of the definitions that were superior to ASTRO are compared.

Table 7-3. Positive and negative predictive values (PV) for three risk groups using two definitions taken from Table 2 [12]

Definition of BF	Risk Group	PV+	PV-
#3	Low	43%	95%
	Intermediate	55%	92%
	High	71%	73%
#4	Low	47%	95%
	Intermediate	58%	89%
	High	74%	71%

The positive predictive values are far from sensational! The maximum in this table is only 74%, i.e. 74% of the group in question who were going to progress to clinical failure had a positive indication of this from the PSA data using the definition of failure indicated. In fact, no definition discussed by Thames *et al* exceeded this value. A more favorable picture emerged for the negative predictive values, i.e. the % where the indication from PSA testing indicated non-progression to clinical failure and the prediction was true, at least at the end of the follow-up. More complete data is available from the paper of Thames *et al* [12].

Thus determining the true state of affairs after RT is simply a probability game with rather unimpressive sensitivity and specificity and while definitions proposed to replace the ASTRO definition offer some improvement, there remains an uncertainty as to the probability of progression to clinically evident failure and thus when to initiate additional treatment. These are, after all, the critical questions from the patient's point of view! The positive predictive values indicate that the probability of being given secondary treatment when it *may* not be necessary is disturbingly large. The data discussed above was based on RT between 1986 and 1995, a period which includes the introduction of 3D-CRT. Life is never simple nor the picture either black or white when dealing with prostate cancer.

The post-RT nadir, the minimum PSA reached after the effects of the radiation have run their course, turns out to be highly predictive of both the probability of developing metastatic disease and also of dying from prostate cancer [13]. This is illustrated in Table 4, which gives the percent of patients having each outcome according to their PSA nadir [13]. This study by Hanlon *et al* involved 615 patients treated with 3D-CRT. Out of this cohort, 186 experienced BF (ASTRO definition), 40 developed distant metastasis (6.5% of those experiencing BF), 18 died of PC. Of those with BF, 48 (26%) were treated with hormone therapy. Noteworthy is both the long follow-up time and the very low rate of distant metastasis (4%) if the nadir is equal to or below 1.0 ng/mL and as well, the low rates of death from prostate cancer (3-4%) for those with a nadir up to 2.0 ng/mL. Their analysis of the data revealed that for patients with BF, freedom from distant metastasis was *independently* predicted by a longer PSA doubling time, a lower PSA nadir, a longer interval from the start of RT to nadir and the use of hormone treatment (androgen deprivation). Similar results for 8-year freedom from metastasis were recently reported by Ray *et al* [14] based on a multi-institutional study.

Table 7-4. Percentage of patients having the indicated outcome stratified according to PSA nadir after radiation therapy [13]

Outcome	PSA Nadir (ng/mL)		
	≤1.0	1.1-2.0	>2.0
8-year freedom from distant metastasis (%)	96	89	61
8-year cancer-specific survival (%)	97	96	78

The decline in PSA post-RT to reach a minimum, i.e. the nadir, and then an increase, passing through the BCR signal point and continuing beyond can be interpreted as a competition between a decrease in PSA due to dying cells in the irradiated region and increasing PSA in regions that were beyond the reach of the beam, this latter possibly reflecting distant or metastatic disease. The ideal outcome is a decline to a plateau where the PSA is very low and constant. Fluctuations about this plateau can occur which in some cases give an ASTRO defined signal because of the simple "three consecutive rises" with no qualifications, but this signal should be viewed with suspicion.

Hanlon *et al* [13] also examined the question as to the influence of the nadir on the probability of BCR. For patients in the nadir range of 0-1.0 ng/mL, they were unable to establish a correlation; a result, which they point out, is in conflict with earlier studies. However, a more recent study by DeWitt *et al* [15] found a statistically significant difference in freedom from PSA failure (BCR—ASTRO definition) as a function of the magnitude of the nadir. Using post-RT nadir quartiles of PSA <0.3, 0.3 to <0.6, 0.6 to <1.2 and 1.2 or more, they estimated 5-year rates of 83%, 72%, 58% and 33%, respectively for freedom from BCR.

Other studies have also pointed not only to the PSA doubling time but also to the time to PSA recurrence as predictors of distant metastasis. In a recent review, Swindle *et al* [2] give less than 12 months to PSA recurrence and less than 6-12 months for the PSA doubling time as indicators of distant metastasis. However, the authors point out that a short time to BCR, a rapid PSA doubling time and also a high Gleason score do not exclude the possibility of the coexistence of local recurrence.

The use of PSA to monitor the success of RT can produce confusing and misleading results because of what is known as the *PSA bounce*. A range of 12-33% of men who receive RT without hormone treatment can experience an increase in PSA followed by a decline sometime after treatment. The increase can exceed the ASTRO definition of BF but the rise does not continue. This bounce can take place over a number of months and can occur within 5 years of treatment, although the mean time to a bounce has been estimated at 9 months. The cause is unknown. The bounce is not predictive of future BF. Its potential to cause alarm, stress, confusion etc. must be considerable.

The use of hormone therapy either just prior to RT (to reduce the prostate size) or immediately after can also distort the PSA picture considerably. Hormone treatment reduces PSA levels and when stopped, there is a PSA bounce. This can significantly complicate the detection of BCR and interfere with secondary treatment decisions.

BIOCHEMICAL RECURRENCE AFTER BRACHYTHERAPY

With external beam RT, when the treatment series is over all that remains is for the cell death to occur as the process of self-destruction of the cancer cells plays out. However, with brachytherapy (BY), the seeds are permanently implanted and the duration of the treatment has no sharp cut-off but is controlled by the half-life of the radioactive isotope used. One of the two commonly used isotopes (palladium) has a half-life of about 17 days (i.e. the radiation intensity decreases to half its value every 17 days), which means that even after about 50 days, the radiation intensity is still approximately 10% of the starting value. Iodine-125, the other commonly used isotope, has a half-life of about 60 days and thus in about 180 days the intensity still being delivered to the prostate is down to approximately 10% of the initial value. When the radiation treatment is over an extended period this impacts the PSA behavior by generally extending the time to nadir.

If one examines recent publications that involve the detection of BCR after BY, the ASTRO definition is most commonly used. However, an absolute cut-off of > 0.5 ng/mL is also used [16]. Radge *et al* [17] compared the ASTRO definition and the use of a cut-off of 0.5 ng/mL and concluded there was no statistically significant difference in the outcomes predicted.

WATCHFUL WAITING OR ACTIVE SURVEILLANCE AFTER BIOCHEMICAL RECURRENCE

Delaying treatment after the occurrence of biochemical recurrence has received little attention. Scardino [11] points out that if a patient's PSA is low and doubling very slowly and the assessment of the nature and extent of the cancer at the time of treatment was favorable, ten or twenty years may elapse before local clinically evident recurrence or metastases causing symptoms actually occurs. Thus the decision regarding watchful waiting will to some extend depend on age, general health, lifestyle and personal preferences. However, as will be discussed below, one of the most important prognostic factors for the success of salvage RT after RP is the PSA at the time of salvage treatment, with strong evidence in favor of a value of less than 1 ng/mL and some evidence favoring ≤ 0.5 ng/mL. Watchful waiting allows the patient to be sure that the elevated value taken as an indication of recurrence is real and not a laboratory error or a meaningless fluctuation. Watchful waiting should really be termed active surveillance with the intent to intervene if such action is intended before the chances of successful salvage diminish. Active surveillance was discussed in detail in Chapter 6 in connection with delaying primary therapy. When the post surgical picture is very unfavorable and the nature of the failure suggests that hormone therapy is appropriate, how long one waits before initiating treatment is debatable, as will be discussed later in this chapter.

SALVAGE AND ADJUVANT THERAPY

ADJUVANT RT AFTER RADICAL PROSTATECTOMY

One of the advantages of RP over RT is that it provides an opportunity to acquire a much more detailed picture of the nature of a patient's cancer, especially if the pelvic lymph nodes are dissected and examined. When the post-surgical pathological picture is unfavorable, there are circumstances where immediate so-called adjuvant treatment may be indicated [18]. The term adjuvant is defined in dictionaries as "assisting in the amelioration, prevention or cure of disease." Ignoring chemotherapy for the moment, the two adjuvant therapies commonly used are external beam radiation therapy and some form of hormone therapy. The potential indications for post-RP adjuvant RT are [18]:

- positive surgical margins found in the prostatectomy specimen;
- seminal vesicle invasion by cancer cells;
- extraprostatic extension.

Contraindications, which suggest disseminated disease, include pelvic lymph nodes positive for cancer, failure of PSA to reach undetectable levels (generally < 0.1 or 0.2 ng/mL) within a week or two or any clinical indications of metastasis such as a positive bone scan. Also, some would reject those with seminal vesicle involvement and those with Gleason 8-10 pathology [19]. In other words, there is no point is radiating the so-called prostate bed and its immediate vicinity if the patient already has disseminated disease present outside the field of radiation. The problem is judging the probability of the risk of recurrent local disease vs. already present metastatic disease. Implicit in this notion is that eliminating the source of the development of local disease will have little effect on cancer specific survival if metastasis is already present, and instead systemic treatment is more appropriate. Treating the situation where the PSA fails to drop below the limit of detectability is generally termed salvage treatment rather than adjuvant. Thus the true adjuvant therapy after RP is not a treatment of local or biochemical recurrence but an attempt to prevent or delay such recurrence.

Historically, the use of adjuvant RT was uncommon, partly due to early studies which showed improved local control but no cause-specific survival advantage [20]. Studies from 1991 to 1999 have been reviewed by Gomella *et al* [20]. When the prognosis was highly unfavorable based on post-surgical pathology, hormone treatment was much more common. Frequently the decision was to wait and see if biochemical or clinically detectable local recurrence (growths in the prostate bed felt with DRE or seen on scans) occurred, and then employs salvage therapy. However, if the residual cancer is indeed localized and can be reached by external beam radiation, adjuvant RT offers a potential cure or long-term freedom from biochemical failure and early treatment associated with true adjuvant therapy may merit consideration, whereas hormone treatment in general merely delays more serious problems and does not offer the possibility for a cure. Men with unfavorable post-surgical pathology need to be aware of recent studies which suggest that considerable benefit may be derived from adjuvant RT. While there are additional side effects added to those from the surgery, the risk of these must be balanced against the high risk of progression and metastasis associated with unfavorable post-surgical pathology. Thus it is appropriate to review the current status of adjuvant RT.

One of the problems associated with studies of adjuvant RT is that it is difficult to have an equivalent comparison group. Thus many studies start with a group of patients some of whom qualify for adjuvant RT while others with more favorable characteristics were treated only with salvage RT after biochemical or local clinical failure. To make comparisons one must assume that if left untreated, both groups would show the same incidence of BCR and receive salvage RT and contribute equally to the failed or successful salvage statistics.

The ideal study involves a randomized clinical trial and several are underway at present but long-term follow-up will take time. However, preliminary results from two randomized trials have been reported, one in the peer review literature [21] and one at the 2005 conference of the American Society of Clinical Oncology (discussed in [22]). Both trials randomized several hundred post surgical patients to either have adjuvant RT or PSA monitoring. Comparison was then made of the incidence of BCR in the two groups as well as cancer specific and overall survival. Patients in the watchful waiting group received treatment once biochemical failure was evident. The results were as follows.

- Bolla *et al* [21] reported in 2005 on preliminary results from the EORTC trial 22911 (European Organization for Research and Treatment of Cancer). Over 1000 patients were randomized to adjuvant RT or PSA monitoring. Patients had to have no distant metastases, negative lymph nodes and at least one of the following risk factors: tumor growth beyond the capsule, positive surgical margins or seminal vesicle invasion. Thus they presented an unfavorable picture after surgery. Adjuvant treatment was begun within 16 weeks of surgery. Only about 70% of the patients had undetectable PSA after surgery. While this appears to be an undesirable aspect of this study [22], the authors claim that this did not significantly distort the results. Five-year clinical progression free survival was significantly improved in the treated over the untreated groups, as was biochemical progression-free survival (74% vs. 52.6%). The treated group also had a longer time to post treatment biochemical failure.

- The second study (reported in [22]) randomized 385 eligible patients between adjuvant RT and watchful waiting. All participants had PSA below the detectable limit. Biochemical progression-free survival favored those receiving adjuvant treatment (81% vs. 60%), which nearly duplicated the EORTC study.

Thus clinicians who have up to now rejected adjuvant RT for patients with unfavorable pathology after RP because of the absence of randomized trials have some preliminary data to consider from studies involving substantial numbers of participants. It is interesting that these results in fact are similar to those obtained in five non-randomized studies published between 2001 and 2005 [23-27]. In all of these studies, patients receiving adjuvant RT fared better, sometimes considerably better, when judged by 5-year freedom from biochemical recurrence than those who waited and then had salvage RT. Of particular interest is a study by Vargas *et al* [23] published in 2005, since it stratified the results by a variety of pathological characteristics. Some of the results are presented in Table 5.

While the results shown in Table 7-5 for those given adjuvant RT may not look spectacular, it must be remembered that these are patients at high risk for recurrence as the biochemical failure rates for those untreated indicate. These results confirm the use of the above pathological characteristics as providing an indication for adjuvant RT immediately after surgery in those at high risk for recurrence rather than waiting for PSA indicated failure or clinically evident local recurrence. A cautionary note, however. The number of treated participants in each of the pathological categories was rather small. Overall survival and cause-specific survival difference were not statistically significant in this study.

Table 7-5 indicates a strong dependence of an improved outcome on the presence of seminal vesicle involvement. This was also observed in two of the recent studies referenced above [25,26], but other studies have failed to reveal a significant difference [24,27,28] even though two of the later studies [24,27] found significant benefit in terms of 5-year biochemical recurrence-free survival associated with adjuvant RT. In connection with one of the randomized trials discussed above [21], the authors state that "treatment benefit was significant in all pathological risk groups." In an editorial [22] accompanying the report of the randomized EORTC trial, the authors comment that the question remains as to whether adjuvant RT is superior in terms of outcomes to early salvage treatment as soon as PSA rises. They point out that in their opinion there is still no direct proof of this hypothesis. Unfortunately the randomized trials did not address this question directly, and it would appear that randomization is necessary for a direct comparison of these two treatment scenarios. As the current randomized trials mature and the outcomes for those treated either with adjuvant or salvage RT after BCR become available for comparison, the resolution of this question may become clear.

Table 7-5. Five-year freedom from biochemical failure* for patients with or without adjuvant radiotherapy following radical prostatectomy, given according to the pathology observed [23]

Pathology	Percent of Patients Free From BCR At 5 Years	
	No Adjuvant RT	Adjuvant RT
Tumor Stage T3	29	56
Extracapsular Extension	30	52
Seminal Vesicle Invasion	18	60
Positive Surgical Margins	27	64

*Biochemical failure was defined as a PSA ≥ 0.1 ng/mL. The differences between the treated and untreated groups were all statistically significant.

TREATMENT OF RECURRENCE OR PERSISTENTLY ELEVATED PSA AFTER RADICAL PROSTATECTOMY

The principal issues are: (a) when and how to treat and how to know when to treat; (b) salvage radiation therapy of the prostate bed (fossa) or hormone treatment or both; (c) conventional chemotherapy; (d) an experimental protocol in the clinical trial stage. The selection of the initial therapy depends on the clinicians judgment as regards the critical question, i.e., is the recurrence real, is it localized or does it represent distant metastasis. This has been discussed above. When the weight of evidence suggests local recurrence after a RP, salvage RT is generally the choice. When metastatic cancer is thought to be present, systemic treatments are indicated such as androgen ablation (castration or hormone therapy—HT) or castration and antiandrogen therapy. Chemotherapy has only become common in recent years and evidence that it may be useful in disseminated cancer is starting to appear. When BCR has just occurred, it may not be clear that it is real rather than a meaningless fluctuation or laboratory error, and even if real, the magnitude of the threat may be debatable, and under these circumstances, watchful waiting or what would probably be active surveillances may in fact be a reasonable initial response since this provides time to obtain additional data which may resolve some of the critical questions. But this option must be weighed against the possible benefit of early intervention. Patient age, comorbidities and life expectancy also are generally considered along with the predicted time to symptomatic metastatic disease.

SALVAGE RADIATION THERAPY

After surgery, radiation therapy can be used to treat biochemical recurrence or clinically identified local recurrence. This is termed salvage radiation therapy. It can also be employed to treat persistently elevated PSA, i.e., the situation where the PSA level fails to become undetectable after surgery. Radiation treatment that is prompted by a detectable (typically 0.2-0.3 ng/mL or more) PSA a month after surgery is termed salvage rather than adjuvant RT by some authors. Salvage radiotherapy is at present the only treatment available after RP that offers the potential for a cure. However, at present in the US less than 50% of men receive salvage RT after biochemical recurrence (BCR—also called biochemical failure) and a majority receive hormone therapy which offers no hope for a cure [29]. Therefore, if a man experiencing BCR is offered only one or more forms of hormone therapy, he should investigate the question—am I a good candidate for salvage RT or do the available indicators point to low probability for success, i.e. the presence of non-localized disease that might indeed better be treated with hormone therapy. Another option is a combination of salvage RT and HT. Thus the question of who is and who is not a good candidate for salvage RT is important and men need to be aware of the results of current research and guidelines. Since salvage radiation is accompanied by non-trivial side effects, men need to be concerned about receiving RT if there is in fact a very high probability that the rising PSA or even the persistently elevated PSA is due at least in part to disseminated disease which will be left untouched by irradiation. Unfortunately, clear-cut differentiation of truly localized disease from metastatic disease still presents a challenge to the clinician and opinions differ as to who is or is not a good candidate for salvage RT.

Part of the problem in diagnosing localized vs. distant disease is that some of the seemingly logical or obvious tools are insensitive, although this is an area where current and future research may yield significant improvements. For the present, however, the DRE, biopsy of the prostate bed, CT, PET or MRI scans, and the ProstaScint scan are all not very sensitive indicators of persistent localized disease [2,30]. In the work-up prior to salvage RT, one or more of these techniques may be employed, but this appears to be a matter of covering all bases rather than relying on the results as definitive if they are strongly positive.

Several recent reviews deal at length with the matter of the appropriate use of salvage RT [2,30-32], These originate from Johns Hopkins, Memorial Sloan-Kettering, Duke University and the Fox Chase Cancer Center. After reviewing the literature running into 2003, Khan and Partin [31] conclude that salvage radiation therapy should be avoided in men with pathological evidence of advanced disease (Gleason score > 7, *or* seminal vesicle *or* lymph node involvement), those who fail to achieve undetectable serum PSA after RP (presumably < 0.2 [33]), those who experience an early initial PSA recurrence and those with serum PSA doubling times of < 6 months. Swindle *et al* [2] concur. As indicators of distant metastasis which would provide a contraindication for salvage RT, Swindel *et al* give a range of 6-10 months for PSA doubling times, a range of < 1 year to < 2years for time to PSA recurrence after surgery, a PSA velocity > 0.75 ng/mL per year, and the same post-surgical pathological characteristics given by Khan and Partin.

In a very recent and comprehensive review covering research reported between 1997 and 2004, Hayes and Pollack from the Fox Chase Cancer Center in Philadelphia also examine in detail the parameters for treatment decisions for salvage RT [30]. They make the following observations (interested readers should consult the full-text since the tables present a detailed analysis):

- The results of salvage RT have been relatively poor. Freedom from biochemical failure rates range between 10% and 66%. (However, if one examines the 5-7 year freedom from biochemical failure in two other reviews [34,35] one gets an average of 45-46% and an even larger range of 10-78%).
- Outcomes are generally worse for patients with persistently detectable PSA post RP (PD-PSA) as compared to those with have a delayed rise after a drop to undetectable levels (DR-PSA).
- Independent of whether the patient can be classified as DR-PSA or PD-PSA, if the PSA doubling time is ≤10 months, occult metastatic disease is likely and salvage RT much less effective. However, they point out that when the PSA level is below 1 ng/mL, estimates of doubling time may be inaccurate and as well, both when to begin the doubling calculation and whether or not it is valid to use only two determinations remain unclear.
- The most consistent predictor of freedom from biochemical failure after salvage RT is the pre-salvage PSA. The best results are seen when the pre-RT PSA is ≤ 1.0 ng/mL and a significant decline in success rates is seen as the cut-off increases to 1.2 to 2 and then > 2 ng/mL.
- A pathological Gleason score of 8-10 consistently indicates a worse prognosis compared to a score of 7 or less.
- Positive surgical margins are a good sign since they indicate that the residual disease is likely to be in the prostate bed and amenable to effective salvage RT.
- Seminal vesicle involvement has in some series been an indicator for an unfavorable outcome measured by post-salvage biochemical failure.
- The authors conclude from their analysis of the relevant literature that the *ideal patient* would have (a) positive surgical margins; (b) a PSA doubling time of > 10 months; (c) a low (<1.0 ng/mL) PSA at the time of salvage radiation therapy; (d) no seminal vesicle involvement; and (e) a Gleason score based on post-RP pathology of ≤ 7. Using these guidelines involves a probability based judgment call that patients with this set of characteristics are likely to have local or locoregional disease recurrence and that distant metastasis is probably absent.

In a recently published study not included in the above reviews, Cheung *et al* [36] found that using just positive margins and a pre-RT PSA ≤ 0.5 ng/mL as criteria for separating a small cohort undergoing salvage RT into favorable vs. unfavorable, that freedom from post-salvage biochemical failure was 83.7% in the former and 61.7% in the latter.

In the context of candidacy for salvage RT, the use of PSA velocity is the subject of a recent study by Patel *et al* [37] from the New York University School of Medicine. The PSA velocity calculations were based on at least 6 months follow-up after PSA recurrence. RT was offered only to patients with PSA remaining below 1.0 ng/mL. Response to salvage RT was defined as maintenance of a post-treatment PSA of < 0.1 ng/mL. The median relapse-free survival time was 28 months for those with a PSA velocity < 0.035 ng/mL per month (0.42 ng/mL per year) and 16 months for those with a velocity greater than 0.035 ng/mL per month. PSA velocity is of course directly related to the doubling time and thus these results are consistent with the poor prognosis associated with short doubling times. Patel *et al* failed to find prediction of failure value for seminal vesicle invasion, surgical margin status, or Gleason score. The authors comment that this may be due to the relatively short follow-up.

Despite considerable research effort over the past decade, the ultimate impact of salvage RT on survival is unknown [32] and no long-term, randomized prospective trial addressing this question appears to have been performed. With patients having multiple adverse indicators, the commonly seen initial PSA response to salvage treatment can be misleading since it is generally short-lived. How this short-lived benefit translates into long-term survival is also unknown.

Finally, it should be kept in mind that the decision to use salvage RT is based on an educated guess as to the status of the disease (local vs. metastatic or both). Thus is to be expected that there will be a large range of study results and that the average success will not be sensational due to a "treat and hope for the best" approach with patients in the grey area between obviously good candidates and obviously poor choices for this type of salvage therapy. Men should also keep in mind that salvage RT after RP failure potentially offers a cure if the recurrence is indeed localized and the residual cancer cells effectively irradiated.

THE SALVAGE RADICAL PROSTATECTOMY

Disease progression after radiation therapy (RT) represents a serious problem for both patients and those involved in their care. Disease progression after RT in the US, based on a 40-60% treatment failure rate, will involve an estimated 30,000 men who will need to be considered for additional treatment (salvage treatment) [38]. Failure to intervene when indicated increases the risk of developing distant metastases or decreases the time to the development of metastatic disease. The mean time interval from untreated biochemical failure after RT to distant metastases is approximately 3 years [39]. While not all men experiencing biochemical failure after RT are good candidates for salvage radical prostatectomy (RP), those who are have the opportunity for a second chance at a cure or at least a long period of freedom from disease progression. In fact, of the available options after the failure of primary RT, salvage RP currently represents the only potentially curative option [40].

Careful selection of candidates for salvage RP is considered essential [41]. This is challenging because, unlike patients failing primary surgical treatment, those failing primary RT do not have nearly as complete a pathological history, i.e. post-surgical staging and Gleason scoring and detailed information regarding seminal vesicle involvement, margin status, and in many case lymph node involvement. The problem of course is to avoid surgically treating patients with metastatic disease unless the goal is simply to decrease the probability of urinary obstruction. Three recent reviews attempt to define the ideal candidate for salvage RP. As with the question of candidates for salvage RT, these criteria attempt to address of the problem of localized vs. metastatic disease.

- Touma *et al* [42] suggest the following: life expectancy of ≥ 10 years; no severe medical comorbidities, patient acceptance of the prospect of surgical morbidity, pre-RT PSA < 10 ng/mL, pre-salvage RP PSA <10 ng/mL, and localized clinical stage both pre-RT and pre-salvage RP.

- Catton *et al* [43] recommend T1-T2 stage both pre-RT and at recurrence, PSA doubling time after recurrence of >6 months, the interval from primary RT to recurrence of > 1 year, pre-salvage RP PSA < 10 ng/mL and an initial Gleason score of ≤ 7.

- Stephenson and Eastham [40] describe the ideal candidate as follows: pre-salvage PSA of < 10, tumor stage of T3a or less, negative imaging results for regional or distant metastasis, absence of voiding symptoms or incontinence (for best functional outcome), and patient recognition that the salvage RP is technically very challenging with the potential for serious complications. Patients with radiation induced cystitis, incontinence or contracted bladder are recommended for cystoprostatectomy and urinary diversion. In an earlier review, Eastham *et al* [41] also list a life-expectancy of at least 10 years, excellent health and a negative result from pelvic lymph node dissection if available.

Two recent reviews summarize the success of salvage RP over the decade 1988-1999. Five- and ten-year progression free survival rates were 58% (4 studies, range 70-55) and 47% (7 studies, range 69-26%), respectively. Ten year prostate cancer specific survival was 80% (3 studies, range 94-60%). These results are similar to those reported in 2005 in two studies, one of which was from the Mayo Clinic [44,45] and one from Memorial Sloan-Kettering Cancer Center [46]. The results are summarized in Table 6.

When the figures in Table 6 are considered along with the averages given above, a fairly consistent picture emerges. Approximately half of all men having a salvage RP experience recurrence over the first 10 years post-operative. However, a much smaller percentage die from prostate cancer over this same period.

Bianco et al [46] also report on the influence of the pre-salvage RP PSA and the pathology observed through examination of the prostate and other tissue on the 5-year progression free survival (PFS) and the 10 year cause specific survival (CSS). The results are shown in Table 7-7.

These figures emphasize the danger of looking at results averaged over a wide range of patient characteristics and indicate that under favorable circumstances, the outcomes can be quite good. Since the pathological features are not known until after the salvage surgery (unless an exploratory lumpectomy provides information on lymph node status), one is left with the PSA level at the time of surgery. It would appear from Table 7-7 that PSA under these circumstances is a good marker for the presence of disseminated disease for which the prostatectomy is ineffective.

Table 7-6. Outcomes for salvage radical prostatectomy after failure of radiotherapy from recently reported studies [44-46]

Study	5 year PFS*	10-year PFS	5-year CCS*	10-year CCS
		OUTCOMES		
Bianco et al [46]	55%	30%	93%	73%
Ward et al [44]**	66%	58%	90%	77%
Amling et al [45]***	66%	43%		

* PFS—Progression free survival, CSS—Cause (PC) specific survival
** From figure in [44]
*** From Figure 3, [45]

Table 7-7. Influence of the pre-salvage PSA and pathological factors found at RP on the outcome of salvage RP after failure of radiotherapy [46]

Parameter	5-year PFS*	10-year CSS*
	OUTCOMES	
Organ confined disease	77%	
Extracapsular extension	71%	
Seminal vesicle invasion	28%	
Lymph node involvement	22%	
Positive surgical margins	38%	
Negative surgical margins	58%	
PSA < 4	86%	
PSA 4-10	55%	
PSA > 10	28%	56%
PSA < 10		95%

* PFS—Progression free survival. CSS—Cancer (PC) specific survival

These observations are more or less consistent with those of Rogers *et al* [47] who found that when the preoperative PSA was < 10 ng/mL, only 15% of patients had advanced pathologic features found at surgery compared with 86% if the PSA level was > 10 ng/mL. It is interesting that the nadir reached after primary RT covers a range that includes values of PSA < 1.0 ng/mL, and with the definitions of failure discussed above intervention should be possible at presalvage PSA levels well below 10 ng/mL for some patients. Thus on the basis of the results described above, if salvage RP is being considered, treatment should obviously be initiated in a timely fashion after failure if the PSA level is < 10 ng/mL.

One of the problems associated with salvage therapy after the failure of radiotherapy is the long time interval after RT before definite indications are available. The cancer may already be advanced by the time many patients and their physicians decide on following the salvage RP route [47]. As discussed above, the PSA only slowly declines to reach a nadir and biopsies are generally not done until about 18 months post-treatment and even then, the interpretation of the histological findings is difficult and requires a high level of experience and expertise. This is in sharp contrast to the situation where the primary treatment was a RP. In this latter case, useful information from PSA measurements becomes available within a few weeks and as well, rather complete pathological data are available immediately after surgery whereas for the patient treated with radiation, what is really going on at the level of cancer pathology is perhaps best described as a black box about which only educated guesses are possible.

Salvage RP has not gained widespread acceptance for men experiencing recurrence after radiotherapy. One reason is the perception of significant morbidity [40]. Eastham *et al* [41] have recently commented on this in a review article. Based on their experience at Memorial Sloan-Kettering Cancer Center, they discuss the changes in intraoperative and postoperative complications and morbidity in the period 1984-1994 as compared to 1995-2002. The early group consisted of 52 subjects, the contemporary group 54. They find a significant improvement in a number of areas as surgical techniques were improved. Rectal injury decreased from 11.5% to 1.9%, urethral injury from 3.8% to 1.9%, hospital stay decreased from 8,7 days to 3.6 days, and the number of postoperative complications went from an incidence rate of 2-4% to zero. Severe incontinence also decreased from 28% to about 12%, but mild incontinence increased from 4.3% to about 28%, and other levels of continence remained about the same. The authors also point out that erectile dysfunction is almost inevitable after salvage RP. Only in selected cases can one or both neurovascular nerve bundles and sexual functionality be preserved. Nerve grafting remains a possibility. These results should prompt a reconsideration of the merits of the salvage RP both by patients and their physicians.

In a recent review dealing in part with the management of treatment failure following brachytherapy, Horwitz *et al* [48] point out that while salvage radical prostatectomy is an option, it should be reserved for patients without significant comorbidities and a life expectancy exceeding 10 years. In addition, patients should have organ-confined disease as indicated by DRE or imaging, a low post-implant PSA of < 10 ng/mL, and favorable pre-implant tumor parameters, and as well, residual urinary or bowel symptoms and radiation cystitis or proctitis should be absent. Patients need to be highly motivated because salvage RP in this setting can be accompanied by a higher level of adverse effects than are experienced in ordinary RPs. These reviewers strongly recommend full pelvic lymph node dissection at the start of the surgery with immediate examination of frozen sections. Positive lymph nodes would be an indication, in their opinion, for considering abandoning the proposed salvage surgery. In addition, brachytherapy may have caused adherence of the front surface of the prostate to the pubis or the back surface to the rectum, and this increases the challenge of the dissection accompanying the gland removal. Nerve preservation is neither advocated nor feasible and thus impotence is inevitable unless nerve grafting is done. Following surgery, there is an increased risk of bladder neck contractures as compared to standard RP. Data from studies of recurrence and its treatment after brachytherapy are limited and some of the considerations and observations in connection with failure of external beam radiation therapy apply also this situation. Patients not meeting the selection criteria are frequently referred for immediate or delayed hormone therapy.

It can be concluded that salvage RP can provide good local control of recurrent prostate cancer and even eradicate the disease in a high proportion of patients when the cancer is confined to the prostate or the immediate surrounding tissue. To achieve this favorable results, patient selection is critical and difficult. The overall picture presented by a suitable candidate is good health with a life expectancy of over 10 years, a local tumor, and no evidence of seminal vesicle involvement or metastatic disease [41]. Operative and postoperative morbidity will depend on the surgical skills available.

OTHER SALVAGE RADIATION TREATMENTS

Brachytherapy has been used after the failure of EBRT, but the literature is very limited with only one small study in the PSA era providing long-term results [49]. Salvage brachytherapy has also been used to treat recurrence after RP and the failure of salvage RT. In this case, there of course must be a tumor present in the prostate bed of suitable size to allow seed implants. Again the literature is extremely limited. Finally, high dose rate brachytherapy (see Chapter 6) has also been used in cases of the failure of salvage RT after RP. In this case, there is a feasibility study [50] with positive results published in 2005.

A salvage option is re-irradiation following brachytherapy failure, but with an external beam using, ideally, 3D-CRT or IMRT. Horwitz *et al* [48] comment that most radiation oncologists use the same selection criteria as described above for salvage RT. A cause for concern is the tolerance of the normal surrounding tissue which has already received radiation from the implants. While there is very limited data from studies, these reviewers conclude that re-irradiation is a feasible option.

The lack of experience with these approaches to salvage treatment, as judged by the extremely limited literature, suggests that they should be regarded as experimental and anyone interested should consider attempting to become part of a clinical trial.

SALVAGE CRYOTHERAPY (CRYOSURGERY)

Therapeutic options for salvage treatment with intent to cure after RT failure are limited to salvage RP, salvage BT and the procedure discussed in this section, salvage cryotherapy. This mode of treatment was introduced in Chapter 6 in the context of primary therapy, but is much more commonly used in the treatment of post-RT recurrence. Clear superiority of any one of these options for the management of locally recurrent prostate cancer after definitive RT has not been demonstrated [51]. The modern 3rd and 4th generation cryosurgery protocols described in Chapter 6 are equally applicable to either primary or salvage therapy. The practice guidelines of 2005 (www.nccn.org) take the position that cryotherapy should be preformed in the context of a clinical trial and that the technique should be considered "investigational." Not everyone agrees. The current status of salvage cryosurgery has recently been reviewed by Touma *et al* [52] and Ahmed *et al* [53].

Four studies utilizing 2nd or 3rd generation cryoablation techniques have appeared recently [54-57]. The majority of these studies involve short follow-up and/or small patient numbers. The study with the longest follow-up (mean 72.5 months) was reported by Bahn *et al* [56] in 2003 and involved 59 patients. The researchers used a biochemical failure definition after cryotherapy of ≥ 0.5 ng/mL for the PSA level. The percentage of patients that remained biochemical failure free was 59%. Shorter duration studies with PSA failure definitions ranging from > 0.3 to > 0.5 ng/mL gave biochemical disease free percentages ranging from 34% to 77% [53]. Morbidity and complications associated with cryosurgery were discussed in Chapter 6.

Comparison between results obtained from salvage RP and salvage cryotherapy are complicated by a number of factors. With salvage RP, the prostate is gone, the PSA should rapidly drop to a very low value, and a rising PSA suggests residual local normal or malignant tissue or disseminated disease. With cryoablation the prostate is still there and studies indicate a significant probability of either residual non-cancerous or cancerous tissue that was not eradicated by freezing, with only the latter presenting a significant risk of prostate cancer progression [51,58]. Thus with cryoablation there will be a nadir followed by either fluctuations or a rise, the latter being the signal of failure although it may be a false signal as regards the risk of cancer progression. With the salvage RP, there is general agreement as to the criterion for failure, i.e. the same as for the primary RP. With cryoablation, there is no agreement and different PSA thresholds yield considerably different rates of failure. Also, the use of pre-cryotherapy hormone therapy is a confounding factor. Thus the problem of making comparisons. Nevertheless, in the studies reviewed by Ahmed *et al* [53] the patient numbers and follow-up times for salvage RP were roughly similar to those for the cryotherapy studies, and the percent remaining biochemically disease free were on average lower for salvage RP than were the results for patients in modern cryotherapy series.

In their review Ahmend *et al* [53] conclude that cryosurgery is a "feasible choice" as a salvage therapy and should be offered to patients with post-radiotherapy recurrence. Touma *et al* [52] suggest the following selection criteria for cryosurgery to be a valid salvage option: life expectancy of at least 10 years, preradiation and preoperative PSA < 10 ng/mL, Gleason score < 8, clinical stage less than T3, and cancer that is hormone sensitive. They regard salvage cryosurgery as especially suited for older patients with some comorbidities who still present a reasonably low anesthetic risk.

However, Stephenson *et al* from Memorial Sloan-Kettering Cancer Center [59] differ. In a recent review (2004) of salvage therapy for locally recurrence after RT they quote evidence that if a similar patient group and definition of failure are used for comparing salvage RP with salvage cryotherapy, the latter is found to be inferior. They quote a study by Leibovich *et al* (the full report does not appear to be published) where 56 salvage RP patients treated at the Mayo Clinic were compared with 60 salvage cryotherapy patients treated at the M.D. Anderson Cancer Center. All patients had pretreatment PSA levels of < 10 ng/mL and biopsy Gleason scores of ≤ 8 and no patient received prior hormone therapy. Biochemical progression occurred in 67% of the cryotherapy cases and only 29% of the salvage RP cases. They conclude from this rather limited study and the absence of long-term survival results for salvage cryotherapy that salvage cryotherapy is inferior to salvage RP. Perhaps eventually there will be data published making such a comparison as that of Leivovich *et al* where all the patients were from the same institution, 3rd or 4th generation cryoablation techniques were employed for all cryotherapy procedures and the follow-up was long enough to examine cancer-specific survival. For now, one must accept the fact that the use of salvage cryotherapy is controversial.

HORMONE THERAPY (ANDROGEN DEPRIVATION)

INTRODUCTION—THE MECHANISM AND PROTOCOLS OF HORMONE THERAPY

Hormone therapy which is really hormone manipulation is most often employed when the patient presents with evidence of non-localized disease after the failure of primary radiotherapy or surgery, i.e. recurrence of the cancer, or when surgery or radiation therapy is not indicated because of age, comorbidities or the high probability or presence of metastatic disease. The use of hormone therapy as a primary modality is uncommon in the post-PSA era when most patients present with T1-T2 disease. Hormone therapy does not offer the potential for a cure. By the time hormone therapy is indicated by most guidelines, delaying progression, controlling pain and ultimately delaying death from prostate cancer are the objectives. In fact, just how the disease results in death, if this does indeed happen, may be not at all clear to the reader.

When prostate cancer initially forms, it is normally organ confined. The natural course then is that the tumor or tumors eventually penetrate the prostate capsule and then proceed to invade the surrounding tissue which then provides a springboard for further spreading and metastasis. At the same time, the seminal vesicles can become involved and provide a route for spreading. Finally, the presence of cancer in the lymph nodes is generally indicative of impending or coexisting metastasis. Progression now includes spreading to bones and to various organs, although the former is the most common. Bone metastases, occurring in a variety of locations, are a major source of pain associated with metastatic cancer, and in addition result eventually in a number of serious problems including cancer related bone weakness, fractures and spinal cord compression. This latter problem then can cause numerous painful symptoms and malfunctioning associated with the impacted nerves. Death can come from comorbidities or be directly caused by the cancer. Scardino *et al* [60] list the following examples where death results from complications directly related to metastatic cancer.

- Weakness or malnutrition leading to impaired ability to deal with infections. This leads to death from pneumonia, sepsis or other generalized infections.
- Tumor induced malnutrition causing electrolyte imbalance, arrhythmias and cardiac death not directly related to acute ischemic disease.
- Urinary, gastrointestinal or biliary (bile tract) obstruction due to tumor mass which results in dementia or coma that in turn gives rise to malnutrition, electrolyte disturbance or pneumonia.

The therapeutic objective of hormone manipulation is to slow the cancer progression once it is outside the area normally subjected to radiation treatment, is not susceptible to surgical excision or where radiation or surgery is not deemed suitable or offering a significant probability of freedom from advanced disease. Hormone therapy is not given with intent to cure, although significant slowing in progression is possible which may, in turn, eventually result in the cause of death being unrelated to the prostate cancer.

Hormone therapy is in fact a complicated subject because it is used under some circumstances as a primary therapy as well as after the failure of other primary treatments. There are several types of drugs used and they can be used as monotherapy or in combination. Surgical castration is also employed. In addition, hormone therapy can be used prior to either radiation therapy or surgery (neoadjuvant therapy), and as well, can be used immediately after these so-called definitive therapies (adjuvant therapy) if, in the opinion of the attending physician, the patient might benefit from systemic therapy. Also, hormone therapy can be either intermittent or constant, and when it is used after primary treatment failure, therapy can be started either immediately or after progression has occurred. Eventually, the prostate cancer cells become resistant to the effects of hormone manipulation and other therapy is called for in the hope of some additional control.

The guidelines of the National Comprehensive Cancer Network (www.nccn.org) are very frequently quoted in the medical literature as a standard of practice. For hormone therapy, the 2005 guidelines for primary therapy indicate the following.

RECURRENCE RISK	HORMONE TREATMENT RECOMMENDATION
Low. T1a-T2a and PSA < 10 and Gleason Score 2-6	Adjuvant HT after RP if lymph nodes positive
Intermediate. T2b-T2c or Gleason score 7 or PSA 10-20	Adjuvant HT after RP if lymph nodes positive
High. T3a or Gleason score 8-10 or PSA >20	HT with RT (3D CRT) or RT with short-term HT for patients with only one adverse high-risk factor. Adjuvant HT or expectant management after RP if lymph nodes positive
Very high. T3b-T4	HT or RT (3D-CRT) plus HT
Metastatic. Any T, N1	HT or RT (3D-cRT) plus HT (N1 = metastasis to the LNs)
Metastatic. Any T Any N, M1	HT (M1 = distant metastasis)

Thus only for those with very high recurrence risk or metastatic cancer do these guidelines indicate HT as a primary monotherapy, but the combination of radiation therapy and HT is recommended for those with high or very high risk or those with only positive lymph node involvement. Adjuvant HT post RP is also indicated when positive lymph nodes are found.

The NCCN also provide guidelines for salvage therapy. After radical prostatectomy, if the PSA fails to fall to undetectable levels and if there is evidence of persistent local tumor, then either HT alone or RT plus HT is indicated. If there is evidence of a persistent local tumor then RT is preferred if the PSA is less than 2 or the surgical margins are positive or the PSA doubling time is greater than 10 months. However, if there were positive lymph nodes or seminal vesicles or the PSA doubling time was less than 3 months, then HT is indicated. If however, the PSA is greater than 0.3 ng/mL and rising on two or more measurements, then the recommendation of either HT plus RT or HT alone depends on evidence of metastatic disease or positive lymph nodes. If absent, the preferred treatment is RT plus HT or HT alone. If present, then the guidelines indicate HT. Observation is given as an alternative to HT in all cases except when there is evidence of local tumor. For post-RT rising PSA or a positive DRE, HT or observation is recommended only if the patient is not a candidate for local therapy or has positive results from tests for metastasis.

The rationale for HT involves the role that the androgen testosterone plays in prostate cancer cell proliferation through its downstream product, dihydrotestosterone. This has in fact been known for over 50 years, and early attempts to take advantage of this involved surgical castration (orchiectomy) to eliminate the principal source of this hormone. Much more recently drugs were found which accomplished testosterone reduction (so-called androgen ablation or androgen deprivation therapy). These are called luteinizing hormone-releasing hormone therapy agents (LHRH agonists e.g. leuprolide and goserelin) and antiandrogen drugs (flutamide, bicalutamide and nilutamide). The LHRH drugs are also called GnRH-A agents. The manner in which these function is illustrated below.

LHRH ACTION

Pathway Which Is Inhibited

Hypothalmus →(*LHRH*) →Pituitary →(*LH*) →Testes →(*Testosterone*) →Prostate cells

In words, the sequence involves the hypothalamus producing LHRH which goes to the pituitary gland (also in the brain) where it induces the production of *luteinizing hormone* (LH) which then triggers the production of testosterone in the testicles. This produces testosterone in the circulation which is picked up by the prostate and binds to androgen receptors on prostate cells. The LHRH agonists decrease the production of LH through the so-called down-regulation of LHRH receptors in the pituitary gland. This breaks the above-diagramed sequence involved in testosterone production in the testes and the serum levels approach surgical castration levels. The term castration in the context of prostate cancer therapy now generally implies either the use of LHRH agonists or surgery. The residual levels of testosterone after either approach should be similar. The net result of LHRH agonist therapy is thus to reduce the serum levels of testosterone in order to prevent its action as a promoter of prostate cancer cell proliferation. It is of incidental interest that estrogen or DES (diethylstilbestrol) will reduce testosterone at the hypothalamus—pituitary stage. DES is not longer available in North America.

ANTIANDROGEN ACTION

Pathway Which Is Inhibited

Circulating testosterone → Prostate Gland → Cell binding of testosterone to androgen receptors

Antiandrogen drugs prevent the binding of testosterone by competitively binding to the receptor sites on prostate cells. This produces the same end result as reducing testosterone in the circulation—no binding of testosterone to androgen receptors. However, an added bonus is related to the fact that about 5% of the circulating testosterone is produced by the adrenal gland. Neither surgical castration or the LHRH agonists interfere with this process and thus there remains a low level of testosterone after either of these approaches. Antiandrogen therapy also eliminates the binding of this residual testosterone and is used as combination therapy with LHRH agonists or as monotherapy. Some call this *total or complete androgen blockage*. The goal of either therapy is to bring the testosterone level to a very low value. There are also drugs that will inhibit the production of testosterone from the adrenal gland. Finally, the 5α-reductase inhibitors such as finasteride (used to treat BPH—see Chapter 4) inhibit the conversion of testosterone to dihydrotestosterone, but as will be discussed below, the use in prostate cancer treatment remains experimental but quite interesting.

Antiandrogens are used as monotherapy or combination therapy. This will be discussed in more detail below. When LHRH agonists are used, there is a testosterone burst that lasts only a couple of weeks followed by a decline in the level of this hormone. For some patients with advanced disease, this burst can cause severe side effects. The use of combined therapy for a few weeks eliminates this problem after which it is common practice to revert to just the LHRH agonist.

At present, androgen agonists are preferred by many men over surgical castration, partly for psychological reasons, but men are generally offered silicone replacement testicles in order that there is no visual evidence of the surgery. Castration and androgen ablation have the same negative sexual side effects—decreased libido and erectile dysfunction.

The term *Androgen Deprivation Therapy* (ADT) is used to describe either LHRH agonist therapy or antiandrogen therapy or combined therapy. However, some authors restrict the term ADT to LHRH agonist therapy. In this chapter will use ADT as indicating LHRH or antiandrogen therapy or both. Thus the term describes a procedure in which the androgen receptor of target cells is not activated either because of a reduction in androgen (testosterone) levels or because of receptor blockage, or both. The term *Combined Androgen Blockage* refers to the combination of LHRH agonist and antiandrogen therapy.

In 2004, the American Society of Clinical Oncology put forward their recommendations for the initial hormonal management of *androgen-sensitive* metastatic, recurrent and progressive prostate cancer [61]. The expert panel considered five questions and provided answers based on their evaluation of available evidence.

- **What are the standard treatment options**? ASCO recommends either surgical or medical (LHRH agonists) castration as the initial treatment for metastatic prostate cancer. They quote evidence that these two approaches to ADT are equally effective, but surgical castration is irreversible and has adverse psychological aspects. LHRH agonists are available in relatively convenient dose protocols and the effects are reversible. DES is not recommended.

- **Are antiandrogens as effective as other androgen deprivation therapies**? The ASCO recommends that antiandrogen monotherapy may be discussed with patients as an alternative to medical or surgical castration. The evidence includes the observed equivalence of survival compared to castration but less toxicity, especially with respect to loss of libido.

- **Which is better, combined androgen blockage or castration (medical or surgical) alone**? It is recommended that a discussion between physician and patient is appropriate given that while there is a small potential gain in overall survival with combined androgen blockage over medical or surgical castration (see [62]), there is also an increase in side effects. However, in a recent paper, Ho *et al* [63] discuss this question and point to studies in the late 1990s that suggest in some cases inferior survival associated with antiandrogen monotherapy vs. castration in metastatic disease. They add, however, that if secondary castration after the failure of antiandrogen monotherapy is employed this might improve the survival statistics. This question comes up in connection with the use of 5-α reductase inhibitors (e.g. Proscar) with antiandrogens, and the indicated action and success of castration as a secondary treatment. This is discussed in some detail below.

- **Are there improved outcomes from early vs. deferred therapy**? The ASCO panel took the position that until data becomes available from studies using modern medical diagnosis and biochemical tests and standardized follow-up schedules, no evidence-based recommendations can be made. This is in fact an interesting question. Ryan and Small [64] limit the term "early" to treatment initiated at the time local therapy is given. They then used "middle" to describe the initiation of ADT at the time of PSA recurrence for patients without clinical evidence of metastatic disease and "late" then refers to starting ADT at the time overt metastatic disease becomes evident. Given these definitions, the argument against early treatment is based on the view that an incomplete cell kill after ADT results in selection pressure. This may fail to prevent and possibly enhance the development of androgen independent disease and hasten death. Those in favor of early treatment point out that the early treatment is working on a lower tumor load and will have a larger relative cell kill and improved disease-specific and overall survival. Ryan and Small [64] discuss evidence for the potential deleterious effects of ADT on the disease biology and in addition point out that there are a number of adverse side effects which must also be considered in the context of early treatment. Ryan and Small also review the situation with regard to the use of ADT at the time of PSA recurrence. Based on preliminary reports, benefits of treating immediately after recurrence include increased overall survival and a delay in the time to metastasis. But the authors point out that prospective studies are required before definitive recommendations can be made. A study not included in the above reviews was published in 2005 [65]. The authors of this study concluded that in their group of patients, which included 20% with lymph node metastasis, that for those who did not undergo potentially curative local treatment, there was no major advantage of immediate vs. delayed treatment. As ASCO concluded, more research is needed.

- **Which is better, intermittent ADT or continuous ADT**? With intermittent hormone therapy, treatment is stopped after PSA drops to undetectable levels and is resumed when PSA rises to some predetermined level. Two reasons for intermittent therapy are frequently presented: (a) intermittent therapy may delay the occurrence of androgen independence (i.e. when ADT stops working) and (b) for part of the period where therapy is suspended, there may be relief from side effects. The ASCO panel withheld making a recommendation due to the unavailability of data from prospective randomized trials. Two such trials are ongoing, but until they report, the panel suggests that intermittent androgen blockage should be considered experimental. Bhandari, Crook and Hussain [66] have also recently reviewed the evidence associated with this question. While they agree with the ASCO panel recommendation, they point out that intermittent ADT is based on substantial preclinical science which supports the possibility of the reduction in both short- and long-term adverse effects while at the same time delaying the development of hormone-refractory disease (androgen independent disease). However, Scardino [11] points out that the relief from sexual side effects as well as weight gain, mood swings. anemia, lethargy and hot flashes may in fact occur only during 10-15% of a patient's remaining lifetime since the time off-treatment decreases with each cycle. He concludes that it is better to simply delay treatment until the PSA reaches the range of 20 ng/mL or there are other signs of overt metastasis. A recently published study from France however comes to a different conclusion. In a study of intermittent ADT after biochemical recurrence post-RP, they found satisfactory long-term oncological results with the intermittent use of antiandrogen monotherapy and LHRH therapy when antiandrogen therapy failed. This study, however, involved only 28 subjects. Nevertheless, there was only a 4% metastatic progression and no cancer specific deaths over a follow-up of over 7 years, and the percentage of each cycle spend in the "off" mode only decreased from 60% to 50% [67].

Thus there are a number of issues associated with the protocol of hormone therapy that remain to be resolved and a number of aspects remain controversial.

COMPLICATIONS AND SIDE EFFECTS OF HORMONE THERAPY

Hormone therapy involves androgen deprivation which translates into the reduction of testosterone to very low levels or blocking the action of testosterone in the prostate. Achieving near zero serum testosterone is currently accomplished by surgical castration or LHRH agonists which block its production. The current method of blocking the action of residual production of testosterone by the adrenal glands is with antiandrogens. When used as a monotherapy, antiandrogens leave the circulating testosterone relatively unchanged, whereas monotherapy with LHRH agonists result in levels that are much lower than found even in the elderly (because of age-related decline). Many of the complications of LHRH agonist or combined therapy result from not only the very low testosterone levels achieved during therapy but also from the prolonged duration of the deprivation. Hormone therapy is being started earlier and used longer, and along with this prolonged use come, in some cases, more severe complications. In addition, in many cases, satisfactory, problem-free therapy to combat these adverse side effects is lacking and the complications, it is argued, are tolerated because they represent the lesser of two evils.

Chen and Petrylak [68] have recently reviewed the subject and provide a number of important insights concerning specific aspects of serious adverse side-effects of the androgen deprivation that results from hormone manipulation.

- **Sexual Side Effects**. While loss of libido and erectile dysfunction are well-recognized adverse side-effects of androgen deprivation therapy (ADT), a significant minority of men are not completely devoid of sexual interest. On the other hand, erectile dysfunction associated with LHRH agonist is present in the majority of men. But because antiandrogen monotherapy does not deplete testosterone, it preserves sexual function to a greater degree.

- **Hot Flashes**. This is the same phenomenon experienced by women going through menopause. Over 50% of men undergoing ADT experience hot flashes and this side effect can have a significant impact on the quality of life. Hormonal agents that might be used to treat hot flashes have the potential for promoting disease progression. There do not appear to be any large or significant trials of agents that solve this problem. Chen and Petrylak comment that alternative hormonal therapies such as high-dose parenteral estrogen should not be used outside of clinical trials.

- **Gynecomastia**. This refers to benign, excessive development of male breast tissue, is commonly associated with pain and can, if prolonged, become irreversible. Either surgical or medical castration or the use of antiandrogens can result in gynecomastia, but the antiandrogens carry a higher incidence. Decreasing the circulating testosterone levels impacts the androgen to estrogen ratio and this can cause gynecomastia. However, the antiandrogens block androgenic activity in breast tissue, thereby removing an inhibitory effect on estrogenic stimulation. In addition, antiandrogens also block androgen receptors in general, and this results in the inhibition of negative feedback of circulating testosterone and causes an increase in testosterone levels. This leads through aromatization (part of the chemistry of the testosterone to estrogen conversion) to an increase in estrogen levels [69]. The incidence of gynecomastia is considerably higher with antiandrogen therapy than with a LHRH agonist. Therapeutic options include prophylactic radiotherapy of the breasts or the use of the drug tamoxifen. A recent randomized trial [70] found tamoxifen effective over the short term in reducing bicalutamide (an antiandrogen) induced gynecomastia. Severe long-standing gynecomastia may merit surgery [71].

- **Adverse effects on metabolism, cardiovascular risk factors and body composition**. ADT has been found to increase weight and body fat mass and decrease lean body mass. This may be related to the role of testosterone in promoting lipolysis (chemical decomposition of fat) in visceral adipose tissue. Metabolic changes include increases in serum levels of insulin and blood lipids such as the various forms of cholesterol and triglycerides. These metabolic changes, taken together, suggest that ADT may increase the risk of cardiovascular disease. In addition, testosterone is thought to be a protective factor against atherosclerosis through immuno-modulation and an influence on plaque development and plaque stability [72]. In addition, large artery stiffening, which has been associated with ADT, may influence adversely the course of vascular disease and explain the possible connection between hormone treatment for prostate cancer and increased mortality from cardiovascular disease [73]. There appear to be no published studies addressing the prevention or management of these metabolic or cardiovascular changes in men receiving ADT.

- **Bone problems**. Bone problems will be discussed below. The current recommendations for the prevention of bone loss in men with prostate cancer include supplementation with both vitamin D and calcium and the avoidance of habits that can exacerbate bone loss such as smoking, excessive alcohol intake and a lack of exercise.

- **Anemia**. Testosterone appears to be involved in the maintenance of normal hemoglobin levels, and ADT can produce significant declines in these levels and produce anemia with concomitant fatigue, shortness of breath and cardiovascular problems. While these problems resolve upon termination of ADT, in many situations the therapy continues for an indefinite time and may compromise patient quality of life over an extended period. Chen and Petrylak discuss only one treatment for ADT induced anemia. It involves administering erythropoietin, a type of protein that occurs naturally in the body, which stimulates the bone marrow to make red blood cells. However, the impact of this therapy on both quality of life and prostate cancer outcomes has not been thoroughly investigated at this point.

- **Cognitive problems**. Testosterone is known to influence mood and cognitive function. This accounts for ADT being implicated in depression and anxiety, i.e. problems with psychological distress and mental health. There is also evidence of cognitive decline, but here there are conflicting studies.

Thus it is clear that in general ADT or complete androgen blockage (LHRH agonist plus antiandrogen) carries considerable risk of adverse side effects which are not fully amenable to therapeutic intervention. In fact, the complications associated with hormone therapy are a frequent reason for patient-initiated discontinuation of treatment.

In the context of the controversy over delayed vs. immediate ADT, these are the side effects that the advocates of delay are trying to avoid for as long as possible. If it turns out to indeed be true that early treatment confers no survival advantage, then avoiding any or all of these side effects for a period of time should gain support. By delaying ADT until it is prudent to initiate treatment, some patients may be spared adverse side effects for a long period, and some may never need hormone treatment, either because of slow progression or death from some other cause.

Androgen deprivation therapy generally leads to so-called hormone or androgen resistant disease. Initially, ADT reduces the serum PSA to a very low value, but eventually the ADT is unable to maintain this state of affairs, the treatment becomes ineffective and other interventions are needed to attempt to slow progression. Thus the effect of ADT is temporary and on average last only 2 years [74]. One theory holds that ADT selectively kills off only a subset of cancer cells, and eventually there remain those that for one reason or another do not respond to the anti-proliferation effects of ADT. This subset eventually becomes dominant and progression resumes and accelerates. The patient now has hormone-resistant prostate cancer and a less hopeful prognosis.

HORMONE THERAPY WITH RADIOTHERAPY

This section deals with the use of androgen deprivation therapy (ADT) along with radiation therapy in either the neoadjuvant or adjuvant setting. This should not be confused with the use of ADT for the treatment of biochemical recurrence (failure) after RT. The subject has recently been reviewed [75,76].

Several randomized trials have shown benefit in overall survival and disease-free survival when ADT is used along with RT with the hormone therapy starting either before, with or immediately after the radiation treatments.

- In a phase III trial conducted by the European Organization for Research and Treatment of Cancer (EORTC) 412 patients with localized or locally advanced disease (T1-T4 without detectable lymph node involvement) were randomized to LHRG agonist therapy alone or started simultaneously with RT [77,78]. The duration of ADT was three years. Five-year overall survival was 78% for the ADT + RT group, 62% for the RT alone group. Five year disease free survival was 74% for the ADT + RT treatment and 40% for the RT alone treatment. Both differences were statistically significant.

- In the Radiation Therapy Oncology Group Trial 85-31, the ADT + RT arm involved starting patients on an LHRH agonist in the last week of RT and continuing indefinitely. The ADT + RT group had 53% overall survival VS. 38% in the RT only group. The cohort was selected for evidence of extracapsular disease or regional lymph node involvement and would be candidates for hormone therapy after recurrence. (see [75,76]).

- D'Amico *et al* [79] reported in 2004 on a randomized trial involving 6-month ADT plus RT vs. RT alone for patients with clinically localized prostate cancer (T1b-T2b, unknown or any lymph node involvement, and no metastasis). RT consisted of 3D-CRT. ADT involved complete androgen blocking with the use of both a LHRH agonist and an antiandrogen, and this treatment was administered two month before RT, during the two months of RT and for two months adjuvant to RT. The 5-year overall survival was 88% for the combined therapy vs. 78% for RT alone. Survival free of salvage ADT (i.e. recurrence free) was 82% for the combined group and 57% for the RT only patients. In an editorial accompanying the report of this trial, DeWeese [80] comments that the results of D'Amico *et al* are similar to those of EORTC trial which used a three-year treatment period. However, he points out that the results from the short-term ADT treatment should not be extrapolated to patients with high-risk locally advanced cancer where long-term ADT has been reported beneficial. In response to questions raised regarding radiation dose and duration of treatment, D'Amico *et al* [81] indicate they believe, given the two-fold reduction in mortality, that the combination of 70 Gy radiation dose and 6 months of ADT represents the preferred therapy for patients with the clinical category T1b to T2b and either a PSA > 10 ng/mL or a Gleason score equal to or greater than 7.

- In a randomized trial very recently reported, Denham *et al* [82] describes the short-term use of ADT for locally advanced prostate cancer. Patients either received RT alone for about 7 weeks, or ADT 2 months before RT for a total of three months, or ADT 5 months before RT for a total of 6 months. ADT consisted of combined LHRH agonist and an antiandrogen. In comparison with the radiation-only group, the 3-month ADT significantly reduced biochemical failure, increased disease-free survival and resulted in less need for salvage treatment. The 6-month protocol augmented these effects and improved cancer-specific survival. The 6-month ADT reduced both local failure and distant failure. However, the authors point out that one shortcoming of this trial is the limitations on the RT equipment (maximum dose 66 Gy) which prevented the use of higher dose levels that have been shown to improve local control. Therefore it is not clear whether the benefits of ADT would have been as great had higher doses of RT been used. The authors are implementing a new study to clarify this and other issues.

- In a randomized trial involving patients with locally advanced cancer (T2c-T4) Hanks *et al* [83], treated all patients with both a LHRH agonist and an antiandrogen for 2 months prior to RT and for 2 months during RT. Both the prostate and the pelvic lymph nodes were irradiated. This cohort was then randomized to receive no additional treatment (the short-term ADT group) or 24 months of a LHRH agonist (the long-term ADT group). The long-term ADT group showed significant improvement in all efficacy endpoints except overall survival (disease free survival, cause specific survival, biochemical failure, distant metastasis, and local progression) compared to the short-term ADT group. Also, in a subgroup with tumors assigned a Gleason score of 8-10, the long-term ADT group also showed significantly better overall survival (81% vs. 70.7%).

- Roach *et al* [84,85] have performed a meta-analysis (data of several studies combined and the data re-analyzed) of four Radiation Therapy Oncology Group studies involving 2742 men treated for clinically localized prostate cancer between 1975 and 1992. Four patient groups were identified: (1) T1-T2 and Gleason score 2-6; (2) T3, Gleason score 2-6 or T1-T2, Gleason score 7; (3) T3, Gleason score 7 or T1-T2, Gleason score 8-10; (4) T3 and Gleason score 8-10. Patients in group 2 (either Gleason 2-6 with bulky tumors or Gleason 7 with organ confined disease) benefited from 4 months (2 months before, two months during) of combined LHRH agonist and antiandrogen therapy plus radiation. Patients in risk groups 3 and 4 benefited from long-term hormonal therapy (adjuvant, continued indefinitely).

These studies are particularly significant because they randomized the patients into two or more study arms. There was clearly a large difference in ADT treatment protocol and duration, and more studies are needed to provide a definitive answer as to what represents the optimum protocol. The 4-6-month protocols used in some of the studies would appear attractive from the standpoint of side effects, since most resolve when ADT is terminated. However, as D'Amico *et al* [81] point out, there are no randomized studies comparing long- and short-term ADT for patients with clinically localized cancer. Nevertheless, the studies listed above suggest benefit from RT with either adjuvant or both neoadjuvant and adjuvant ADT for men with clinically localized and locally advanced prostate cancer. As discussed above, the NCCN recommends HT plus RT as an option for patients with high-risk disease but not for those who fall into the intermediate risk category [86]. In the D'Amico *et al* study [79], only 15% of participants had a Gleason score of 8-10 and 13% had PSA > 20 ng/mL, characteristics that would put them in the NCCN high risk category. Finally, it should be noted that most studies involving RT do not have an ADT-only arm but instead compare RT only with RT plus ADT.

ADJUVANT HORMONE THERAPY WITH RADICAL PROSTATECTOMY

There is a very limited literature on the benefits of immediate hormone therapy after radical prostatectomy and very little guidance is available concerning either the optimum form of therapy or the protocol (intermittent or continuous) [31,87]. Three studies are of interest:

- Messing *et al* [88] randomized 98 men with T1-T2 disease and with nodal metastases found at the time of RP to immediate LHRH agonist therapy (goserelin) or surgical castration or observation. The median follow-up was 7.1 years. The 5-year progression free survival was 87% in the immediate therapy group vs. 40% in the observation group. Prostate cancer-specific survival at 5 years was 96 % vs. 80% when the immediate ADT group was compared with the observation group left untreated until distant metastases were found (from their Fig. 1, B, C). Overall 10-year survival rates were 72% vs. 49% (see [89]).

- Prayer-Galetti *et al* (see [87]) found a 25.4% improvement in 5-year disease-free survival for a group of 201 patients (T3) given post-RP LHRH agonist therapy (goserelin).

- In a study that used the antiandrogen bicalutamide for immediate adjuvant therapy (in the first 16 weeks), 8113 patients were randomized to receive an antiandrogen plus standard care (RT or RP) or watchful waiting vs. a placebo and standard care. The patient population had localized and locally advanced disease (T1-T4, any lymph node involvement, and no metastasis). At 5.4 years median follow-up, adjuvant antiandrogen treatment significantly reduced the risk of progression by 29% compared to RP alone in patients with locally advanced disease, but no effect was found with localized disease. Longer follow-up will not be available because the trial was terminated [31].

- In a study from the Mayo Clinic reported [90] in 2001, a group of 707 patients with pathologically staged cancer who were seminal vesicle positive were treated with RP. Of these, 157 received adjuvant hormonal therapy. Progression-free survival was significantly better in the hormone therapy group (67%) compared to those who had only surgery (23%). Cancer-specific survival was also improved in the adjuvant hormone group as compared to the surgery only group (95% vs. 87%) and the percentage systemic progression-free also favored hormonal treatment (90% vs. 78%).

- The combination of LHRH agonists and antiandrogens in the above context has received limited study and the results were conflicting [31].

Thus for patients treated by radical prostatectomy as the primary therapy, both randomized and other studies suggest that there is a significantly improved recurrence-free and disease-specific survival with the use of adjuvant medical or surgical castration for those with lymph node metastases or seminal vesicle invasion. An obvious question concerns a comparison between the adjuvant ADT discussed above vs. adjuvant RT or with or without ADT after progression is evident. Waiting for progression obviously provides a side effect free window in time but there is need for randomized study data to judge the relative merits of these two intervention protocols especially since post-recurrence RT is a standard interventional response to progression after RP.

There is also the natural history of progression to consider. Pound *et al* [1] reported that the median time for the development of metastasis and the median time to prostate-specific death were 8 and 13 years respectively, both measured from the time of PSA increase (failure) after radical prostatectomy. Therefore, Khan *et al* [31] suggest that a delay in hormonal therapy beyond the point of PSA elevation can be considered for men with significant comorbidities, slow disease progression and in older men.

NEOADJUVANT HORMONE THERAPY BEFORE RADICAL PROSTATECTOMY OR RADIOTHERAPY

The use of ADT before prostate cancer surgery has been the subject of a limited number of studies. Short-term endpoints such as tumor volume or surgical margin status were positively influenced, but when PSA progression was examined (the longest for a median of 6.8 years follow-up) no significant benefit was found. Thus the utility of neoadjuvant hormone therapy prior to RP remains unproven [87,89].

Two studies are also of interest in connection with neoadjuvant hormone therapy.

- In a recently published study by Laverdiere *et al* [91] the comparison between RT only compared to (a) 3 months of neoadjuvant therapy with both a LHRH agonist and an antiandrogen prior to RT or (b) either this neoadjuvant treatment followed by concomitant ADT therapy or (c) RT with concomitant and then adjuvant hormone therapy for a total of 10 months. Patients had T2-T3 cancer.

The only significant result was an increase in the 7-year biochemical free survival of 66% vs. 42% when neoadjuvant treatment was compared to RT alone. Hormone treatment during or after RT resulted in no improvement.

• In a similar study [92], 2 months of neoadjuvant hormone treatment with combined LHRH agonist and an antiandrogen followed by hormone treatment during RT proved effective for the overall cohort for a number of endpoints including local control, reduction in metastasis, disease-free survival, PSA disease free survival and cancer specific mortality. Patients were grade T2-T4 with or without lymph node involvement but without evidence of distant metastases. However, the most significant beneficial results were obtained with a subgroup characterized by a Gleason score of 2-6. For patients with Gleason score 7-10 tumors, the treatment protocol did not result in enhancement in either locoregional control or survival. This is particularly interesting since for patients with high Gleason scores (8-10) another study [93] found that the result of adjuvant ADT was effective whereas patients with low Gleason Scores experienced little benefit from post-RT ADT.

Miljenko et al [92] point out that different strategies appear to be required for different subsets of patients and those with high Gleason scores, 4 months of androgen deprivation before RT is not adequate whereas for those with Gleason scores 2-6, such treatment exerts a major beneficial effect on all endpoints and should be considered as a standard of care.

HORMONE TREATMENT UPON RECURRENCE AFTER RADIOTHERAPY

As discussed above, one option after primary RT has failed is the salvage radical prostatectomy or cryotherapy. Another option is hormone therapy, and for patients who are not considered suitable for surgery or cryotherapy, it is the only option in standard practice. Uncertainties concerning the treatment protocols were discussed above in connection with the ASCO panel views.

COMBINING HORMONE THERAPY WITH THE 5-α REDUCTASE INHIBITORS

The class of drug, known as 5-α reductase inhibitors (finasteride or dutasteride), is widely used in the medical treatment of benign prostatic hyperplasia (BPH—see Chapter 2). This enzyme inhibitor acts to prevent the conversion of testosterone to dihydrotestosterone. Since this is one of the objectives of hormone therapy, it is not surprising that its role in treating advanced cancer has been investigated. In addition, it has been recognized for some time that intraprostatic dihydrotestosterone levels remain high despite androgen deprivation and it has been suggested that adding a 5-α reductase inhibitor may enhance intracellular androgen blockage and augment disease control [94]. While large or long-term or even randomized studies are lacking, several interesting and encouraging research findings have in fact appeared in the last few years.

As discussed in Chapter 4, a recent study found in a much-publicized trial that finasteride (Proscar) appeared to prevent prostate cancer, but there was some concern that it promoted advanced cancer. There is considerable current debate regarding this latter aspect, with evidence accumulating that this latter result may be an artifact. Finasteride has also been used as monotherapy for the treatment of recurrence after RP with results suggesting that finasteride delays but does not prevent the rise in serum PSA after failed surgery [95]. Two other approaches using this 5α-reductase inhibitor involve either combining it with an antiandrogen (flutamide or bicalutamide) or using it with both an antiandrogen and a LHRH agonist. Studies of the first protocol were in the setting of either a pilot or Phase II study and provided positive results as regards both minimal side effects and a greater decrease in PSA (lower nadir) when finasteride is added to the antiandrogen treatment. In addition, this treatment did not appear to interfere with subsequent LHRH use when indicated [63,94,96,97]. These studies involved small numbers of participants, short follow-up, and no opportunity to compare with other protocols.

An interesting case study [96] followed the treatment of a patient with RT failure (PSA detected) who was initially treated with an antiandrogen (bicalutimide) for approximately 15 months until a nadir was established. At this point finasteride was added to the therapy producing a lower and undetectable PSA ≤ 0.05 ng/mL which was durable for 2 years (the end of the follow-up). The authors discuss a hypothesized biological basis for 5-α reductase inhibitors to delay or arrest the progression to androgen independent disease.

Two studies have addressed the use of finasteride combined with so-called complete androgen blockage. Strum and Pogliano [98] describe a study which employed combined intermittent LHRH and antiandrogen therapy plus finasteride (Proscar 5 mg twice a day) which was used during both the on and off phases of the ADT. This study is quite interesting because patients on this protocol were compared with those just on the intermittent ADT. For the ADT plus Proscar group, the median off-phase time was 44 months compared to 17 months for the ADT group. When a subgroup of those showing only recurrence detected by PSA failure, the ADT median off-phase time was 24 months and for the ADT plus Proscar group a median had not been reached in 60 months. This subgroup had had recurrence after RP or RT or both and elected the ADT plus Proscar treatment after PSA recurrence. The long off-phase times allowed patients to recover testosterone function and many of the side effects resolved.

In another study using ADT plus Proscar, Leibowitz and Tucker [99] retrospectively evaluated 110 consecutive patients. Proscar (5 mg) was given once daily along with an antiandrogen and a LHRH agonist on an intermittent protocol. Proscar was continued during the off-phase which started when the serum PSA reached a nadir. All patients were T1-T3 (clinically localized or locally advanced) who had refused any form of local therapy. Over half were low-risk by the usual definitions. After a median follow-up of 36 months, 105 of 110 patients (95.5%) had stable PSA levels. The study recruited between 1990 and 1999 and at the time of submission of the manuscript (2000) no patient had received a second cycle of ADT, i.e. they were still in the first "off" phase. As Strum and Pogliano point out, both this study and theirs are provocative enough to encourage a large scale trial of ADT vs. ADT plus a 5-α reductase inhibitor.

Some men with advanced or recurrent disease may find this an interesting option to consider and discuss with their attending physician, just on the basis of these studies, especially if they are considering intermittent therapy. It may be some time before randomized, large-scale long-term studies will be done and reported. A fairly detailed discussion is presented by Strum and Pogliano in the recent edition of the book *A Primer on Prostate Cancer* [98].

HORMONE RESISTANT (ANDROGEN INDEPENDENT) DISEASE

For the NCCN high-risk category as well as for those failing salvage therapy the most common treatment involves androgen deprivation, either with LHRH agonists or in combination with antiandrogens. The assumption is that the cancer has metastasized and that only systemic treatment is indicated. The hormone therapy generally results in a low PSA value, a result that may give rise to false hope that the progression has been permanently arrested. However, over a period of several years, the effectiveness generally diminishes, PSA starts to increase, clinical evidence of renewed tumor growth and metastasis may appear and eventually the state of affairs is described as *hormone-refractory, hormone-resistant* or *androgen-independent* disease. This is also termed PSA failure after hormone ablation. It is not known whether this is due to clonal selection, simply adaptation or one or more other mechanisms. The lack of detailed mechanistic understanding is an impediment to the development of effective therapeutic agents. But progress has been reported on various fronts [100]. Discussion of the mechanism is beyond the scope of this work.

Once the cancer has become androgen-independent, there is a huge range of cancer-specific survival times observed in patients given no chemotherapy or cytotoxic treatment. Shulman and Benaim [101] have recently reported on a study that attempts to quantify this aspect of advanced disease. Failure of hormone therapy was detected by increasing PSA (2 consecutive increases each 25% of nadir), and the time between the start of treatment and failure was termed the recurrence time. PSA doubling times were calculated from the time of failure. With these parameters they found that the cohort divided into three risk groups stratified according to cancer specific survival. The low-risk group had a doubling time of > 6 months. The intermediate group had a doubling time of < 6 months, time to recurrence > than 7 months, and a nadir while on hormone therapy of ≤ 0.5 ng/mL. The high-risk group has one of the following two combinations; (1) doubling time of < 6 months and time to recurrence of ≤ 7 months or (2) doubling time of < 6 months, time to recurrence of > 7 months and a nadir during treatment of > 0.5 ng/mL. The cancer specific survival times for these three groups cover a remarkable range as indicated in Table 8.

Table 7-8. Median prostate cancer specific survival times with androgen independent disease by risk grouping (see text) [101]

Risk Grouping	Median Time of Ca-Specific Survival (Months)
Low	89.1
Intermediate	38.4
High	14.0

The important aspect of this study is the result that risk stratification was on the basis of PSA history alone. The low-risk group had a median cancer-specific survival time that was over 7 years. None of the patients in this study had chemotherapy. Thus according to the authors, these results accurately describe the true natural history of androgen-independent prostate cancer. Men may find these results of considerable interest when considering chemotherapy vs. other options.

One of the other options involves changing the nature and protocol of the hormone treatment. Scardino [11] discusses modifications and variations of the hormone treatment that are apparently used at Memorial Sloan-Kettering Cancer Center when evidence of treatment failure appears. For example, if a patient has been on only a LHRH agonist, an antiandrogen is added, but if both were already being used, the antiandrogen might be stopped. They also substitute adrenal-blocking drugs like ketoconazole or aminogluterthamide for an antiandrogen (e.g. bicalutamide). Corticosteroids like hydrocortisone or prednisone are effective according to Scardino [11] and they are often added to adrenal-blocking drugs to prevent adrenal insufficiency. They also use high-dose estrogens, recognizing that there is an increased risk of blood clots. These are delaying tactics used in the hope of extending the symptom-free period as long as possible. Similar recommendations can be found in the NCCN 2005 Guidelines [86]. A recent Phase III trial of ketoconazole in hormone-resistant prostate cancer patients also found that the use of this adrenal-blocking agent at the time of antiandrogen withdrawal is a reasonable, well tolerated treatment option with moderate success in this group of patients who develop androgen independent disease [102].

CHEMOTHERAPY

Traditionally, when hormone and steroid treatment fail, the final act involves trying to keep the patient comfortable, i.e. palliative care. This involves dealing with the pain of bone metastases and general pain control and generally ultimately requires opiates. However, recently there has been a flurry of activity in the development and testing chemotherapeutic agents as a potential therapy for hormone-resistant prostate cancer. Historically, chemotherapeutic agents offered benefits that did not balance the associated risks and the low rate of response resulted in a lack of enthusiasm among urologists and medical oncologists for this approach to treating advanced hormone-resistant disease. Since 1999 the drug combination of mitoxantrone and prednisone/hydrocortisone has served as the standard of care for hormone refractory prostate cancer. This combination was shown to improve symptom control and quality of life compared to steroid therapy alone, but offered no survival advantage [103]. Now we are seeing medical journal articles concerning chemotherapy containing phrases or sub-titles such as "Emerging from the Shadows," "Finally an Effective Chemotherapy," and "Finally an Advance!" The research behind this apparent enthusiasm is of interest. The drug responsible is called docetaxel (Taxotere).

Two studies reported in the New England Journal of Medicine in 2004 are currently regarded as of particular significance in this context. The first, the so-called TAX 327 study [104], was an international, multicenter randomized Phase III trial that used various protocols for the drug docetaxel combined with prednisone as compared to the older combination mitoxantrone and prednisone. The best results yielded survival rates of 18.9 month (95% confidence limits of 17-21.2 months) vs. 16.5 months (95% confidence limits of 15.7-19.0) for the comparison group and docetaxel with prednisone produced better pain control. Adverse events were common. The docetaxel-prednisone group on the dose protocol giving the best survival had somewhat higher serious adverse effects than the mitoxantrone-prednisone control, and also had higher low-grade adverse events such as fatigue, nausea/vomiting, alopecia, diarrhea, neuropathy, stomatitis, dyspnea, tearing, peripheral edema and epistaxis than the mitoxantrone group. Note that there was no placebo control and the randomization was between the treatment groups, one of which was considered to offer no survival advantage. However, since some form of treatment is necessary, the use of a placebo would probably have been considered unethical. Thus if one ignores the life extension of about 2 months with the strongly overlapping 95% confidence limits, then some would argue that better pain reduction is the only basis for truly justified enthusiasm, and this can be a bit subjective.

The second study [105], denoted SWOG 9916, combined docetaxel and estramustine (thought to be an antineoplastic agent operating by an unknown mechanism) compared to mitoxantrone and prednisone. The median overall survival for docetaxel-estramustine vs. mitoxantrone was 17.5 months vs. 15.6 months. Side effects that were greater in the docetaxel-estramustine group compared to the mitoxantrone-prednisone group included cardiovascular events, nausea and vomiting, metabolic disturbances and neurological changes. Again there was no placebo control. Thus both of these studies of docetaxel vs. the older treatment yielded only about two months additional survival. The fact that these differences were statistically significant may carry more weight with oncologists than with patients, especially since these numbers are averages with some variation. The challenge is to balance the benefits vs. the side effects and quality of life, which is not simple and to some extent requires more data, especially concerning quality of life. Also, these chemotherapy trials have been criticized as enrolling younger men who are not representative of the principal population with hormone-resistant prostate cancer. While some think docetaxel provides "effective" chemotherapy, there does not appear to be a randomized trial where just prednisone was the control.

Many journals now require a declaration of potential conflicts of interest. Some of the investigators in one of the above docetaxel studies, and all but one investigator in the other had financial ties or financial interests of one form or another with the maker of docetaxel. One of the studies was financially supported by the drug company, the other both by the National Cancer Institute (US) and the drug manufacturer. This opportunity for a conflict of interest is both common and normal today, and is an integral part of the functioning of the drug development, testing and approval system, at least in the US [106]. There has in fact been a flood of books in the past two years detailing the pros and cons of this phenomenon. The array of literature for the general audience can be viewed by putting the key phrase "drug companies" into the book search feature of Amazon.com. Two of the recent books are in fact written by past editors of the *New England Journal of Medicine!*

Thus men offered chemotherapy may wish to think about what "significant" survival extension really means for them and ask for the basis on which the use of a new chemotherapeutic agent is being recommended and how significant is the improvement in palliation and survival extension vs. the older combination in use for the last decade. Quality of life and success of palliation are not easy to measure and depend on a number of factors including age, comorbidities etc. The results quoted above suggest that side effects were more serious for the new chemotherapy protocols. In particular, men may wish to probe aggressively into what is the attending physician's own experience with the actual protocol being suggested. This is not a simple matter and it would seem that the benefits aside from what some would term a very small life extension must clearly exceed downside of the side effects of the treatment, given that if pain is the problem, an alternative involves opiates or the older mitoxantrone and prednisone therapy, and it appears unrealistic to be concerned with addiction problems if life expectancy is short. Also, men must be wary of the promotional aspect of the drop in PSA with chemotherapy if it has no real significance in overall survival.

The search for a chemotherapeutic approach to advanced prostate cancer will continue to be pursued. The financial rewards are substantial, given the prevalence of the disease and the associated demographics. But it may be that small effects on life expectancy are greeted and promoted with unreasonable enthusiasm. It seems that one of the characteristics of the practice of oncology is enthusiasm for small benefits, but in all fairness, it is not uncommon that this is all that can be offered. Some patients reject chemotherapy for this reason, arguing that the decrease in their quality of life and in some cases, an increased risk of treatment induced mortality, when compared to an increase in *estimated* survival measured in weeks or at best a month or two, results, for them, in a negative risk-reward indication.

New drugs of course mean new clinical trials, and patients with little hope remaining may have the option of enrolling in such a trial if it is locally available. Some trials may involve drugs with low levels of side effects and perhaps approaches other than the use of cytotoxic drugs. As well the so-called alternative treatments discussed in Chapter 8 can be considered.

BONE METASTASES

Metastases to bone are a very common complication of advanced prostate cancer and are responsible for significant morbidity. Two recent reviews [107,108] help to put the need for effective treatment in perspective. The authors make the following points.

- Three factors put prostate cancer patients at risk for skeletal morbidity. These are advanced age at diagnosis, hormonal therapy and the development of bone metastases.
- Bone metastases will typically develop in 65-100% of patients during the natural course of the disease. The spine, pelvis and rib cage are the common sites involved.
- Patients with bone metastases will exhibit skeletal complications such as fractures of pathological origin, spinal cord compression and severe bone pain. Relief of the bone pain can require palliative radiation therapy.
- Low bone mineral density (BMD) is found in patients with prostate cancer who are given hormone therapy. Long-term hormone therapy (androgen deprivation therapy) can lead to a significant and even severe decrease in BMD.
- Advanced metastatic cancer develops most frequently in the bone.
- Spinal cord compression occurs in 7% of all patients with malignant bone disease associated with prostate cancer. Devastating neurologic consequences which can result from nerve compression, including paralysis of both lower extremities, require immediate intervention.
- In a recent study of bisphosphonate therapy (see below) in men with hormone-refractory prostate cancer and bone metastasis, the placebo arm revealed that nearly 50% of untreated patients experienced skeletal complications within two years of the start of the study.
- Long-term hormone therapy (ADT) and bone metastases can have a significant impact on the quality of life. In addition, fractures associated with this pathology have been shown to reduce overall survival. Many metastases-related bone fractures fail to heal and require orthopedic surgery with an attendant morbidity and small but finite mortality rate.

This is a very long litany of bone-related problems associated with advanced prostate cancer. Detailed citations can be found in the cited reviews. Clearly, this is a large, complex and important problem. All men, having failed primary and salvage treatment, should consider confronting this problem and acquiring knowledge regarding the important aspects of prevention and treatment.

It is well known that aging is associated with decreased bone mineral density (BMD), a skeletal feature than can be measured by x-ray techniques. As BMD decreases the risk of fracture increases. Thus even before primary or secondary treatment, some men are at risk of bone-related problems. Deficiencies in vitamin D and calcium are common throughout this population and are frequently unrecognized and untreated. In fact, it is not unusual for studies of the efficacy of a proposed treatment of prostate cancer related bone problems to include supplementation with both calcium and vitamin D in *both* the placebo and treatment arms even though it is acknowledged that this may decrease the observed benefit (vs. the placebo) of the drug being tested.

Bone is not an inert structural unit like the framework of a house. Rather, bone resorption and formation are ongoing processes of considerable complexity. It has been repeatedly suggested that the growth-factor rich environment in the bone provides an attractive "soil" for the seeding of certain tumor cells and tumor breakdown of bone stimulates further cancer cell growth which leads to further increases in bone resorption, i.e. a classical vicious cycle [109]. Prostate bone metastases can frequently be seen on radiographs and as well can be imaged by radioactive tracer techniques (the bone scan). Multiple sites of metastasis are common, and an increasing number of sites on repeated examination is indicative of a poor prognosis.

The treatment of bone problems associated with advanced prostate cancer has centered on a class of drugs called *bisphosphonates*. These drugs are potent inhibitors of tumor-induced softening, absorption and destruction of bony tissue. They are not only used in the context of prostate cancer but also for breast cancer and multiple myeloma [108]. Historically a number of different bisphosphonates were evaluated and used but with little durable success. However, one drug in this class, zoledronic acid, has emerged as a potentially effective agent for treating both pain and skeletal morbidity and as well, may have significant preventive applications. Of three randomized Phase III studies of bisphosphonate therapy, two were negative [110] but a third, which involved zoledronic acid, merits discussion.

The first results of this trial were published in 2002 by Saad *et al* [111] with a follow-up published [112] in 2004. Subjects (643) were randomized to receive a double-blind treatment of intravenous zoledronic acid or a placebo every 3 weeks for 15 months. The dose dictated by renal safety was 4 mg. The study showed that patients receiving 4 mg of zoledronic acid experienced 22% fewer events that were skeletal-related as compared to the placebo group. The median time to the first skeletal-related event was extended by more than 5 months in the drug group. Higher pain and analgesic use were found in the placebo group as compared to the drug group. However, while there was also an extension of overall survival of 77 days, this effect lacked statistical significance.

In a mini-review in *BJU international* [110] Parker examines the question of whether or not these results justify the routine use of zoledronic acid in this setting. He makes three points. First, statistical significance does not equal clinical significance. He comments that the improvement among treated patients in pain control, while statistically significant, may not be clinically relevant. Second, he questions the clinical significance of the observed reduction in the need for bone radiation. Finally, he reviews the adverse effects of the trial. These were, in comparison to the placebo group, a 32.7% vs. 25.5% increase in fatigue, a 26.6% vs. 17.8% increase in anemia, a 24.8% vs. 17% increase in myaliga, a 20.1% vs. 13% increase in fever, a 19.2% vs. 13% increase in edema, and a 16.8% vs. 12.5% weight loss. In the opinion of Parker, there was no increase in quality of life in the treatment arm. Thus one is left with a complicated risk-reward equation. Parker concludes that the current evidence does not support the use of bisphosphonates in the standard management of bone problems in hormone-resistant prostate cancer. However, others who have reviewed the use of zoledronic acid do not take as negative a view [108,109].

As pointed out above, hormone therapy has adverse bone effects. In a recent study, Smith *et al* [113] examined the effect of zoledronic acid therapy on bone mineral density (BMD) in patients without metastatic prostate cancer who were just starting androgen deprivation therapy (LHRH agonist with or without an antiandrogen). The trial was randomized and placebo controlled. The primary efficacy parameter was the change in BMD from baseline to 1 year in the lumbar spine as measured by x-ray analysis. BMD changes were also measured in the neck, hip and as well in the bony prominences near the upper end of the femur. It was found that treatment with zoledronic acid promoted increased BMD whereas those on the placebo experienced decreases. The differences were statistically significant and adverse effects did not appear to be an issue. The design of the protocol, study conduct and monitoring, data collection and statistical analysis were all performed by the drug company that manufactures zoledronic acid [113].

PAIN MANAGEMENT

The first line of action in direct pain management in patients with advanced prostate cancer generally involves analgesics. The most common source of pain is from bone metastases. Analgesics can be ranked as non-opioids, weak opioids (e.g. codeine) and strong opioids (e.g. morphine and hydromorphone). The opioids are of course potentially addictive. From time to time, the question of undertreatment of pain has been raised and recently two papers have appeared that relate to this question.

Yau *et al* [114] provide an interesting picture based on a Canadian study from the Toronto Sunnybrook Regional Cancer Center. From January 1999 to January 2002, a total of 534 patients were referred to the Rapid Response Radiotherapy Program for pain associated with bone metastasis. While only 23% had metastasis related to prostate cancer, the overall results nevertheless reflect a pattern of under-treatment. After exclusions, 518 patients formed the study group. Of these, 31% had moderate pain and 45% had severe pain at the initial consultation. However, 34% of the 398 patients with moderate to severe pain were not prescribed adequate pain-control medication. The authors suggest that barriers to treatment with stronger opioids may come from health care providers with misconceptions about medications and side effects or insufficient knowledge and training in pain management. Potential patient/provider contributions to under-medication were suggested as well and included concerns about addiction, poor communication, wanting to be a "good" patient, and misconceptions about the inevitability of pain. Only fifty-one patients (9.8%) appeared to be adequately palliated with strong opioids. Finally the authors comment that in an earlier study the prevalence of under-medication for bone pain found similar results, and that they detect no improvement in the situation. When concerns about addiction come from the health care providers, one can wonder about how realistic this is if the patient is in moderate to severe pain and is probably terminal.

A second multicenter study focused on the under-treatment of pain in African American and Hispanic cancer patients [115]. The main concern of the study was the effectiveness of patient education which had a limited impact on what the authors call underserved minority patients. But in the context of this section, the point is that there was under-treatment of cancer-related pain, and this study quotes earlier work which suggests that this is not just a problem common to minority patients.

It is not consistent with the theme of this book to discuss in any depth the pros and cons of analgesic options. However, it should be mentioned that radiotherapy directed at bone metastases is both commonly employed and can be temporarily effective in pain modification in some patients. Yau *et al* [114] indicate that about 80% of patients derive benefit from this approach to pain control.

| CONCLUSIONS |

Recurrence after definitive primary treatment is unfortunately not uncommon. In fact it is in part the inevitable result of local treatment for disseminated disease which was either thought to be absent or merely recognized as a possibility at the time of therapy. Men must realize that recurrence does not mean that the prognosis has turned hopeless. Quite the contrary, in favorable cases, salvage therapy can result in what amounts to a cure or at least a very long disease-free survival period. The possibility of this outcome should encourage men to persist in following the course of their disease after primary definitive treatment, an action that will of course be strongly recommended by the physician involved in the case. Even when progression cannot be halted and eventually metastatic cancer occurs, the process may be slow, treatments with objectionable side effects can in some cases be delayed, and the progression can be retarded by various treatment modalities. In the treatment of prostate cancer there will always be winners and losers.

As discussed in this chapter, a number of options exist for how hormone treatment is implemented, and at this writing no real consensus appears to exist due to the absence of compelling evidence favoring any one protocol. This is an area where rapid change can be expected as regards favored options as larger and longer-term studies are reported. To the man considering the recommendation of hormone therapy, the protocol can be very important because of the inevitable side effects which impact the quality of life. It is important that he discuss with his physician the various options such as delayed vs. immediate treatment, intermittent vs. constant dosing, LHRH agonists vs. antiandrogens vs. combined therapy, etc. One protocol may emerge at any time as clearly favored for his clinical presentation. For example, the intermittent use of hormone therapy combined with long term use of one of the 5-α reductase inhibitors, in this case finasteride (Proscar), has shown promise in producing remarkably long "off" periods with stable PSA and the attendant increase in the period where side effects are less severe. This particular protocol is still experimental, but more studies will no doubt soon appear, and already there is probably enough data to satisfy some physicians that this protocol has merit.

While little progress appears to have occurred in the treatment of the hormone resistant stage of the disease, this is an area of active research which may soon yield important new approaches. As discussed above, even simple alterations in the protocol used for hormone sensitive advanced disease have yielded promising results when one protocol has ceased to work. The merits of chemotherapy will remain controversial due to the small absolute increase in survival with the current protocols. There are alternative treatments discussed in Chapter 8 which have yielded significant and in some cases remarkable life extension in cases declared terminal and untreatable except with pain management. Finally, men in the latter stages of this disease should be forceful in demanding pain control when confronted with care givers who take too conservative an approach or for one reason or another fail to aggressively treat this aspect of the disease. There is after all evidence that under-treatment of pain is common and unnecessary, and to put it bluntly, if the prognosis is terminal, the risk of addiction to strong narcotic-type drugs would seem at the very least, irrelevant.

Chapter 8

Alternative and Complementary Therapies

Hans R. Larsen MSc ChE

INTRODUCTION

Prostate cancer is conventionally treated with surgery, radiation, hormone therapy or, to a lesser extent, chemotherapy. In some cases the results of these treatments are spectacular, in other cases they are pretty dismal and the accompanying adverse effects, particularly incontinence and impotence may, in the minds of many men, negate the fact that the cancer is no longer growing, at least for a time. Not surprisingly, this state of affairs has led to a search for other approaches and this is where alternative and complementary therapies come in. A clear distinction should be made between alternative and complementary therapies. Alternative therapies are those that stand on their own without the involvement of conventional medicine, whereas complementary therapies are essentially alternative ones that complement conventional therapies.

To most of the world's population, alternative medicine is not 'alternative' at all, but rather the basis of the health care system. To western-trained physicians alternative medicine is "something not taught in medical schools" and a field that allopathic doctors don't practice and, one could add, generally know little about.

The use of alternative and complementary therapies in the treatment of prostate cancer will be discussed under the following headings:

- Alternative Medicine – An Overview
- Alternative Therapies
- Complementary Therapies
- Cancer Clinics
- Pharmaceutical Drugs

ALTERNATIVE MEDICINE – AN OVERVIEW

Alternative medicine is no longer a "fringe phenomenon". It is estimated, by none other than the Harvard Medical School, that one out of every two persons in the United States between the ages of 35 and 49 years used at least one alternative therapy in 1997. The users were primarily well-educated, affluent baby boomers.[1] The trend to alternative medicine is repeated throughout Western society. In Australia 57% of the population now use some form of alternative medicine; in Germany 46% do, and in France 49%. Alternative medicine encompasses a very large array of different systems and therapies ranging from Ayurvedic medicine to vitamin therapy.[1-3]

Ayurvedic medicine has been practiced in India for the past five thousand years and has recently undergone a renaissance in the West due, in no small measure, to the work and lectures of Dr. Deepak Chopra, MD. Ayurvedic medicine is a very comprehensive system that places equal emphasis on body, mind, and spirit and uses a highly personalized approach to return an individual to a state where he or she is again in harmony with their environment. Ayurvedic medicine uses diet, exercise, yoga, meditation, massage, herbs, and medication and, despite its long lineage, is as applicable today as it was 5000 years ago. For example, the seeds of the *Mucuna pruriens* plant have long been used to treat Parkinson's disease in India; it is now receiving attention in conventional circles as it is more effective than l-dopa and has fewer side effects.[4]

Traditional Chinese medicine has been practiced for over 3000 years and over one quarter of the world's population now uses one or more of its component therapies. TCM combines the use of medicinal herbs, acupuncture, and the use of therapeutic exercises such as Qi Gong. It has proven to be effective in the treatment of many chronic diseases including cancer, allergies, heart disease and AIDS. As does Ayurvedic medicine, TCM also focuses on the individual and looks for and corrects the underlying causes of imbalance and patterns of disharmony.

Herbal medicine was the mainstay of European and North American medicine until the advent of the pharmaceutical industry in the mid 19th century. Herbal medicines are still used extensively in Germany and France, sometimes in the form of prescription medicines. However, their use in North America declined fairly rapidly once the products of the pharmaceutical industry became widely accepted and prescribed exclusively by physicians. In recent years, herbal medicine has experienced a remarkable renaissance. Between 1991 and 1997 the use of herbal medicines in the United States grew by 380%.[1]

Homeopathy, developed in the early 1800s by the German physician Samuel Hahnemann, is a low-cost, non-toxic health care system now used by hundreds of millions of people around the world. It is particularly popular in South America and the British Royal Family has had a homeopathic physician for the last four generations. Homeopathy is an excellent first-aid system and is also superb in the treatment of minor ailments such as earaches, the common cold, and flu. Homeopathy is again based on the treatment of the individual and when used by a knowledgeable practitioner can also be very effective in the treatment of conditions such as hay fever, digestive problems, rheumatoid arthritis, and respiratory infections.

Chiropracty primarily involves the adjustment of spine and joints to alleviate pain and improve general health. It was practiced by the early Egyptians and was developed into its present form by the American Daniel David Palmer in 1895. It is now the most common form of alternative medicine in the United States. Chiropractors not only manipulate spine and joints, but also advise their patients on lifestyle and diet matters. They believe that humans possess an innate healing potential and that all disease can be overcome by properly activating this potential.

Naturopathic medicine also strongly believes in the body's inherent ability to heal itself. Naturopathy emphasizes the need for seeking and treating the causes of a disease rather than simply suppressing its symptoms. Naturopaths use dietary modifications, herbal medicines, homeopathy, acupuncture, hydrotherapy, massage, and lifestyle counselling to achieve healing.

Vitamin therapy or orthomolecular medicine uses vitamins, minerals, and amino acids to return a diseased body to wellness in the belief that the average diet today is often woefully inadequate in providing needed nutrients and that the need for specific nutrients is highly individual. Conditions as varied as hypertension, depression, cancer, and schizophrenia can all benefit enormously from vitamin therapy.

Biofeedback, bodywork, massage therapy, reflexology, hydrotherapy, aromatherapy, and various other forms of energy medicine round out the vast spectrum of alternative medicine modalities. There are indeed major differences between conventional and alternative medicine.

- Conventional medicine is largely organ specific, hence ophthalmologists, cardiologists, nephrologists, neurologists, etc. Alternative medicine, without exception, considers each person as a unique individual and uses a holistic approach in treatment.

- Conventional medicine believes in aggressive intervention to treat disease. It revels in terms such as "magic bullet" and "war" ("the war on cancer"), and prefers quick fixes (as do many patients). Alternative medicine believes in gentle, long-term support to enable the body's own innate powers to do the healing.

- Conventional medicine's main "arsenal" consists of surgery, chemotherapy, radiation, and powerful pharmaceutical drugs. Alternative medicine uses time-tested, natural remedies and gentle, hands-on treatments.

- Conventional medicine practitioners are guided in their treatment by strict rules set out by the Colleges of Physicians and Surgeons. This often leads to a "one size fits all" approach. Practitioners of alternative medicine, on the other hand, treat each patient as an individual and do what, in their opinion, is best rather than what is specified in a "rule book".

- Both conventional and alternative medicine subscribe to the principle "Do no harm". However, while alternative medicine is essentially achieving this goal, conventional medicine seems to have almost totally lost sight of it. Hospitals are now the third largest killer in Australia and over one million people are seriously injured in American hospitals every year. Blood infections acquired in American hospitals cause 62,000 fatalities every year and bypass surgery results in 25,000 strokes a year. Two million patients experience adverse drug reactions in hospitals in the United States every year; of these, over 100,000 die making hospital-induced adverse drug reactions the fourth leading cause of death after heart disease, cancer, and stroke.[5-11]

- The practice of conventional medicine is intimately tied in with the whole medico-pharmaceutical-industrial complex whose first priority is to make a profit. Although most conventional physicians have "healing the patient" as their first priority, they find it increasingly difficult to do so while operating within the system with its pharmaceutical salesmen, its rule books, its fear of malpractice suits, its endless paperwork to satisfy bureaucrats and insurance companies, and its time pressures. Most alternative medicine practitioners have no such constraints and pressures and can give the patient their undivided attention.

The conventional, Western allopathic medical system is unequalled when it comes to trauma and emergency. After all, you don't call an herbalist if you get hit by a car. However, it is less effective when it comes to prevention, chronic disease, and in addressing the mental, emotional and spiritual needs of an individual. Thus, it is not surprising that alternative medicine is rapidly gaining a foothold, not only in the prevention, but also in the treatment of prostate cancer.

ALTERNATIVE THERAPIES

Clearly the question uppermost in the mind of any man diagnosed with prostate cancer is, "What are my options?" Again, it must be emphasized that, by far, the majority of prostate cancers are slow-growing thus leaving ample time for research and deliberation before making the decision on how to proceed. It should also be kept in mind that urologists, radiologists, and oncologists all have different agendas and preferred therapies. Thus, it is incumbent on the patient to educate himself thoroughly before proceeding with any treatment. This book and the books listed in Appendix D provide good starting points. I can also recommend *The Moss Report on Prostate Cancer* available at www.cancerdecisions.com.

Whether or not to choose alternative therapy is clearly a highly individual decision. A robust, healthy man of 60 years of age with strictly localized cancer may well select radical prostatectomy as the best option. On the other hand, a 75-year-old with heart disease may decide to go with alternative therapies in order to maintain a reasonable quality of life in his remaining years, as may a man diagnosed with incurable, hormone refractory cancer. Some men may also choose to use alternative therapies in combination with watchful waiting, or expectant management (active surveillance). A factor which may weigh heavily in the decision is the unfortunate fact that there is little, if any, long-term data regarding the expected survival time for men using alternative therapies. This compares unfavourably with the situation in regard to conventional treatments (radical prostatectomy and radiation therapy) where reasonably reliable 5- and 10-year survival data are available.

Irrespective of the option chosen, it is important to begin as early as possible to support the immune system which, after all, is carrying the "brunt of the burden". So, unless your doctor advises otherwise, begin boosting your immune system immediately. The late Dr. Linus Pauling recommended that all cancer patients start vitamin supplementation as early as possible. The preferred regimen, formulated by Canadian Dr. Abram Hoffer, MD PhD involves a daily intake of 12,000 mg vitamin C, 800 IU vitamin E, 1500 mg vitamin B3 (nicotinic acid or nicotinamide), 25 or 50 times the RDA (Recommended Daily Allowance) of other B vitamins, and 200 micrograms of selenium. It is necessary to begin with smaller amounts of the supplements and build up gradually.[1]

Once this is underway, you can then select the appropriate alternative therapy, be it Ayurvedic medicine, Traditional Chinese medicine, vitamin therapy (orthomolecular medicine), or phytotherapy (herbal medicine). A description of cancer protocols used in Ayurvedic and Traditional Chinese medicine is beyond the scope of this book, but several effective protocols are available involving vitamin therapy and phytotherapy.

When it comes to distinguishing between prevention (prophylactic) and treatment (therapeutic) effects of supplements and botanical medicines in prostate cancer things become a little blurred. Vitamin D, lycopene, isoflavones (genistein), red clover, and pomegranate juice have all been proven to retard cancer growth (as measured by increased PSA doubling time or reduction in PSA level) and would thus be therapeutic as well as prophylactic. Many other supplements and herbs have proven preventive properties, but no evidence is available to prove or disprove whether they also have therapeutic effects. It is likely that products that have been found to induce apoptosis, reduce proliferation of malignant cells, and inhibit PSA secretion would have therapeutic effects, whereas products that primarily owe their preventive effect to strong antioxidant properties, or their ability to inhibit the aromatase and 5-alpha reductase enzymes would be less likely to have therapeutic effects. Thus, it is unlikely that saw palmetto would be effective in the treatment of prostate cancer. However, it is certainly possible that garlic, green tea, flaxseed, beta-sitosterol, silymarin (silibinin), quercetin, resveratrol, pycnogenol, grape seed extract, coenzyme Q10, boron, selenium, and zinc may some day prove to be effective in halting, or at least slowing, the progression of prostate cancer.

At this time, vitamin D, isoflavones (genistein), lycopene, red clover, pomegranate juice, and several combination protocols have been proven to able to slow the progression of prostate cancer. Other vitamins (vitamin C and alpha-tocopheryl succinate) and phytochemicals (mistletoe extract, thymic extracts, Maitake mushroom extract) have also been found useful in cancer treatment, but have not been specifically evaluated in the treatment of prostate cancer.

VITAMIN THERAPY AND PHYTOTHERAPY

Vitamin D
One small study carried out at the University of Toronto involved 15 prostate cancer patients whose PSA levels had begun to increase after seemingly successful treatment with surgery or radiation. The men were given 2000 IU (50 micrograms) of vitamin D3

daily and monitored every 2-3 months. In 9 of the 15 patients the PSA increase was halted or even reversed for periods as long as 21 months. The median PSA doubling time (an important marker of cancer progression) increased from 14.3 months prior to the start of supplementation to 25 months after beginning the program. Fourteen out of the 15 patients experienced a lengthening of doubling time. There were no side effects of the therapy. The observed prolongation of doubling time is very significant in view of the fact that studies have shown that the risk of developing metastasis within 5 years is 65-75% when PSA doubling time is less than 10 months, but only 10-20% when PSA doubling time exceeds 10 months. The Toronto researchers recommend further studies to confirm their findings and point out that the cost of the vitamin D supplementation was only $2.00 a month.[2]

Isoflavones
Inspired by studies showing a preventive effect of soy products and isoflavones (their active components), several studies have been undertaken to investigate if isoflavones are effective in halting the progression of clinically diagnosed cancer.

Hussain, et al at Wayne State University have found that a twice-daily intake of 100 mg of soy isoflavone (*Novasoy*) stabilized or at least markedly reduced the rise in PSA levels in three groups of men who had been diagnosed with prostate cancer. The average serum level of genistein rose from 0.11 microM to 0.65 microM during the 5.5-month supplementation period.[3] The same group of researchers more recently reported that genistein may inhibit prostate cancer bone metastasis by regulating metastasis-related genes.[4]

Researchers at the University of South Florida evaluated the effect of daily supplementation with 60 mg of soy isoflavones in a group of 59 men diagnosed with early-stage prostate cancer. At the end of the 12-week trial period serum free testosterone was reduced or unchanged in 61% of the members of the isoflavone group as compared to 33% in the placebo group. PSA levels declined by 2 points or more in 19% of the patients supplementing with isoflavones.[5]

Dalais, et al at Monash University in Australia randomized 29 men scheduled for prostatectomy to one of 3 groups. Group 1 (placebo group) supplemented their diet with 4 slices of regular wheat bread daily. Group 2 added 4 slices of a special bread containing 50 grams of heat-treated soy grit to their diet, and group 3 consumed 4 slices daily of a bread containing 50 grams of soy grit and 20 grams of flaxseed. Just before their prostatectomy the members of the soy grit group (group 2) had experienced an 11% drop in total PSA level, while the wheat group had experienced a 22% increase. Free/total PSA ratio increased by 30% in the soy grit group, but decreased by 18% in the wheat group. Statistically significant differences were also observed between the soy grit group (group 2) and the soy grit plus flaxseed group (group 3). The free androgen index increased by 9% in group 2 versus a decrease of 18% in group 3. Blood levels of genistein rose from 4 to 221 nanograms/micromol creatinine in the soy grit group, from 5 to 124 in the soy grit plus flaxseed group, and decreased from 7 to 3 in the wheat group. The researchers conclude that adding 4 slices of soy-enriched bread to the daily diet favourably influences PSA level and free/total PSA ratio in men diagnosed with prostate cancer.[6]

Thus, there is some evidence that including soy products or isoflavones in the diet may slow or perhaps even halt the progression of localized prostate cancer; however, much larger and lengthier studies are clearly required to conclusively prove this.

Lycopene

There is substantial evidence that processed (cooked) tomato products help protect against the development of prostate cancer. It is believed that the protective effect is due to the high concentration of lycopene in tomato products. Several studies have found that supplementation is also effective in increasing lycopene levels in both blood serum and prostate tissue.

An obvious question is does lycopene have a role in the treatment of already existing prostate cancer? A clinical trial of lycopene supplementation was carried out by an international team of researchers from Wayne State University, McGill University, University of Maryland, and the University of Hawaii. The study included 26 men with clinically localized prostate cancer who were scheduled to undergo radical prostatectomy (removal of the prostate gland). The men were randomized into a control group and an intervention group. The intervention group received one 15-mg lycopene capsule (*Lyc-O-Mato*) with breakfast and dinner for three weeks prior to surgery. Blood samples were taken before the start of supplementation and three weeks later just before surgery. The removed tumors and surrounding tissue were examined by pathologists. The researchers conclude that lycopene supplementation lowers PSA levels; they observed an average 18 per cent decrease in the lycopene group as compared to a 14 per cent increase in the control group. The level of the tumor suppressing protein Cx43 in the malignant part of the tumor was found to be substantially higher in the lycopene group. It was also apparent that tumors tended to be smaller and more sharply defined (less encroachment into surrounding healthy tissue) in the lycopene group. No adverse effects of the lycopene supplementation were reported by the patients or their physicians. The researchers conclude that lycopene is likely to be beneficial for both prevention and treatment of prostate cancer, but urge larger trials to confirm this.[7,8]

Researchers at the University of Illinois report that tomato sauce is effective in slowing down and perhaps even reversing existing prostate cancer. Their study involved 32 patients with prostate cancer who were scheduled to undergo a radical prostatectomy. The participants underwent a baseline examination to determine their lycopene levels, their PSA (prostate specific antigen) level, and the level of oxidative damage to their DNA (in leukocytes). They were then fed a pasta dish with tomato sauce (3/4 of a cup of commercial spaghetti sauce) once a day for three weeks. The additional daily lycopene intake from the sauce was 30 mg. At the end of the three-week period lycopene levels in the blood serum had doubled and lycopene levels in prostate tissue had tripled. The average PSA level had declined from 10.9 ng/mL to 8.7 ng/mL – a drop of 17.5 per cent. The DNA damage indicator in leukocytes dropped by 21.4% after the intervention. The DNA damage level in actual prostate tissue (removed during surgery) was found to be 28.3% lower in the tomato sauce group than in a reference group of seven prostate cancer patients who had not consumed the tomato sauce diet. The researchers conclude that their study "suggests a role for tomato sauce and possibly for lycopene in the prevention and treatment of prostate cancer."[9,10]

Thus, both tomato sauce and a commercially available lycopene supplement (*Lyc-O-Mato*) have shown considerable promise not only in prevention, but also in the treatment of localized prostate cancer. It is, unfortunate, but certainly understandable from an ethical point of view, that the trials involving prostate cancer patients were not continued beyond 3 weeks to see if the cancer would regress further with continued lycopene treatment. Future, larger studies will, hopefully, investigate this.

Red Clover

Trifolium pratense is a potent source of the phytoestrogens genistein, daidzein, and biochanin A. Several studies have found that phytoestrogens, more specifically genistein, inhibit the activity of aromatase and 5-alpha reductase (the enzyme responsible for converting testosterone to dihydrotestosterone). Genistein has also been associated with a general regulatory effect on sex hormone receptors and is believed to induce apoptosis and inhibit angiogenesis in cancer cells.[11,12]

Studies have confirmed that supplementation with red clover substantially raises the levels of genistein and daidzein in blood serum and prostate tissue. Finnish researchers observed a 29-fold increase in serum level of genistein after supplementation for 2 weeks with 240 mg/day of red clover (*Trinovin*). Daidzein concentration showed a 28-fold increase and equol (a phytoestrogen) went up 22-fold. Levels in prostate tissue also increased significantly – by a factor of 23 for genistein and a factor of 7 for daidzein.[11] It is thus clear that oral supplementation with red clover is highly effective in raising genistein and daidzein levels in both prostate and blood serum. The fact that genistein inhibits aromatase and 5-alpha reductase, would make it an excellent candidate for the prevention and treatment of benign prostatic hyperplasia (BPH or enlarged prostate). At least 2 studies have shown that red clover does indeed reduce prostate size – at least in mice.[13,14] Korean researchers have observed that men with BPH have significantly lower levels of genistein in their prostate tissue than do men with normal-sized prostates.[12]

Red clover has been found effective in the treatment of prostate cancer. The first report of its amazing effects came in 1997 when Professor Frederick Stephens of the University of Sydney reported a case where a 66-year-old physician with prostate cancer took a concentrated phyto-estrogen based on red clover for just one week and thereby caused his tumour to regress. The patient had been diagnosed with a high PSA level (13.1 ng/mL) in March 1996 and a subsequent needle biopsy had confirmed the presence of a low-grade adenocarcinoma. He was scheduled for a radical (suprapubic) prostatectomy and, on his own initiative, decided to take a daily dose of 160 mg of a phyto-estrogen product based on red clover (*Promensil* tablets - 4 X 40 mg/day) for the seven days preceding his operation. After the operation the biopsy tissue and the tumour tissue were compared. It was clear that the tumour tissue showed a high degree of apoptosis (cell death) resembling the effect of high-dose estrogen therapy and consistent with tumour regression. Professor Stephens concludes that this case provides further evidence that phyto-estrogens may prevent prostate cancer. He also points out that there were no adverse effects of the phyto-estrogen treatment.[15]

Following up on Professor Stephens' initial observation, Australian researchers evaluated red clover in 38 patients scheduled for prostate cancer surgery. They observed that red clover supplementation markedly increased apoptosis in cancer cells and conclude that supplementation with dietary isoflavones such as red clover may halt the progression of prostate cancer by inducing apoptosis (cell death) in low- to moderate-grade tumours.[16]

The Australian-produced red clover extract *Trinovin* is probably the most widely available product. It contains the four important isoflavones – genistein, daidzein, formonoetin, and biochanin A.[17]

Green Tea

Green tea has been found to inhibit the negative effects of prostate specific antigen (PSA) on cell migration, metastasis and degradation of type IV collagen. A team of Italian researchers has found that even the ingestion of one cup of green tea a day has a significant beneficial effect and concludes that green tea, or epigallocatechin gallate (EGCG) specifically, may serve as a natural inhibitor of prostate cancer progression.[18]

The Canadian Breast Cancer Research Initiative after a thorough review of published literature concluded that there is enough evidence of the beneficial effects of green tea to warrant further, properly conducted, full-scale clinical evaluation.[19] Green tea extract capsules are now available with an EGCG content corresponding to 6 or more cups of green tea per capsule.

Pomegranate Juice

The fruit of the pomegranate tree (*Punica granatum*) has been used medicinally for thousands of years. It is a powerful source of phenolic antioxidants and is estimated to have about 3 times the antioxidant activity of green tea and red wine.

In 2004 Israeli researchers discovered that pomegranate juice is effective in removing atherosclerotic deposits in patients suffering from carotid artery stenosis. They also found that pomegranate consumption reduced systolic blood pressure by 21%. Maximum effect was obtained after one year of supplementation.[20] Researchers at Boston University have found that pomegranate juice is more effective than red wine, blueberry juice, cranberry juice, and green tea in preventing LDL oxidation and suggest that pomegranate juice may be useful in reversing erectile dysfunction.[21]

American, German and Israeli researchers have concluded that pomegranate juice and extracts are highly effective in halting growth of both androgen-dependent and androgen-independent prostate cancer cells, and also significantly inhibits PSA secretion by these cells.[22-24]

More recently, researchers from the University of California reported that pomegranate juice is effective in markedly increasing PSA doubling time, a measure of tumor progression. Their clinical trial involved 48 prostate cancer patients who were experiencing a rise in PSA level following radical prostatectomy. The PSA doubling time prior to the trial averaged 15 months. Daily consumption of 8 oz of pomegranate juice increased the doubling time to 37 months – a gain of almost 2 years. *In vitro* testing showed decreased cancer cell proliferation combined with increased apoptosis.[25]

The findings that pomegranate juice prevents the proliferation of cancer cells, induces apoptosis, and inhibits PSA secretion certainly makes it a good candidate for both the prevention and treatment of prostate cancer. A phase III clinical trial is currently underway.[25]

Combination Protocols

Dutch researchers have evaluated an antioxidant combination in prostate cancer patients with rising PSA levels. The combination consisted of vitamin C (750 mg before breakfast), selenium (200 micrograms before breakfast), vitamin E (350 mg before breakfast), and coenzyme Q10 (100 mg before breakfast and 100 mg before dinner). The 70 study participants were randomized to receive a placebo or the antioxidant combination for a total of 21 weeks. The researchers found that plasma levels of vitamin E, selenium and coenzyme Q10 increased significantly over the treatment period, but found no statistically significant differences in serum levels of testosterone, dihydrotestosterone (DHT), or luteinizing hormone sex hormone binding globulin. They also found that PSA levels continued to rise in both controls and treated patients. They conclude that the antioxidant combination does not affect PSA or hormone levels in patients with hormonally untreated prostate cancer.[26]

The results of the Dutch study are not too surprising. Antioxidants help prevent the *initiation* of prostate cancer by protecting cells from free radical attacks, but there is no evidence that they might also be effective in altering hormone levels or inhibiting PSA secretion at the dosages used in this trial.

Another group of Dutch researchers has developed a **soy-based combination** protocol that combines soy isoflavones, lycopene, silymarin, and antioxidants. The active ingredients in the supplement are as follows (per daily dose of 4 tablets):

Soy isoflavone aglyconces (*ADM Novasoy*)	62.5	mg
Lycopene (*Lyc-O-Mato*)	15	mg
Silymarin (Milk thistle)	160	mg
Ascorbic acid	225	mg
Alpha-tocopherol	75	mg
Carotenoids	3	mg
Bioflavonoids	19	mg
Ubiquinol (Co Q10)	4	mg
Selenium	128	mcg
Zinc	18	mg
Copper	2.7	mg
Manganese	5	mg
Riboflavin	2.5	mg
Pyridoxine	2.6	mg
Cyanocobalamin (vitamin B12)	3	mcg
Folic acid	400	mcg
N-acetyl-L-cysteine	500	mg

The researchers tested the combination in a randomized, double-blind, placebo-controlled crossover study involving prostate cancer patients who were experiencing rising PSA levels after prostatectomy or radiotherapy. The clinical trial consisted of two

10-week supplementation or placebo periods separated by a 4-week washout period. The researchers noted a very significant difference in PSA doubling time between period when the men were on placebo and when they were taking the supplement. The average PSA doubling time when on placebo was 445 days (1.2 months) versus 1150 days (3.2 months) when taking the supplement. This translates into a very significant 2.6-fold increase in doubling time. The researchers also observed a substantial increase in plasma levels of genistein and daidzein among supplement users (genistein – from 0 mcg/L to 491 mcg/L and daidzein – from 0 mcg/L to 273 mcg/L). Supplementation was also associated with a highly significant 30% drop in homocysteine level (from an average of 13.3 micromol/L to 9.3 micromol/L). The researchers conclude that the soy-based supplement substantially increased PSA doubling time and warrants further study.[27]

PC-SPES

The first herbal combination specifically formulated to combat prostate cancer was probably PC-SPES. PC-SPES had a short, but fascinating career. It is a combination of eight herbs - chrysanthemum, isatis, licorice, *Ganoderma lucidum, Panax pseudo-ginseng, Rabdosia rubescens*, saw palmetto, and scutellaria (skullcap). The combination was tested on eight patients with biopsy-proven prostate cancer. The patients took PC-SPES for at least one month (four 320 mg capsules /day). Their blood levels of testosterone and prostate-specific antigen (PSA) were measured before, during and two to six weeks after taking the preparation. Testosterone levels decreased markedly in all eight patients during treatment (to an average 225 ng/dL), but increased again (to an average 879 ng/dL) within three weeks after the PC-SPES was discontinued. PSA levels also decreased markedly in all eight patients after treatment with PC-SPES, but increased again (although not to original levels) within three weeks of discontinuing treatment. In one patient, PSA levels decreased from 122 ng/mL to 1.2 ng/mL during treatment with PC-SPES. Side effects were similar to those observed with conventional estrogen therapy (loss of libido and breast tenderness).[28]

The initial trial was followed by at least three other somewhat larger trials. One major trial included 33 patients with androgen-dependent (AD) prostate cancer and 37 patients with androgen-independent (AI) disease (a more severe form). The patients received three capsules of PC-SPES three times a day. Patients with AD disease saw an average 80 per cent decrease in PSA levels over a 23-week period - two patients experienced a reduction in bone metastasis. All patients experienced loss of libido, impotence and a precipitous fall in testosterone levels. PSA levels also declined in the AI group, but to a somewhat lesser degree (greater than 50 per cent). Another study of patients with AI disease concluded that PC-SPES significantly reduced pain and improved quality of life scores. Dr. John Pirani of Clinical Urology Associates concluded that PC-SPES is a valid therapy option for prostate cancer. However, it is not entirely benevolent. It can cause nipple tenderness and breast enlargement. If taken in excessive dosages it can cause internal bleeding because of its content of warfarin-like compounds. Medical doctors at the University of Washington warned that PC-SPES should only be taken under the supervision of a physician and dosages in excess of six capsules a day should be avoided.[29,30]

Then the balloon burst. By the summer of 2001 reports began to appear on the Internet of possible contamination with diethylstilbestrol, a synthetic form of estrogen. The

California Department of Health Services tested several lots of PC-SPES and found that they were contaminated with diethylstilbestrol and warfarin. In February 2002 the Health Services issued a warning about the product and its manufacturer, BotanicLab, voluntarily recalled it. BotanicLab went out of business in June 2002 and PC-SPES is no longer commercially available.[31]

Researchers at the University of California obtained several lots of PC-SPES manufactured between 1996 and 2001. They tested them and found that they, particularly the early lots, were effective in killing prostate cancer cells. They also found that the early lots were heavily contaminated with diethylstilbestrol and the anti-inflammatory drug indomethacin (Indocin). In July 1998, warfarin, an anticoagulant began to appear in the product in quantities that could affect blood clotting. The researchers conclude that phytochemical (herbal) compounds may well have a place in the treatment of prostate cancer, but that manufacturing practices and quality control procedures need to be vastly improved before such compounds can be reliably tested in clinical trials.[32,33]

Despite the negative press researchers are still experimenting with PC-SPES. In September 2004 researchers at the Dana-Farber Cancer Institute reported that PC-SPES supplementation (3 capsules/day) had resulted in average PSA reductions of 50% in a group of patients with diagnosed androgen-independent prostate cancer. They confirmed that the PC-SPES contained small quantities of diethylstilbestrol and observed side effects including gynecomastia, mastodynia, and mild fatigue.[34]

Although the PC-SPES fiasco injected a note of caution against the use of herbal combinations in prostate cancer treatment, it also showed that such combinations might have considerable potential.

HP8
An Australian team of scientists from the Centre for Phytochemistry in New South Wales set out to pick through the ashes of PC-SPES and eventually came up with a new, patented combination of selenium and standardized extracts of saw palmetto, bromelain, licorice root, willow herb leaf, grape seed and skin, hibiscus and passion fruit seed. The product, HP8, has been found to prevent prostate cancer cells from dividing and multiplying. The product was tested in 14 patients with diagnosed prostate cancer or elevated PSA levels. Seventy per cent of the patients experienced a drop in PSA levels ranging from 15 to 87% after using HP8 for 6 months. The PSA levels in patients discontinuing HP8 began to increase again. None of the study participants experienced side effects and some reported significant improvements in their BPH symptoms and a general feeling of well-being.[35] Clearly, much larger, well-controlled clinical trials are required to determine the merits of HP8 in the prevention and treatment of prostate cancer. It is likely that the product could be useful in dealing with urinary symptoms arising from an enlarged prostate (BPH). However, it is quite expensive and less expensive solutions to BPH are certainly readily available.

Zyflamend
Dr. Aaron Katz, MD, a urologist and researcher at New York's Columbia-Presbyterian Medical Center recently began investigating a new product, *Zyflamend*, reputed to be effective in the treatment of BPH and in the prevention and treatment of prostate

cancer.[36] Brazilian researchers have already established that at least two of the components of *Zyflamend* are effective in inhibiting the growth of prostate cancer cells.[37]

Zyflamend is a standardized combination of carbon dioxide (supercritical) extracts of turmeric, ginger, Holy Basil, green tea, rosemary, skullcap, and oregano. All of these components have proven antioxidant, anti-inflammatory or cancer preventing properties. Dr. Katz's team has confirmed that *Zyflamend* is a strong COX-2 inhibitor in prostate cancer cell lines. Whether it will actually prevent the progression of prostate cancer in humans remains to be seen. However, Dr. Katz and his team are in the process of finding out. They have started a 3-year trial that will follow 100 prostate cancer patients treated with *Zyflamend*, assessing disease status via biopsies every 6 months.[36]

Zyflamend clearly looks promising and is likely to be entirely safe, although it may induce diarrhea in sensitive people. For those wishing to prevent prostate cancer and BPH, through supplementation with herbs and plant extracts, it would be a good alternative to taking all its components separately. It is also likely to help ameliorate arthritis and other inflammatory disease symptoms.

Lifestyle Changes

A group of American researchers report that intensive lifestyle changes may be effective in slowing the progression of early, low-grade, localized prostate cancer. Their 1-year trial involved 93 volunteers with an average age of 65 years (range of 58-72 years) who had been diagnosed with prostate cancer, but had decided on watchful waiting rather than prostatectomy, radiotherapy, or hormone treatment. At baseline the mean PSA level among the men averaged 6.3 ng/mL with a range of 4 to 10 ng/mL. The average Gleason score was 5.7 and all participants had a score below 7. Study participants were randomized to a usual care group or to a group that was advised and agreed to make extensive lifestyle modifications. The changes included adhering to a vegan diet providing less than 10% of calories as fat, walking 30 minutes 6 days a week, engaging regularly in stress management (meditation, yoga, progressive relaxation, etc. for 60 minutes daily), and participation in a 1-hour support group discussion once a week. The intensive lifestyle intervention group also adhered to a special supplementation regimen including one daily serving of tofu plus 58 grams of soy protein, 3 grams of fish oil, 400 IU of vitamin E, 200 mcg of selenium, and 2000 mg of vitamin C daily.

At the end of the 1-year study period, the average PSA level in the usual care group had increased by 0.38 ng/mL versus a decrease of 0.25 ng/mL in the lifestyle change group. The researchers also observed that blood serum from the lifestyle group inhibited the growth of LNCaP prostate cancer cells by 70% versus 9% inhibition with serum from the usual care group. Other noteworthy, beneficial changes in the lifestyle modification group were a 16% drop in total cholesterol, a 23% drop in LDL cholesterol, and an average weight loss of 10 lbs (4 kg). The researchers conclude that intensive lifestyle changes may slow the progression of early, localized, low-grade prostate cancer.[38]

There are numerous other vitamin- and herbal-based cancer treatments. However, most of them have not been discussed in peer-reviewed medical journals nor are they specific to prostate cancer.

METABOLIC, HERBAL AND IMMUNE THERAPIES

These therapies aim at cleansing the body, boosting the immune system, and assisting the body in ridding itself of the cancer and toxins created by the breakdown of the tumor.

The **Gerson therapy**, formulated by Dr. Max Gerson, a German physician who came to the United States just before World War II, believed that cancer results from a faulty metabolism and long- term exposure to pesticides and other environmental pollutants. His treatment involves a detoxification program and a meat-free, salt-free, and low-fat diet along with copious quantities of fresh fruit and vegetable juices as well as various supplements. The Gerson program is purportedly particularly effective for melanoma, lymphomas, and cancers of the liver, pancreas and colon.[39] Success has also been achieved with inoperable brain cancer, metastasized breast cancer, and prostate cancer.

The **Hoxsey therapy**, was developed by a self-taught American healer, Harry Hoxsey. By the 1950s, the Hoxsey Cancer Clinic in Dallas was the world's largest private cancer clinic. In 1960, however, the American Medical Association, the National Cancer Institute, and the Food and Drug Administration managed to close down the clinic. It later reopened in Tijuana, Mexico as the Bio-Medical Center. The clinic treats all kinds of cancer on an out-patient basis only; best results have been achieved with lymphoma, melanoma, and skin cancer; however, patients with breast, cervical, prostate, colon, and lung cancers have also been successfully treated. The Hoxsey therapy includes the total avoidance of pork, vinegar, tomatoes, carbonated drinks, alcohol, bleached flour, and refined sugar. Various supplements are also given with the main component of the treatment being the Hoxsey tonic which consists of several different herbs, many with potent anti-cancer effects.[40]

Immune therapies are used in both conventional and alternative treatment protocols. The Livingston Foundation Medical Center in San Diego treats cancer patients with various individually-tailored vaccines, gamma globulin, and a vegetarian diet with vitamin and mineral supplements. The Immunology Research Center in Freeport, Bahamas uses injections of immune substances to augment the body's own immune system and claims good success with breast, colon, kidney, and bladder cancer. The Burzynski Research Institute in Houston, Texas uses injections or supplements of peptides and amino acid derivatives occurring naturally in the body to augment the body's biochemical defense system and reprogram cancer cells so that they revert to normal development.[41,42] Several clinics use the Breuss fasting cure as part of their treatment. The Breuss Cure can also be done at home under the guidance of a knowledgeable holistic health care practitioner.[43]

It is clear that there is a wide range of alternative therapies available to aid in the fight against cancer. The challenge is to find the right one, one you believe will work for you, and then commit to it. Your conventional doctor may have told you that your illness is terminal and that nothing can be done, but this is really irrelevant. It just means that conventional medicine cannot help you, but it is certainly no reason to give up. Remember though, just as conventional treatments should only be carried out by professionals, so should alternative treatments. Self-diagnosis and self-medication have no place when it comes to fighting cancer.

COMPLEMENTARY THERAPIES

A recent survey of 110 prostate cancer patients revealed that 18.2% of them were currently using a complementary therapy, while 23.5% had done so in the past. Patients who were undergoing conventional hormone therapy or had been assigned to "watchful waiting" were the most likely to use complementary therapies. The use was more widespread among well-educated, high-income patients. About 90% of all users believed that the therapy would help them live longer, 47% thought it would eliminate the prostate cancer, and 60% believed it would relieve symptoms. The study participants were only asked about their use of dietary changes or supplements. The most common therapy was a low-fat diet (35.2%) followed by multivitamins (30.5%), green tea (21.8%), and selenium (21.4%). Only 18.2% of the participants had discussed the use of complementary therapies with their family physician, while 35.5% had discussed it with their urologist.[1]

The line between alternative and complementary therapies is somewhat blurred. Some approaches that have primarily been evaluated in combination with conventional therapy may actually be highly beneficial in their own right and thus could also be classified as alternative therapies – vitamin C and European mistletoe are good examples of this. None of the complementary therapies discussed have been specifically evaluated for prostate cancer, but some are likely to be beneficial.

MEGADOSE VITAMIN THERAPY

Megadose vitamin therapy involves the infusion or ingestion of large amounts of vitamins. This treatment has been extensively evaluated at the Vale of Leven Hospital in Scotland under the supervision of Drs. Cameron and Pauling. The experiments found that terminal cancer patients who received large, daily doses of vitamin C along with their regular treatment lived significantly longer than patients who did not receive vitamin C; they also had less pain and in general, a much improved quality of life.[2]

The Vale of Leven clinical trial involved 1100 patients with terminal cancer. One hundred of the patients were treated with 10 grams of sodium ascorbate (vitamin C) per day, for the first 10 days in the form of an infusion and then by oral supplementation. They also received standard, conventional treatment, as did the other 1000 patients who served as a control group. Each ascorbate-treated patient was matched with 10 control patients with the same cancer diagnosis, sex and age. These matched controls made up the total control group of 1000 patients. After one year, 22% of the patients in the vitamin C group were still alive as compared to 0.4% in the control group. Overall, the ascorbate-treated patients were found to have a survival time about 300 days longer than controls. There were only two prostate cancer patients in the vitamin C group, a 48-year-old man and a 68-year-old man. They survived for 255 days and 122 days respectively as compared to 77 days and 15 days for matched controls, or in other words, a 3- to 8-fold increase in survival. The authors of the study suggest that if vitamin C treatment had been started before the patient was declared "untreatable" (terminal) the survival advantage would have been even more impressive.[2]

Vitamin C has many properties which makes it an excellent cancer fighter. It is a detoxifying agent, an antioxidant, and helps to produce antibodies. It is also very important in preventing growing tumors from invading adjacent tissue.[3]

Dr. Abram Hoffer, MD PhD of Victoria, Canada later expanded on the Pauling/Cameron treatment protocol by adding large amounts of vitamin E, vitamin B-3, other B vitamins, beta-carotene, and some minerals. Those of Dr. Hoffer's cancer patients who followed this regimen lived, on the average, about 16 times longer than those who did not.[4]

In January 1994, Dr. Donald Lamm and his colleagues at the West Virginia University School of Medicine reported that daily megadose vitamin therapy significantly lessens the risk of recurrence in bladder cancer patients. Patients who received the therapy, on the average, had less than half the tumor recurrence rate than did patients who did not receive it. Dr. Lamm's vitamin combination included multivitamins (RDA dosages) plus 40,000 IU vitamin A, 100 mg vitamin B-6, 2,000 mg vitamin C, 400 IU vitamin E, and 90 mg zinc.[5]

The megadose vitamin therapy, so far, has only been evaluated in combination with conventional cancer treatments. Mainstream medicine has long been adamantly opposed to megadose vitamin therapy and, in particular, therapy with large does of vitamin C.

THE VITAMIN C STORY

Thirty years ago, Dr. Linus Pauling, a two-time Nobel Prize winner, and Dr. Ewan Cameron, a Scottish physician, evaluated vitamin C in the treatment of terminal cancer. They found that daily intravenous infusions of mega doses (10 grams) of vitamin C for 10 days followed by continuing oral administration resulted in a 5-6 times longer survival time than that experienced by matched controls.[2]

After much cajoling and presentation of convincing research data, the Mayo Clinic finally agreed to evaluate mega doses of vitamin C in the treatment of cancer. However, over Dr. Pauling's strenuous protests the Mayo researchers decided to administer the 10 grams of vitamin C by mouth rather than intravenously. Not too surprisingly, their trial concluded that mega doses of vitamin C were worthless in cancer treatment.[6,7] Nevertheless, many progressive alternative and complementary physicians continued to use intravenous infusions of vitamin C in cancer treatment with good results. Additional research also confirmed that vitamin C is highly toxic to cancer cells in vitro in blood plasma concentrations of 1000 micromol/L or greater. There is no indication that it is toxic to normal cells.

Twenty-five years after Dr. Pauling's initial discovery, researchers at the National Institutes of Health took a second look at the possibility of using intravenous vitamin C in cancer treatment. The first phase of their work did not involve a clinical trial to determine if vitamin C combats cancer, but rather a detailed comparison of the blood plasma concentrations achievable with oral and intravenous administration of vitamin C. The study involved 17 healthy young men and women who were hospitalized for 3-6 months in order to keep their environment and dietary intake under strict control. Over the trial period, the researchers administered various doses of vitamin C either orally or intravenously and measured the resulting plasma concentration. Among the highlights of their findings:

- Plasma concentrations achieved through intravenous infusion were at least 8 times higher than those achieved through oral administration of equivalent amounts.

- The maximum achievable plasma concentration via the oral route was 220 micromol/L and was obtained by supplementing with 3 grams of vitamin C every 4 hours. In contrast, administration of 3 grams intravenously produced a plasma concentration of 1760 micromol/L.

- Intravenous infusion of 10, 50, and 100 grams produced plasma concentrations of 5580, 13,350 and 15,380 micromol/L respectively. Thus it is possible to attain plasma levels of vitamin C via intravenous administration that are 70 times higher than what is obtainable through oral supplementation. Doses of 60 grams, given intravenously, are used for cancer treatment by complementary and alternative medicine practitioners.

- A diet rich in fruit and vegetables may provide as much as 200 mg/day of vitamin C and this would result in a plasma concentration of about 90 micromol/L. Plasma concentration can be further increased by oral supplementation. Peak plasma concentration increased to 187 micromol/L after supplementing with 1.25 grams (1250 mg) and to 220 micromol/L after ingesting 3 grams every 4 hours. The researchers suggest that 220 micromol/L may be about the highest plasma concentration achievable through oral supplementation.

- Vitamin-C, whether administered orally or intravenously, is rapidly excreted in the urine, essentially returning plasma concentration to baseline levels in 4-6 hours.

The researchers conclude that the plasma level necessary to kill cancer cells (1000 micromol/L or greater) can only be achieved through intravenous administration. They further state that intravenous vitamin C would be expected to have little toxicity compared with conventional chemotherapy agents. They conclude that, "the role for intravenous vitamin C in cancer treatment should be reevaluated".[8]

The re-evaluation has already begun. Jeanne Drisko and colleagues at the University of Kansas Medical Center report the case of two women with advanced ovarian cancer who received intravenous vitamin C (60 grams a day for a week or 60 grams twice a week) in combination with standard chemotherapy. The women also supplemented with oral vitamin C, beta-carotene, vitamin E, coenzyme Q10, and a multivitamin/mineral complex. Both women experienced complete remission of their cancer and have remained cancer-free for at least 3 years.[9]

Sebastian Padayatty and colleagues at the National Institutes of Health and McGill University recently reported on 3 cases of patients with advanced cancer (renal cancer, bladder cancer, and lymphoma). All patients refused chemotherapy and instead opted for high-dose (15-65 grams) vitamin C infusions at regular intervals for periods up to a year. The patients also took a wide range of oral supplements like N-acetylcysteine, niacinamide, vitamin C, alpha-lipoic acid, selenium, magnesium, coenzyme Q10, and others. All 3 patients improved significantly, showed clear signs of tumor regression, and survived far longer than expected.[10,11]

The use of megadose vitamin therapy or, more specifically, antioxidant infusions in combination with radiation and chemotherapy is a highly controversial subject. One camp maintains that the antioxidants interfere with the cytoxic actions of radiation and chemotherapy, while the other camp maintains that high-dose antioxidants, vitamin C in particular, actually help protect healthy cells and also, in themselves, have powerful cytoxic properties that help kill cancer cells. Says Jeanne Drisko in a recent article, "Despite the fact that chemotherapy-induced formation of free radicals is well demonstrated, chemotherapy-induced cytotoxicity in general does not seem to depend on formation of reactive oxygen species; thus, the concept that antioxidants are contraindicated during most chemotherapy regiments is no longer valid."[12] Many other researchers strongly support Dr. Drisko's position.[13-20]

A study published in the *Journal of Orthomolecular Medicine* painstakingly reviews the medical literature dealing with the use of vitamin C as an adjunct to chemotherapy. A total of 36 studies or reviews conclude that vitamin C is beneficial, three that it could be harmful, while one is neutral on the subject. Overall, the author of the study concludes that the use of vitamin C during chemotherapy results in:

- An increase in survival time
- Enhancement of the effect of chemotherapy
- Inhibition of tumor growth
- A decrease in toxicity
- An increase in cell death

Dr. K.N. Prasad of the University of Colorado Health Sciences Center sums up the benefits of combining chemotherapy with vitamin C supplementation in these words. ".... Antioxidants (including vitamin C) do not protect cancer cells against free radical and growth-inhibitory effects of standard therapy. On the contrary, they enhance its growth-inhibitory effects on tumor cells, but protect normal cells against its adverse effects."[21]

Hopefully, this emerging body of substantial evidence will eventually make antioxidant infusions standard practice in radiation and chemotherapy. And, the myth that high doses of vitamin C cause kidney stones is just that – a myth.[22]

ALPHA-TOCOPHEROL SUCCINATE

Alpha-tocopheryl succinate (ATS) is a reaction product of alpha-tocopherol (vitamin E) and succinic acid. In 1982 it was reported that ATS is highly effective in inhibiting proliferation of melanoma cells in culture. Alpha-tocopherol and alpha-tocopherol acetate, the most common forms of vitamin E, do not share this desirable trait. Animal experiments later confirmed the tumor-killing effect of ATS and also noted that ATS is easily hydrolyzed in the human intestinal tract, so needs to be given intravenously for maximum effect. Further experiments have shown that ATS alone, or in combination with vitamin A, vitamin C and carotenoids, is effective in reducing proliferation of tumor cells in culture and also enhances the effects of radiation therapy and some chemotherapy protocols.[23,24] A very recent experiment elucidated the way ATS causes apoptosis in prostate cancer cells.[25] Hopefully, ATS will continue to receive the attention it seemingly deserves, but full scale clinical trials are, no doubt, a ways away.

EUROPEAN MISTLETOE EXTRACT

Mistletoe extract (*Viscum album L.*) was prescribed as a natural remedy by Hippocrates, by the Druids, and by Arabian physicians long before the German physician Rudolph Steiner in 1920 introduced its aqueous extract in the treatment of cancer. It is estimated that about one-third of German doctors now use mistletoe in their practices.[26] Mistletoe extract has been found to kill cancer cells, induce apoptosis, stabilize DNA, and modulate and stimulate the immune system.[27] A recent study carried out at the University of Freiburg in Germany concluded that European fermented mistletoe is very effective in preventing metastasis and improving survival in patients who have had a melanoma surgically removed.[28]

A clinical study carried out in Switzerland in 2004 involved 1442 breast cancer patients who were randomized to receive either standard chemotherapy or chemotherapy plus mistletoe extract. Only 16.3% of the patients in the mistletoe group developed adverse effects as compared to 54.1% in the chemotherapy only group. The survival rate in the mistletoe group was also significantly longer.[29] Another trial in China also showed considerable benefits of adding mistletoe to conventional treatment.[30]

The most commonly used brand of mistletoe is Iscador, which is prepared by fermenting an aqueous extract of the whole mistletoe plant with *Lactobacillus plantarum* bacteria. It is injected subcutaneously into the abdominal wall or directly into the tumor. A course of treatment may last several weeks and involves injections 3 to 7 times a week. Iscador is compatible with chemotherapy and radiation and no toxic effects have been reported when used as directed. There are, however, reports of serious side effects if the plant or extract is taken orally or injected intravenously. Iscador can be legally prescribed in South Africa, Germany and several other European countries, but is generally not available in North America.[31]

SODIUM SELENITE

The optimum form of selenium for cancer **prevention** is selenomethionine, an organic nutritional form of selenium. However, for **therapeutic** applications the inorganic form, sodium selenite, is the preferred form. Sodium selenite is primarily used as a complementary therapy to reduce the side effects of chemotherapy and radiation. It can be administered either orally or intravenously, and the usual dose is 300-1000 micrograms a day of selenium prior to and during conventional treatment followed by 100 micrograms a day as a maintenance dose. Sodium selenite has been found to reduce inflammatory reactions to chemotherapy drugs, help protect against radiation damage, enhance the function of the immune system, and in general, tends to improve the quality of life in patients undergoing radiation or chemotherapy. Sodium selenite is reduced to elemental selenium by vitamin C, so their administration should be at least two hours apart.[32]

PROTEOLYTIC ENZYMES

Proteolytic enzymes such as papain, chymotrypsin, and trypsin are effective in reducing the side effects of radiation and chemotherapy. They are believed to work through modulation and stimulation of the immune system and also have anti-tumor and anti-metastatic effects. A study involving 650 patients with non-metastasizing breast cancer undergoing conventional therapy found that those who also received proteolytic enzymes had far fewer side effects (25% vs 45%) and also were less likely to experience metastasis and death. Another clinical trial found 1242 patients with colorectal cancer also found that those receiving complementary proteolytic enzyme therapy experienced fewer side effects from conventional therapy and survived longer. [33]

THE AESKULAP PROTOCOL

Professor Ben Pfeifer, MD and colleagues at the Aeskulap Clinic in Switzerland have developed an effective complementary protocol for the treatment of advanced hormone refractory prostate cancer. The protocol consists of a combination of phytotherapy, immune therapy, and antioxidative/orthomolecular therapy. The protocol has four specific components – *Prostasol*, curcumin complex, Biobran, and IMUPROS.

Prostasol is available in both Europe and the US as a food supplement and contains the following ingredients: - sitosterols, quercetin, pygeum, saw palmetto, ginseng, ginger, stinging nettle, scull cap, and Reishi mushroom. A clinical trial involving 194 hormone refractory cancer patients found that taking 900-2800 mg/day of *Prostasol* for 2-3 months resulted in an average 50% drop in PSA value among 70% of the 194 patients and also led to a decline in metastatic pain and a general improvement in quality of life. Shrinkage of the primary tumor was observed in about a third of the patients and no significant adverse events occurred.

The **curcumin complex** contains curcumin, bioperin (black pepper extract), and resveratrol. Research has shown that it inhibits the division of cancer cells.

IMUPROS us available in Europe and the UK as a food supplement. It is supplied in a time-release formula and contains vitamin E, selenium, ginseng, lycopene, green tea extract, vitamin D3, vitamin C, calcium citrate, and zinc citrate.

Biobran is an immunostimulant made by treating rice bran with enzymes extracted from Shitake mushrooms. Its main component, arabinoxylan causes a significant rise in the number and activity of T and B cells, as well as natural killer cells (NK cells).

Physicians at the Aeskulap Clinic have used the combination therapy in the treatment of several patients with metastatic prostate cancer with excellent results.[34,35]

CACHEXIA (MALNUTRITION)

Cachexia (general weakness and loss of weight and appetite) is a major problem in many forms of cancer. Fish oils and hydrazine sulfate have both been found effective in its alleviation. Preliminary research has shown that supplementing the diet with **fish oils**, about 2.2 grams of EPA (eicosapentaenoic acid) and 1.4 grams of DHA (docosahexaenoic acid) daily will stabilize weight in patients with inoperable pancreatic cancer. Researchers at the Royal Infirmary of Edinburgh found that patients with pancreatic cancer can actually gain weight by consuming a nutritional supplement fortified with fish oils. The experiment involved 20 patients with inoperable pancreatic cancer (aged 18 to 80 years). The participants were asked to ingest two cans of fish oil-enriched nutritional supplement per day in addition to their normal food intake. The nutritional supplement provided 310 kcal per can and contained 16.1 g protein, 49.7 g carbohydrate, 6.5 g fat, 1.09 g EPA, 0.46 g DHA, and 28 essential vitamins and minerals. After three weeks the patients had gained an average (median) of 1 kg in weight and at seven weeks an average of 2 kg. A significant improvement in performance status and appetite was also noted after three weeks on the supplement. Other research has shown that EPA inhibits the growth of pancreatic cancer cells *in vitro*. It is therefore of interest to note that the average survival time among the patients was over eight months. This compares very favourably with the normal survival time of 4.1 months and is at least as good as the survival time that can be obtained with aggressive chemotherapy. The researchers conclude that a fish oil-enriched nutritional supplement has the potential to be a safe and effective means of preventing weight loss in cancer patients and may even increase survival time in patients with cancer of the pancreas.[36]

There is also evidence that **hydrazine sulfate** given orally or by injection may reduce the severity of cachexia and improve the quality of life in cancer patients. There are also some still controversial indications that hydrazine sulfate may inhibit tumor growth and improve survival. The use of hydrazine sulfate in cancer therapy was first proposed by Dr. Joseph Gold, an oncologist at the Syracuse Cancer Research Institute. Since Dr. Gold's discovery extensive research on hydrazine sulfate has been carried out in Russia and the United States. The Russian studies report significant improvements in well-being and survival while the results of the American studies are more ambiguous.

Hydrazine sulfate is legally available to physicians in both Canada and the United States. It is usually given orally (60 mg three times daily) over a period of 30-45 days followed by a rest period of two to six weeks. There are no serious side effects but Dr. Gold cautions that alcohol, barbiturates, and tranquillizers (particularly benzodiazepines) interfere with the effectiveness of hydrazine sulfate. Because hydrazine sulfate is a monoamine oxidase inhibitor it is also advisable to avoid foods rich in tyramine (aged cheese, beer, leftovers, MSG, over-ripe fruits and vegetables, pickled and smoked foods, red wine, and soy products) during therapy. This therapy is compatible with and may enhance conventional therapies, especially chemotherapy.[37]

OTHER COMPLEMENTARY THERAPIES

Preliminary studies indicate that thymic peptides, probiotics, quercetin, Panax ginseng, and Maitake mushrooms also may be useful in alleviating the effects of chemotherapy and radiation. However, much more research is needed before their use can be advocated.[38-43]

CANCER CLINICS

Several of the alternative and complementary therapies described in previous sections involve proprietary formulations, difficult to obtain medications, or the need for intravenous infusions or injections. This has spawned the creation of specialized cancer clinics where patients go for an extended stay (usually 3 weeks) to receive intensive treatment and counselling on how to stay cancer-free after leaving the clinic.

Some of the largest and most successful cancer clinics used to operate in the United States, but have gradually been closed down or forced to move by the combined efforts of the American Medical Association, the National Cancer Institute, and the Food and Drug Administration.

No doubt, some of the clinics were fraudulent, but the effort to shut them down was likely motivated more by a desire to eliminate competition than by a desire to protect the welfare of the patients. There is really no good reason why a fully qualified medical doctor operating a cancer clinic should be less trustworthy, caring and concerned about their patients than an urologist making his living from performing biopsies and radical prostatectomies. Nevertheless, mainstream medicine in North America has been very successful in imparting to alternative cancer clinics an aura of sleaziness and potential danger. While there are, no doubt, clinics that deserve this perception, there are many more that do not.

A few clinics still operate in the United States, and other successful clinics are operated by caring, highly qualified physicians in northern Europe and Mexico where the attitude towards alternative methods tends to be more liberal. A small selection of these clinics is presented below:

Burzynski Clinic, Houston, TX
Medical Director – Stanislaw R. Burzynski, MD PhD
Therapies used – Antineoplastons
Specializes in brain cancer and non-Hodgkin's lymphoma
Address – 9432 Old Katy Road, Suite 200, Houston, Texas
Web site – www.cancermed.com

Aeskulap Klinik, Brunnen, Switzerland
Medical Director – Dr. Med Marcel G. Brander
Prostate Problems Contact – Professor, Dr. Med Ben L. Pfeifer
Clinic established – 1990 (40 rooms)
Therapies used – A wide range of conventional, alternative and complementary therapies
Address – Gersauer strasse 8, CH-6440 Brunnen, Switzerland
Web site – www.aeskulap.com

Humlegaarden, Humlebaek, Denmark
Medical Director – Finn Skott Andersen, MD
Clinic established – 1979
Therapies used – Hyperthermia, light therapy, vitamins and minerals, mistletoe extract, photodynamic therapy, magnet field therapy
Address – Ny Strandvej 11, 3050 Humlebaek, Denmark
Web site – www.humlegaarden.com/english/index.html

Bio Med Klinik, Bad Bergzabern, Germany
Medical Director – Dieter Hager, MD PhD
Clinic established – 1989 (125 beds)
Therapies used – Conventional therapies, hyperthermia, immune therapy, diet and vitamin therapy, mistletoe and thymic peptide therapy, enzyme therapy, photodynamic therapy
Address – Bio Med-Klinik GmbH, Tischberger Str. 5-8, 76887 Bad Bergzabern, Germany
Web site – www.biomed-klinik.de/bm1en-bza.htm

Hufeland Klinik, Bad Mergentheim, Germany
Medical Director – Wolfgang Woeppel, MD
Clinic established – 1985 (53 beds)
Therapies used – Detoxification, hyperthermia, mistletoe extract, holistic dentistry, immunotherapy (Josef Issels protocol)
Address – Hufeland Klinik, Loeffelstelzer Str. 1-3, Bad Mergentheim, Germany
Web site – www.hufeland.com

International Bio Care, Tijuana, Mexico
Medical Director – Rodrigo Rodriguez, MD
Clinic established – 1975 (32 beds)
Therapies used – Nutrition, rest, exercise, detoxification, immune therapy, hyperthermia
Address – No. 15 Azucenas St., Tijuana, Mexico
Web site – www.ibchospital.com

Baja NutriCare (Gerson Institute), Tijuana, Mexico
Director – Charlotte Gerson
Clinic established – 2002
Therapies used – Gerson dietary program
Address – The Gerson Institute, 1572 Second Ave., San Diego, CA 92101
Web site – www.gerson.org

There are numerous other cancer clinics especially in Germany, Mexico and Switzerland. However, it is very difficult to evaluate them without actually going there. The clinics mentioned above have all been personally inspected and evaluated by Ralph Moss, PhD, a leading American cancer researcher and have been discussed in his newsletters (www.cancerdecisions.com). Dr. Moss' evaluations are thorough and clinics not meeting his standards are listed as "not recommended". If you are seriously considering travelling to an alternative clinic, it may be worthwhile consulting with Dr. Moss before making your choice. Another good source for finding alternative cancer clinics is The Cancer Cure Foundation at www.cancure.org.

| PHARMACEUTICAL DRUGS |

Apart from drugs used in hormone therapy (see Chapter 7) and standard chemotherapy drugs, there are no pharmaceutical drugs specifically approved for the treatment of prostate cancer. Calcitriol (1,25-dihydroxycholecalciferol), a vitamin D metabolite and fenretinide, an analogue of vitamin A, are currently being investigated for their possible benefits in the treatment of prostate cancer.[44,45]

Chapter 9

The Future--Diagnosis, Staging, Novel Therapies

William R. Ware PhD and Hans R. Larsen MSc ChE

INTRODUCTION

Worldwide there is a large research effort directed at novel solutions, both at the diagnosis and treatment of prostate cancer. However, the process of technology transfer from "bench to bedside", as professionals call it, depends on regulatory approval. To get to this point randomized clinical trials are generally required that demonstrate benefit. But many treatment protocols do not lend themselves to placebo control or randomized studies. In fact, there is considerable freedom in connection with surgical techniques and other invasive procedures as regards the necessity of trials, and those trials that are conducted frequently involve comparisons between techniques. But new drugs or diagnostic tests are another matter. There is a long, torturous and unbelievably expensive path between a brilliant idea and the approval of a drug, and the acceptance of a diagnostic procedure requires fairly large studies intended to provide proof of adequate safety, sensitivity and specificity before clinicians are willing to adopt the procedure for routine use.

For example, the PSA test has been subjected to so many investigations that practically everything that one might want to know has been studied. But for non-PSA markers that might provide improved specificity and sensitivity, the challenge to have similar evidence-based data will be difficult to meet. And along with this state of affairs no doubt comes a reluctance on the part of clinicians to rely on new diagnostic markers that are by comparison relatively untested and lack extensive data regarding to benchmarks. Academic physicians may use relatively new diagnostic tests in their clinics, but it takes a long time and considerable publicity before new diagnostic or screening tests are widely adopted. Thus new biomarkers will face an uphill battle against a marker such as PSA that is, to put it mildly, firmly entrenched and both its merits and its shortcomings well documented. This is in spite of the fact that PSA is really a rather unsatisfactory marker except when used for identifying progression after treatment, sounding an alarm when the level is above 10 or 20 ng/mL, or identifying what is *probably* metastatic cancer when the value is, for example, very high such as 50 or 100 ng/mL.

Drug approval involves Phase I, II and III studies and even though only limited numbers of participants are required, the cost in money and time is huge. Drug companies must demonstrate to the satisfaction of the regulatory agency that the drug is safe, establish optimum dose levels, and show in randomized controlled clinical trials that their drug works better than a placebo for the predetermined endpoints related to the proposed use. Clinical trials of non-patentable substances are generally left to governments or private foundations to support, since the drug companies have little interest in anything they cannot patent. When a natural product looks interesting, they try to produce a modified substance that is patentable. As bad experiences with drugs after introduction multiply, regulatory agencies are under increased pressure to be conservative in the approval process or face trouble from those elected to represent the consumers. Thus to hope that in the next few years new drugs to treat BPH and the various aspects of prostate cancer will be approved and generally available is perhaps unrealistic.

The good news is that trials need subjects, and if a new drug is being tested for advanced prostate cancer, and especially hormone refractory cancer, then being a part of the trial has some merit since the outlook is dismal for advanced, hormone refractory PC, and the notion that "I have nothing to loose" is probably close to reality. There are of course risks, and these are probably greatest in trials attempting to establish adverse effects and effective vs. harmful doses. Once these are out of the way, the risk may be more in keeping with the potential benefit for those with advanced cancer. In addition, a man with clinically evident metastatic prostate cancer does not have time to wait until novel treatments are approved by the regulatory agency in his jurisdiction. He will almost certainly be dead unless approval and introduction are imminent. Men considering participating in a trial should realize that if it is a randomized, placebo-controlled study, then half the participants will receive a placebo which is unlikely to alter the course of a terminal disease. He will never know if he is actually receiving treatment.

There can be little doubt that if the mechanisms of prostate carcinogenesis and metastasis were fully understood, successful and durable interventions which utilize this knowledge would not be far behind. Unfortunately this does not appear to be the case, but the research effort aimed at this goal is mind boggling, at least as judged by the number of scientific papers appearing each month that relate to fundamental questions, and progress appears to be rapid. There has also been a huge change over the last decade or so in the level of sophistication associated with research in this area, in keeping with the rapid advances in the understanding of the role of genetics, signaling pathways, control mechanisms, etc., at a molecular and genome level. In the following sections, some new developments in diagnosis and treatment will be discussed and in addition, what improvements if any might be expected in the various treatment options currently available will be reviewed.

BENIGN PROSTATIC HYPERPLASIA

Significant progress at this point in time in dealing with benign prostatic hyperplasia (BPH) would involve advances in three areas: (1) differentiating the four possibilities, BPH alone, prostate cancer alone, or both present or both absent; (2) preventing the onset of BPH rather than treating symptoms or delaying progression after it is present and (3) reversing prostate growth due to BPH without producing undesirable or unacceptable adverse effects.

Progress in the first area involves developing a diagnostic protocol for prostate cancer that has a high level of specificity since the simplest solution to the diagnostic problem is to rule out prostate cancer with certainty equal to or greater than 90%, preferable without requiring a biopsy. While this is the subject of intense research, the goal does not as yet appear to be in sight. In fact the debate over screening, which involves the same problems of cancer testing, goes on unabated.

The second area will require years of testing of a variety of approaches including lifestyle and diet, phytotherapy and prescription drugs. Since BPH develops slowly, studying long-term prevention will take years of follow-up. Using what is currently known about risk factors and preventive measures (see Chapters 2 and 5) allows one to outline a lifestyle, diet and supplement program that might minimize the risk, but how significant this will turn out to be in the long run is unknown and may never be known, since studies in this area are easily confounded, and it is unlikely that comprehensive risk reduction programs will ever be adequately tested. Compliance, follow-up and confounding would also be serious problems in a trial of a really comprehensive primary prevention program that lasted 20 years and started when men were 40 years of age.

As regards reversing BPH, it is now known that the 5-alpha-reductase inhibitors (e.g. finasteride and dutasteride) will reduce the size of the prostate along with providing symptomatic relief for many men with BPH. Whether drug treatment will return the prostate to the size it had prior to the onset of BPH appears unknown, but it can be argued that these drugs are indeed reversing BPH. The challenge is in the development of new drugs or the discovery of phytochemicals that will accomplish the same result without the adverse effects. Saw Palmetto, for example, is a weak 5-alpha-reductase inhibitor which in many studies has been found to be as effective as the 5-alpha-reductase class of drugs, but there do not appear to be studies starting with men with normal-sized prostates and examining the question of the efficacy of saw palmetto in preventing BPH, a study that would probably require many years of follow-up. The pessimistic view is that such studies will never be done. Saw palmetto is not a patentable drug. Also, there is need for long-term studies of low dose prescription 5-alpha-reductase inhibitors to determine just how low a dose will result in reversal of prostate growth, and in addition, will low doses given to asymptomatic men with prostates of normal size maintain the status-quo with no significant side effects. It may turn out that ultra-sensitive PSA measurements can be used as a surrogate for prostate volume in men entering the age period when the prostate starts to grow. This could provide tentative answers to the efficacy question over a shorter period.

New approaches to the problem of severe obstruction, a condition for the most part treated by surgery (TURP), are under active development. These are less invasive procedures and are receiving considerable attention, and some may eventually become part of standard practice. At present, only transurethral microwave thermotherapy (TUMT) has been studied extensively. TUMT has in fact undergone a significant evolution, mainly through improvements in the equipment, the use of thermal sensors and computer assisted treatment planning. Further advances aimed at perfecting TUMT may eventually lead to a protocol that will become as widely used as TURP. Nevertheless, all invasive or minimally invasive approaches will probably still have side effects, some quite undesirable. The male anatomy practically guarantees this, given the position of the urethra within the prostate and the close proximity of the prostate to the bladder neck, rectum, the neurovascular nerve bundle and the urine flow control sphincters.

Many individuals with BPH symptoms are also thought to perhaps have what is called an overactive bladder. A drug is currently in trials that would address this as well as the irritative symptoms. However, as discussed in Chapter 2, the class of drug known as alpha-blockers appears to address this problem. Other approaches being suggested include alcohol (ethanol) or botulinum toxin (Botox) injections. Both are experimental, but the latter appears very interesting and merits further discussion.

BOTULINUM TOXIN (BOTOX) FOR BPH

The Holy Grail for BPH treatment might be described as therapy that is completely devoid of side effects, dramatically reduces symptoms and results in large and significant decreases in prostate volume and serum PSA. Preliminary results from studies that employed the injection of botulinum toxin (Botox or Dysport) directly in both lobes of the prostate indicate that this treatment protocol may possess the above ideal characteristics.

Botulinum toxin (BT) is produced by the gram-positive rod-shaped anaerobic bacterium *Clostridium botulinum* which is widely distributed in soil and water. Of the seven distinct neurotoxins produced by this bacterium, type A is currently of interest in the context of BPH. The common name of one of the commercial products is Botox, a name made famous by the cosmetic use of this toxin. Botox is a purified natural product. The preparation strength is measured units, one unit being the amount required to kill half of a group of injected mice. The biological activity as given in units is not in general comparable or transferable to other botulinum toxin products.

Chuang *et al* [1] have recently reviewed the relevant studies published or in press up to 2006. Eight studies involving 172 patients with follow-up ranging from 3 to 19.6 months were reviewed. Two were double blind, and one placebo controlled (saline injection). These studies cover men with both large and small prostates. Injection was either transrectal, transperineal or transurethral. Points of injection were established by simultaneous transrectal ultrasound. This is an outpatient procedure requiring only a short procedural time. Some physicians use antibiotics for several days as a precaution. All studies showed improvements, many dramatic, in most but not all of the following outcomes: symptom score, quality-of-life score, maximum flow rate, residual urine volume, prostate volume and PSA. The pioneering study by Maria *et al* [2] randomized 30 patients to 100 U of Botox in each lobe or a saline injection. Patients treated with Botox experienced a 52% improvement in maximum urinary flow rate, a 65% decrease in symptom score (AUA) and an 83% decrease in residual urine volume. Mean prostate volumes decreased from 52.6 to 16.8 mL (68%) and mean PSA from 3.7 to 1.8 ng/mL (51%). Values of these parameters were virtually unchanged in the controls. The authors point out that these changes were similar to those achieved by surgery (TURP, see Chapter 2) and were durable for up to a year. There were no complications or systemic side effects over the mean follow-up of 19.6 months. Similar results were obtained in the other studies reviewed by Chuang *et al*. At this point, it is unknown how long the results of a single application of BT therapy will remain durable.

In a study by Kuo reviewed by Chuang *et al* which enrolled 10 patients with severe BPH related LUTS who were not considered suitable candidates for surgery, the use of a single botulinum toxin injection resulted in the resumption of efficient voiding in 100% of the patients with voiding dysfunction. The mean follow-up was 9 months. No patient had a recurrence of urinary retention and the voiding condition in all patients remained at the post-treatment status. Mean prostate volume decreased from 65.5 to 49.6 mL at 6 months follow-up. No adverse effects were observed.

The mechanism whereby BT therapy results in these remarkable results is not clear. Apostolidis *et al* [3] have discussed possible mechanisms in the context of the overactive bladder, but the effects on BPH are probably multifactorial since neurotoxic effects which influence both the sympathetic and parasympathetic nerves and the effect of a decrease in prostate size must both be considered.

While there do not appear to be any published studies involving the effect of botulinum toxin on prostate cancer, the large decreases in prostate size obtained over a short period would suggest that botulinum toxin could replace hormone therapy as a pre-treatment method for reducing prostate size. The absence of side effects would make this attractive, as would the large percentage changes possible in prostate gland volume.

This use of botulinum toxin is experimental and is not approved at present by the FDA—a so-called off-label use, generally restricted to men where currently available medical treatments have proven ineffective and who are not candidates for surgery. Also, dose as a function of prostate size has not been optimized. Men interested in this therapy may have difficulty obtaining it. The ideal solution would involve participation in a clinical trial. The patient's urologist should be able to advise as to this possibility in the local area, but since the procedure requires only one short outpatient visit, traveling some distance might even be considered worthwhile by some men.

PROSTATE CANCER

GENETICS AND DIAGNOSIS OR TREATMENT

The rapid advances and the high level of research activity in the genetics of prostate cancer provides justification for optimism in connection with treatments geared to an individual's own genetic makeup. However, the current indications are that the matter is highly complex. While there is a large body of evidence indicating that prostate cancer has a strong genetic basis, it is now thought that susceptibility is likely caused by multiple genes possibly interacting with each other and with environmental factors [4,5]. One recent review [6] lists ten genes associated with hereditary prostate cancer and fifty-four genes where polymorphisms significantly associated with increased risk of prostate cancer have been identified. Thus while the vision of some in medical genetics of obtaining a genetic profile of a patient which would then dictate targeted therapy appears, in the case of prostate cancer, to be just that, a vision. At this point in time, substituting a careful history for a genetic profile is probably more effective in identifying individuals with hereditary predisposition. But even when these men are identified, there are at present only a limited number of preventive interventions. These have been discussed in Chapter 5, but they are not interventions that are dictated specifically by detailed genetic knowledge of the patient in question. Thus while the hope that genetics holds the ultimate answers to prostate cancer therapy may be justified, at present it appears that this approach is only in its infancy. However, the connection between Hedgehog signaling pathway and advanced prostate cancer which is discussed below is an example where a proposed intervention, in this case pathway blocking, can be traced back to genetic-related research and the over-expression of a particular gene. Also, the UPM3 urine test and the use of the hypermethylation of the GSTP1 gene described below both detect prostate-specific genes that are over-expressed in cancer cells.

DIAGNOSIS

The challenge in prostate cancer diagnosis is the same as already discussed above in the context of BPH. At present, the only way to diagnose prostate cancer with a very low level of false negative results is a biopsy involving at least 11-12 needles, and to further decrease the probability of missing cancers, a second biopsy is indicated. Even two biopsies will not reduce the probability of missing a cancer to a value below 10-12%, but those cancers that are missed are probably very small and perhaps insignificant. The need to do biopsies to answer the question, "do I have cancer," emphasizes the failure of other tests, and in particular the PSA test, to provide adequate specificity. While there is active research aimed at finding a blood or urine marker that is both prostate and cancer specific with very high sensitivity and specificity, even if one of great promise is developed, it will be quite some time before sufficient clinical experience and data are acquired. For example, to determine the specificity of a new blood test for detecting prostate cancer, biopsies would be required, probably for a large group of patients exhibiting various levels of the marker. It may be very difficult to recruit for a trial large numbers of asymptomatic men, i.e. good screening candidates, who are willing to undergo the discomfort and risk the low but finite morbidity of the 12 (or more) needle biopsy. However, large numbers of men undergo biopsies each year because of an abnormal DRE and/or elevated PSA. Studies involving blood or urine tests done prior to these biopsies should not be difficult to implement, but this population is not equivalent to the asymptomatic population with PSA below the standard cut-off for triggering a biopsy.

uPM3, A NEW URINE BASED PROSTATE CANCER TEST

This new approach employs a urine test to detect a gene over-expressed in prostate cancer cells. Urine is collected immediately after a prostate massage, i.e. a prolonged palpation (massage) of the prostate as during a DRE. The gene, called PSA3[DD3] is one of the most prostate cancer-specific genes described to date. To detect it under the circumstances of this test requires an assay of great sensitivity, in this case a so-called reverse transcriptase polymerase chain reaction, which provides a high level of amplification. The proposed test also has a built-in control since PSA is assayed at the same time to confirm the presence of prostate cells in the urine sample. [7]

A multi-center study from Quebec, Canada recently reported by Fradet *et al* [8] was designed to establish the sensitivity and specificity of the uPM3 test as a function of the cut-off in a parameter that was obtained by detailed analysis of the assay kinetics. In this study 443 patients undergoing biopsy had prior to the procedure submitted to a prostate massage and provided a useable sample of urine. Both the biopsy results and the PSA were known which provided an opportunity to stratify the sensitivity and specificity according to the PSA range. The results, based on an assay cut-off that gave the best compromise between sensitivity and specificity, are given in Table 1. Similar results were reported by Hessels *et al* [9] in a single institution study from the Netherlands.

Table 9-1. Sensitivity and specificity of the uPM3 test for prostate cancer stratified by PSA level [8].

tPSA range (ng/mL)	Sensitivity (%)	Specificity (%)
<4	74	91
4-10	58	91
>10	79	90
Overall	66	89

Values of specificity in the low 90s are comparable to what is obtained with two biopsies or a saturation biopsy (see chapter 4). When the positive and negative predictive values for the uPM3 test were compared with PSA, for a PSA level above 4, the positive predictive values were 38% for PSA and 75% for uPM3, whereas the negative predictive values were 80% for PSA and 84% for uPM3. The test also performed well in a subset of patients undergoing subsequent biopsies after one or more previous negative biopsies. In this group, the observed sensitivity and specificity were 74 and 87% respectively. The authors comment that the positive predictive value of the uPM3 test appears better than risk factors such as PIN (see Chapter 4) which is commonly used to justify repeat biopsies.

Fradet *et al* suggest that this new test may provide some of the answers to the current dilemmas of early cancer detection. In addition, the test may be particularly useful in monitoring men with previously negative biopsies. Finally, they point out that this test may become one of the first new molecular diagnostic tools to aid in prostate cancer detection [7,8]. However, the downside is that the test requires more sophisticated data analysis than would be necessary for the measurement of a simple concentration.

GSTP1 HYPERMETHYLATION

The silencing of the glutathione-S-transferase P1 gene (GSTP1) by what is called hypermethylation is the most common genetic alteration so far reported in prostate cancer. Hypermethylation involves the bonding of a number of methyl (CH_3) groups. By detecting this gene in body fluids (serum, plasma, urine and ejaculate) it is possible to detect the presence of cancer with specificity near 100%. This hypermethylated gene can also be assayed in prostate tissue recovered from biopsy. The very high specificity can be utilized to differentiate benign tissue such as in BPH from cancerous tissue in cores recovered in biopsy. The use of this assay is also being suggested to reduce the number of repeat biopsies. This test may well provide a general solution to the low specificity of the PSA test and provide a powerful tool for both diagnosis and treatment management [10-12].

THE TREATMENT FRONTIER

WATCHFUL WAITING—ACTIVE SURVEILLANCE

If a physician were to tell a patient that he had a low-grade non-aggressive cancer and was able to say this with a very high level of certainty, then the option of active surveillance would probably hold great appeal. If a man was also convinced that if his cancer became aggressive, this could be detected early enough to assure timely and effective treatment, the merits of active surveillance would be reinforced. It will probably be a while before much data is available that address the merits of this option. As discussed in Chapter 6, criteria have been proposed for both initiation and terminating active surveillance, patients are being offered this option, and some encouraging data regarding outcomes have been collected. Since the active surveillance program was started at Hopkins, only approximately 1% of newly diagnosed prostate cancer patients have enrolled. However, Hopkins scientists have just reported the results of a small study which compared the outcome of immediate surgical treatment performed on 150 men who would have been eligible for active surveillance according to the Hopkins criteria [13] with 38 patients electing this form of watchful waiting. When noncurable cancer was defined as less than a 75% chance of remaining disease-free for ten years, there was no advantage found for immediate treatment over active surveillance [14].

As discussed in Chapters 4 and 6, the clinical observations on which the criteria for eligibility for active surveillance are based are subject to uncertainty. Of particular concern are the clinical Gleason scores. It is well known among pathologists and urologists that both upgrading and downgrading is common when clinical Gleason scores are compared with what is considered an accurate assessment based on the examination of the prostate after surgery. There are also rather large variations in scoring when two or more pathologists examine the slides, and also variability when a pathologist reexamines slides without being aware of having seen them before. PSA and PSA velocities are also not infallible guides to how serious the cancer is. Thus an area of great interest involves improving the tools for making the clinical judgment with a high level of certainty regarding the presence of aggressive vs. indolent cancer. This problem will almost certainly be solved, probably sooner rather than later and then many men, by choosing active surveillance, will avoid immediate treatment and perhaps never need to be treated. The Hedgehog signaling pathway research described below is but one example of the quest for better ways to ascertain the true nature of a man's cancer without taking out his prostate.

The fact that biopsies miss cancers is another concern since the institutions promoting active surveillance use biopsy results as an integral component of their criteria, both for suggesting the option and for triggering the advice to have definitive treatment. The group at Johns Hopkins recently advanced data supporting saturation biopsies as a solution in this context [15]. The extent to which this will discourage men form electing this option remains to be seen, but men should recognize that the slight added discomfort and morbidity associated with the saturation technique, which in fact seem to be declining as the technique is perfected, may still be preferable to immediate radical prostatectomy or radiation therapy, given that there is a significant likelihood of avoiding definitive treatment altogether.

Thus men should recognize that in the PSA era the chances are that their T1c (elevated PSA with normal DRE) cancer may in fact pose no immediate danger. The problem is that they may not be offered the active surveillance option based on the criteria being used at leading institutions. In fact, no mention of it may be made at all. Men who think they might be eligible based on the criteria being used at Hopkins or Memorial Sloan Kettering (see Chapter 6) should consider forcing the issue with the physician in charge of their treatment since considerable benefit might accrue and unnecessary treatment avoided.

INTERFERENCE WITH SIGNALING—THE *HEDGEHOG* PATHWAY

If a scientist was searching for the Holy Grail in prostate cancer treatment, discovering a single weak link in the cell proliferation mechanism that was unique to these cancer cells and then finding a way to break this unique link such that proliferation was stopped completely would seemingly qualify. Such a pathway appears to have been discovered and there are even known inhibitors.

The pathway in question goes by the name the *Hedgehog* or *Sonic Hedgehog signaling* pathway. It has been known for some time that the Hedgehog family of growth factors activate signaling systems for cell-cell communication that regulate cell proliferation and differentiation during development. The proliferation and invasive behavior of tumor cells have now been shown to partly involve the molecular mechanisms and pathway components that have been uncovered in biochemical, genetic and molecular studies of Hedgehog signaling. When there is continuous pathway activation, prostate cells become tumorigenic. In addition, elevated pathway activity distinguishes localized prostate from metastatic cancer. In fact it is thought that the Hedgehog activity is both a necessary and sufficient factor for metastatic behavior. Cell culture and animal studies have confirmed that inhibition of prostate cancer proliferation by blocking this pathway is possible with existing agents such as the plant alkaloid cyclopamine or anti-Hedgehog antibodies. There seems to be general agreement that herein lies a novel therapeutic approach, at least for advanced cancer [16-18]. It has also recently been suggested that Hedgehog signaling requires lipoprotein particles, which might explain the long-standing recognition of the connection between cholesterol levels and the risk of prostate cancer, although this work, which used fruit flies, needs to be extended at, least initially, to animal models [16,19].

Thus there are both diagnostic (staging) and therapeutic aspects associated with the discovery of the involvement of the Hedgehog signaling pathway and prostate cancer. An assay that measured Hedgehog signaling activity in biopsy tissue would have the potential for identifying patients with advanced aggressive cancer and would also aid in deciding whether active surveillance would be an appropriate option if the assay indicated only slow-growing localized cancer [16,18].

The therapeutic aspect involves inhibition of the pathway in an attempt to both halt proliferation and metastasis and cause tumor regression. The natural product cyclopamine, which curiously enough was first identified in connection with the one-eyed sheep mutation, is one possibility, but because it is not patentable, there is currently effort to produce small molecule Hedgehog signaling antagonists based on the cyclopamine function. One of these candidate pharmaceuticals is expected to undergo Phase I testing in 2006. However attractive this approach is theoretically, there may be problems associated with the fact that Hedgehog signaling is not unique to the prostate, but is to some extent ubiquitous in cell development and stem cell maintenance [16]. Even mature adults rely on stem cell proliferation, for example, to replace blood cells, and maintain both the functional integrity of the intestines and skin. Also, hedgehog pathways are present in the mature brain, and blockage might, through the inhibition of stem cell renewal, decrease the cerebral stem cell pools and result in cognitive or other disturbances that might even appear long after the use of this therapy [20]. Thus it is possible that the success of Hedgehog signaling inhibition therapy will depend on targeting and eliminating prostate cells while having a minimal impact on normal stem cell populations and their function. This promises to be an active area of research, given the potential for such therapy to drastically decrease the probability of localized cancer progression towards advanced stages. Greater understanding of the molecular and genetic complexities of this signaling process will no doubt give rise to a variety of therapeutic possibilities.

Recent discoveries regarding the role of Hedgehog signaling in prostate cancer are related to the hypothesis that stem cells are involved in carcinogenesis by a mechanism that is theorized to involve the failure of control mechanisms that govern tissue repair and stem cell self-renewal. Hedgehog signaling pathways are involved in tissue regeneration, stem cell renewal and cancer growth, suggesting a mechanism for what goes wrong when uncontrolled proliferation occurs and focusing attention on either stem cells or other similar cells [20].

It is also well known that chronic tissue injury caused by acid reflux, the action of toxins, chronic infection and such conditions as inflammatory bowel disease can result in cancer. Presumably, not all of these adverse interactions involved mutagenic agents, and thus there is the question of the mechanism relating tissue injury to carcinogenesis. The repair process involves the production of cells that can differentiate to form the specialized cells needed to repair the injured tissue. The source of these differentiated cells is stem cells. Thus the hypothesis that cancer is due to unregulated tissue repair associated with chronic activation of pathways such as the Hedgehog. In other words, the repair process fails to stop when the repair is complete. The mechanism involved in sustaining stem cells in an activated state could be due to genetic changes as well as influences from surrounding cells. Also, the motile behavior of cells which are activated to repair injury induced defects might account in part for the highly invasive nature of some cancers [21]. While this is only a hypothesis and many aspects of the underlying pathology are not well understood at this time, nevertheless this will no doubt prove to be an active area of research that may significantly influence of the future development of theories of carcinogenesis and novel therapeutic approaches.

ONCOLYTIC ADENOVIRUS THERAPY

Oncolytic adenoviruses specifically replicate in and lyse (destroy) cells of prostate epithelial origin. These include prostate adenocarcinoma cells. Prostate cancer specific adenoviruses are engineered to seek out prostate cells that produce PSA. Furthermore, their replication is controlled by prostate-specific regulatory mechanisms. They not only kill prostate cancer cells, but replicate and infect other cancer cells which lead to a controlled virus spread, thus amplifying the therapeutic effect. There have been only limited Phase I/II clinical trials which, while failing to yield complete tumor regression, nevertheless have provided evidence of the safety and therapeutic potential of these viruses. In cell culture studies, some of these viruses show a very high ratio of cancer cells to normal cells killed, ratios that are in fact much higher than found with commonly used chemotherapeutic agents. There is currently interest in combining adenoviruses with chemo- and radiotherapy to increase the potential for destroying cancer cells. The oncolytic adenoviruses satisfy some of the requirements associated with the so-called magic bullet [22,23].

CHEMOTHERAPY

The search for new and better cytotoxic chemotherapeutic agents will no doubt continue indefinitely. As discussed in Chapter 7, those currently used for prostate cancer provide, from the patient's point of view, what may seem to be very little advantage when measured by absolute life extension. Critics of chemotherapy point out that this is a common characteristic of currently popular agents. A very recent meta analysis of Morgan *et al* [24] is of interest, It was based on randomized-controlled trials that reported statistically significant increases in 5-year survival due solely to cytotoxic chemotherapy from 1990 to 2004. The authors found that the overall contribution of curative and adjuvant cytotoxic chemotherapy to 5-year survival in adults was 2.1% in the USA. This very low result is somewhat misleading since the included a number of cases even when no 5-year data was available. In addition, the analysis represents an average over a set of cancers which included some that show quite large responses. Another way to analyze their data is to look at only those sites with the percentage of 5-year survivors due to chemotherapy low, i.e. less than 8%. This assumes that when the number is this large or larger, there is much less debate as to the merits of chemotherapy. This leaves head and neck (1.9%), esophagus (4.9%), stomach (0.7%), colon (1.0%), rectum (3.4%), lung (2.0%), breast (1.4%) and brain (3.7%). The percentages are calculated for each site from the number of cases eligible for inclusion and the absolute number of 5-year survivors due to chemotherapy. The total cancers in this subgroup equaled 84,828 and the absolute number of 5-year survivors due to chemotherapy was 1458, or 1.7%. Put another way, 98.3% of individuals with this subgroup of cancers who received chemotherapy achieved no improvement in their 5-year survival. Cancer sites where there was much larger benefit were cervix (12%), testis (37.7%), Non-Hodgkin's lymphoma (10.5%) and Hodgkin's disease (40.3%). Thus blanket rejection of chemotherapy, as suggested by the overall results calculated by the authors of 2.1%, seems to lack justification since clearly those with certain cancers appear to benefit, some substantially, and in fact this was presumably already well known.

For prostate cancer, Morgan *et al* [24] identified 23,242 US cases that qualified, but report that there was no evidence that cytotoxic chemotherapy improved 5-year survival. Two recent short-term studies were described in Chapter 7. Both gave percentage reductions in risk of death of 24-28%, but the absolute increases in survival time were only 2.4 and 2 months. The disparity between the impression given by the percentage decrease in risk of death and the actual life extension merits discussion.

One of the problems with chemotherapy is that it is promoted to patients (and even physicians) on the basis of relative rather than absolute changes in outcome. For example, an average change in life expectancy of from 4 months to 2 months represents a large and impressive percentage change (50%) and when quoted to patients as a percentage can be convincing and result in acceptance of treatment, but the absolute change of 2 month may be viewed as more or less irrelevant by many patients, given the severe morbidity and non-zero mortality that generally accompany this therapy. Also, the change being quoted is an average, and some will be on the low side with even less life extension. Another problem involves the use of surrogate endpoints. This can seriously confuse the issue of efficacy. Progression-free survival, disease-free survival or recurrence-free survival may reflect only a temporary lull after chemotherapy and may last only a few months. Progression resumes, sometimes with renewed vigor, and the impact on survival can be minimal. Thus the potential for these surrogate endpoints creating an illusion of benefit when none exists.

It is also important to always keep in mind that statistically significant differences or results in clinical studies are not always clinically significant. The word significant is almost always used in epidemiology as a statistical term, and the everyday usage may not be at all appropriate. The fact that a difference, say between cases and controls, has less than a 5% chance of having occurred randomly (the normally used cut-off for statistical significance) does not mean that the difference is clinically important. It is important to look at the actual numbers, especially when deciding for or against a treatment that carries high risk of adverse events.

Actually, the problems facing a man considering the offer of cytotoxic chemotherapy are even more complex than indicated above. As Clarke and Wylie [25] point out, the majority of patients in the two chemotherapy studies for prostate cancer that form the basis for current recommendations and enthusiasm involved a patient population with advanced cancer that was significantly younger than that encountered in practice and probably had fewer comorbidities. Thus there is the uncertainty associated with the use of these agents on older patients, especially those with comorbidities and in fact, according to Clarke and Wylie, some would not be considered eligible in many centers. It is almost impossible for men to evaluate new chemotherapy agents being offered to them without examining the data at a level that may in fact not be available or comprehensible to them.

As new chemotherapeutic agents appear and are suggested for the treatment of advanced prostate cancer, men who might qualify as candidates should at least insist on being provided with absolute life extension information before making a decision. They also need to beware of unbridled enthusiasm common in this field. While it can be understood that small increases in efficacy would be greeted as breakthroughs, given the dismal performance of chemotherapy for many cancers and historically for prostate cancer, men must apply their own standards, which may mean weighing improvement in life expectancy against the morbidity and potential mortality associated with the treatment. The possibility of participating in a cytotoxic chemotherapy trial may also be offered. This has its own set of obvious pros and cons, especially if the risk and nature of adverse reactions as well as the risk of mortality are not well defined, which will be the case almost by definition if the trial is Phase I or Phase II.

The conclusion is not that cytotoxic chemotherapy for prostate cancer should be rejected out of hand, but that when new agents are offered they should be scrutinized carefully with the issues discussed above in mind.

OTHER THERAPEUTIC APPROACHES UNDER DEVELOPMENT

- Drugs that enhance apoptosis in precancerous and cancerous tissue without harming healthy tissue offer interesting possibilities.
- Immunologic therapies that stimulate the immune system to attack and kill cancer cells. In one approach, particular cells are isolated from a blood sample, activated for this task, and then infused back into the patient's body.
- Anti-angiogenesis has for many years been considered an attractive approach to cancer therapy—cut of the blood supply to the tumor and it dies. Many drugs are now in clinical trials, some of which involve prostate cancer.
- Manipulating cell regulators that protect cancer cells from apoptosis (cell death).

This list is far from complete but is intended to illustrate the directions being taken. What is clear from the big picture is that most of the effort is being directed toward pharmaceutical drug solutions to the treatment of prostate cancer.

SURGERY

It would appear that the so-called open radical prostatectomy has reached what is close to a state of perfection in the hands of surgeons who have concentrated on this aspect. Measured either by outcomes, complications or long-term adverse effects, it appears to the experts that there is little room for improvement. Thus the challenge of the future is not to improve on the surgical technique as practiced and promoted by such surgeons as Dr. Patrick Walsh, but is rather for more surgeons to rise to this level of perfection.

A new and exciting approach involves robotic laparoscopic radical prostatectomies. Robotic surgery was discussed in Chapter 6. Champions of this procedure point to a number of aspects where robotic surgery is superior to open surgery, but those who are less enthusiastic suggest that many of the advantages offer only a marginal improvement over the best open surgery, but agree nevertheless, that the enhanced ability to visualize the surgical field with magnification offers the robotic surgeon the opportunity to refine both the nerve sparing aspects of the operation and in addition, achieve better surgical margins. In addition, some surgeons who achieve only average results with open surgery may obtain better outcomes with the robotic approach. Thus, robotic laparoscopic prostate surgery may indeed be the way of the future, in spite of the large capital investment and significant learning curve. Centers where this technique is well established and which have a good track record find that the majority of men, when given the option of robotic vs. open surgery, will select the former. With time, the number of centers offering robotic prostate surgery will no doubt expand dramatically. The procedure has everything going for it—it is very fashionable, works very well indeed in the hands of experts, is less invasive, and has a shorter hospital stay with less post-operative pain.

As with open surgery, the robotic laparoscopic prostate surgery may already, in the hands of the best practitioners, have reached the point where improvements will be of marginal significance, and the next big advance will probably require radical innovation.

RADIATION

External beam radiation therapy (EBRT) has also evolved rapidly with the development of 3D-confocal techniques (3D-CRT), the further modification involving intensity modulation of the beam (IMRT) and finally accurate repositioning of the patient during daily treatments. Also, treatment planning has been elevated to a high level of sophistication. Thus within the constraints of using linear accelerators as radiation sources, EBRT would appear to be approaching a level where improvements may now be marginal. Even the question of optimum dose seems to be rapidly clarifying now that modern techniques allow higher doses without concomitant higher morbidity and complications.

Brachytherapy has also been perfected over a considerable time span, and now involves sophisticated techniques for treatment planning and seed implantation. The so-called high-density radiation brachytherapy represents a significant innovation which has also undergone considerable evolution. While incremental improvements will no doubt take place, real advances will require radical innovation.

Waiting in the wings for prime-time status are other types of external beams, and in particular proton beams. Protons are positively charged particles that together with neutrons make up almost all the mass of the atom. The nucleus of the hydrogen atom consists of only one proton. Heavier isotopes of hydrogen will have neutrons along with the lone proton. As one moves up the periodic chart, both the number of nuclear protons and neutrons systematically increases. High-energy proton beams are generally generated by either cyclotrons or synchrotrons. Both imply large accelerator facilities, which in contrast to the compact linear accelerators used in EBRT, are exceedingly expensive to acquire and maintain. These accelerators occupy whole buildings, not just part of a treatment room. At present only a small number of centers offer proton beam therapy, and this number is unlikely to experience more than slow growth due to financial constraints. Nevertheless, the proton beam offers unique advantages. Accelerators employed for proton beam therapy generate protons with energies up to well over 200 MEV. These high-energy protons deposit low energies at entrance to the irradiated volume and a maximal dose at a user-defined depth (called the *Bragg peak*). The exit dose following the deposition of most of the energy in the target region is also low. These unique properties due to the Bragg peak allow a high dose to be delivered to the prostate while sparing nearby structures including the bladder and rectum. Thus charged particle irradiation provides a significant dose-distribution advantage over standard 3D-CRT employing high-energy electromagnetic radiation.

There are relatively few studies concerning the efficacy of proton beam therapy, but the technique has been in use for a considerable period of time and long-term studies are starting to appear. The Department of Radiation Oncology at Loma Linda University Medical Center in California has been a leader in this area. They employ a 70-250 MEV proton synchrotron with four treatment rooms adjacent to the accelerator. In a recent report [26] from this institution, the results from 1255 patients treated between 1991 and 1997 are summarized. Long-term biochemical disease-free survival rates were comparable with those reported for other modalities where there was the intent to cure, and they observed minimal morbidity. Dose escalation strategies are currently under investigation which may provide even better long-term results. To quote Dr. Peter Scardino [27], "If you happen to live near one of the twenty or so centers worldwide that has a proton beam unit, it can provide good state-of-the-art therapy."

CRYOTHERAPY

The frontier in cryotherapy appears to involve achieving better temperature control within the ice ball (the frozen prostate) while minimizing the damage to adjacent structures and maximizing the prostate cancer cell kill. A big advance involved the use of a number of temperature sensors in order to monitor not only the thermal gradients within the prostate but also the temperatures of such vulnerable structures as the rectum. It is reasonable to expect that this technique will experience continued innovation and will advance in sophistication along with an associated increase in the power of computer assisted treatment planning and execution. Also, it seems predictable that equipment which includes multiple thermal sensors will replace cryotherapy machines that lack this refinement. Improvements associated with the duration and number of freeze-thaw cycles would, at this stage in the development of the technique, appear to offer only minimal opportunity for further perfection. However, there may be breakthroughs in methods for cooling and warming. Men wishing to undergo cryotherapy should seek out centers where the latest equipment with real-time multiple temperature measurements is in routine use.

In the above discussion of the common approaches to therapy for localized prostate cancer, it has been suggested that some procedures like the radical prostatectomy, 3D-conformal radiation therapy, intensity modulated radiation therapy, and modern cryotherapy with temperature sensing have been perfected to the point where there is little room for improvement. This is obviously a dangerous position to adopt, and historical examples of similar positions can be found which proved to be terribly wrong. However, it would seem that for really significant breakthroughs to occur it is necessary for innovation to represent fairly radical changes in general approach since extensive fine-tuning of the present techniques has already largely taken place.

PHOTODYNAMIC THERAPY

Photodynamic therapy (PDT) uses visible light at the red end of the spectrum to selectively kill cancer cells. This is accomplished by first administering a so-called sensitizer which has the following properties. This chemical must preferentially seek out cancer tissue and concentrate there in preference to anywhere else. It must absorb the light at the wavelength being used for the therapy, and it must, when activated by light, generate cytotoxic substances which kill cancer cells. Compounds have been synthesized that possess the required properties, but the problem is to get the light energy at the proper dose into the desired locations in the prostate. Thus far the only satisfactory way to accomplish this is with light conducting fibers that are inserted through the perineum using a procedure similar to that employed in the ultrasound guided seed placement in brachytherapy. Both light conducting fibers and light sensing fibers are inserted and an attempt is made to monitor the light distribution and prevent collateral damage. The light source is a laser which employs a beam splitter to distribute the energy to the set of fibers [28,29]. Advantages include the harmless nature of the radiation, the potential for differential necrosis for tumor vs. normal tissue, and the fact that the procedure can be repeated.

Prostate cancer is a multifocal disease and the many tumors are difficult or impossible to image. Thus PDT must irradiate the glandular prostate completely, which somewhat reduces the utility of the selective uptake of the sensitizer. Transurethral light delivery is not satisfactory and the sources of light and their special distribution must be tailored to each patient. The course of the treatment cannot be satisfactorily followed with ultrasound because the contrast between treated and untreated tissue is unsatisfactory. Thus the effectiveness of PTD at present cannot be effectively monitored during therapy, and treatment plans are executed with computer software based on the ultrasound image of the gland. Other Difficulties with this technique involve depth of light penetration estimates and thus probe placement, and this impacts dose determinations. The central problem is that prostates have a range of light transmission properties [28,30].

To be accepted as a viable treatment modality, PDT must compete favorably with cryotherapy, brachytherapy and perhaps eventually high-intensity ultrasound. The first two are of similar invasiveness but neither is potentially as selective as PDT. Thus far there have been only a limited number of small clinical trials, mostly reported at conferences, and it is much too early to have useful information on comparative effectiveness and morbidity. These studies employed a diverse patient groups (after TURP, after RT, and primary treatment) and have been of the pilot or phase I/II design [28,31]. They have provided proof in principle of the technique with demonstrated PSA drops, evidence of tissue necrosis, and a preliminary indication of side effects and complications. Clearly, much research will be necessary before PDT is accepted as an option for either primary or salvage therapy.

PDT has been most successful with tumors that are easily accessible with an optical fiber or some form of light pipe. These include esophageal, cervical and bladder cancers. Unfortunately, the location of the prostate renders the use of PDT much more difficult as compared to the above sites.

HIGH-INTENSITY FOCUSED ULTRASOUND (HIFU)

This technique was developed about 10 years ago and has undergone testing in France, Germany and Japan. Ultrasound is produced by a transducer which generates a beam of sound waves which can be used for imaging, a valuable technique of long standing for diagnosis and for guiding such procedures as biopsies. If this beam is unfocused, heat is more or less uniformly distributed along the path with minimal temperature elevation. However, if a spherical-shaped transducer is used, the beam will have a focal point where tissue heating will reach a maximum. For example, a focused beam can generate tissue temperatures of 85°C at the focal point and yet the temperature 5 mm removed from this point can beat near normal body temperature. Ultrasonic machines used for this purpose are designed to emit pulsed beams. During the firing sequence, the heat-generated lesion of a distorted elliptical shape grows with a greater volume in the direction of the transducer. Modern machines designed for prostate cancer treatment are computer controlled from information obtained from a transrectal ultrasonic probe which is combined with the focused transducer. The patient is immobilized and the computer operates a mechanical system which moves the focusing transducer from one point to the next in order to carry out the planned tumor tissue ablation while avoiding surrounding tissue [32]. Given the size of the prostate and the intention to only treat certain areas, precise control is essential.

In theory, HIFU would seem to be an ideal solution to the problem of killing tumor tissue. It is minimally invasive—no incisions are made nor are probes inserted through the perineum or rectal wall. But effective ablation of tumor tissue requires precise location of the focal point relative to the prostate, precise relocation at each step in the treatment process, and a reproducible or controllable ablation volume, while avoiding as much as possible thermal damage to the external sphincter, the neurovascular bundles, the bladder neck and the rectum. It is common practice to attempt the ablation of the entire gland while preserving the rectal wall and surrounding tissues. An advantage of this technique is that it is repeatable.

Two machines are currently in use and being promoted for HIFU, a French device named *Ablatherm* and a U.S. machine called *Sonablat*. Except for studies from the University of Tokia Hachioju in Japan which employed the Sonablat, all the studies reported so far have been from Europe and used the Ablatherm. Five studies are of interest in the context of this section [33-37]. They involve over 900 subjects but have limited follow-up averaging typically only 1-2 years, although a very recent report from Japan had a 3-year follow-up. Most patients had Gleason scores ≤ 7 and but the PSA range went up to 20 ng/mL.

These studies naturally address two issues—side-effects and complications and oncological outcomes. The latter were generally assessed by the same standard as used in judging radiotherapy failure, the ASTRO definition (see Chapter 7) or by biopsy. Using negative biopsy as a criterion, typical disease-free survival over the periods studied was close to 86-87%. In the most recently reported study by Uchida *et al* [33] the 3-year disease-free survival stratified by recurrence risk yielded 84%, 69% and 51% for low-, moderate- and high-risk disease, respectively. Gianduzzo *et al* [38] point out that these oncological results compare very unfavorably with even their first 100 laparoscopic radical prostatectomies, where the comparative survival figures were 96.7%, 87.5% and 72.7%, and they express particular concern at what they consider poor performance in the low-risk group with good prognostic features who were in their opinion "eminently curable." They also comment on the use of the sextant biopsy as a criterion for identifying disease-free survival, remind readers of the high (23%) false negative cancer detection rate of this procedure, and suggest that the actual number of patients who were cancer free was lower than found.

The overall side-effect and complications picture is somewhat confused because in Europe it is becoming common practice [35,37] to add either a transurethral resection of the prostate (TURP) or a bladder neck incision prior to the HIFU procedure. The objective is to decrease the probability of post-HIFU urinary retention, but the practice implies that this is obviously a major problem. In the study of Uchida *et al* [33], neither TURP or bladder neck incisions were employed prior to HIFU, but Gianduzzo *et al* [38] point that 24% of the patients experienced urethral stricture and required either surgical treatment or mechanical dilation. In the study that compared HIFU alone to HIFU combined with TURP [37], the former yielded incontinence rates up to about 9% whereas with the combined therapy it was 4.6%. Uchida *et al* reported a 25% rate of erectile dysfunction, but the percentage where this was permanent was not given.

It will no doubt be some time before HIFU is accepted in North America. A trial involving the Ablatherm machine was suspended in 2001 for lack of timely accrual of participants [39]. What appears to be a rather unfavorable comparison between the oncological outcomes achieved by HIFU and the major accepted treatments with intent to cure currently in use may dampen enthusiasm. However, HIFU is an accepted and widely used treatment in Europe and as long-term studies are reported, it may turn out that HIUF will compete favorably with RP and RT both for primary and salvage treatment. Also, some men may consider that the absence of any incision provides a powerful motivation for this approach.

The principal researchers and centers in HIFU appear to be:

- Stefan Thüroff, Krankenhaus München-Haarlaching, München, Germany
- Guy Vallancien, Institut Montsouris, Paris, France
- Toyoaki Uchida, University of Tokai Hachioji Hospital, Hachioji, Japan

MICROWAVE THERMOTHERAPY

This technique involves the implantation of small microwave antennas in the tumor. The area is subjected to microwave radiation resulting in heating of the cancerous tissue and subsequent death of the cancer cells. Microwave thermotherapy for prostate cancer is still very much in the trial phase, but initial results are promising. The lead researcher in this field would appear to be Dr. Michael D. Sherar at the Princess Margaret Hospital in Toronto, Canada [40-43].

HYPERTHERMIA

The observation that cancer cells are significantly more sensitive to heat than are normal cells has led to the development of several minimally-invasive protocols designed to raise tumor temperature to a lethal level (to the cancer cells), while keeping surrounding normal tissue relatively cool. The heat can be applied by ultrasound (HIFU), microwaves, or through the heating of implanted rods of a ferromagnetic alloy (interstitial hyperthermia). Many cancer clinics in Europe also use whole body hyperthermia where the entire body is heated to 42° C (108° F) or higher either by immersion in a water bath or by circulating the blood through an external heater. Whole body hyperthermia is used mainly for systemic and metastasized cancers. Hyperthermia can be used as a stand-alone procedure or in combination with radiation or chemotherapy.

INTERSTITIAL HYPERTHERMIA

Interstitial hyperthermia involves the placement of small rods of a ferromagnetic alloy (7% cobalt and 93% palladium) near the cancerous tissue, somewhat similar to the technique used in brachytherapy (implantation of radioactive iodine pellets). By applying an external magnetic field to the pelvic area the rods heat up to a preset (maximum) temperature of 70° C (158° F) and, in the process, kill cancer cells within a 1-2 cm radius from the rods. The treatment takes about 60 minutes, is well tolerated, and is done in one outpatient session. The rods are left in place so that treatment can be repeated if the cancer recurs. This treatment has not been formally approved as yet, but is being evaluated in several clinical trials. The lead researcher in the field would seem to be Dr. R.D. Tucker at the University of Iowa [44-47]. Interstitial hyperthermia is also being used in combination with conventional external beam irradiation (radiotherapy) as studies have shown that even mild hyperthermia markedly increases the effectiveness of the radiotherapy application. The technique, known as thermoradiotherapy, is not yet commercial, but is being actively investigated in at least three centers: [48-51]

- Department of Urology, Humboldt University of Berlin – lead researcher is Dr. D. Deger
- University Medical Center, Utrecht, The Netherlands – lead researcher is Dr. M. van Vulpen
- Division of Radiation Oncology, Northwestern University, Chicago, IL – lead researcher is Dr. J.A. Kalapurakal

A clinical trial of interstitial hyperthermia was recently carried out by Dr. Tucker and colleagues at the University of Iowa. The trial involved 20 patients with biopsy-confirmed stage T1 or T2 prostate cancer. The average age of the patients was 71 years, their pre-treatment PSA levels varied between 2.5 and 10.7 ng/mL, and their Gleason scores ranged from 3 to 7. The patients were exposed to one 60-minute session of interstitial hyperthermia using implanted alloy rods placed in the prostate in a procedure similar to the one used for brachytherapy. After one year, 5 of the patients had relapsed and showed positive biopsies. These patients, however, had had significantly fewer rods implanted than the others. Eight patients developed erectile dysfunction, but none reported incontinence. With a one-year cure rate of 75% the researchers conclude that the technique is well tolerated and safe and may be useful in certain patients with T1 or T2 stage prostate cancer. Larger trials are planned [52].

A group of researchers at the Charite Hospital in Berlin recently reported the first experimental trial of interstitial hyperthermia using magnetic nanoparticles instead of alloy rods. The nanoparticle suspensions were injected transperineally into the prostate under ultrasound and fluoroscopy guidance. The patients underwent 6 weekly hyperthermia sessions of 60 minutes each during which the areas around the nanoparticles were heated to between 40-48.5° C (104-119° F) in the first session and to between 39.4-42.5° C (103-108° F) in the last session. The heating was induced by a 100 kHz alternating current magnetic field and the nanoparticles were retained in the prostate during the 6-week treatment period. A specially designed cooling device was used and the treatment was well tolerated without anaesthesia. The patients included in the trial had all experienced biopsy-proven recurrence after radiation therapy. The German researchers now plan a phase I trial of interstitial hyperthermia using magnetic nanoparticles suspensions in the treatment of recurrent prostate cancer [53].

ENHANCEMENT OF HYPERTHERMIA

Cell culture experiments have shown that alpha-tocopheryl succinate enhances the effects of hyperthermia and thus allows the use of lower temperatures while achieving equivalent cancer cell destruction. There is also evidence that quercetin dramatically amplifies the tumor killing effect of hyperthermia [54,55].

CONCLUSION

Several hyperthermia protocols have shown considerable promise in the treatment of certain types of prostate cancer. The finding that the efficacy of the procedures can be significantly enhanced (at least in cell cultures) by concomitant administration of such natural compounds as quercetin and alpha-tocopheryl succinate makes the research in this area all the more exciting. Hyperthermia procedures are minimally invasive, have few side effects, and likely require significantly less surgical skills than do a radical prostatectomy. Although still in their infancy, interstitial hyperthermia, and perhaps microwave thermotherapy, would seem to have a bright future and may well eventually become a viable choice in prostate cancer therapy.

Appendix A

Glossary Of Terms

(See also Glossary of Abbreviations – Appendix B)

ABDOMEN: The part of the body above the pelvic bone but below the ribs. Contains the intestines and organs such as liver, kidneys and stomach.

ABLATION: Refers to removal or destruction of tissue or blocking the effects of the binding of chemicals to cell receptors.

ACTIVE SURVEILLANCE: Monitoring a condition such as prostate cancer with the intent to intervene if and when appropriate treatment intended to cure is indicated.

ACUTE URINARY RETENTION: Complete inability to urinate due to obstruction or constriction.

ADENOCARCINOMA: Cancer that develops from a malignant abnormality in the epithelial cells in a glandular organ. Almost all prostate cancers are of this type.

ADJUVANT: Auxiliary. Treatment given in addition or auxiliary to the primary one.

AGONIST: A drug or substance capable of combining with receptors to influence biochemical activity.

ALPHA-BLOCKER: Prescription drugs that block alpha-receptors in the prostate and bladder. The net result is smooth muscle relaxation which improves voiding. Used to treat BPH

and prostatitis. Historically used to treat hypertension, but recently alpha-blockers which are prostate-specific have come into common usage.

ANABOLIC: Promoting or relating to anabolism.

ANABOLISM: The building up of complex molecules from simpler ones, e.g. proteins from amino acids. The opposite of catabolism.

ANASTOMOSIS: The site where the urethra is connected to the bladder neck after the prostate has been removed.

ANDROGEN DEPRIVATION THERAPY: Treatment that prevents the body from making or using androgens. Includes castration as well as drug therapy.

ANDROGEN: A hormone that promotes the development of male sexual characteristics and stimulates the activity of male sex organs.

ANTHROPOMETRIC: Relating to anthropometry.

ANTHROPOMETRY: The branch of anthropology concerned with comparative measurements related to the human body.

ANTIANDROGEN: A drug that blocks the effect of testosterone at the cellular level.

APEX: The lower end of the prostate where the urethra exits.

APOPTOSIS: Programmed cell death. This is a natural process where cells self-destruct and are replaced by new cells. Cancer cells have defects in this process which allow uncontrolled proliferation.

AUA SCORE: American Urological Association score. A measure of adverse urinary symptoms based on answers to a number of questions related to urination.

AUTONOMIC: Relating to the autonomic nervous system.

AUTONOMIC NERVOUS SYSTEM: The part of the nervous system that represents the motor innervation of smooth muscle, cardiac muscle and gland cells.

BASELINE: In a study, the characteristics of the participants are termed *baseline* if established at the start of the study.

BENIGN: Non-cancerous. Applied to growths and tumors.

BENIGN PROSTATIC HYPERPLASIA: The enlargement (hypertrophy) of the prostate.

BILATERAL: Occurring on both sides. Bilateral tumor growth would involve both lobes of the prostate.

BIOCHEMICAL FAILURE: The failure of definitive treatment to eradicate prostate cancer as indicated by PSA levels rather than by clinically evident symptoms.

BIOMARKER: A tissue, cellular or serum indicator of biological activity that can be used to monitor the state of health or disease. Generally a chemical compound.

BIOPSY: Removal and microscopic examination of tissue to establish the presence or absence of disease.

BISPHOSPHONATES: A class of drugs that stop bone loss (resorption).

BLADDER NECK: The portion of the bladder that attaches to the prostate.

BODY MASS INDEX: A numerical measure of being underweight, normal weight, overweight obese. BMI = weight (kg) divided by height (m) squared (or 703 X weight in pounds divided by height in inches squared).

BONE SCAN: A radioactive isotope based procedure used to detect prostate cancer activity in bones. Abnormal concentrations of the isotope detected in the scan indicate potential cancer sites.

BRACHYTHERAPY: The use of implanted radioactive seeds or pellets as a radiation source for therapy.

BUMP: In the context of prostate cancer, a rise and fall of the serum level of PSA after therapy.

CAPSULE: The outer layer or "skin" of the prostate.

CARCINOGENESIS: The process whereby cancer is initiated.

CASTRATE: To remove the testicles surgically.

CATHETER: A thin flexible tube. In the context of urology, it is used to drain the bladder.

CAVERNOUS NERVES: The erectile nerves that run along each side of the prostate and control erections.

CENTRAL ZONE: See transition zone.

CLINICAL STAGE: Clinical staging of prostate cancer involves estimating how advanced the cancer is based only on clinical information available prior to treatment, as distinct from information gained after surgery through pathological examination of tissues removed.

COLLIMATOR: A device or system of baffles designed to shape a beam of radiation.

COMORBIDITY: Coexisting health problems.

COMPUTERIZED TOMOGRAPHY: An x-ray imaging technique employing computer software that facilitates the presentation of the images as slices through selected sections of the body. The so-called CT scan.

CONFORMAL: Conforming to the shape of an object, such as a conformal radiation beam with a field shape matching that of the prostate with controlled margins.

CONFOUNDING: A situation where the effects of two or more processes are not separated or the distortion of the apparent effects of a factor related to risk brought about by an association with other factors that can influence the outcome. For example, the effect of heavy drinking on the incidence of lung cancer must be corrected for confounding associated with the high prevalence of smoking among heavy drinkers.

CRYOSURGERY: Freezing of an organ to kill tissue including tumor tissue.

CRYOTHERAPY: See Cryosurgery.

CYROABLATION: See Cryosurgery.

CYSTITIS: Inflammation of the bladder.

CYSTOSCOPY: A procedure where the interior of the bladder is examined visually with an instrument called a cystoscopy inserted through the urethra.

DETRUSOR: Smooth muscle in the wall of the bladder that contracts the bladder and expels the urine.

DIFFERENTIATION: Relates to the morphology of cells with normal cells being well differentiated whereas primitive and aggressive cancer cells are much less differentiated.

DOWNSTAGING: In the context of prostate cancer, a decrease in the stage and thus the predicted seriousness of the cancer that can occur when pathological samples are compared with biopsy tissue.

EMBOLISM: A blood clot. For example pulmonary embolism involves a blood clot moving generally from the leg to the lung.

ENZYME: A protein produced by cells which influences the rate of biochemical reactions without undergoing a change itself, i.e. a biological catalyst.

EPITHELIAL: Relating to or consisting of the epithelium.

EPITHELIUM: Cells covering all surfaces.

ESTROGEN: Predominantly female hormone produced mainly in the ovaries. It is also present in males.

ETIOLOGY: The science and study of the causes of disease or the science of causes and causality.

EXTRACAPSULAR EXTENSION: The situation where cancer has spread beyond the prostatic capsule.

EXTERNAL URINARY SPHINCTER: The valve at the exit end of the prostate which controls the flow of urine. The simultaneous opening of this sphincter and the closing of the internal urinary sphincter allows for ejaculation through the urethra.

GENE: A hereditary unit. A sequence of chromosomal DNA involved in the cellular production of a biochemically functional product.

GENOME: The complete DNA sequence containing the entire genetic information of an individual or population.

GLEASON SCORE: A system for classifying cells seen in prostate tissue samples according to the extent of cell differentiation. Used both with biopsy specimens and in scoring tumor tissue in prostates removed at radical prostatectomy or tissue recovered during transurethral resection.

GRAY SCALE: An energy scale used for high-energy radiation. Abbreviated GY.

GYNECOMASTIA: Excessive development of male breasts. A frequent side effect associated with hormone treatment for prostate cancer.

HALF-LIFE: The time for some quantity to decline to half its value. Used to quantify the rate of decay of radioactive (unstable) isotopes and the rate of disappearance of substances such as drugs in the circulation system. A constant half-life, which is characteristic of radioactive isotopes, implies exponential decay.

HEMATOSPERMIA: Blood in the seminal fluid.

HEMATURIA: Blood in the urine.

HESITANCY: Delay or difficulty in starting the urinary stream.

HIGH-GRADE PIN (PROSTATIC INTRAEPITHELIAL NEOPLASIA): Clusters of cells in the prostate thought to be premalignant, the presence of which increases the probability of future prostate cancer. High-grade PIN cells also occur along with established prostate cancer.

HORMONE: A chemical produced in one organ that regulates the functions of another, i.e. a signaling chemical.

HORMONE REFRACTORY: Prostate cancer that does not respond to androgen deprivation (hormone therapy).

HORMONE SENSITIVE: In the case of prostate cancer, the cancer cell growth is dependent on testosterone.

HORMONE THERAPY: Manipulation of the testosterone levels in the circulation and the blocking of testosterone binding sites in the prostate in order to prevent its action associated with cell proliferation.

HYPERLIPIDEMIA: Elevated serum cholesterol and/or triglycerides.

INCONTINENCE: Inability to retain urine or control its flow.

INDOLENT CANCER: A tiny cancer that is thought to pose no immediate threat.

INNERVATE: To supply a body part, tissue or organ with nerves or nervous stimulation.

INTENSITY MODULATED RADIATION THERAPY (IMRT): A modification of 3D-conformal radiation therapy. The intensity of the beam is variable throughout the irradiated area as dictated by the treatment plan and controlled by the operator.

INTERMITTENCY: A urination dysfunction where the attempt to completely empty the bladder is described as accomplished in spurts.

INTERNAL URINARY SPHINCTER: Muscular valve structure in the bladder neck that retains urine until it is voluntarily released.

ISOTOPE: Isotopes of a given element have the same atomic number (nuclear charge and thus chemistry) but different atomic masses. Most elements have both stable and unstable isotopes, the latter being radioactive.

LAPRASCOPIC SURGERY: Surgical technique employing small incisions through which a laprascope and other instruments are inserted.

LOBE: A subdivision of an organ or body part bounded by fissures or other structural boundaries.

LOCALIZED: Restricted to a defined region, as for example a tumor localized inside the prostate.

LYMPH NODES: Small glands located throughout the body that are associated with the immune system and are involved in protection from infection and the spread of disease.

MALIGNANT: Cancerous, having the invasive and metastatic characteristics of cancer.

MARGIN: In the context of the prostate, margin generally refers to "surgical margin" which is the outer edge of the tissue removed at surgery. If cancer cells are found at the margin, the implication is that some were on the other side of the margin and that not all the cancer cells were removed.

MAXIMUM ANDROGEN BLOCKAGE: The combined use of both androgen agonists and antiandrogen drugs to minimize both the levels and the activity of androgens in the prostate.

MEATUS: Opening

MEDICAL CASTRATION: Drug use accomplishing the same effect on testosterone production as achieved with surgical castration.

METASTASIS: A secondary tumor formed elsewhere and originating from a primary tumor. Plural-metastases. Also, a term denoting the process of spreading of cancer from the primary site.

METASTATIC: Adjective referring to metastasis.

MORBIDITY: A diseased state or the frequency of appearance of complications following surgical or other treatment.

MORTALITY: Death rate or fatal outcome.

MYOFASCIAL PAIN: Chronic pain in muscle tissues.

NADIR: The lowest value a marker reaches after treatment.

NEOADJUVANT: A therapy that precedes the definitive therapy.

NEOPLASM: An abnormal tissue exhibiting more rapid growth through proliferation which continues to grow after the stimuli that initiate new growth are no longer present.

NEUROVASCULAR BUNDLE: Cordlike structures attached to the surface of the prostate and containing microscopic nerves that are involved in the erection process. Included in these bundles are both arteries and veins. Preserved in the so-called nerve sparing radical prostatectomy.

NOCTURIA: Frequent need to urinate during the night.

NOMOGRAM: A graphic representation of a set of variables associated with an outcome such that weighting factors can be graphically determined and then summed to get the probability of the outcome. Can be automated for on-line use where the parameters are specified and the program calculates the probability of a given outcome.

NON-INVASIVE: Not involving the insertion of an instrument into the body or the use of an incision.

NUCLEAR MEDICINE: The use of radioactive isotopes for diagnosis and treatment.

OBSTRUCTIVE SYMPTOMS: Symptoms of difficulties associated with obstruction of urine flow such as intermittency, hesitancy etc.

ODDS RATIO: Odds ratio. The probability that a particular event (e.g. a disease) will occur divided by the probability that the event will not occur.

ONCOLITIC: Pertaining to, causing or characterized by oncolysis, a process which involves the destruction of a neoplasm.

ORCHIECTOMY: Surgical castration

ORGAN CONFINED DISEASE: Physical manifestation of the disease confined to the organ in question, e.g. localized prostate cancer.

OVERSTAGING: Determining the stage of a disease which later turns out to be overly pessimistic.

P-VALUE: The probability that a difference observed in a study is in fact due to chance and no difference really exists. The usual cut-off for statistical significance is a p value of > 0.05, i.e. a chance of 1 in 20 that an observed difference has occurred by chance.

PALLIATION: Alleviation of symptoms, e.g. pain, without curing the disease.

PALPABLE: In the context of prostate cancer, a lump, lesion or nodule that can be felt during the digital rectal examination.

PALPATE: Process of feeling for palpable features.

PARASYMPATHETIC: Pertaining to a division of the autonomic nervous system into opposing sympathetic and parasympathetic functions.

PERINEUM: Region between the scrotum and the anus.

PERIPHERAL ZONE: The part of the prostate immediately inside the capsule. The peripheral zone surrounds the transitional zone.

PHYTOCHEMICAL: A chemical substance having its origin in natural sources such as plants.

PHOTODYNAMIC THERAPY: A mode of treatment where light is used to activate a chemical to become toxic or produce a cytotoxic product. Forms of the chemical are used which preferentially accumulate in tumors after which light directed to the tumor (frequently with a laser and a flexible light pipe) is used to activate the cytotoxic process.

PHYTOTHERAPY: Therapeutic use of phytochemicals.

POLYMORPHISM: Occurrence together in a population of two or more alternative genotypes, each at a prevalence greater than that which could be maintained by recurrent mutation.

POSITIVE SURGICAL MARGINS: See margins.

POSITRON EMISSION TOMOGRAPHY: A radioactive isotope is taken up by tissue (e.g. tumor tissue) and highlighted in a scan that detects the two gamma rays emitted when the positron from the initial decay of the isotope is annihilated (so-called *positron annihilation radiation*). Great sensitivity and high signal-to-noise is provided by the fact that the two gamma rays are emitted simultaneously and at 180 degrees from each other and have identical energies. Radiation detection systems can be designed to detect only these gamma rays (a PET scan). The positron is really antimatter and it interacts after emission from the nucleus with a nearby electron followed by conversion of mass completely into energy, yielding two gamma rays of 0.51 MEV energy.

POST-VOID RESIDUAL VOLUME: The amount of urine remaining in the bladder at the end of urination. Can be imaged by ultrasound.

PROCTITIS: Inflammation of the mucus membrane of the rectum. An adverse effect that sometimes is associated with damage from radiation therapy.

PROSTATECTOMY: The surgical removal of the prostate and seminal vesicles.

PROSTATITIS: Infection or inflammation of the prostate.

PROTOCOL: A well-defined set of methods or rules by which a procedure or study is executed.

RADIATION CYSTITIS: Inflammation of the bladder caused by radiation.

RADIATION PROCTITIS: See Proctitis.

RADIATION THERAPY: The use of radiation to kill cancer cells and other tissue.

RADIATION URETHRITIS: Radiation induced inflammation of the urethra.

RADICAL: Relating to or directed at eliminating the root cause of a disease. Also, in chemistry, a molecule with an unpaired electron which makes it highly reactive (also termed a free radical).

RADIOACTIVE: Applies to unstable isotopes which decay with the emission of radiation.

RELATIVE RISK: The likelihood of the occurrence of a particular event among persons exposed to a given risk divided by the corresponding likelihood among persons unexposed to the same risk.

RESIDUAL VOLUME: In the context of BPH, the amount of urine remaining in the bladder after urination.

RESORPTION: Loss of bone through breakdown with the resultant reduction in bone mass.

RETROGRADE EJACULATION: Ejaculation into the bladder. Can be partial or complete.

SALVAGE THERAPY: A procedure carried out after the failure of a definitive therapy in the hope of accomplishing what the failed therapy attempted to do. The term is used with both radiation therapy and radical prostatectomy.

SATURATION BIOPSY: Prostate biopsy involving generally twenty or more cores, performed to reduce the probability of missing cancer when fewer cores are taken. The procedure rarely uses more than 40 cores.

SCREENING: Testing asymptomatic individuals in the hope of early detection of a health problem. Prime examples are the use of mammography for breast cancer and serum PSA for prostate cancer.

SEMINAL VESICLE: Structures located above and behind the prostate that secrete and store seminal fluid.

SENSITIVITY: In epidemiology, a statistical parameter. The probability that a diagnostic test will correctly identify the presence of a disease.

SENSITIZER: In photochemistry, a chemical which absorbs light and then because it is in an activated or excited state, initiates a physical or chemical process

SEXTANT: As applied to the biopsy, a technique that employs six needles, i.e. collects six cores.

SPECIFICITY: In epidemiology, a statistical parameter. The probability that a test will correctly identify the absence of a disease.

SPHINCTER: A muscle that encircles a duct, tube or orifice and can act as a valve or control flow.

STRICTURE: A narrowing, for example of the urethra, which can be caused by scar tissue.

SYMPATHETIC: See parasympathetic.

TESTOSTERONE: Male sex hormone, produced mainly by the testicles with small amounts produced by the adrenal glands.

THERMAL THERAPY: Use of heat to kill tissue, including tumor tissue.

TRANSITION ZONE: The part of the prostate immediately surrounding the urethra. BPH occurs in the transition zone, although cancer can also arise there, it is more commonly found in the peripheral zone.

TRANSRECTAL ULTRASOUND: The use of an ultrasound probe inserted into the rectum for the purpose of imaging the prostate and adjacent structures, and guiding the placement of biopsy needles and the infusion of local anesthetic.

TRANSRECTAL: Generally applied to describe a procedure carried out through the rectum, such as a biopsy.

TRANSURETHRAL: A procedure carried out by inserting instruments or probes into the urethra for the purpose of diagnosis or surgery associated with the prostate or bladder.

TRANSURETHRAL MICROWAVE THERAPY (TUMT): A treatment for BPH that involves heating prostate tissue with a microwave antenna inserted in the urethra.

ULTRASOUND: High-frequency (inaudible) sound waves. Note that sound waves require a medium for propagation whereas electromagnetic waves such as x-rays and gamma rays and light do not.

UNDERSTAGING: See Overstaging.

URETER: Tube that carries urine from the kidneys to the bladder.

URETHRA: Tube from the bladder, which passes through the prostate, and carries urine from the bladder to the outside.

URETHRAL: Of or pertaining to the urethra.

URGE INCONTINENCE: A strong, sudden urge to urinate which may or may not be controllable.

URINARY RETENTION: Generally refers to the complete inability to urinate. Also termed an acute urinary retention episode.

VASECTOMY: A male birth-control procedure involving the surgical cutting of the vas deferens (the secretory duct of the testicle) in order to prevent sperm from the testicles reaching the prostate.

WATCHFUL WAITING: In general, leaving a patient untreated and observing the progression, if any, of a disease, and offering only palliation. Can also involve observation and testing with the intent to intervene with treatment when with the intent to cure is indicated. This latter usage is being replaced by the term *active surveillance* or the equivalent.

Appendix B

Glossary Of Abbreviations

(See also the Glossary of Terms – Appendix A)

< : Less than

> : Greater than

≤ : Equal to or less than

≥ : Equal to or greater than

≈ : Approximately equal to

3D-CRT: Three-dimensional conformal radiation therapy. A modern version of EBRT where the radiation field precisely matches the shape of the organ or tumor.

5ARI: 5-alpha-reductase inhibitor. An inhibitor of the enzyme that converts testosterone to dihydrotestosterone.

%fPSA: Percent free PSA. The serum free PSA divided by the total PSA, expressed as a percentage.

ADT: Androgen deprivation therapy. Therapy that prevents androgens from activating androgen receptors, either by blocking or by reducing androgen concentrations.

ANS: Autonomic nervous system.

AS: Active surveillance.

ASTRO: American Society for Therapeutic Radiology and Oncology.

AUA: American Urological Association.

AUR: Acute urinary retention.

BCR: Biochemical recurrence. See Biochemical failure in Appendix A.

BF: Biochemical failure. Recurrence of cancer after treatment detected by an elevated or increasing PSA.

BMD: Bone mineral density. Measured by x-ray techniques to establish bone health and the extent of resorption.

BMI: Body mass index.

BPH: Benign prostatic hyperplasia (hypertrophy).

CAT: Computerized axial tomography. This imaging technique allows combining of images from multiple x-rays through computer control to produce cross-sectional or three-dimensional pictures of internal organs.

CI: A statistical confidence limit. For example the 95% CI provides a range in which 95% of additional measurements would be expected to fall.

COX: Cyclooxygenase, an enzyme involved in the conversion of long-chain fatty acids in the cell walls of white blood cells into pro- and anti-inflammatory substances. Targets for non-steroidal anti-inflammatory drugs such as ibuprofen and Celebrex. There are two forms, COX-1 and COX-2.

CP: Chronic prostatitis.

CPPS: Chronic pelvic pain syndrome.

DES: Diethylstilbestrol. A synthetic

estrogen no longer used in North America.

DHEA: Dehydroepiandrosterone. An adrenal androgen precursor produced by the adrenal cortex. It is converted to testosterone in the prostate.

DHT: Dihydrotestosterone, an androgen derived from testosterone through a chemical reaction involving the enzyme 5-alpha-reductase.

DRE: Digital rectal exam where the physician palpates the prostate through the rectal wall using a finger. Abnormalities which can be felt suggest the possibility of cancer.

EAU: European Association of Urology.

EBRT: External beam radiation therapy. Irradiation from outside the body, generally with a collimated or focused beam.

EPS: Expressed prostatic secretion. A fluid sample obtained by repeated massage of the prostate.

fPSA: Free PSA, as distinguished from complexed PSA.

GS: Gleason score.

Gy: Abbreviation of the unit of radiation called "Gray" used with the Gray Scale.

HDR: High density radiation. A term generally used with brachytherapy to denote high doses for short periods.

HIFU: High-intensity focused ultrasound. Can refer to a treatment procedure that uses heat produced by high-frequency ultrasound to kill prostate cells including tumor cells.

IMRT: Intensity modulated radiation therapy. A form of 3D-CRT where the intensity within the field of radiation can be varied to suit a predetermined irradiation protocol.

IPPS: International prostate symptom score. Equivalent to the AUA symptom score.

LE: Life expectancy.

LH: Luteinizing hormone. Production of testosterone in the testicles is stimulated by this pituitary hormone.

LHRH: Luteinizing hormone-releasing hormone (GnRH or gonadotrophin releasing hormone). Hypothalamus generated hormone that interacts with the LHRH receptor in the pituitary gland to release LH which then stimulates testosterone production in the testicles.

LRP: Laparoscopic radical prostatectomy.

LUTS: Lower urinary tract symptoms. Symptoms associated with difficulties of urination.

MEV: Million electron volts. An energy unit commonly used to characterize high-energy radiation.

mL: abbreviation for milliliter, 1/1000 of a liter.

ng: abbreviation for nanogram, one billionth of a gram.

NCCN: National Comprehensive Cancer Network.

NSAID: Non-steroidal anti-inflammatory. A class of over-the-counter and prescription drugs that treat inflammation. Most act on one or both of the forms of the enzyme cyclooxygenase (COX) to decrease the production of inflammatory substances derived from long-chain fatty acids in the cell walls of white blood cells.

OR: Odds ratio. See Appendix A

p: So-called p-value. See Appendix A

PSAD: PSA density. Serum PSA value divided by the prostate volume in cc.

PC: Prostate cancer.

PDT: Photodynamic therapy.

PET: Positron emission tomography.

PIN: Prostatic intraepithelial neoplasia. Abnormal cells believed to be precursors to prostate cancer.

PNS: Parasympathetic nervous system.

PSATZD: PSA transition zone density. Serum PSA level divided by the volume of the prostate transition zone.

PSAV: PSA velocity. The rate of change of PSA level with time, generally measured in months or years.

RP: Radical prostatectomy. A surgical procedure to remove the entire prostate gland and seminal vesicles.

RR: Relative risk. See Appendix A

RT: Radiation therapy. The use of radiation to kill malignant cells.

SD: Standard deviation. A statistical index of the degree of deviation from a mean or median. For example, the square root of the average of the squared deviations from a mean.

SNS: Sympathetic nervous system.

TNM: Tumor, Nodes, Metastasis. A popular system for staging prostate cancer which takes into account the extent and location of the tumor (T) and the presence and extent of lymph note invasion (N) and metastasis (M). E.g. T1c—detected by elevated PSA with a normal DRE.

tPSA: Total serum PSA—the PSA normally measured.

TRUS: Transrectal ultrasound.

TUIP: Transurethral incision of the prostate. Used to treat BPH.

TUMT: Transurethral Microwave Thermotherapy. Used to treat BPH.

TURP: Transurethral resection of the prostate. The so-called roto-rooter operation. A surgical procedure where tissue obstructing the urethra is removed. Used to treat BPH.

TUVP: Transurethral electrovaporization. Used to treat BPH.

TWOC: Trial without catheter. A test of an individual's ability to urinate successfully when the catheter is removed after relieving an acute urinary retention episode.

TZ: Transition zone.

UTI: Urinary tract infection.

Appendix C

Glycemic Loads

FOOD	Serving Size	Glycemic Index	Carbohydrates per serving, g	Glycemic Load /serving	Glycemic Load per 100 g
GRAINS & BREADS					
Bagel	1 medium	72	56	40	38
Pasta, cooked	1 cup	60	57	34	15
White rice, cooked	1 cup	64	53	34	19
Breakfast cereals	2/3 cup	75	44	33	60
Brown rice, cooked	1 cup	55	45	25	13
Whole wheat bread	2 slices	71	26	18	33
White bread	2 slices	73	25	18	37
Rye bread	2 slices	53	31	16	25
Oatmeal porridge	1 cup	58	25	15	6
Oatmeal, dry	½ cup	50	27	14	34
Cornflakes	2/3 cup	81	16	13	70
Rice cakes (brown)	2 cakes	82	15	12	67
Whole-grain bread	2 slices	45	24	11	21
Popcorn	2 cups	72	12	9	56
Crackers, *Ryvita*	2 slices	69	10	7	37
FRUITS					
Raisins	½ cup	64	58	37	51
Banana	1 medium	60	28	17	14
Watermelon	1 wedge	72	21	15	5
Prunes	6 only	39	32	12	25
Pear, fresh	1 medium	38	25	10	6
Apple, raw	1 medium	38	21	8	6
Orange	1 medium	42	16	7	5
Pineapple, fresh	1 slice	59	10	6	7
Peach, fresh	1 medium	42	11	5	5
Blueberries	½ cup	40	10	4	6
Grapes	½ cup	46	8	4	8
Plum, fresh	1 medium	39	9	4	5
Raspberries	½ cup	40	7	3	5
Grapefruit	½ medium	25	10	3	2
Strawberries	½ cup	40	6	2	3
LEGUMES					
Garbanzo beans	½ cup	28	27	8	6
Lima beans, cooked	½ cup	32	20	6	8
Kidney beans, cooked	½ cup	28	20	6	6
Green peas	½ cup	48	11	5	7
Lentils, red, cooked	½ cup	26	20	5	3
Soy beans, cooked	½ cup	18	10	2	2
Green beans, cooked	½ cup	29	5	1	2
Tofu, firm	½ cup	35	4	1	5

FOOD	Serving Size	Glycemic Index	Carbohydrates per serving, g	Glycemic Load /serving	Glycemic Load per 100 g
VEGETABLES					
French fries	20 pieces	75	31	23	23
Potato, baked	1 medium	60	34	20	13
Sweet potato, cooked	1 medium	61	28	17	8
Potato, boiled	1 medium	50	27	14	10
Corn, cooked	1 ear	54	19	10	14
Yam, cooked	½ cup	37	19	7	10
Beets, cooked	2 medium	64	10	6	6
Carrots, cooked	½ cup	60	8	5	6
Onion, raw*	1 medium	50	9	5	5
Squash, cooked*	½ cup	15	11	2	2
Broccoli, cooked*	1 med. stalk	15	9	1	1
Tomatoes, raw*	1 medium	15	7	1	1
Carrot, raw	1 medium	16	6	1	2
Asparagus, cooked*	4 spears	20	3	1	1
Kale, cooked*	½ cup	15	4	1	1
Lettuce, raw*	1 cup	15	1	0	0
NUTS & SEEDS					
Almonds*	½ cup	25	14	4	5
Sesame seeds*	½ cup	20	17	3	5
Peanuts*	½ cup	20	12	2	3
Walnuts*	½ cup	20	8	2	3
Sunflower seeds*	½ cup	20	5	1	1
DAIRY PRODUCTS					
Ice cream	½ cup	50	17	9	12
Yoghurt	½ cup	36	8	3	3
Milk	8 oz glass	27	11	3	1
Cheese	1 oz	25	0.5	0	1
MISCELLANEOUS					
Orange juice	8 oz glass	52	26	14	5
Sugar, refined	1 tablespoon	99	12	12	99
Carrot juice	8 oz glass	43	22	9	4
Honey	1 tablespoon	55	17	9	45
Maple syrup	1 tablespoon	55	13	7	37
Tomato juice	8 oz glass	38	10	4	2
Protein (soy) powder*	2 oz	15	4	1	1
Protein (whey) " *	2 oz	15	2	0	0
Green tea*	1 cup	10	1	0	0
Stevia sweetener*	1 teaspoon	0	-	0	0

The glycemic index is based on glucose=100. Values (except as indicated) are from the International Table of Glycemic Index and Load published in the *American Journal of Clinical Nutrition* (July 2002, pp. 5-56)

* Glycemic index value from *The Food Connection* by Sam Graci (pp. 170-72)

Appendix D

Grading Prostatitis Symptoms

National Institutes of Health Chronic Prostatitis Symptom Index (1)

Pain or Discomfort

1. In the last week, have you experienced any pain or discomfort in the:

		Yes	No
a.	area between rectum and testicles (perineum)?	1	2
b.	testicles?	1	2
c.	tip of the penis (not related to urination)?	1	2
d.	below your waist, in your pubic or bladder area?	1	2

2. In the past week, have you experienced:

		Yes	No
a.	pain or burning during urination?	1	2
b.	pain or discomfort during or after sexual climax (ejaculation)?	1	2

3. How often have you had pain or discomfort in any of these areas over the last week?

> 0 Never
> 1 Rarely
> 2 Sometimes
> 3 Often
> 4 Usually
> 5 Always

4. Which number best describes your **average** pain or discomfort on the days that you experienced it over the last week?

> 0* 1 2 3 4 5 6 7 8 9 10**

> * No pain
> ** Extreme pain

Urination

5. How often have you had a sensation of not emptying your bladder completely after you finished urinating over the last week?

> 0 Not at all
> 1 Less than 1 time in 5
> 2 Less than half the time
> 3 About half the time
> 4 More than half the time
> 5 Almost always

6. How often have you had to urinate again less than 2 hours after you finished urinating over the last week?

        0   Not at all
        1   Less than 1 time in 5
        2   Less than half the time
        3   About half the time
        4   More than half the time
        5   Almost always

Impact of Symptoms

7. How much have your symptoms kept you from doing the kinds of things you would usually do over the last week?

    0 None
    1 Only a little
    2 Some
    3 A lot

8. How much did you think about your symptoms over the last week?

    0 None
    1 Only a little
    2 Some
    3 A lot

Quality of Life

9. If you were to spend the rest of your life with your symptoms just the way they have been during the last week, how would you feel about that?

    0 Delighted
    1 Pleased
    2 Mostly satisfied
    3 Mixed (about equally satisfied and dissatisfied)
    4 Mostly dissatisfied
    5 Unhappy
    6 Terrible

Scoring the NIH-Chronic Prostatitis Symptom Index Domains

Pain – Total of items 1a, 1b, 1c, 1d, 2a, 2b, 3 and 4 = _____

Urinary Symptoms – Total of items 5 and 6 = _____

Quality of Life Impact – Total of items 7, 8 and 9 = _____

(1) Journal of Urology, Vol. 162, 1999, pp. 369-75

Appendix E

Grading BPH Symptoms

American Urological Association (AUA) Symptom Index for BPH (1)

Score

1. Over the past month, how often have you experienced a sensation of not emptying your bladder completely after you finished urinating? _____

2. Over the past month, how often have you had to urinate again less than 2 hours after you finished urinating? _____

3. Over the past month, how often have you stopped and started again several times when you urinated? _____

4. Over the past month, how often have you found it difficult to postpone urination? _____

5. Over the past month, how often have you experienced a weak urinary stream? _____

6. Over the past month, how often have you had to push or strain to begin urination? _____

0 = not at all   3 = about half the time
1 = less than 1 time in 5   4 = more than half the time
2 = less than half the time   5 = almost always

7. Over the past month, how many times did you most typically get up to urinate from the time you went to bed at night until the time you got up in the morning? _____

0 = none   3 = 3 times
1 = 1 time   4 = 4 times
2 = 2 times   5 = 5 or more times

TOTAL SYMPTOM SCORE _____

(1) Journal of Urology, Vol. 170, No. 2, Pt. 1, 2003, pp. 530-47

Appendix F

Bibliography

BOOKS – THE PROSTATE

- Arnot, Robert. *The Prostate Cancer Protection Plan*, Little, Brown and Company, NY, 2000
- Grimm, Peter D, et al. eds. *The Prostate Cancer Treatment Book*, McGraw-Hill, NY, 2004
- Jones, J. Stephen. *The Complete Prostate Book*. Prometheus Book, Amherst, NY, 2005
- Scardino, Peter T. and Kelman, Judith. *Dr. Peter Scardino'a Prostate Book*, Penguin Group, NY, 2005
- Simone, Charles B. *The Truth About Prostate Health* – Prostate Cancer, Princeton Institute, Princeton, NJ, 2005
- Strum, Stephen B. and Pogliano, Donna. *A Primer on Prostate Cancer*. Life Extension Foundation, Hollywood, FL, 2nd edition, 2005
- Walsh, Patrick C. and Worthington, Janet Farrar. *Dr. Patrick Walsh's Guide to Surviving Prostate Cancer*. Warner Book, NY, 2001

BOOKS – CANCER (GENERAL)

- Blaylock, Russell L. *Natural Strategies for Cancer Patients*, Kensington Publishing Corp., NY, 2003
- Beuth, Josef and Moss, Ralph W. *Complementary Oncology*, Thieme, NY, 2006
- Breuss, Rudolf. *The Breuss Cancer Cure*. Alive Books, Vancouver, Canada, 1995
- Cameron, Ewan and Pauling, Linus. *Cancer and Vitamin C*, Camino Books Inc., Philadelphia, PA, 1993
- Diamond, W. John, et al. *An Alternative Medicine Definitive Guide to Cancer*, Future Medicine Publishing, Inc., Tiburon, CA, 1997
- Passwater, Richard A. *Cancer Prevention and Nutritional Therapies*, Keats Publishing, New Canaan, CT, 1993
- Simone, Charles B. *Cancer and Nutrition*, Avery Publishing Group, Garden City Park, NY, 1994
- Walters, Richard. *Options: The Alternative Cancer Therapy Book*, Avery Publishing Group, Garden City Park, NY, 1993

BOOKS – ALTERNATIVE MEDICINE

- Burton Goldberg Group. ***Alternative Medicine: The Definitive Guide***. Future Medicine Publishing, Inc., Puyallup, WA, 1993
- Life Extension Foundation. ***Disease Prevention and Treatment***. LEF, Hollywood, FL, 4th edition, 2003
- Murray, Michael T. ***Encyclopedia of Nutritional Supplements***. Prima Publishing, Rocklin, CA, 1996
- Murray, Michael T. and Pizzorno, Joseph E. ***Encyclopedia of Natural Medicine.*** Prima Publishing, Rocklin, CA, 2nd edition, 1998
- Rona, Zoltan P. editor. ***Encyclopedia of Natural Healing***. Alive Books, Vancouver, Canada, 1997

HELPFUL WEB SITES

- CANHELP, INC. – Personalized information about the latest alternative and conventional cancer treatments is available (for a fee) from this site.
  http://www.canhelp.com/

- *The Moss Reports* – Dr. Ralph Moss' site is an excellent starting point for people looking for advice concerning alternative cancer treatments.
  http://www.cancerdecisions.com/

- American Cancer Society   http://www.cancer.org/

- Canadian Cancer Society   http://www.cancer.ca/

- *International Health News*   www.yourhealthbase.com

- Life Extension Foundation   www.lef.org

- Dr. Julian Whitaker   www.drwhitaker.com

- National Comprehensive Cancer Network (NCCN) – Guidelines for treatment of cancer.
  http://nccn.org/professionals/physician_gls/f_guidelines.asp?button=1

- Memorial Sloan-Kettering Cancer Center. Nomogram webpage and online calculator to predict treatment outcome probabilities based on either clinical or pathological data.
  http://www.mskcc.org/mskcc/html/10088.cfm

- PubMed – National Library of Medicine
  http://www.ncbi.nlm.nih.gov/entrez/query.fcgi?DB=pubmed

- *Johns Hopkins Prostate Bulletin*
  http://www.hopkinsprostate.com

- Partin Tables – Tables and online calculator for the probability of organ-confined disease, extraprostatic extension, seminal vesicle invasion and lymph node involvement, based on the clinical presentation.
  http://urology.jhu.edu/prostate/partintables.php

- *Medical News Today.* The latest prostate news and prostate article, updated daily.
  http://www.medicalnewstoday.com/medicalnews.php?category=92

- National Cancer Institute (U.S. National Institutes of Health) – Prostate cancer website.
  http://www.cancer.gov/cancertopics/types/prostate

- Centers for Disease Control (U.S.) – Prostate cancer control initiatives webpage.
  http://www.cdc.gov/cancer/prostate/index.htm

References

CHAPTER 1 - Prostatitis

1. Campbell's Urology, Saunders, Philadelphia, PA, 8th edition, 2002, pp. 603-30
2. Clemens, JQ, et al. Incidence and clinical characteristics of National Institutes of Health type III prostatitis in the community. Journal of Urology, Vol. 174, December 2005, pp. 2319-22
3. Ku, JH, et al. Epidemiologic risk factors for chronic prostatitis. International Journal of andrology, Vol. 28, 2005, pp. 317-27
4. Habermacher, GM, et al. Prostatitis/chronic pelvic pain syndrome. Annu. Rev. Med, Vol. 57, 2006, pp. 10.1-10.12
5. Sindhwani, P and Wilson, CM. Prostatitis and serum prostate-specific antigen. Current Urology Reports, Vol. 6, 2005, pp. 307-12
6. Smith's General Urology, McGraw-Hill, NY, 15th edition, 2000, pp. 254-59
7. Shoskes, DA. Phytotherapy in chronic prostatitis. Urology, Vol. 60, Suppl 6A, December 2002, pp. 35-37
8. Murray, Michael T. and Pizzorno, Joseph E. Encyclopedia of Natural Medicine, Prima Publishing, Rocklin, CA, revised 2nd edition, 1998, pp. 300-02
9. Scardino, Peter T. and Kelman, Judith. Dr. Peter Scardino's Prostate Book, Penguin Group, NY, 2005, pp. 49-63
10. Jones, J. Stephen. The Complete Prostate Book. Prometheus Books, Amherst, NY, 2005, pp. 87-103
11. Nickel, JC, et al. Repetitive prostatic massage therapy for chronic refractory prostatitis: the Philippine experience. Tech Urol, Vol. 5, No. 3, September 1999, pp. 146-51
12. Cohen, JS. Peripheral neuropathy associated with fluoroquinolones. The Annals of Pharmacotherapy, Vol. 35, December 2001, pp. 1-7
13. Van der Linden, PD, et al. Increased risk of Achilles tendon rupture with quinolone antibacterial use, especially in elderly patients taking oral corticosteroids. Archives of Internal Medicine, Vol. 163, August 11/25, 2003, pp. 1801-07
14. Pontari, MA and Ruggieri, MR. Mechanisms in prostatitis/chronic pelvic pain syndrome. Journal of Urology, Vol. 172, September 2004, pp. 839-45
15. Shoskes, DA, et al. Diagnosis and management of acute and chronic prostatitis. Urologic Nursing, Vol. 21, August 2001, pp. 255-62
16. Yaman, O, et al. Increased prostate-specific antigen in subclinical prostatitis: the role of aggressiveness and extension of inflammation. Urol Int, Vol. 71, No. 2, 2003, pp. 160-64
17. Bozeman, CB, et al. Treatment of chronic prostatitis lowers serum prostate specific antigen. Journal of Urology, Vol. 167, April 2002, pp. 1723-26
18. Neal, DE, et al. Prostate-specific antigen and prostatitis I: effect of prostatitis on serum PSA in the human and nonhuman primate. Prostate, Vol. 20, 1992, pp. 105-11
19. Porter, CR, et al. Absence of lower urinary tract symptoms is an independent predictor for cancer at prostate biopsy, but prostate-specific antigen is not: results from a prospective series of 569 patients. Clin Prostate Cancer, Vol. 4, No. 1, June 2005, pp. 50-54
20. Shoskes, DA and Katz, E. Multimodal therapy for chronic prostatitis/chronic pelvic pain syndrome. Current Urology Reports, Vol. 6, 2005, pp. 296-99
21. Collins, Mary McNaughton, et al. Prevalence and correlates of prostatitis in the Health Professionals Follow-Up Study cohort. Journal of Urology, Vol. 167, March 2002, pp. 1363-66
22. Doggweiler-Wiygul, R. Prostatitis: epidemiology of inflammation. Current Urology Report, Vol. 6, 2005, pp. 282-89
23. Ullrich, PM, et al. Stress is associated with subsequent pain and disability among men with nonbacterial prostatitis/pelvic pain. Annals of Behavioral Medicine. Vol. 30 No. 2, 2005, pp. 112-18
24. Tripp, DA, et al. Predictors of quality of life and pain in chronic prostatitis/chronic pelvic pain syndrome: findings from the National Institutes of Health Chronic Prostatitis Cohort Study. BJU Int, Vol. 94, 2004, pp. 1279-82
25. Berger, RE. Journal of Urology, Vol. 174, November 2005, p. 1843 (editorial comment)

26. Shoskes, DA, et al. Anti-nanobacterial therapy for men with chronic prostatitis/chronic pelvic pain syndrome and prostatic stones: preliminary experience. Journal of Urology, Vol. 173, February 2005, pp. 474-77

27. Bedir, S, et al. Endoscopic treatment of multiple prostatic calculi causing urinary retention. International Journal of Urology, Vol. 12, 2005, pp. 693-95

28. Leibovitch, I and Mor, Y. The vicious cycling: bicycling related urogenital disorders. European Urology, Vol. 47, March 2005, pp. 277-87

29. Edorh, AP, et al. Magnesium content in seminal fluid as an indicator of chronic prostatitis. Cell Mol Biol (Noisy-le-Grand), Vol. 49, 2003, pp. 419-23

30. Alexander, RB, et al. Ciprofloxacin or tamsulosin in men with chronic prostatitis/chronic pelvic pain syndrome. Annals of Internal Medicine, Vol. 141, October 19, 2004, pp. 581-89

31. Kaplan, SA, et al. A prospective, 1-year trial using saw palmetto versus finasteride in the treatment of category III prostatitis/chronic pelvic pain syndrome. Journal of Urology, Vol. 171, January 2004, pp. 284-88

32. Shoskes, DA, et al. Quercetin in men with category III chronic prostatitis: a preliminary prospective, double-blind, placebo-controlled trial. Urology, Vol. 54, No. 6, 1999, pp. 960-63

33. Buck, AC, et al. Treatment of chronic prostatitis and prostatodynia with pollen extract. British Journal of Urology, Vol. 64, No. 5, November 1989, pp. 496-99

34. Buck, AC, et al. Treatment of outflow tract obstruction due to benign prostatic hyperplasia with the pollen extract, cernilton: a double-blind, placebo-controlled study. British Journal of Urology, Vol. 66, No. 4, October 1990, pp. 398-404

35. Rugendorff, EW, et al. Results of treatment with pollen extract (Cernilton N) in chronic prostatitis and prostatodynia. British Journal of Urology, Vol. 71, No. 4, April 1993, pp. 433-38

36. Gordon, AE and Shaughnessy, AF. Saw palmetto for prostate disorders. American Family Physician, Vol. 67, March 15, 2003, pp. 1281-83

37. Yang, J and Te, AE. Saw palmetto and finasteride in the treatment of category-III prostatitis/chronic pelvic pain syndrome. Current Urology Reports, Vol. 6, 2005, pp. 290-95

38. Treben, Maria. Health Through God's Pharmacy. Wilhelm Ennsthaler, Steyr, Austria, 13th edition, 1989, pp. 47-49

39. Steenkamp, V, et al. Studies on antibacterial, anti-inflammatory and antioxidant activity of herbal remedies used in the treatment of benign prostatic hyperplasia and prostatitis. Journal of Ethnopharmacology, Vol. 103, January 3, 2006, pp. 71-75

40. Walling, A. Therapeutic modulation of the psychoneuroimmune system by medical acupuncture creates enhanced feelings of well-being. J Am Acad Nurse Pract, Vol. 18, April 2006, pp. 135-43

41. Huang, ST, et al. Increase in the vagal modulation by acupuncture at Neiguan point in healthy subjects. American Journal of Chinese Medicine, Vol. 33, No. 1, 2005, pp. 157-64

42. Agelink, MW, et al. Does acupuncture influence the cardiac autonomic nervous system in patients with minor depression or anxiety disorders? Fortschr Neurol Psychiatr, Vol. 71, March 2003, pp. 141-49 [article in German] (abstract only)

43. Chen, R and Nickel, JC. Acupuncture ameliorates symptoms in men with chronic prostatitis/chronic pelvic pain syndrome. Urology, Vol. 61, June 2003, pp. 1156-59

44. Honjo, H, et al. Effects of acupuncture for chronic pelvic pain syndrome with intrapelvic venous congestion: preliminary results. International Journal of Urology, Vol. 11, August 2004, pp. 607-12

45. Yu, Y and Kang, J. Clinical studies on treatment of chronic prostatitis with acupuncture and mild moxibustion. Journal of Traditional Chinese Medicine, Vol. 25, No. 3, September 2005, pp. 177-81

46. Ye, ZQ, et al. Biofeedback therapy for chronic pelvic pain syndrome. Asian J Androl, Vol. 5, No. 2, June 2003, pp. 155-58

47. Clemens, JQ, et al. Biofeedback, pelvic floor re-education, and bladder training for male chronic pelvic pain syndrome. Urology, Vol. 56, No. 6, December 20, 2000, pp. 951-55

48. John, H, et al. A new high frequency electrostimulation device to treat chronic prostatitis. Journal of Urology, Vol. 170, October 2003, pp. 1275-77

49. Rowe, E, et al. A prospective, randomized, placebo controlled, double-blind study of pelvic electromagnetic therapy for the treatment of chronic pelvic pain syndrome with 1 year of followup. Journal of Urology, Vol. 173, June 2005, pp. 2044-47

50. Zvara, P, et al. Minimally invasive therapies for prostatitis. Current Urology Reports, Vol. 5, 2004, pp. 320-26

51. Nickel, JC and Sorenson, R. Transurethral microwave thermotherapy of nonbacterial prostatitis and prostatodynia: initial experience. Urology, Vol. 44, No. 3, September 1994, pp. 458-60

52. Nickel, JC and Sorenson, R. Transurethral microwave thermotherapy for nonbacterial prostatitis: a randomized double-blind sham controlled study using new prostatitis specific assessment questionnaires. Journal of Urology, Vol. 155, June 1996, pp. 1950-55

53. Choi, NG, et al. Clinical experience with transurethral microwave thermotherapy for chronic nonbacterial prostatitis and prostatodynia. Journal of Endourology, Vol. 8, No. 1, February 1994, pp. 61-64

54. Chiang, PH and Chiang, CP. Therapeutic effect of transurethral needle ablation in non-bacterial prostatitis: chronic pelvic pain syndrome type IIIa. International Journal of Urology, Vol. 11, February 2004, pp. 97-102

55. Kee, KC, et al. Transurethral needle ablation for chronic nonbacterial prostatitis. BJU International, Vol. 89, No. 3, February 2002, pp. 226-29

56. Leskinen, MJ, et al. Transurethral needle ablation for the treatment of chronic pelvic pain syndrome (category III prostatitis): a randomized, sham-controlled study. Urology, Vol. 60, No. 2, August 2002, pp. 300-4

57. Shoskes, DA, et al. Long-term results of multimodal therapy for chronic prostatitis/chronic pelvic pain syndrome. Journal of Urology, Vol. 169, April 2003, pp. 1406-10

CHAPTER 2 – Benign Prostatic Hyperplasia

1. Scardino PTKJ, Dr. Peter Scardino's Prostate Book. Avery/Penguin Group, New York, 2005.
2. Djavan B et al., 2004. Benign prostatic hyperplasia progression and its impact on treatment. Curr.Opin.Urol. 14(1):45-50.
3. Murphy LJT, The History of Urology. Charles C. Thomas, Springfield, Ill, 1972.
4. Carter HB, Coffey DS, 1990. The prostate: an increasing medical problem. Prostate. 16(1):39-48.
5. Jacobsen SJ, Girman CJ, Lieber MM, 2001. Natural history of benign prostatic hyperplasia. Urology. 58(6 Suppl 1):5-16.
6. Naderi N, Mochtar CA, de la Rosette JJ, 2004. Real life practice in the management of benign prostatic hyperplasia. Curr.Opin.Urol. 14(1):41-44.
7. Bhargava S, Canda AE, Chapple CR, 2004. A rational approach to benign prostatic hyperplasia evaluation: recent advances. Curr.Opin.Urol. 14(1):1-6.
8. Lanes SF et al., 1996. A cost density analysis of benign prostatic hyperplasia. Clin.Ther. 18(5):993-1004.
9. Shibata Y et al., 2000. Changes in the endocrine environment of the human prostate transition zone with aging: simultaneous quantitative analysis of prostatic sex steroids and comparison with human prostatic histological composition. Prostate. 42(1):45-55.
10. Neuhouser ML, Kristal AR, Penson DF, 2004. Steroid hormones and hormone-related genetic and lifestyle characteristics as risk factors for benign prostatic hyperplasia: review of epidemiologic literature. Urology. 64(2):201-211.
11. Walsh PC, Hutchins GM, Ewing LL, 1983. Tissue content of dihydrotestosterone in human prostatic hyperplasis is not supranormal. J Clin.Invest. 72(5):1772-1777.
12. Roberts RO et al., 2004. Serum sex hormones and measures of benign prostatic hyperplasia. Prostate. 61(2):124-131.
13. Sciarra F, Toscano V, 2000. Role of estrogens in human benign prostatic hyperplasia. Arch.Androl. 44(3):213-220.
14. Yun AJ, Doux JD, 2006. Opening the floodgates: Benign prostatic hyperplasia may represent another disease in the compendium of ailments caused by the global sympathetic bias that emerges with aging. Med Hypotheses. January 19, 2006 [Epub ahead of print]

15. Lee PY, Yun AJ, Bazar KA, 2004. Conditions of aging as manifestations of sympathetic bias unmasked by loss of parasympathetic function. Med Hypotheses. 62(6):868-870.
16. Yun AJ, Lee PY, Bazar KA, 2004. Temporal variation of autonomic balance and diseases during circadian, seasonal, reproductive, and lifespan cycles. Med Hypotheses. 63(1):155-162.
17. Lee PY, Yun AJ, Bazar KA, 2004. Acute coronary syndromes and heart failure may reflect maladaptations of trauma physiology that was shaped during pre-modern evolution. Med Hypotheses. 62(6):861-867.
18. Yun AJ, Lee PY, Bazar KA, 2004. Many diseases may reflect dysfunctions of autonomic balance attributable to evolutionary displacement. Med Hypotheses. 62(6):847-851.
19. Yun AJ, Lee PY, Bazar KA, 2005. Can thromboembolism be the result, rather than the inciting cause, of acute vascular events such as stroke, pulmonary embolism, mesenteric ischemia, and venous thrombosis?: a maladaptation of the prehistoric trauma response. Med Hypotheses. 64(4):706-716.
20. McVary KT et al., 2005. Autonomic nervous system overactivity in men with lower urinary tract symptoms secondary to benign prostatic hyperplasia. J Urol. 174(4 Pt 1):1327-1433.
21. Ullrich PM et al., 2005. Stress, hostility, and disease parameters of benign prostatic hyperplasia. Psychosom.Med. 67(3):476-482.
22. Malloy BJ et al., 1998. Alpha1-adrenergic receptor subtypes in human detrusor. J Urol. 160(3 Pt 1):937-943.
23. Schwinn DA, Michelotti GA, 2000. alpha1-adrenergic receptors in the lower urinary tract and vascular bed: potential role for the alpha1d subtype in filling symptoms and effects of ageing on vascular expression. BJU Int. 85 Suppl 2:6-11.
24. Chapple CR et al., 2005. The role of urinary urgency and its measurement in the overactive bladder symptom syndrome: current concepts and future prospects. BJU Int. 95(3):335-340.
25. Takahashi S et al., 2006. Clinical efficacy of an alpha1A/D-adrenoceptor blocker (naftopidil) on overactive bladder symptoms in patients with benign prostatic hyperplasia. Int.J Urol. 13(1):15-20.
26. Nishino Y et al., 2006. Comparison of two alpha1-adrenoceptor antagonists, naftopidil and tamsulosin hydrochloride, in the treatment of lower urinary tract symptoms with benign prostatic hyperplasia: a randomized crossover study. BJU Int. 97(4):747-51, discussion.
27. Kramer G, Marberger M, 2006. Could inflammation be a key component in the progression of benign prostatic hyperplasia? Curr Opin.Urol. 16(1):25-29.
28. Vela NR et al., 2003. BPH and inflammation: pharmacological effects of Permixon on histological and molecular inflammatory markers. Results of a double blind pilot clinical assay. Eur.Urol. 44(5):549-555.
29. Sears B, The Anti-inflammation Zone. Harper Collins--Regan Books, New York, 2005.
30. Berger AP et al., 2005. Vascular damage induced by type 2 diabetes mellitus as a risk factor for benign prostatic hyperplasia. Diabetologia. 48(4):784-789.
31. Kang D et al., 2004. Risk behaviours and benign prostatic hyperplasia. BJU.Int. 93(9):1241-1245.
32. Platz EA et al., 2000. Race, ethnicity and benign prostatic hyperplasia in the health professionals follow-up study. J Urol. 163(2):490-495.
33. Denis L, Morton MS, Griffiths K, 1999. Diet and its preventive role in prostatic disease. Eur.Urol. 35(5-6):377-387.
34. Pearson JD et al., 2003. Familial aggregation of bothersome benign prostatic hyperplasia symptoms. Urology. 61(4):781-785.
35. Negri E et al., 2005. Family history of cancer and the risk of prostate cancer and benign prostatic hyperplasia. Int.J Cancer. 114(4):648-652.
36. Suzuki S et al., 2002. Intakes of energy and macronutrients and the risk of benign prostatic hyperplasia. Am.J Clin.Nutr. 75(4):689-697.
37. Meigs JB et al., 2001. Risk factors for clinical benign prostatic hyperplasia in a community-based population of healthy aging men. J.Clin.Epidemiol. 54(9):935-944.
38. Yang YJ et al., 1999. Comparison of fatty acid profiles in the serum of patients with prostate cancer and benign prostatic hyperplasia. Clin.Biochem. 32(6):405-409.
39. Bravi F et al., 2006. Food groups and risk of benign prostatic hyperplasia. Urology. 67(1):73-79.

40. Lagiou P et al., 1999. Diet and benign prostatic hyperplasia: a study in Greece. Urology. 54(2):284-290.
41. Crispo A et al., 2004. Alcohol and the risk of prostate cancer and benign prostatic hyperplasia. Urology. 64(4):717-722.
42. Gass R, 2002. Benign prostatic hyperplasia: the opposite effects of alcohol and coffee intake. BJU.Int. 90(7):649-654.
43. Vliegenthart R et al., 2004. Alcohol consumption and coronary calcification in a general population. Arch.Intern.Med. 164(21):2355-2360.
44. Platz EA et al., 1999. Alcohol consumption, cigarette smoking, and risk of benign prostatic hyperplasia. Am.J Epidemiol. 149(2):106-115.
45. Rohrmann S et al., 2004. Association between serum concentrations of micronutrients and lower urinary tract symptoms in older men in the Third National Health and Nutrition Examination Survey. Urology. 64(3):504-509.
46. Brossner C et al., 2004. Phytoestrogen tissue levels in benign prostatic hyperplasia and prostate cancer and their association with prostatic diseases. Urology. 64(4):707-711.
47. Morton MS et al., 1999. Can dietary factors influence prostatic disease? BJU.Int. 84(5):549-554.
48. Hathcock JN et al., 2005. Vitamins E and C are safe across a broad range of intakes. Am.J Clin.Nutr. 81(4):736-745.
49. Hammarsten J, Hogstedt B, 1999. Clinical, anthropometric, metabolic and insulin profile of men with fast annual growth rates of benign prostatic hyperplasia. Blood Press. 8(1):29-36.
50. Hammarsten J, Hogstedt B, 2001. Hyperinsulinaemia as a risk factor for developing benign prostatic hyperplasia. Eur.Urol. 39(2):151-158.
51. Michel MC et al., 2000. Effect of diabetes on lower urinary tract symptoms in patients with benign prostatic hyperplasia. J.Urol. 163(6):1725-1729.
52. Sandfeldt L, Hahn RG, 2003. Cardiovascular risk factors correlate with prostate size in men with bladder outlet obstruction. BJU.Int. 92(1):64-68.
53. Weisman KM et al., 2000. Relationship between benign prostatic hyperplasia and history of coronary artery disease in elderly men. Pharmacotherapy. 20(4):383-386.
54. Burke JP et al., 2006. Diabetes and benign prostatic hyperplasia progression in Olmsted County, Minnesota. Urology. 67(1):22-25.
55. Berger AP et al., 2003. Increased growth factor production in a human prostatic stromal cell culture model caused by hypoxia. Prostate. 57(1):57-65.
56. Ghafar MA et al., 2002. Does the prostatic vascular system contribute to the development of benign prostatic hyperplasia? Curr.Urol.Rep. 3(4):292-296.
57. Moyad MA, 2003. Lifestyle changes to prevent BPH: heart healthy = prostate healthy. Urol.Nurs. 23(6):439-441.
58. Dahle SE et al., 2002. Body size and serum levels of insulin and leptin in relation to the risk of benign prostatic hyperplasia. J Urol. 168(2):599-604.
59. Gades NM et al., 2005. Prevalence of conditions potentially associated with lower urinary tract symptoms in men. BJU Int. 95(4):549-553.
60. 2003. AUA guideline on management of benign prostatic hyperplasia (2003). Chapter 1: Diagnosis and treatment recommendations. J.Urol. 170(2 Pt 1):530-547.
61. Madersbacher S et al., 2004. EAU 2004 guidelines on assessment, therapy and follow-up of men with lower urinary tract symptoms suggestive of benign prostatic obstruction (BPH guidelines). Eur.Urol. 46(5):547-554.
62. Denmeade SR, Isaacs JT, 2004. The role of prostate-specific antigen in the clinical evaluation of prostatic disease. BJU.Int. 93 Suppl 1:10-15.
63. Thompson IM et al., 2004. Prevalence of prostate cancer among men with a prostate-specific antigen level < or =4.0 ng per milliliter. N.Engl.J Med. 350(22):2239-2246.
64. Eastham JA et al., 2003. Variation of serum prostate-specific antigen levels: an evaluation of year-to-year fluctuations. JAMA: The Journal of the American Medical Association. 289(20):2695-2700.
65. Walsch P, 2004. Editorial comment on N Eng J Med,2004; 350:2239. J Urol. 172:550.
66. Stamey TA et al., 2004. The prostate specific antigen era in the United States is over for prostate cancer: what happened in the last 20 years? J.Urol. 172(4 Pt 1):1297-1301.

67. Martinez-Pineiro L et al., 2004. Probability of prostate cancer as a function of the percentage of free prostate-specific antigen in patients with a non-suspicious rectal examination and total prostate-specific antigen of 4-10 ng/ml. World J Urol. 22(2):124-131.

68. Roehrborn CG et al., 1997. Correlation between prostate size estimated by digital rectal examination and measured by transrectal ultrasound. Urology. 49(4):548-557.

69. Bartsch G et al., 2004. Consensus statement: the role of prostate-specific antigen in managing the patient with benign prostatic hyperplasia. BJU.Int. 93 Suppl 1:27-29.

70. Nickel JC, 2006. The overlapping lower urinary tract symptoms of benign prostatic hyperplasia and prostatitis. Curr Opin.Urol. 16(1):5-10.

71. Krieger JN, Nyberg L, Jr., Nickel JC, 1999. NIH Consensus Definition and Classification of Prostatitis. JAMA: The Journal of the American Medical Association. 282(3):236-237.

72. Nickel JC, 2004. The three As of chronic prostatitis therapy: antibiotics, alpha-blockers and anti-inflammatories. What is the evidence? BJU Int. 94(9):1230-1233.

73. Shoskes DA et al., 2003. Long-term results of multimodal therapy for chronic prostatitis/chronic pelvic pain syndrome. J Urol. 169(4):1406-1410.

74. Nickel JC et al., 2004. Failure of a monotherapy strategy for difficult chronic prostatitis/chronic pelvic pain syndrome. J Urol. 172(2):551-554.

75. Shoskes DA et al., 1999. Quercetin in men with category III chronic prostatitis: a preliminary prospective, double-blind, placebo-controlled trial. Urology. 54(6):960-963.

76. Desgrandchamps F, Mongiat-Artus P, 2006. Dosage and duration of medication for men with lower urinary tract symptoms: two questions without definitive answers. Curr Opin.Urol. 16(1):37-39.

77. Milani S, Djavan B, 2005. Lower urinary tract symptoms suggestive of benign prostatic hyperplasia: latest update on alpha-adrenoceptor antagonists. BJU.Int. 95 Suppl 4:29-36.

78. Nordling J, 2005. Efficacy and safety of two doses (10 and 15 mg) of alfuzosin or tamsulosin (0.4 mg) once daily for treating symptomatic benign prostatic hyperplasia. BJU Int. 95(7):1006-1012.

79. McVary KT, 2006. Alfuzosin for symptomatic benign prostatic hyperplasia: long-term experience. J Urol. 175(1):35-42.

80. Chang DF, Campbell JR, 2005. Intraoperative floppy iris syndrome associated with tamsulosin. J Cataract Refract.Surg. 31(4):664-673.

81. Lawrentschuk N, Bylsma GW, 2006. Intraoperative 'floppy iris' syndrome and its relationship to tamsulosin: a urologist's guide. BJU Int. 97(1):2-4.

82. Nguyen DQ, Sebastian RT, Philip J, 2006. Intraoperative floppy iris syndrome associated with tamsulosin. BJU Int. 97(1):197.

83. Desgrandchamps F, 2004. Who will benefit from combination therapy? The role of 5 alpha reductase inhibitors and alpha blockade: a reflection from MTOPS. Curr.Opin.Urol. 14(1):17-20.

84. Lepor H et al., 1996. The Efficacy of Terazosin, Finasteride, or Both in Benign Prostatic Hyperplasia. The New England Journal of Medicine. 335(8):533-540.

85. Kirby RS et al., 2003. Efficacy and tolerability of doxazosin and finasteride, alone or in combination, in treatment of symptomatic benign prostatic hyperplasia: the Prospective European Doxazosin and Combination Therapy (PREDICT) trial. Urology. 61(1):119-126.

86. Sandhu JS, Te AE, 2004. The role of 5-alpha-reductase inhibition as monotherapy in view of the MTOPS data. Curr.Urol.Rep. 5(4):274-279.

87. Simone CB, The Truth About Prostate Health, Prostate Cancer. Princeton Institute, Princeton, NJ, 2005.

88. McConnell JD et al., 1998. The effect of finasteride on the risk of acute urinary retention and the need for surgical treatment among men with benign prostatic hyperplasia. Finasteride Long-Term Efficacy and Safety Study Group. N.Engl.J.Med. 338(9):557-563.

89. Roehrborn CG et al., 2004. Sustained decrease in incidence of acute urinary retention and surgery with finasteride for 6 years in men with benign prostatic hyperplasia. J.Urol. 171(3):1194-1198.

90. McConnell JD et al., 2003. The Long-Term Effect of Doxazosin, Finasteride, and Combination Therapy on the Clinical Progression of Benign Prostatic Hyperplasia. The New England Journal of Medicine. 349(25):2387-2398.

91. Souverein PC et al., 2005. Treatment of benign prostatic hyperplasia and occurrence of prostatic surgery and acute urinary retention: a population-based cohort study in the Netherlands. Eur.Urol. 47(4):505-510.

92. Debruyne FM et al., 1998. Sustained-release alfuzosin, finasteride and the combination of both in the treatment of benign prostatic hyperplasia. European ALFIN Study Group. Eur.Urol. 34(3):169-175.

93. Clark RV et al., 2004. Marked suppression of dihydrotestosterone in men with benign prostatic hyperplasia by dutasteride, a dual 5alpha-reductase inhibitor. J Clin.Endocrinol Metab. 89(5):2179-2184.

94. Debruyne F et al., 2004. Efficacy and safety of long-term treatment with the dual 5 alpha-reductase inhibitor dutasteride in men with symptomatic benign prostatic hyperplasia. Eur.Urol. 46(4):488-494.

95. Schulman C et al., 2006. Long-term therapy with the dual 5alpha-reductase inhibitor dutasteride is well tolerated in men with symptomatic benign prostatic hyperplasia. BJU Int. 97(1):73-79.

96. Thompson IM et al., 2003. The influence of finasteride on the development of prostate cancer. N.Engl.J.Med. 349(3):215-224.

97. Andriole G et al., 2005. The effects of 5alpha-reductase inhibitors on the natural history, detection and grading of prostate cancer: current state of knowledge. J Urol. 174(6):2098-2104.

98. Buck AC, 1996. Phytotherapy for the prostate. Br.J Urol. 78(3):325-336.

99. Bales GT et al., 1999. Phytotherapeutic agents in the treatment of lower urinary tract symptoms: a demographic analysis of awareness and use at the University of Chicago. Urology. 54(1):86-89.

100. Boyle P et al., 2004. Updated meta-analysis of clinical trials of Serenoa repens extract in the treatment of symptomatic benign prostatic hyperplasia. BJU.Int. 93(6):751-756.

101. Gerber GS, Fitzpatrick JM, 2004. The role of a lipido-sterolic extract of Serenoa repens in the management of lower urinary tract symptoms associated with benign prostatic hyperplasia. BJU.Int. 94(3):338-344.

102. Wilt T, Ishani A, MacDonald R, 2005. Serenoa repens for benign prostatic hyperplasia. The Cochrane Library.(1).

103. Fong YK, Milani S, Djavan B, 2005. Role of phytotherapy in men with lower urinary tract symptoms. Curr Opin.Urol. 15(1):45-48.

104. Djavan, B, Seitz, C, Dobrovits, M, and et al. Multicenter European prospectdive comparative study of phytotherapy and watchfuyl waiting in men with mild symptoms of bladder outle obstruction. Can progression be delayed or prevented. J Urol 171, 244. 2005.

105. Sokeland J, 2000. Combined sabal and urtica extract compared with finasteride in men with benign prostatic hyperplasia: analysis of prostate volume and therapeutic outcome. BJU.Int. 86(4):439-442.

106. Popa G, Hagele-Kaddour H, Walther C, 2005. [Efficacy of a combined Sabal-urtica preparation in the symptomatic treatment of benign prostatic hyperplasia. Results of a placebo-controlled double-blind study]. MMW.Fortschr.Med. 147 Suppl 3:103-108.

107. Lopatkin N et al., 2005. Long-term efficacy and safety of a combination of sabal and urtica extract for lower urinary tract symptoms--a placebo-controlled, double-blind, multicenter trial. World J Urol. 23(2):139-146.

108. Debruyne F et al., 2002. Comparison of a phytotherapeutic agent (Permixon) with an alpha-blocker (Tamsulosin) in the treatment of benign prostatic hyperplasia: a 1-year randomized international study. Eur.Urol. 41(5):497-506.

109. Bent S et al., 2006. Saw palmetto for benign prostatic hyperplasia. The New England Journal of Medicine. 354(6):557-566.

110. DiPaola RS, Morton RA, 2006. Proven and Unproven Therapy for Benign Prostatic Hyperplasia. The New England Journal of Medicine. 354(6):632-634.

111. Buck AC, 2004. Is there a scientific basis for the therapeutic effects of serenoa repens in benign prostatic hyperplasia? Mechanisms of action. J.Urol. 172(5 Pt 1):1792-1799.

112. Marks LS et al., 2001. Tissue effects of saw palmetto and finasteride: use of biopsy cores for in situ quantification of prostatic androgens. Urology. 57(5):999-1005.

113. Raynaud JP, Cousse H, Martin PM, 2002. Inhibition of type 1 and type 2 5alpha-reductase activity by free fatty acids, active ingredients of Permixon. J.Steroid Biochem.Mol.Biol. 82(2-3):233-239.

114. Di Silverio F et al., 1998. Effects of long-term treatment with Serenoa repens (Permixon) on the concentrations and regional distribution of androgens and epidermal growth factor in benign prostatic hyperplasia. Prostate. 37(2):77-83.

115. Tunuguntla HS, Evans CP, 2002. Minimally invasive therapies for benign prostatic hyperplasia. World J.Urol. 20(4):197-206.

116. Vela NR et al., 2003. BPH and inflammation: pharmacological effects of Permixon on histological and molecular inflammatory markers. Results of a double blind pilot clinical assay. Eur.Urol. 44(5):549-555.

117. Djavan B, 2003. Lower urinary tract symptoms/benign prostatic hyperplasia: fast control of the patient's quality of life. Urology. 62(3 Suppl 1):6-14.

118. Glemain P et al., 2002. [Tamsulosin with or without Serenoa repens in benign prostatic hyperplasia: the OCOS trial]. Prog.Urol. 12(3):395-403.

119. 2002. Pygeum africanum (Prunus africanus) (African plum tree). Monograph. Altern.Med Rev. 7(1):71-74.

120. Ishani A et al., 2000. Pygeum africanum for the treatment of patients with benign prostatic hyperplasia: a systematic review and quantitative meta-analysis. Am.J Med. 109(8):654-664.

121. Wilt.T et al., 2005. Pygeum africanujm for benign prostatic hyperplasia. The Cochrane Library.(1).

122. Levin RM, Das AK, 2000. A scientific basis for the therapeutic effects of Pygeum africanum and Serenoa repens. Urol.Res. 28(3):201-209.

123. Wilt TJ, MacDonald R, Ishani A, 1999. beta-sitosterol for the treatment of benign prostatic hyperplasia: a systematic review. BJU Int. 83(9):976-983.

124. Berges RR et al., 1995. Randomised, placebo-controlled, double-blind clinical trial of beta-sitosterol in patients with benign prostatic hyperplasia. Beta-sitosterol Study Group. Lancet. 345(8964):1529-1532.

125. Iguchi K et al., 2001. Myristoleic acid, a cytotoxic component in the extract from Serenoa repens, induces apoptosis and necrosis in human prostatic LNCaP cells. Prostate. 47(1):59-65.

126. Sokeland J, 2000. Combined sabal and urtica extract compared with finasteride in men with benign prostatic hyperplasia: analysis of prostate volume and therapeutic outcome. BJU International. 86(4):439-442.

127. Koch E, 2001. Extracts from fruits of saw palmetto (Sabal serrulata) and roots of stinging nettle (Urtica dioica): viable alternatives in the medical treatment of benign prostatic hyperplasia and associated lower urinary tracts symptoms. Planta Med. 67(6):489-500.

128. MacDonald R et al., 2000. A systematic review of Cernilton for the treatment of benign prostatic hyperplasia. BJU Int. 85(7):836-841.

129. Wilt TJ et al., 2000. Phytotherapy for benign prostatic hyperplasia. Public Health Nutr. 3(4A):459-472.

130. Comhaire F, Mahmoud A, 2004. Preventing diseases of the prostate in the elderly using hormones and nutriceuticals. Aging Male. 7(2):155-169.

131. Friederich M, Theurer C, Schiebel-Schlosser G, 2000. [Prosta Fink Forte capsules in the treatment of benign prostatic hyperplasia. Multicentric surveillance study in 2245 patients]. Forsch.Komplementarmed.Klass.Naturheilkd. 7(4):200-204.

132. Lynch M, Anson K, 2006. Time to rebrand transurethral resection of the prostate? Curr Opin.Urol. 16(1):20-24.

133. Mayo Clinic On Prostate Health. Mayo Clinic Health Information, Rochester, MN, 2003.

134. Djavan B, 2005. Benign prostatic hyperplasia in the new millennium. Curr Opin.Urol. 15(1):33-34.

135. Hoffman RM et al., 2004. Transurethral microwave thermotherapy vs transurethral resection for treating benign prostatic hyperplasia: a systematic review. BJU Int. 94(7):1031-1036.

136. Wagrell L et al., 2004. Three-year follow-up of feedback microwave thermotherapy versus TURP for clinical BPH: a prospective randomized multicenter study. Urology. 64(4):698-702.

137. Alivizatos G et al., 2005. Feedback microwave thermotherapy with the ProstaLund Compact Device for obstructive benign prostatic hyperplasia: 12-month response rates and complications. J Endourol. 19(1):72-78.

138. David RD et al., 2004. Multicenter initial U.S. experience with CoreTherm-monitored feedback transurethral microwave thermotherapy for individualized treatment of patients with symptomatic benign prostatic hyperplasia. J Endourol. 18(7):682-685.

139. Huidobro C et al., 2004. Evaluation of microwave thermotherapy with histopathology, magnetic resonance imaging and temperature mapping. J Urol. 171(2 Pt 1):672-678.

140. Naspro R et al., 2005. Update of the minimally invasive therapies for benign prostatic hyperplasia. Curr Opin.Urol. 15(1):49-53.

141. Naderi N, Mochtar CA, de la Rosette JJ, 2004. Real life practice in the management of benign prostatic hyperplasia. Curr Opin.Urol. 14(1):41-44.

142. van Melick HH, van Venrooij GE, Boon TA, 2003. Long-term follow-up after transurethral resection of the prostate, contact laser prostatectomy, and electrovaporization. Urology. 62(6):1029-1034.

143. Djavan B, Seitz C, Marberger M, 2003. Heat versus drugs in the treatment of benign prostatic hyperplasia. BJU.Int. 91(2):131-137.

144. Hargreave TB, McNeill AS, 2005. Acute urinary retention in men: the risks and outcomes with medical therapy. Curr Urol Rep. 6(4):263-270.

145. McNeill SA, Hargreave TB, Roehrborn CG, 2005. Alfuzosin 10 mg once daily in the management of acute urinary retention: results of a double-blind placebo-controlled study. Urology. 65(1):83-89.

146. Slawin KM et al., 2006. Development of nomogram to predict acute urinary retention or surgical intervention, with or without dutasteride therapy, in men with benign prostatic hyperplasia. Urology. 67(1):84-88.

147. Fong YK, Milani S, Djavan B, 2005. Natural history and clinical predictors of clinical progression in benign prostatic hyperplasia. Curr.Opin.Urol. 15(1):35-38.

148. Djavan B et al., 2004. Longitudinal study of men with mild symptoms of bladder outlet obstruction treated with watchful waiting for four years. Urology. 64(6):1144-1148.

149. Wasson JH et al., 1995. A comparison of transurethral surgery with watchful waiting for moderate symptoms of benign prostatic hyperplasia. The Veterans Affairs Cooperative Study Group on Transurethral Resection of the Prostate. N.Engl.J.Med. 332(2):75-79.

150. Flanigan RC et al., 1998. 5-year outcome of surgical resection and watchful waiting for men with moderately symptomatic benign prostatic hyperplasia: a Department of Veterans Affairs cooperative study. J.Urol. 160(1):12-16.

151. Brown CT, Emberton M, 2004. Could self-management challenge pharmacotherapy as a long-term treatment for uncomplicated lower urinary tract symptoms? Curr.Opin.Urol. 14(1):7-12.

CHAPTER 3 – Prostate Cancer: Causes and Risk Factors

Causes

1. National Cancer Institute (US), Genetics of Prostate Cancer, July 14, 2005
   www.nci.nih.gov/cancertopics/pdq/genetics/prostate/healthprofessional/allpages

2. Levy, IG, et al. Prostate cancer: 1. The descriptive epidemiology in Canada. Canadian Medical Association Journal, Vol. 159, September 8, 1998, pp. 509-13

3. Stadtman, ER. Protein oxidation and aging. Science, Vol. 257, August 28, 1992, pp. 1220-24

4. Walsh, Patrick C. and Worthington, JF. Dr. Patrick Walsh's Guide to Surviving Prostate Cancer. NY, Time Warner Book Group, 2001, pp. 46-47

5. Franklin, RB, et al. hZIP1 zinc uptake transporter down regulation and zinc depletion in prostate cancer. Molecular Cancer, Vol. 4, 2005 http://www.molecular-cancer.com/content/4/1/32

6. Costello, LC and Franklin, RB. Novel role of zinc in the regulation of prostate citrate metabolism and its implications in prostate cancer. Prostate, Vol. 35, No. 4, June 1, 1998, pp. 285-96

7. Costello, LC, et al. Zinc and prostate cancer: a critical scientific, medical, and public interest issue (USA). Cancer Causes and Control, Vol. 16, 2005, pp. 901-15

8.   Lehrer, S, et al. C-reactive protein is significantly associated with prostate-specific antigen and metastatic disease in prostate cancer. BJU Int., Vol. 95, No. 7, May 2005, pp. 961-62

9.   Wang, W, et al. Cyclooxygenase-2 expression correlates with local chronic inflammation and tumor neovascularization in human prostate cancer. Clin Cancer Res., Vol. 11, No. 9, May 1, 2005, pp. 3250-56

10.   Tkacz, VL, et al. Cyclooxygenase-2 and angiogenesis in prostate cancer. Cancer Biol Ther., Vol. 4, No. 8, August 11, 2005

11.   Pathak, SK, et al. Oxidative stress and cyclooxygenase activity in prostate carcinogenesis: targets for chemopreventive strategies. European Journal of Cancer, Vol. 41, January 2005, pp. 61-70

12.   Basler, JW and Piazza, GA. Nonsteroidal anti-inflammatory drugs and cyclooxygenase-2 selective inhibitors for prostate cancer chemoprevention. Journal of Urology, Vol. 171, February 2004, pp. S59-S63

13.   Cohen, P, et al. Prostate-specific antigen (PSA) in an insulin-like growth factor binding protein-3 protease found in seminal plasma. Journal of Clinical Endocrinology and Metabolism, Vol. 75, No. 4, October 1992, pp. 1046-53

14.   Diamandis, EP. Prostate-specific antigen: a cancer fighter and a valuable messenger? Clinical Chemistry, Vol. 46, No. 7, 2000, pp. 896-900

Age, Nationality, Hereditary Factors

1.   Bostwick, DG, et al. Human prostate cancer risk factors. Cancer, Vol. 101, Suppl. 10, November 15, 2004, pp. 2371-2490

2.   Gronberg, H. Prostate cancer epidemiology. The Lancet, Vol. 361, March 8, 2003, pp. 859-64

3.   Scardino PT, Kelman J, Dr. Peter Scardino's Prostate Book. Avery/Penguin Group, New York, 2005, p. 95

4.   Sonn, Ga, et al. Impact of diet on prostate cancer: a review. Prostate Cancer and Prostatic Diseases, Vol. 8, 2005, pp. 304-10

5.   Cerhan, JR, et al. Family history and prostate cancer risk in a population-based cohort of Iowa men. Cancer Epidemiology, Biomarkers & Prevention, Vol. 8, January 1999, pp. 53-60

6.   Walsh, Patrick C. and Worthington, JF. Dr. Patrick Walsh's Guide to Surviving Prostate Cancer. NY, Time Warner Book Group, 2001, pp. 52-54

7.   Presti, JC. Neoplasms of the prostate gland. In Smith's General Urology, 15th edition, 2000, Lange Medical Books/McGraw-Hill, NY, p. 406

8.   National Cancer Institute (US), Genetics of Prostate Cancer, July 14, 2005 www.nci.nih.gov/cancertopics/pdq/genetics/prostate/healthprofessional/allpages

9.   Zeegers, MPA, et al. Empiric risk of prostate carcinoma for relatives of patients with prostate carcinoma. Cancer, Vol. 97, April 15, 2003, pp. 1894-1903

10.   Carter, BS, et al. Mendelian inheritance of familial prostate cancer. Proceedings of the National Academy of Sciences (USA), Vol. 89, April 1992, pp. 3367-71

11.   Hemminki, K and Czene, K. Attributable risk of familial cancer from the family-cancer database. Cancer Epidemiology, Biomarkers & Prevention, Vol. 11, December 2002, pp. 1638-44

12.   Gronberg, H, et al. Age specific risks of familial prostate carcinoma. Cancer, Vol. 86, August 1, 1999, pp. 477-83

13.   Keetch, DW, et al. Clinical and pathological features of hereditary prostate cancer. Journal of Urology, Vol. 155, June 1996, pp. 1841-42

14.   Bratt, O. Hereditary prostate cancer: clinical aspects. Journal of Urology, Vol. 168, September 2002, pp. 906-13

15.   Gronberg, H, et al. Cancer risk in families with hereditary prostate carcinoma. Cancer, Vol. 89, September 15, 2000, pp. 1315-21

16.   Valeri, A. Genetic, epidemiologic and clinical study of familial prostate cancer. Bull Acad Natl Med, Vol. 186, No. 4, 2002, pp. 779-88 [article in French]

Diet

1.   Hebert, James R., et al. Nutritional and socioeconomic factors in relation to prostate cancer mortality: a cross-national study. Journal of the National Cancer Institute, Vol. 90, November 4, 1998, pp. 1637-47

2.   Deneo-Pellegrini, H., et al. Foods, nutrients and prostate cancer: a case- control study in Uruguay. British Journal of Cancer, Vol. 80, No. 3/4, May 1999, pp. 591-97

3.   Whittemore, Alice S., et al. Prostate cancer in relation to diet, physical activity, and body size in blacks, whites, and Asians in the United States and Canada. Journal of the National Cancer Institute, Vol. 87, No. 9, May 3, 1995, pp. 652-61

4.   Gann, Peter H., et al. Prospective study of plasma fatty acids and risk of prostate cancer. Journal of the National Cancer Institute, Vol. 86, No. 4, February 16, 1994, pp. 281-86

5.   Gronberg, H. Prostate cancer epidemiology. The Lancet, Vol. 361, March 8, 2003, pp. 859-64

6.   Ghosh, Jagadananda and Myers, Charles E. Inhibition of arachidonate 5- lipoxygenase triggers massive apoptosis in human prostate cancer cells. Proceedings of the National Academy of Sciences USA, Vol. 95, No. 22, October 27, 1998, pp. 13182-87

7.   Xu, J., et al. Serum levels of phytanic acid are associated with prostate cancer risk. Journal of Urology, Vol. 174, November 2005, p. 1824

8.   Chan, JM, et al. Role of diet in prostate cancer development and progression. Journal of Clinical Oncology, Vol. 23, No. 32, November 10, 2005, pp. 8152-60

9.   Jian, L, et al. Do preserved foods increase prostate cancer risk? British Journal of Cancer, Vol. 90, No. 9, May 4, 2004, pp. 1792-95

10.   Giovannucci, Edward, et al. Calcium and fructose intake in relation to risk of prostate cancer. Cancer Research, Vol. 58, February 1, 1998, pp. 442- 47

11.   Chan, June M., et al. Dairy products, calcium, and prostate cancer risk in the Physicians' Health Study. American Journal of Clinical Nutrition, Vol. 74, October 2001, pp. 549-54

12.   Tseng, M. et al. Dairy, calcium, and vitamin D intakes and prostate cancer risk in the National Health and Nutrition Examination Epidemiologic Follow-up Study cohort. American Journal of Clinical Nutrition, Vol. 81, May 2005, pp. 1147-54

13.   Qin, LQ, et al. Milk consumption is a risk factor for prostate cancer: meta-analysis of case-control studies. Nutr Cancer, Vol. 48, No. 1, 2004, pp. 22-27

14.   Qin, LQ, et al. Estrogen: one of the risk factors in milk for prostate cancer. Medical Hypotheses, Vol. 62, No. 1, 2004, pp. 133-42

15.   Baron, JA, et al. Risk of prostate cancer in a randomized clinical trial of calcium supplementation. Cancer Epidemiol Biomarkers Prev, Vol. 14, March 2005, pp. 586-89

16.   Schuurman, AG, et al. Animal products, calcium and protein and prostate cancer risk in the Netherlands Cohort Study. British Journal of Cancer, Vol. 80, No. 7, June 1999, pp. 1107-13

17.   Rodriguez, C, et al. Calcium, dairy products, and risk of prostate cancer in a prospective cohort of United States men. Cancer Epidemiol Biomarkers Prev, Vol. 12, July 2003, pp. 597-603

18.   Giovannucci, E, et al. A prospective study of calcium intake and incident and fatal prostate cancer. Cancer Epidemiol Biomarkers Prev, Vol. 15, February 2006, pp. 203-10

19.   Fleshner, N, et al. Dietary fat and prostate cancer. Journal of Urology, Vol. 171, February 2004, pp. S19-24

20.   Attar-Bashi, NM, et al. Alpha-linolenic acid and the risk of prostate cancer. What is the evidence? Journal of Urology, Vol. 171, April 2004, pp. 1402-07

21.   Astorg, P. Dietary N-6 and N-3 polyunsaturated fatty acids and prostate cancer risk: a review of epidemiological and experimental evidence. Cancer Causes and Control, Vol. 15, May 2004, pp. 367-86

22.   Leitzmann, MF, et al. Dietary intake of n-3 and n-6 fatty acids and the risk of prostate cancer. American Journal of Clinical Nutrition, Vol. 80, July 2004, pp. 204-16

23.   Astorg, P. Dietary fatty acids and colorectal and prostate cancers: epidemiological studies. Bull Cancer, Vol. 92, July 2005, pp. 670-84

24.   Demark-Wahnefried, W, et al. Pilot study to explore effects of low-fat, flaxseed-supplemented diet on proliferation of benign prostatic epithelium and prostate-specific antigen. Urology, Vol. 63, May 2004, pp. 900-04

Occupation and Lifestyle

1.	Bostwick, DG, et al. Human prostate cancer risk factors. Cancer, Vol. 101, Suppl. 10, November 15, 2004, pp. 2371-2490
2.	Agalliu, I, et al. Prostate cancer incidence in relation to time windows of exposure to metalworking fluids in the auto industry. Epidemiology, Vol. 16, No. 5, September 2005, pp. 664-71
3.	Seidler, A, et al. Association between diesel exposure at work and prostate cancer. Scand J Work Environ Health, Vol. 24, No. 6, December 1998, pp. 486-94
4.	Ritchie, JM, et al. Organochlorines and risk of prostate cancer. J Occup Environ Med., Vol. 45, July 2003, pp. 692-702
5.	Plaskon, LA, et al. Cigarette smoking and risk of prostate cancer in middle-aged men. Cancer Epidemiology, Biomarkers & Prevention, Vol. 12, July 2003, pp. 604-09
6.	Lotufo, PA, et al. Cigarette smoking and risk of prostate cancer in the physicians' health study (US). International Journal of Cancer, Vol. 87, No. 1, July 1, 2000, pp. 141-44
7.	Giovannucci, E, et al. Smoking and risk of total and fatal prostate cancer in the United States health professionals. Cancer Epidemiology, Biomarkers & Prevention, Vol. 8, Pt. 1, April 1999, pp. 277-82
8.	Rodriguez, C, et al. Smoking and fatal prostate cancer in a large cohort of adult men. American Journal of Epidemiology, Vol. 145, No. 5, March 1, 1997, pp. 466-75
9.	Yu, GP, et al. Smoking history and cancer patient survival: a hospital cancer registry study. Cancer Detection and Prevention, Vol. 21, No. 6, 1997, pp. 497-509
10.	Schoonen, WM, et al. Alcohol consumption and risk of prostate cancer in middle-aged men. International Journal of Cancer, Vol. 113, 2005, pp. 133-140

Nutritional Deficiencies

1.	van der Wielen, Reggy P.J., et al. Serum vitamin D concentrations among elderly people in Europe. The Lancet, Vol. 346, July 22, 1995, pp. 207-10
2.	Gloth, F. Michael and Tobin, Jordan D. Vitamin D deficiency in older people. Journal of the American Geriatrics Society, Vol. 43, No. 7, July 1995, pp. 822-28
3.	Tangpricha, V, et al. Vitamin D insufficiency among free-living healthy young adults. American Journal of Medicine, Vol. 112, June 1, 2002, pp. 659-62
4.	Rucker, D, et al. Vitamin D insufficiency in a population of healthy western Canadians. Canadian Medical Association Journal, Vol. 166, June 11, 2002, pp. 1517-24
5.	Vieth, R and Fraser, D. Vitamin D insufficiency: no recommended dietary allowance exists for this nutrient. Canadian Medical Association Journal, Vol. 166, June 11, 2002, pp. 1541-42
6.	Garland, Frank C., et al. Geographic variation in breast cancer mortality in the United States: A hypothesis involving exposure to solar radiation. Preventive Medicine, Vol. 19, 1990, pp. 614-22
7.	Fraser, D.R. Vitamin D. The Lancet, Vol. 345, January 14, 1995, pp. 104-07
8.	Webb, Ann R., et al. An evaluation of the relative contributions of exposure to sunlight and of diet to the circulating concentrations of 25-hydroxyvitamin D in an elderly nursing home population in Boston. American Journal of Clinical Nutrition, Vol. 51, 1990, pp. 1075-81
9.	Larsen, Hans R. Sunscreens: Do they cause skin cancer? International Journal of Alternative and Complementary Medicine, Vol. 12, No. 12, December 1994, pp. 17-19
10.	Matsuoka, Lois Y., et al. Sunscreens suppress cutaneous vitamin D-3 synthesis. Journal of Clinical Endocrinology and Metabolism, Vol. 64, No. 6, 1987, pp. 1165-68
11.	Matsuoka, Lois Y., et al. Chronic sunscreen use decreases circulating concentrations of 25-hydroxyvitamin D. Archives of Dermatology, Vol. 124, December 1988, pp. 1802-04
12.	Holick, Michael F. Environmental factors that influence the cutaneous production of vitamin D. American Journal of Clinical Nutrition, Vol. 61, No. 3, March 1995, pp. 638S-45S
13.	Matsuoka, Lois Y., et al. Clothing prevents ultraviolet-B radiation-dependent photosynthesis of vitamin D-3. Journal of Clinical Endocrinology and Metabolism, Vol. 75, No. 4, 1992, pp. 1099-1103

14. Lamberg-Allardt, Christel, et al. Low serum 25-hydroxyvitamin D concentrations and secondary hyperparathyroidism in middle-aged white strict vegetarians. American Journal of Clinical Nutrition, Vol. 58, No. 5, November 1993, pp. 684-89

15. Holick, Michael F., et al. The vitamin D content of fortified milk and infant formula. The New England Journal of Medicine, Vol. 326, April 30, 1992, pp. 1178-81

16. Chen, Tai C., et al. An update on the vitamin D content of fortified milk from the United States and Canada. The New England Journal of Medicine, Vol. 329, No. 20, November 11, 1993, p. 1507

17. Garland, Cedric F. and Garland, Frank C. Do sunlight and vitamin D reduce the likelihood of colon cancer? International Journal of Epidemiology, Vol. 9, No. 3, September 1980, pp. 227-31

18. Gorham, Edward D., et al. Acid haze air pollution and breast and colon cancer mortality in 20 Canadian cities. Canadian Journal of Public Health, Vol. 80, March/April 1989, pp. 96-100

19. Ainsleigh, H. Gordon. Beneficial effects of sun exposure on cancer mortality. Preventive Medicine, Vol. 22, 1993, pp. 132-40

20. Schneider Lefkowitz, Ellen and Garland, Cedric F. Sunlight, vitamin D, and ovarian cancer mortality rates in US women. International Journal of Epidemiology, Vol. 23, No. 6, December 1994, pp. 1133-36

21. Tolstoi, Linda G. and Levin, Robert M. Osteoporosis - The treatment controversy. Nutrition Today, July/August 1992, pp. 6-12

22. Tilyard, Murray W., et al. Treatment of postmenopausal osteoporosis with calcitriol or calcium. The New England Journal of Medicine, Vol. 326, February 6, 1992, pp. 357-62 and 406-07 (editorial)

23. Guillemant, Josette, et al. Age-related effect of a single oral dose of calcium on parathyroid function: Relationship with vitamin D status. American Journal of Clinical Nutrition, Vol. 60, No. 3, September 1994, pp. 403-07

24. Dawson-Hughes, Bess, et al. Rates of bone loss in postmenopausal women randomly assigned to one of two dosages of vitamin D. American Journal of Clinical Nutrition, Vol. 61, May 1995, pp. 1140-45

25. Jacobsen, Steven J., et al. Seasonal variation in the incidence of hip fracture among white persons aged 65 years and older in the United States, 1984-1987. American Journal of Epidemiology, Vol. 133, No. 10, 1991, pp. 996-1004

26. Chapuy, Marie C., et al. Vitamin D-3 and calcium to prevent hip fractures in elderly women. The New England Journal of Medicine, Vol. 327, No. 23, December 3, 1992, pp. 1637-42

27. Chapuy, Marie C., et al. Effect of calcium and cholecalciferol treatment for three years on hip fractures in elderly women. British Medical Journal, Vol. 308, April 23, 1994, pp. 1081-82

28. Skowronski, R.J., et al. Actions of vitamin D-3, analogs on human prostate cancer cell lines: Comparison with 1,25-dihydroxyvitamin D-3. Endocrinology, Vol. 136, No. 1, January 1995, pp. 20-26

29. Ahonen, MH, et al. Prostate cancer risk and prediagnostic serum 25-hydroxyvitamin D levels (Finland). Cancer Causes Control, Vol. 11, No. 9, October 2000, pp. 847-52

30. Chen, TC and Holick, MF. Vitamin D and prostate cancer prevention and treatment. Trends Endocrinol Metab, Vol. 14, No. 9, November 2003, pp. 423-30

31. Willett, WC, et al. Prediagnostic serum selenium and risk of cancer. Lancet, July 16, 1983, pp. 130-34

32. Yoshizawa, K, et al. Study of prediagnostic selenium level in toenails and the risk of advanced prostate cancer. Journal of the National Cancer Institute, Vol. 90, No. 16, August 19, 1998, pp. 1219-24

33. Giovannucci, Edward. Selenium and risk of prostate cancer. The Lancet, Vol. 352, September 5, 1998, pp. 755-56

34. Brooks, James D., et al. Plasma selenium level before diagnosis and the risk of prostate cancer development. Journal of Urology, Vol. 166, December 2001, pp. 2034-38

35. Vogt, TM, et al. Serum selenium and risk of prostate cancer in US blacks and whites. International Journal of Cancer, Vol. 103, No. 5, February 20, 2003, pp. 664-70

36. Li, H, et al. A prospective study of plasma selenium levels and prostate cancer risk. Journal of the National Cancer Institute, Vol. 96, May 5, 2004, pp. 696-703

37. Taylor, PR, et al. Science peels the onion of selenium effects on prostate carcinogenesis. Journal of the National Cancer Institute, Vol. 96, May 5, 2004, pp. 645-47

38. van den Brandt, PA, et al. Toenail selenium levels and the subsequent risk of prostate cancer. Cancer Epidemiology, Biomarkers & Prevention, Vol. 12, September 2003, pp. 866-71

39. Ghadirian, P, A case-control study of toenail selenium and cancer of the breast, colon, and prostate. Cancer Detection and Prevention, Vol. 24, No. 4, 2000, pp. 305-13

40. Allen, NE, et al. A case-control study of selenium in nails and prostate cancer risk in British men. British Journal of Cancer, Vol. 90, No. 7, April 5, 2004, pp. 1392-96

41. Lipsky, K, et al. Selenium levels of patients with newly diagnosed prostate cancer compared with control group. Urology, Vol. 63, May 2004, pp. 912-16

42. Longtin, Robert. Selenium for prevention: Eating your way to better DNA repair? Journal of the National Cancer Institute, Vol. 95, January 15, 2003, pp. 98-100

Hormones

1. Wilson, Jean D. and Foster, Daniel W., eds. Williams Textbook of Endocrinology, 8th edition, London, W.B. Saunders Company, 1992, pp. 1096-1106

2. Cohen, Pinchas, et al. Insulin-like growth factors (IGFs), IGF receptors, and IGF-binding proteins in primary cultures of prostate epithelial cells. Journal of Clinical Endocrinology and Metabolism, Vol. 73, No. 2, 1991, pp. 401-07

3. Rudman, Daniel, et al. Effects of human growth hormone in men over 60 years old. New England Journal of Medicine, Vol. 323, July 5, 1990, pp. 1-6

4. LeRoith, Derek, moderator. Insulin-like growth factors in health and disease. Annals of Internal Medicine, Vol. 116, May 15, 1992, pp. 854-62

5. Rosenfeld, R.G., et al. Insulin-like growth factor binding proteins in neoplasia (meeting abstract). Hormones and Growth Factors in Development and Neoplasia, Fogarty International Conference, June 26-28, 1995, Bethesda, MD, 1995, p. 24

6. Lippman, Marc E. The development of biological therapies for breast cancer. Science, Vol. 259, January 29, 1993, pp. 631-32

7. Papa, Vincenzo, et al. Insulin-like growth factor-I receptors are overexpressed and predict a low risk in human breast cancer. Cancer Research, Vol. 53, 1993, pp. 3736-40

8. Stoll, B.A. Breast cancer: further metabolic-endocrine risk markers? British Journal of Cancer, Vol. 76, No. 12, 1997, pp. 1652-54

9. LeRoith, Derek, et al. The role of the insulin-like growth factor-I receptor in cancer. Annals New York Academy of Sciences, Vol. 766, September 7, 1995, pp. 402-08

10. Mantzoros, C.S., et al. Insulin-like growth factor 1 in relation to prostate cancer and benign prostatic hyperplasia. British Journal of Cancer, Vol. 76, No. 9, 1997, pp. 1115-18

11. Cascinu, S., et al. Inhibition of tumor cell kinetics and serum insulin growth factor I levels by octreotide in colorectal cancer patients. Gastroenterology, Vol. 113, September 1997, pp. 767-72

12. Chan, June M., et al. Plasma insulin-like growth factor I and prostate cancer risk: a prospective study. Science, Vol. 279, January 23, 1998, pp. 563-66

13. Kaaks, R. and Lukanova, A. Energy balance and cancer: the role of insulin and insulin-like growth factor-1. Proc Nutr Society, Vol. 60, No. 1, February 2001, pp. 91-106

14. Epstein, Samuel S. Unlabeled milk from cows treated with biosynthetic growth hormones: a case of regulatory abdication. International Journal of Health Services, Vol. 26, No. 1, 1996, pp. 173-85

15. Chan, June M., et al. Insulin-like growth factor-1 (IGF-1) and IGF binding protein-3 as predictors of advanced-stage prostate cancer. Journal of the National Cancer Institute, Vol. 94, July 17, 2002, pp. 1099-1106

16. Chan, June M. Insulin-like growth factor-1 (IGF-1) and IGF binding protein-3 as predictors of advanced- stage prostate cancer. Journal of the National Cancer Institute, Vol. 94, December 18, 2002, pp. 1893- 94

17. Ironman, November 1998, pp. 54-6, 192

18. Rudman, Daniel, et al. Effects of human growth hormone in men over 60 years old. New England Journal of Medicine, Vol. 323, July 5, 1990, pp. 1-6

19. Harrison's Principles of Internal Medicine, 12th edition, McGraw-Hill, NY, 1991, pp. 1660-82

20. Williams Textbook of Endocrinology, 8th edition, W.B. Saunders Company, 1992, pp. 175-77 and 1096-1106

21. Larsen, Hans. Conversation with Dr. Samuel Epstein on September 28, 1998

22. Gould, DC and Kirby, RS. Testosterone replacement therapy for late onset hypogonadism: what is the risk of inducing prostate cancer? Prostate Cancer and Prostatic Diseases, November 1, 2005 (advance online publication)

23. Heikkila, R, et al. Serum testosterone and sex hormone-binding globulin concentrations and the risk of prostate carcinoma. Cancer, Vol. 86, July 15, 1999, pp. 312-15

24. Prehn, Richmond T. On the prevention and therapy of prostate cancer by androgen administration. Cancer Research, Vol. 59, September 1, 1999, pp. 4161-64

25. Parsons, JK, et al. Serum testosterone and the risk of prostate cancer: potential implications for testosterone therapy. Cancer Epidemiol Biomarkers Prev, Vol. 14, September 2005, pp. 2257-60

26. Barqawi, A and Crawford, ED. Testosterone replacement therapy and the risk of prostate cancer: Is there a link? International Journal of Impotence Research, November 10, 2005 (advance online publication)

27. National Institute on Drug Abuse. Steroids (Anabolic-Androgenic), March 2005 http://www.nida.nih.gov/Infofacts/Steroids.html

28. Hickson, RC, et al. Adverse effects of anabolic steroids. Med Toxicol Adverse Drug Exp, Vol. 4, No. 4, July-August 1989, pp. 254-71

29. Hartgens, F and Kuipers, H. Effects of androgenic-anabolic steroids in athletes. Sports Medicine, Vol. 34, No. 8, 2004, pp. 513-54

30. Pepping, Joseph. DHEA: dehydroepiandrosterone. American Journal of Health-Systems Pharmacy, Vol. 57, November 15, 2000, pp. 2048-56

31. Rao, KVN, et al. Chemoprevention of rat prostate carcinogenesis by early and delayed administration of dehydroepiandrosterone. Cancer Research, Vol. 59, No. 13, July 1, 1999, pp. 3084-89

32. Morales, AJ, et al. Effects of replacement dose of dehydroepiandrosterone in men and women of advancing age. Journal of Clinical Endocrinology and Metabolism, Vol. 78, June 1994, pp. 1360-67

33. Chen, F, et al. Direct agonist/antagonist functions of dehydroepiandrosterone. Endocrinology, Vol. 146, November 2005, pp. 4568-76

34. Arnold, JT and Blackman, MR. Does DHEA exert direct effects on androgen and estrogen receptors, and does it promote or prevent prostate cancer? Endocrinology, Vol. 146, December 2005, pp. 4565-67

35. Bartsch, C, et al. Evidence for modulation of melatonin secretion in men with benign and malignant tumors of the prostate: relationship with the pituitary hormones. J Pineal Res, Vol. 2, No. 2, 1985, pp. 121-32

36. Bartsch, C, et al. Melatonin and 6-sulfatoxymelatonin circadian rhythms in serum and urine of primary prostate cancer patients: evidence for reduced pineal activity and relevance of urinary determinations. Clin Chim Acta, Vol. 209, August 31, 1992, pp. 153-67

37. Erren, TC and Piekarski, C. Does winter darkness in the Arctic protect against cancer? The melatonin hypothesis revisited. Med Hypotheses, Vol. 53, July 1999, pp. 1-5

38. Moretti, RM, et al. Antiproliferative action of melatonin on human prostate cancer LNCaP cells. Oncol Rep, Vol. 7, March-April 2000, pp. 347-51

39. Marelli, MM, et al. Growth-inhibitory activity of melatonin on human androgen-independent DU 145 prostate cancer cells. Prostate, Vol. 45, No. 3, November 1, 2000, pp. 238-44

40. Shiu, SY, et al. Melatonin slowed the early biochemical progression of hormone-refractory prostate cancer in a patient whose prostate tumor tissue expressed MT1 receptor subtype. J Pineal Res, Vol. 35, October 2003, pp. 177-82

41. Sainz, RM, et al. Melatonin reduces prostate cancer cell growth leading to neuroendocrine differentiation via a receptor and PKA independent mechanism. Prostate, Vol. 63, No. 1 April 1, 2005, pp. 29-43

42. Molis, TM, et al. Melatonin modulation of estrogen-regulated proteins, growth factors, and proto-oncogenes in human breast cancer. J Pineal Res, Vol.18, March 1995, pp. 93-103

43. Davis, S, et al. Residential magnetic fields, light-at-night, and nocturnal urinary 6-sulfatoxymelatonin concentration in women. American Journal of Epidemiology, Vol. 154, October 1, 2001, pp. 591-600

44. Kliukiene, J, et al. Residential and occupational exposures to 50-Hz magnetic fields and breast cancer in women: a population-based study. American Journal of Epidemiology, Vol. 159, May 1, 2004, pp. 852-61

45. Davis, S, et al. Effects of 60-Hz magnetic field exposure on nocturnal 6-sulfatoxymelatonin, estrogens, luteinizing hormone, and follicle-stimulating hormone in healthy reproductive-age women: results of a crossover trial. Ann Epidemiol, January 31, 2006

46. Feychting, M and Forssen, U. Electromagnetic fields and female breast cancer. Cancer Causes Control, Vol. 17, No. 4, May 2006, pp. 553-8

47. Hansen, J. Increased breast cancer risk among women who work predominantly at night. Epidemiology, Vol. 12, January 2001, pp. 74-77

48. Jasser, SA, et al. Light during darkness and cancer: relationships in circadian photoreception and tumor biology. Cancer Causes Control, Vol. 17, No. 4, May 2006, pp. 515-23

49. Stevens, RG. Artificial lighting in the industrialized world: circadian disruption and breast cancer. Cancer Causes Control, Vol. 17, No. 4, May 2006, pp. 501-07

50. Bartsch, C and Bartsch, H. The anti-tumor activity of pineal melatonin and cancer enhancing life styles in industrialized societies. Cancer Causes Control, Vol. 17, No. 4, May 2006, pp. 559-71

51. U.S. Department of Energy. Environment, Safety, and Health Manual. Document 20.7 – Nonionizing Radiation and Fields (Electromagnetic Fields and Radiation with Frequencies Below 300 GHz), April 5, 2005, Appendix A
http://www.llnl.gov/es_and_h/hsm/doc_20.07/doc20-07.pdf

Medical History

1. Whitaker, Julian. Reversing Diabetes. Warner Books, NY, 2001, pp. 19-27

2. Polonsky, KS. Evolution of beta-cell dysfunction in impaired glucose tolerance and diabetes. Exp Clin Endocrinol Diabetes, Vol. 107, Suppl. 4, 1999, pp. S124-S127

3. Giovannucci, E, et al. Diabetes mellitus and risk of prostate cancer (United States). Cancer Causes Control, Vol. 9, January 1998, pp. 3-9

4. Zhu, K, et al. History of diabetes mellitus and risk of prostate cancer in physicians. American Journal of Epidemiology, Vol. 159, No. 10, May 15, 2004, pp. 978-82

5. Rodriguez, C, et al. Diabetes and risk of prostate cancer in a prospective cohort of US men. American Journal of Epidemiology, Vol. 161, No. 2, January 15, 2005, pp. 147-52

6. Gonzalez-Perez, A and Garcia Rodriguez, LA. Prostate cancer risk among men with diabetes mellitus (Spain). Cancer Causes and Control, Vol. 16, 2005, pp. 1055-58

7. Will, JC, et al. Is diabetes mellitus associated with prostate cancer incidence and survival? Epidemiology, Vol. 10, No. 3, May 1999, pp. 313-18

8. Tavani, A, et al. Diabetes mellitus and the risk of prostate cancer in Italy. European Urology, Vol. 47, March 2005, pp. 313-37

9. Chan, JM, et al. History of diabetes, clinical features of prostate cancer, and prostate cancer recurrence-data from CaPSURE (United States). Cancer Causes Control, Vol. 16, No. 7, September 2005, pp. 789-97

10. Laukkanen, JA, et al. Metabolic syndrome and the risk of prostate cancer in Finnish men: a population-based study. Cancer Epidemiology, Biomarkers & Prevention, Vol. 13, October 2004, pp. 1646-50

11. Wuermli, L, et al. Hypertriglyceridemia as a possible risk factor for prostate cancer. Prostate Cancer and Prostatic Diseases, September 13, 2005 (advance online publication)

12. Bravi, F, et al. Self-reported history of hypercholesterolemia and gallstones and the risk of prostate cancer. Annals of Oncology, April 12, 2006 (published online)

13. Kris-Etherton, PM, et al. Fish consumption, fish oil, onega-3 fatty acids, and cardiovascular disease. Circulation, Vol. 106, November 19, 2002, pp. 2747-57

14. Walsh, Patrick C. and Worthington, JF. Dr. Patrick Walsh's Guide to Surviving Prostate Cancer. NY, Time Warner Book Group, 2001, p. 76
15. Bostwick, DG, et al. Human prostate cancer risk factors. Cancer, Vol. 101, Suppl. 10, November 15, 2004, pp. 2371-2490
16. Chokkalingam, AP, et al. Prostate carcinoma risk subsequent to diagnosis of benign prostatic hyperplasia. Cancer, Vol. 98, No. 8, October 15, 2003, pp. 1727-34
17. Hammarsten, J and Hogstedt, B. Calculated fast-growing benign prostatic hyperplasia. Scand J Urol Nephrol, Vol. 36, 2002, pp. 330-38
18. Dennis, LK, et al. Epidemiologic association between prostatitis and prostate cancer. Urology, Vol. 60, No. 1, July 2002, pp. 78-83
19. Roberts, RO, et al. Prostatitis as a risk factor for prostate cancer. Epidemiology, Vol. 15, January 2004, pp. 93-99
20. Platz, EA and De Marzo, AM. Epidemiology of inflammation and prostate cancer. Journal of Urology, Vol. 171, No. 2, Pt. 2, February 2004, pp. S36-S40
21. Nelson, WG, et al. The role of inflammation in the pathogenesis of prostate cancer. Journal of Urology, Vol. 172, No. 5, Pt. 2, November 2004, pp. S6-S12
22. Hammarsten, J, et al. Does transurethral resection of a clinically benign prostate gland increase the risk of developing clinical prostate cancer? A 10-year follow-up study. Cancer, Vol. 74, No. 8, October 15, 1994, pp. 2347-51
23. Holman, CD, et al. Mortality and prostate cancer risk in 19,598 men after surgery for benign prostatic hyperplasia. BJU Int., Vol. 84, No. 1, July 1999, pp. 37-42
24. Rohrmann, S, et al. Association of vasectomy and prostate cancer among men in a Maryland cohort. Cancer Causes and Control, Vol. 16, 2005, pp. 1189-94
25. Dennis, LK, et al. Vasectomy and the risk of prostate cancer: a meta-analysis examining vasectomy status, age at vasectomy, and time since vasectomy. Prostate Cancer and Prostatic Diseases, Vol. 5, No. 3, 2002, pp. 193-203
26. Sunny, L. Is it reporting bias doubled the risk of prostate cancer in vasectomised men in Mumbai, India? Asian Pacific Journal of Cancer Prevention, Vol. 6, No. 3, July-September 2005, pp. 320-25
27. Lynge, E. Prostate cancer is not increased in men with vasectomy in Denmark. Journal of Urology, Vol. 168, No. 2, August 2002, pp. 488-90
28. Stanford, JL, et al. Vasectomy and risk of prostate cancer. Cancer Epidemiology, Biomarkers & Prevention, Vol. 8, October 1999, pp. 881-86
29. Cox, B, et al. Vasectomy and risk of prostate cancer. JAMA, Vol. 287, June 19, 2002, pp. 3110-15
30. Zhu, K, et al. Vasectomy and prostate cancer: a case-control study in a health maintenance organization. American Journal of Epidemiology, Vol. 144, October 15, 1996, pp. 717-22
31. Emard, JF, et al. Vasectomy and prostate cancer in Quebec, Canada. Health Place, Vol. 7, No. June 2001, pp. 131-39
32. Lightfoot, N, et al. Prostate cancer risk: medical history, sexual, and hormonal factors. Annals of Epidemiology, Vol. 10, No. 7, October 1, 2000, p. 470
33. Wildschut, HI and Monincx, W. Vasectomy and the risk of prostate cancer. Bulletin of the World Health Organization, Vol. 72, No. 5, 1994, pp. 777-78
34. Nie, Y, et al. A survey of the long-term incidence rate of benign prostate hyperplasia after vasectomy. Zhonghua Yi Xue Za Zhi, Vol. 83, No. 15, August 10, 2003, pp. 1303-05 [English abstract only]

CHAPTER 4 - Diagnosis and Staging of Prostate Cancer

1. 2003. AUA guideline on management of benign prostatic hyperplasia (2003). Chapter 1: Diagnosis and treatment recommendations. J.Urol. 170(2 Pt 1):530-547.
2. Scardino PT, Kelman J, Dr. Peter Scardino's Prostate Book. Avery/Penguin Group, New York, 2005.
3. Philip J et al., 2005. Is a digital rectal examination necessary in the diagnosis and clinical staging of early prostate cancer? BJU Int. 95(7):969-971.

4. Crawford ED et al., 1999. Efficiency of prostate-specific antigen and digital rectal examination in screening, using 4.0 ng/ml and age-specific reference range as a cutoff for abnormal values. Prostate. 38(4):296-302.
5. Murthy GD, Byron DP, Pasquale D, 2004. Underutilization of digital rectal examination when screening for prostate cancer. Arch Intern Med. 164(3):313-316.
6. Thompson IM et al., 2004. Prevalence of prostate cancer among men with a prostate-specific antigen level < or =4.0 ng per milliliter. N.Engl.J Med. 350(22):2239-2246.
7. Thompson IM et al., 2003. The influence of finasteride on the development of prostate cancer. The New England Journal of Medicine. 349(3):215-224.
8. Walsh P, 2004. Editorial comment on N Eng J Med,2004; 350:2239. J Urol. 172:550.
9. Barry MJ, 2006. The PSA Conundrum. Arch Intern Med. 166(1):7-8.
10. Shah JB et al., 2005. PSA updated: still relevant in the new millennium? Eur.Urol. 47(4):427-432.
11. Crawford ED, 2005. PSA testing: what is the use? Lancet. 365(9469):1447-1449.
12. Mitka M, 2004. Is PSA testing still useful? JAMA: The Journal of the American Medical Association. 292(19):2326-2327.
13. Eisenberger M, Partin A, 2004. Progress toward identifying aggressive prostate cancer. The New England Journal of Medicine. 351(2):180-181.
14. Oottamasathien S, Crawford ED, 2003. Should routine screening for prostate-specific antigen be recommended? Arch Intern Med. 163(6):661-662.
15. Hoffman RM, 2003. An argument against routine prostate cancer screening. Arch Intern Med. 163(6):663-665.
16. van der Cruijsen-Koeter IW et al., 2005. Comparison of screen detected and clinically diagnosed prostate cancer in the European randomized study of screening for prostate cancer, section rotterdam. J Urol. 174(1):121-125.
17. Etzioni R et al., 2002. Overdiagnosis due to prostate-specific antigen screening: lessons from U.S. prostate cancer incidence trends. JNCI Cancer Spectrum. 94(13):981-990.
18. Epstein JI et al., 2005. Utility of saturation biopsy to predict insignificant cancer at radical prostatectomy. Urology. 66(2):356-360.
19. Baxter NN et al., 2005. Increased risk of rectal cancer after prostate radiation: a population-based study. Gastroenterology. 128(4):819-824.
20. D'Amico AV, 2005. Screening for prostate carcinoma: prostate-specific antigen--friend or foe? Cancer. 103(5):881-883.
21. Damber JE, 2004. Decreasing mortality rates for prostate cancer: possible role of hormonal therapy? BJU Int. 93(6):695-701.
22. Labrie F et al., 2004. Screening decreases prostate cancer mortality: 11-year follow-up of the 1988 Quebec prospective randomized controlled trial. Prostate. 59(3):311-318.
23. Elwood M, 2004. A misleading paper on prostate cancer screening. Prostate. 61(4):372-374.
24. Bartsch G et al., 2001. Prostate cancer mortality after introduction of prostate-specific antigen mass screening in the Federal State of Tyrol, Austria. Urology. 58(3):417-424.
25. Ballentine H, 2001. Editorial comment. Urology. 58:242.
26. Lu-Yao G et al., 2002. Natural experiment examining impact of aggressive screening and treatment on prostate cancer mortality in two fixed cohorts from Seattle area and Connecticut. BMJ. 325(7367):740.
27. Thompson IM et al., 2005. Operating characteristics of prostate-specific antigen in men with an initial PSA level of 3.0 ng/ml or lower. JAMA: The Journal of the American Medical Association. 294(1):66-70.
28. Shannon J et al., 2005. Statins and prostate cancer risk: a case-control study. Am.J Epidemiol. 162(4):318-325.
29. Bill-Axelson A et al., 2005. Radical prostatectomy versus watchful waiting in early prostate cancer. The New England Journal of Medicine. 352(19):1977-1984.
30. Kopec JA et al., 2005. Screening with prostate specific antigen and metastatic prostate cancer risk: a population based case-control study. J Urol. 174(2):495-499.
31. Grubb RL et al., 2005. Results of compliance with prostate cancer screening guidelines. J Urol. 174(2):668-672.
32. Neulander EZ, Soloway MS, 2003. Failure after radical prostatectomy. Urology. 61(1):30-36.

33. Krygiel JM et al., 2005. Intermediate term biochemical progression rates after radical prostatectomy and radiotherapy in patients with screen detected prostate cancer. J Urol. 174(1):126-130.

34. Antenor JA et al., 2005. Preoperative PSA and progression-free survival after radical prostatectomy for Stage T1c disease. Urology. 66(1):156-160.

35. Freedland SJ et al., 2004. Biochemical outcome after radical prostatectomy among men with normal preoperative serum prostate-specific antigen levels. Cancer. 101(4):748-753.

36. Lu-Yao GL, Yao SL, 1997. Population-based study of long-term survival in patients with clinically localised prostate cancer. Lancet. 349(9056):906-910.

37. Oesterling JE et al., 1993. Serum prostate-specific antigen in a community-based population of healthy men. Establishment of age-specific reference ranges. JAMA: The Journal of the American Medical Association. 270(7):860-864.

38. Catalona WJ et al., 1994. Selection of optimal prostate specific antigen cutoffs for early detection of prostate cancer: receiver operating characteristic curves. J Urol. 152(6 Pt 1):2037-2042.

39. Veltri RW et al., 2002. Impact of age on total and complexed prostate-specific antigen cutoffs in a contemporary referral series of men with prostate cancer. Urology. 60(4 Suppl 1):47-52.

40. Mayo Clinic On Prostate Health. Mayo Clinic Health Information, Rochester, MN, 2003.

41. Walsh PC, Worthington JF, Dr. Patrick Walsh's Guide to Surviving Prostate Cancer. Warner Books, New York, N.Y., 2001.

42. Khan MA et al., 2003. Long-term cancer control of radical prostatectomy in men younger than 50 years of age: update 2003. Urology. 62(1):86-91.

43. Carter HB, Epstein JI, Partin AW, 1999. Influence of age and prostate-specific antigen on the chance of curable prostate cancer among men with nonpalpable disease. Urology. 53(1):126-130.

44. Aleman M et al., 2003. Age and PSA predict likelihood of organ-confined disease in men presenting with PSA less than 10 ng/mL: implications for screening. Urology. 62(1):70-74.

45. Smith CV et al., 2000. Prostate cancer in men age 50 years or younger: a review of the Department of Defense Center for Prostate Disease Research multicenter prostate cancer database. J Urol. 164(6):1964-1967.

46. Datta MW et al., 2005. Prostate cancer in patients with screening serum prostate specific antigen values less than 4.0 ng/dl: results from the cooperative prostate cancer tissue resource. J Urol. 173(5):1546-1551.

47. Carter HB, 2004. Prostate cancers in men with low PSA levels–must we find them? The New England Journal of Medicine. 350(22):2292-2294.

48. Bosch JL et al., 2006. Establishing normal reference ranges for PSA change with age in a population-based study: The Krimpen study. Prostate. 66(4):335-343.

49. Krumholtz JS et al., 2002. Prostate-specific antigen cutoff of 2.6 ng/mL for prostate cancer screening is associated with favorable pathologic tumor features. Urology. 60(3):469-473.

50. Catalona WJ, Smith DS, Ornstein DK, 1997. Prostate cancer detection in men with serum PSA concentrations of 2.6 to 4.0 ng/mL and benign prostate examination. Enhancement of specificity with free PSA measurements. JAMA: The Journal of the American Medical Association. 277(18):1452-1455.

51. Welch HG, Schwartz LM, Woloshin S, 2005. Prostate-specific antigen levels in the United States: implications of various definitions for abnormal. JNCI Cancer Spectrum. 97(15):1132-1137.

52. Parsons JK, Partin AW, 2004. Applying complexed prostate-specific antigen to clinical practice. Urology. 63(5):815-818.

53. Roddam AW et al., Use of Prostate-Specific Antigen (PSA) Isoforms for the Detection of Prostate Cancer in Men with a PSA Level of 2-10 ng/ml: Systematic Review and Meta-Analysis. European Urology. In Press, Corrected Proof.

54. Martinez-Pineiro L et al., 2004. Probability of prostate cancer as a function of the percentage of free prostate-specific antigen in patients with a non-suspicious rectal examination and total prostate-specific antigen of 4-10 ng/ml. World J Urol. 22(2):124-131.

55. Lein M et al., 2003. A multicenter clinical trial on the use of complexed prostate specific antigen in low prostate specific antigen concentrations. J Urol. 170(4 Pt 1):1175-1179.

56. Rowe EW et al., 2005. Prostate cancer detection in men with a 'normal' total prostate-specific antigen (PSA) level using percentage free PSA: a prospective screening study. BJU Int. 95(9):1249-1252.

57. Epstein JI et al., 1998. Nonpalpable stage T1c prostate cancer: prediction of insignificant disease using free/total prostate specific antigen levels and needle biopsy findings. J Urol. 160(6 Pt 2):2407-2411.

58. Southwick PC et al., 1999. Prediction of post-radical prostatectomy pathological outcome for stage T1c prostate cancer with percent free prostate specific antigen: a prospective multicenter clinical trial. J Urol. 162(4):1346-1351.

59. Aus G et al., 2003. Free-to-total prostate-specific antigen ratio as a predictor of non-organ-confined prostate cancer (stage pT3). Scand.J Urol Nephrol. 37(6):466-470.

60. Grossklaus DJ et al., 2002. The free/total prostate-specific antigen ratio (%fPSA) is the best predictor of tumor involvement in the radical prostatectomy specimen among men with an elevated PSA. Urol Oncol. 7(5):195-198.

61. Kobayashi T et al., 2005. Volume-adjusted prostate-specific antigen (PSA) variables in detecting impalpable prostate cancer in men with PSA levels of 2-4 ng/mL: transabdominal measurement makes a significant contribution. BJU Int. 95(9):1245-1248.

62. Horninger W et al., 1998. Improvement of specificity in PSA-based screening by using PSA-transition zone density and percent free PSA in addition to total PSA levels. Prostate. 37(3):133-137.

63. Djavan B et al., 1998. Prostate specific antigen density of the transition zone for early detection of prostate cancer. J Urol. 160(2):411-418.

64. Sung DJ et al., 2004. Comparison of prostate-specific antigen adjusted for transition zone volume versus prostate-specific antigen density in predicting prostate cancer by transrectal ultrasonography. J Ultrasound Med. 23(5):615-622.

65. Moon DG et al., 1999. Prostate-specific antigen adjusted for the transition zone volume versus free-to-total prostate-specific antigen ratio in predicting prostate cancer. Int.J Urol. 6(9):455-462.

66. Ferreira MD, Koff WJ, 2005. Assessment of serum level of prostate-specific antigen adjusted for the transition zone volume in early detection of prostate cancer. Int.Braz.J Urol. 31(2):137-145.

67. Ohi M et al., 2004. Diagnostic significance of PSA density adjusted by transition zone volume in males with PSA levels between 2 and 4ng/ml. Eur.Urol. 45(1):92-96.

68. Djavan B et al., 1999. PSA, PSA density, PSA density of transition zone, free/total PSA ratio, and PSA velocity for early detection of prostate cancer in men with serum PSA 2.5 to 4.0 ng/mL. Urology. 54(3):517-522.

69. Berger AP et al., 2005. Longitudinal PSA changes in men with and without prostate cancer: Assessment of prostate cancer risk. Prostate. 64(3):240-245.

70. Carter HB et al., 1992. Longitudinal evaluation of prostate-specific antigen levels in men with and without prostate disease. JAMA: The Journal of the American Medical Association. 267(16):2215-2220.

71. Smith DS, Catalona WJ, 1994. Rate of change in serum prostate specific antigen levels as a method for prostate cancer detection. J Urol. 152(4):1163-1167.

72. Fang J et al., 2002. PSA velocity for assessing prostate cancer risk in men with PSA levels between 2.0 and 4.0 ng/ml. Urology. 59(6):889-893.

73. Anscher MS, 2005. PSA Kinetics and Risk of Death From Prostate Cancer: In Search of the Holy Grail of Surrogate End Points. JAMA: The Journal of the American Medical Association. 294(4):493-494.

74. D'Amico AV et al., 2005. Pretreatment PSA Velocity and Risk of Death From Prostate Cancer Following External Beam Radiation Therapy. JAMA: The Journal of the American Medical Association. 294(4):440-447.

75. Freedland SJ et al., 2005. Risk of Prostate Cancer-Specific Mortality Following Biochemical Recurrence After Radical Prostatectomy. JAMA: The Journal of the American Medical Association. 294(4):433-439.

76. Riffenburgh RH, Amling CL, 2003. Use of early PSA velocity to predict eventual abnormal PSA values in men at risk for prostate cancer. Prostate Cancer Prostatic.Dis. 6(1):39-44.

77. Roobol MJ et al., 2004. Prostate-specific antigen velocity at low prostate-specific antigen levels as screening tool for prostate cancer: results of second screening round of ERSPC (ROTTERDAM). Urology. 63(2):309-313.

78. Raaijmakers R et al., 2004. Prostate-specific antigen change in the European Randomized Study of Screening for Prostate Cancer, section Rotterdam. Urology. 63(2):316-320.

79. Boddy JL et al., 2004. Intra-individual variation of serum prostate specific antigen levels in men with benign prostate biopsies. BJU Int. 93(6):735-738.

80. Eastham JA et al., 2003. Variation of serum prostate-specific antigen levels: an evaluation of year-to-year fluctuations. JAMA: The Journal of the American Medical Association. 289(20):2695-2700.

81. Lechevallier E et al., 1999. Effect of digital rectal examination on serum complexed and free prostate-specific antigen and percentage of free prostate-specific antigen. Urology. 54(5):857-861.

82. Herschman JD, Smith DS, Catalona WJ, 1997. Effect of ejaculation on serum total and free prostate-specific antigen concentrations. Urology. 50(2):239-243.

83. Link RE et al., 2004. Variation in prostate specific antigen results from 2 different assay platforms: clinical impact on 2304 patients undergoing prostate cancer screening. J Urol. 171(6 Pt 1):2234-2238.

84. Etzioni RD et al., 2005. Long-term effects of finasteride on prostate specific antigen levels: results from the prostate cancer prevention trial. J Urol. 174(3):877-881.

85. Cyrus-David MS et al., 2005. The effect of statins on serum prostate specific antigen levels in a cohort of airline pilots: a preliminary report. J Urol. 173(6):1923-1925.

86. Graaf MR et al., 2004. The Risk of Cancer in Users of Statins. Journal of Clinical Oncology. 22(12):2388-2394.

87. Moyad MA, 2005. Heart healthy equals prostate healthy equals statins: the next cancer chemoprevention trial. Part II. Curr Opin.Urol. 15(1):7-12.

88. Barqawi AB et al., 2005. Observed effect of age and body mass index on total and complexed PSA: analysis from a national screening program. Urology. 65(4):708-712.

89. Jemal A et al., 2002. Cancer Statistics, 2002. CA: A Cancer Journal for Clinicians. 52(1):23-47.

90. Patel U, 2004. TRUS and prostate biopsy: current status. Prostate Cancer Prostatic.Dis. 7(3):208-210.

91. Djavan B, Milani S, Remzi M, 2005. Prostate biopsy: who, how and when. An update. Can.J Urol. 12 Suppl 1:44-48.

92. Roehl KA, Antenor JA, Catalona WJ, 2002. Serial biopsy results in prostate cancer screening study. J Urol. 167(6):2435-2439.

93. Ochiai A, Babaian RJ, 2004. Update on prostate biopsy technique. Curr Opin.Urol. 14(3):157-162.

94. Presti JC, Jr. et al., 2003. Extended peripheral zone biopsy schemes increase cancer detection rates and minimize variance in prostate specific antigen and age related cancer rates: results of a community multi-practice study. J Urol. 169(1):125-129.

95. Philip J et al., 2004. Effect of peripheral biopsies in maximising early prostate cancer detection in 8-, 10- or 12-core biopsy regimens. BJU Int. 93(9):1218-1220.

96. Addla SK et al., 2003. Local anaesthetic for transrectal ultrasound-guided prostate biopsy: a prospective, randomized, double blind, placebo-controlled study. Eur.Urol. 43(5):441-443.

97. Berger AP et al., 2003. Periprostatic administration of local anesthesia during transrectal ultrasound-guided biopsy of the prostate: a randomized, double-blind, placebo-controlled study. Urology. 61(3):585-588.

98. Alavi AS et al., 2001. Local anesthesia for ultrasound guided prostate biopsy: a prospective randomized trial comparing 2 methods. J Urol. 166(4):1343-1345.

99. Matlaga BR, Lovato JF, Hall MC, 2003. Randomized prospective trial of a novel local anesthetic technique for extensive prostate biopsy. Urology. 61(5):972-976.

100. Ragavan N et al., 2005. A randomized, controlled trial comparing lidocaine periprostatic nerve block, diclofenac suppository and both for transrectal ultrasound guided biopsy of prostate. J Urol. 174(2):510-513.

101. Soloway MS, Obek C, 2000. Periprostatic local anesthesia before ultrasound guided prostate biopsy. J Urol. 163(1):172-173.

102. Fried S, Bitter Pills. Inside the hazadrousworld of legal drugs. Bantam, New York, 2005.
103. Ghani KR, Dundas D, Patel U, 2004. Bleeding after transrectal ultrasonography-guided prostate biopsy: a study of 7-day morbidity after a six-, eight- and 12-core biopsy protocol. BJU Int. 94(7):1014-1020.
104. Djavan B et al., 2001. Safety and morbidity of first and repeat transrectal ultrasound guided prostate needle biopsies: results of a prospective European prostate cancer detection study. J Urol. 166(3):856-860.
105. Epstein JI, 2000. Gleason score 2-4 adenocarcinoma of the prostate on needle biopsy: a diagnosis that should not be made. Am.J Surg.Pathol. 24(4):477-478.
106. Makarov DV et al., 2002. Gleason score 7 prostate cancer on needle biopsy: is the prognostic difference in Gleason scores 4 + 3 and 3 + 4 independent of the number of involved cores? J Urol. 167(6):2440-2442.
107. Montironi R et al., 2005. Gleason grading of prostate cancer in needle biopsies or radical prostatectomy specimens: contemporary approach, current clinical significance and sources of pathology discrepancies. BJU Int. 95(8):1146-1152.
108. Sved PD et al., 2004. Limitations of biopsy Gleason grade: implications for counseling patients with biopsy Gleason score 6 prostate cancer. J Urol. 172(1):98-102.
109. Lattouf JB, Saad F, 2002. Gleason score on biopsy: is it reliable for predicting the final grade on pathology? BJU Int. 90(7):694-698.
110. Gonzalgo ML et al., 2006. Relationship between primary Gleason pattern on needle biopsy and clinicopathologic outcomes among men with Gleason score 7 adenocarcinoma of the prostate. Urology. 67(1):115-119.
111. Steiner MS, 2003. High-grade prostatic intraepithelial neoplasia and prostate cancer risk reduction. World J Urol. 21(1):15-20.
112. Epstein JI, Potter SR, 2001. The pathological interpretation and significance of prostate needle biopsy findings: implications and current controversies. J Urol. 166(2):402-410.
113. Gokden N et al., 2005. High-grade prostatic intraepithelial neoplasia in needle biopsy as risk factor for detection of adenocarcinoma: current level of risk in screening population. Urology. 65(3):538-542.
114. Lefkowitz GK et al., 2002. Followup interval prostate biopsy 3 years after diagnosis of high grade prostatic intraepithelial neoplasia is associated with high likelihood of prostate cancer, independent of change in prostate specific antigen levels. J Urol. 168(4 Pt 1):1415-1418.
115. Rosser CJ et al., 1999. Detection of high-grade prostatic intraepithelial neoplasia with the five-region biopsy technique. Urology. 54(5):853-856.
116. Lefkowitz GK et al., 2001. Is repeat prostate biopsy for high-grade prostatic intraepithelial neoplasia necessary after routine 12-core sampling? Urology. 58(6):999-1003.
117. Zwergel U et al., 2004. Lymph node positive prostate cancer: long-term survival data after radical prostatectomy. J Urol. 171(3):1128-1131.
118. Ward JF, Zincke H, 2003. Radical prostatectomy for the patient with locally advanced prostate cancer. Curr Urol Rep. 4(3):196-204.
119. Ward JF et al., 2005. Radical prostatectomy for clinically advanced (cT3) prostate cancer since the advent of prostate-specific antigen testing: 15-year outcome. BJU Int. 95(6):751-756.
120. Pollack A, Horwitz EM, Movsas B, 2003. Treatment of prostate cancer with regional lymph node (N1) metastasis. Semin.Radiat.Oncol. 13(2):121-129.
121. Bhatta-Dhar N et al., 2004. No difference in six-year biochemical failure rates with or without pelvic lymph node dissection during radical prostatectomy in low-risk patients with localized prostate cancer. Urology. 63(3):528-531.
122. Weckermann D, Wawroschek F, Harzmann R, 2005. Is there a need for pelvic lymph node dissection in low risk prostate cancer patients prior to definitive local therapy? Eur.Urol. 47(1):45-50.
123. Palapattu GS et al., 2004. Prostate specific antigen progression in men with lymph node metastases following radical prostatectomy: results of long-term followup. J Urol. 172(5 Pt 1):1860-1864.
124. Harisinghani MG et al., 2003. Noninvasive detection of clinically occult lymph-node metastases in prostate cancer. The New England Journal of Medicine. 348(25):2491-2499.

125. Lee N et al., 2000. Which patients with newly diagnosed prostate cancer need a radionuclide bone scan? An analysis based on 631 patients. Int.J Radiat.Oncol Biol.Phys. 48(5):1443-1446.

126. Yanke BV et al., 2005. Validation of a nomogram for predicting positive repeat biopsy for prostate cancer. J Urol. 173(2):421-424.

127. Kattan MW et al., 2003. Counseling men with prostate cancer: a nomogram for predicting the presence of small, moderately differentiated, confined tumors. J Urol. 170(5):1792-1797.

128. Cagiannos I et al., 2003. A preoperative nomogram identifying decreased risk of positive pelvic lymph nodes in patients with prostate cancer. J Urol. 170(5):1798-1803.

129. Di Blasio CJ et al., 2003. Predicting clinical end points: treatment nomograms in prostate cancer. Semin.Oncol. 30(5):567-586.

130. Kattan MW, 2003. Nomograms are superior to staging and risk grouping systems for identifying high-risk patients: preoperative application in prostate cancer. Curr Opin.Urol. 13(2):111-116.

131. Boddy JL et al., 2005. An elevated PSA, which normalizes, does not exclude the presence of prostate cancer. Prostate Cancer Prostatic.Dis.

132. Allaf ME, Carter HB, 2004. Update on watchful waiting for prostate cancer. Curr Opin.Urol. 14(3):171-175.

CHAPTER 5 – Prevention of Prostate Cancer

Introduction

1. Strum, Stephen B. and Pogliano, Donna. A Primer on Prostate Cancer. Life Extension Foundation, Hollywood, FL, 2nd edition, 2005, pp. 75-81

2. Klein, Eric A. Chemoprevention of prostate cancer. Critical Reviews in Oncology/Hematology, Vol. 54, 2005, pp. 1-10

3. Arnot, Robert. The Prostate Cancer Protection Plan. Little, Brown and Company, 1st edition, 2000, p. 11

Pharmaceutical Drugs

1. Cote, R.J., et al. The effect of finasteride on the prostate gland in men with elevated serum prostate-specific antigen levels. British Journal of Cancer, Vol. 78, No. 3, August 1998, pp. 413-18

2. Thompson, I.M., et al. The influence of finasteride on the development of prostate cancer. New England Journal of Medicine, Vol. 349, July 17, 2003, pp. 215-24

3. Zuger, A. A big study yields big questions. New England Journal of Medicine, Vol. 349, July 17, 2003, pp. 213-14

4. Scardino, PT. The prevention of prostate cancer – The dilemma continues. New England Journal of Medicine, Vol. 349, July 17, 2003, pp. 297-99

5. Burke, HB. Prevention of prostate cancer with finasteride. New England Journal of Medicine, Vol. 349, October 16, 2003, p. 1570 (letter to the editor)

6. Ross, RK, et al. Prevention of prostate cancer with finasteride. New England Journal of Medicine, Vol. 349, October 16, 2003, p. 1571 (letter to the editor)

7. Andriole, GL, et al. Effect of the dual 5-alpha-reductase inhibitor dutasteride on markers of tumor regression in prostate cancer. Journal of Urology, Vol. 172, September 2004, pp. 915-19

8. Iczkowski, KA, et al. The dual 5-alpha-reductase inhibitor dutasteride induces atrophic changes and decreases relative cancer volume in human prostate. Urology, Vol. 65, January 2005, pp. 76-82

9. Andriole, G, et al. Chemoprevention of prostate cancer in men at high risk: rationale and design of the REDUCE trial. Journal of Urology, Vol. 172, October 2004, pp. 1314-17

10. Perron, L, et al. Dosage, duration and timing of nonsteroidal antiinflammatory drug use and risk of prostate cancer. International Journal of Cancer, Vol. 106, No. 3, September 1, 2003, pp. 409-15

11. Garcia Rodriguez, LA and Gonzalez-Perez, A. Inverse association between nonsteroidal anti-inflammatory drugs and prostate cancer. Cancer Epidemiol Biomarkers Prev, Vol. 13, April 2004, pp. 649-53

12. Platz, EA, et al. Nonsteroidal anti-inflammatory drugs and risk of prostate cancer in the Baltimore Longitudinal Study of Aging. Cancer Epidemiol Biomarkers Prev, Vol. 14, February 2005, pp. 390-96

13. Jacobs, EJ, et al. A large cohort study of aspirin and other nonsteroidal anti-inflammatory drugs and prostate cancer incidence. Journal of the National Cancer Institute, Vol. 97, No. 13, July 6, 2005, pp. 975-80

14. Royle, S, et al. Nitric oxide donating nonsteroidal anti-inflammatory drugs induce apoptosis in human prostate cancer cell systems and human prostatic stroma via caspase-3. Journal of Urology, Vol. 172, July 2004, pp. 338-44

15. Coogan, PF, et al. Statin use and the risk of breast and prostate cancer. Epidemiology, Vol. 13, May 2002, pp. 262-67

16. Cyrus-David, MS, et al. The effect of statins on serum prostate specific antigen levels in a cohort of airline pilots: a preliminary report. Journal of Urology, Vol. 173, June 2005, pp. 1923-25

17. Strandberg, TE, et al. Mortality and incidence of cancer during 10-year follow-up of the Scandinavian Simvastatin Survival Study (4S). The Lancet, Vol. 364, August 28, 2004, pp. 771-77

18. Kaye, JA and Jick, H. Statin use and cancer risk in the General Practice Research Database. British Journal of Cancer, Vol. 90, No. 3, 2004, pp. 635-37

19. Graaf, MR, et al. The risk of cancer in users of statins. Journal of Clinical Oncology, Vol. 22, June 15, 2004, pp. 2388-94

20. Shannon, J, et al. Statins and prostate cancer risk: a case-control study. American Journal of Epidemiology, Vol. 162, No. 4, 2005, pp. 318-25

Fruits and Vegetables

1. Giovannucci, Edward, et al. Calcium and fructose intake in relation to risk of prostate cancer. Cancer Research, Vol. 58, February 1, 1998, pp. 442-47

2. Hebert, James R., et al. Nutritional and socioeconomic factors in relation to prostate cancer mortality: a cross-national study. Journal of the National Cancer Institute, Vol. 90, November 4, 1998, pp. 1637-47

3. Key, TJA, et al. A case-control study of diet and prostate cancer. British Journal of Cancer, Vol. 76, No. 5, September 1997, pp. 678-87

4. Cohen, Jennifer, et al. Fruit and vegetable intakes and prostate cancer risk. Journal of the National Cancer Institute, Vol. 92, January 5, 2000, pp. 61-68

5. Giovannucci, E, et al. A prospective study of cruciferous vegetables and prostate cancer. Cancer Epidemiol Biomarkers Prev, Vol. 12, December 2003, pp. 1403-09

6. Wang, L, et al. Targeting cell cycle machinery as a molecular mechanism of sulforaphane in prostate cancer prevention. International Journal of Oncology, Vol. 24, January 2004, pp. 187-92

7. Singh, SV, et al. Sulforaphane-induced cell death in human prostate cancer cells is initiated by reactive oxygen species. Journal of Biol Chem, Vol. 280, No. 20, May 20, 2005, pp. 19911-24

8. Brooks, JD, et al. Potent induction of phase 2 enzymes in human prostate cells by sulforaphane. Cancer Epidemiol Biomarkers Prev, Vol. 10, September 2001, pp. 949-54

9. Zhang, J, et al. Indole-3-carbinol induces a G1 cell cycle arrest and inhibits prostate-specific antigen production in human LNCaP prostate carcinoma cells. Cancer, Vol. 98, No. 11, December 1, 2003, pp. 2511-20

10. Hsu, JC, et al. Indole-3-carbinol inhibition of androgen receptor expression and Downregulation of androgen responsiveness in human prostate cancer cells. Carcinogenesis, Vol. 26, November 2005, pp. 1896-904

11. Sarkar, FH and Li, Y. Indole-3-carbinol and prostate cancer. Journal of Nutrition, Vol. 134, 2004, pp. 3493S-98S

12. Fahey, Jed W., et al. Broccoli sprouts: An exceptionally rich source of inducers of enzymes that protect against chemical carcinogens. Proceedings of the National Academy of Sciences USA (Medical Sciences), Vol. 94, No. 19, September 16, 1997, pp. 10367-72

13. Gill, CIR, et al. The effect of cruciferous and leguminous sprouts on genotoxicity, in vitro and in vivo. Cancer Epidemiology, Biomarkers & Prevention, Vol. 13, July 2004, pp. 1-7

14. Microwave cooking zaps nutrients. New Scientist, October 25, 2003, p. 14
15. McCann, SE, et al. Intakes of selected nutrients, foods, and phytochemicals and prostate cancer risk in western New York. Nutrition and Cancer, Vol. 53, No. 1, 2005, pp. 33-41
16. Le Marchand, L, et al. Animal fat consumption and prostate cancer: a prospective study in Hawaii. Epidemiology, Vol. 5, No. 3, May 1994, pp. 276-82
17. Schuurman, AG, et al. Vegetable and fruit consumption and prostate cancer risk: a cohort study in The Netherlands. Cancer Epidemiol Biomarkers Prev, Vol. 7, August 1998, pp. 673-80
18. Key, TJ, et al. Fruits and vegetables and prostate cancer: no association among 1104 cases in a prospective study of 130,544 men in the European Prospective Investigation into Cancer and Nutrition (EPIC). International Journal of Cancer, Vol. 109, No. 1, March 2004, pp. 119-24

Tomato Products
1. Giovannucci, Edward, et al. Intake of carotenoids and retinol in relation to risk of prostate cancer. Journal of the National Cancer Institute, Vol. 87, No. 23, December 6, 1995, pp. 1767-76
2. Giovannucci, Edward, et al. A prospective study of tomato products, lycopene, and prostate cancer risk. Journal of the National Cancer Institute, Vol. 94, No. 5, March 6, 2002, pp. 391-98
3. Wu, K, et al. Plasma and dietary carotenoids, and the risk of prostate cancer: a nested case-control study. Cancer Epidemiology, Biomarkers & Prevention, Vol. 13, February 2004, pp. 260-69
4. Lagiou, A, et al. Are there age-dependent effects of diet on prostate cancer risk? Soz Praventivmed, Vol. 46, No. 5, 2001, pp. 329-34
5. Mucci, LA, et al. Are dietary influences on the risk of prostate cancer mediated through the insulin-like growth factor system? BJU Int, Vol. 87, No. 9, June 2001, pp. 814-20
6. Gann, Peter H., et al. Lower prostate cancer risk in men with elevated plasma lycopene levels: results of a prospective analysis. Cancer Research, Vol. 59, March 15, 1999, pp. 1225-30
7. Etminan, M, et al. The role of tomato products and lycopene in the prevention of prostate cancer: a meta-analysis of observational studies. Cancer Epidemiology, Biomarkers & Prevention, Vol. 13, March 2004, pp. 340-45
8. Agarwal, Sanjiv and Rao, AV. Tomato lycopene and its role in human health and chronic diseases. Canadian Medical Association Journal, Vol. 163, September 19, 2000, pp. 739-44
9. Campbell, JK, et al. Tomato phytochemicals and prostate cancer risk. Journal of Nutrition, Vol. 134, 2004, pp. 3486S-92S
10. Stacewicz-Sapuntzakis, M and Bowen, PE. Role of lycopene and tomato products in prostate health. Biochim Biophys Acta, Vol. 1740, No. 2, May 30, 2005, pp. 202-05
11. Rao, AV. Processed tomato products as a source of dietary lycopene: bioavailability and antioxidant properties. Can J Diet Pract Res, Vol. 65, No. 4, Winter 2004, pp. 161-65
12. Mohanty, NK, et al. Lycopene as a chemopreventive agent in the treatment of high-grade prostate intraepithelial neoplasia. Urol Oncol, Vol. 23, No. 6, Nov-Dec. 2005, pp. 383-85
13. Forbes, K, et al. Lycopene increases urokinase receptor and fails to inhibit growth or connexion expression in a metastatically passaged prostate cancer cell line: a brief communication. Exp Biol Med, Vol. 228, 2003, pp. 967-71
14. Kim, HS, et al. Effects of tomato sauce consumption on apoptotic cell death in prostate benign hyperplasia and carcinoma. Nutr Cancer, Vol. 47, No. 1, 2003, pp. 40-47
15. Gartner, Christine, et al. Lycopene is more bioavailable from tomato paste than from fresh tomatoes. American Journal of Clinical Nutrition, Vol. 66, July 1997, pp. 116-22
16. Stahl, W and Sies, H. Uptake of lycopene and its geometrical isomers is greater from heat-processed than from unprocessed tomato juice in humans. Journal of Nutrition, Vol. 122, 1992, pp. 2161-66
17. Rissanen, TH, et al. Low serum lycopene concentration is associated with an excess incidence of acute coronary events and stroke: the Kuopio Ischaemic Heart Disease Risk Factor Study. British Journal of Nutrition, Vol. 85, June 2001, pp. 749-54

18. Erhardt, JG, et al. Lycopene, beta-carotene, and colorectal adenomas. American Journal of Clinical Nutrition, Vol. 78, December 2003, pp. 1219-24

19. Gaziano, JM, et al. Discrimination in absorption or transport of beta-carotene isomers after oral supplementation with either all-trans- or 9-cisbeta-carotene. American Journal of Clinical Nutrition, Vol. 61, 1995, pp. 1248-52

20. Micozzi, MS, et al. Plasma carotenoid response to chronic intake of selected foods and beta-carotene supplements in men. American Journal of Clinical Nutrition, Vol. 55, June 1992, pp. 1120-25

21. Paetau, I, et al. Chronic ingestion of lycopene-rich tomato juice or lycopene supplements significantly increases plasma concentrations of lycopene and related tomato carotenoids in humans. American Journal of Clinical Nutrition, Vol. 68, December 1998, pp. 1187-95

22. Walfisch, Y, et al. Lycopene in serum, skin and adipose tissues after tomato-oleoresin supplementation in patients undergoing haemorrhoidectomy or peri-anal fistulotomy. British Journal of Nutrition, Vol. 90, No. 4, October 2003, pp. 759-66

Fish and Fish Oils

1. Yang, Yoon Jung, et al. Comparison of fatty acid profiles in the serum of patients with prostate cancer and benign prostatic hyperplasia. Clinical Biochemistry, Vol. 32, August 1999, pp. 405-09

2. Norrish, A.E., et al. Prostate cancer risk and consumption of fish oils: a dietary biomarker-based case-control study. British Journal of Cancer, Vol. 81, No. 7, December 1999, pp. 1238-42

3. Terry, Paul, et al. Fatty fish consumption and risk of prostate cancer. The Lancet, Vol. 357, June 2, 2001, pp. 1764-66

4. Leitzmann, MF, et al. Dietary intake of n-3 and n-6 fatty acids and the risk of prostate cancer. American Journal of Clinical Nutrition, Vol. 80, July 2004, pp. 204-16

5. Simopoulos, Artemis. Omega-3 fatty acids in health and disease and in growth and development. American Journal of Clinical Nutrition, Vol. 54, 1991, pp. 438-63

6. Pepping, Joseph. Omega-3 essential fatty acids. American Journal of Health-System Pharmacy, Vol. 56, April 15, 1999, pp. 719-24

7. Uauy-Dagach, Ricardo and Valenzuela, Alfonso. Marine oils: the health benefits of n-3 fatty acids. Nutrition Reviews, Vol. 54, November 1996, pp. S102-S108

8. Connor, William E. Importance of n-3 fatty acids in health and disease. American Journal of Clinical Nutrition, Vol. 71 (suppl), January 2000, pp. 171S-75S

9. Daviglus, Martha L., et al. Fish consumption and the 30-year risk of fatal myocardial infarction. New England Journal of Medicine, Vol. 336, April 10, 1997, pp. 1046-53

10. Simon, Joel A., et al. Serum fatty acids and the risk of coronary heart disease. American Journal of Epidemiology, Vol. 142, No. 5, September 1, 1995, pp. 469-76

11. Flaten, Hugo, et al. Fish-oil concentrate: effects of variables related to cardiovascular disease. American Journal of Clinical Nutrition, Vol. 52, 1990, pp. 300-06

12. Levine, Barbara S. Most frequently asked questions about DHA. Nutrition Today, Vol. 32, November/December 1997, pp. 248-49

13. Kalmijn, S., et al. Polyunsaturated fatty acids, antioxidants, and cognitive function in very old men. American Journal of Epidemiology, Vol. 145, January 1, 1997, pp. 33-41

14. Kalmijn, S., et al. Dietary fat intake and the risk of incident dementia in the Rotterdam Study. Annals of Neurology, Vol. 42(5), November 1997, pp. 776-82

15. Yehuda, S., et al. Essential fatty acids preparation (SR-3) improves Alzheimer's patients quality of life. International Journal of Neuroscience, Vol. 87(3-4), November 1996, pp. 141-9

16. Edwards, R., et al. Omega-3 polyunsaturated fatty acid levels in the diet and in red blood cell membranes of depressed patients. Journal of Affective Disorders, Vol. 48, March 1998, pp. 149-55

17. Hibbeln, Joseph R. Fish consumption and major depression. The Lancet, Vol. 351, April 18, 1998, p. 1213 (correspondence)

18. Hibbeln, Joseph R. and Salem, Norman. Dietary polyunsaturated fatty acids and depression: when cholesterol does not satisfy. American Journal of Clinical Nutrition, Vol. 62, July 1995, pp. 1-9

19. Stoll, Andrew L., et al. Omega 3 fatty acids in bipolar disorder. Archives of General Psychiatry, Vol. 56, May 1999, pp. 407-12 and pp. 415-16 (commentary)
20. Calabrese, Joseph R., et al. Fish oils and bipolar disorder. Archives of General Psychiatry, Vol. 56, May 1999, pp. 413-14 (commentary)
21. Laugharne, J.D.E., et al. Fatty acids and schizophrenia. Lipids, Vol. 31 (suppl), 1996, pp. S163-S65
22. Appel, Lawrence J., et al. Does supplementation of diet with "fish oil" reduce blood pressure? Archives of Internal Medicine, Vol. 153, June 28, 1993, pp. 1429-38
23. Radack, Kenneth, et al. The effects of low doses of n-3 fatty acid supplementation on blood pressure in hypertensive subjects. Archives of Internal Medicine, Vol. 151, June 1991, pp. 1173-80
24. Morris, Martha Clare, et al. Does fish oil lower blood pressure? A meta-analysis of controlled trials. Circulation, Vol. 88, No. 2, August 1993, pp. 523-33
25. Andreassen, A.K., et al. Hypertension prophylaxis with omega-3 fatty acids in heart transplant recipients. J Am Coll Cardiol, Vol. 29, May 1997, pp. 1324-31
26. Cobiac, L., et al. Effects of dietary sodium restriction and fish oil supplements on blood pressure in the elderly. Clin Exp Pharmacol Physiol, Vol. 18, May 1991, pp. 265-68
27. Toft, Ingrid, et al. Effects of n-3 polyunsaturated fatty acids on glucose homeostasis and blood pressure in essential hypertension. Annals of Internal Medicine, Vol. 123, No. 12, December 15, 1995, pp. 911-18
28. Kremer, Joel M., et al. Fish-oil fatty acid supplementation in active rheumatoid arthritis: A double-blinded, controlled, crossover study. Annals of Internal Medicine, Vol. 106, April 1987, pp. 497-503
29. Kremer, Joel M. n-3 fatty acid supplements in rheumatoid arthritis. American Journal of Clinical Nutrition, Vol. 71 (suppl), January 2000, pp. 349S-51S
30. Fortin, Paul R., et al. Validation of a meta-analysis: the effects of fish oil in rheumatoid arthritis. Journal of Clinical Epidemiology, Vol. 48, 1995, pp. 1379-90
31. Kremer, J.M., et al. Effects of high-dose fish oil on rheumatoid arthritis after stopping nonsteroidal anti-inflammatory drugs - clinical and immune correlates. Arthritis and Rheumatology, Vol. 38, August 1995, pp. 1107-14
32. Geusens, P., et al. Long-term effect of omega-3 fatty acid supplementation in active rheumatoid arthritis: a 12-month, double-blind, controlled study. Arthritis and Rheumatology, Vol. 37, June 1994, pp. 824-29
33. Navarro, Elisabet, et al. Abnormal fatty acid pattern in rheumatoid arthritis - A rationale for treatment with marine and botanical lipids. Journal of Rheumatology, Vol. 27, February 2000, pp. 298-303
34. Aslan, Alex and Triadafilopoulos, George. Fish oil fatty acid supplementation in active ulcerative colitis: A double-blind, placebo-controlled, crossover study. American Journal of Gastroenterology, Vol. 87, April 1992, pp. 432-37
35. Salomon, P., et al. Treatment of ulcerative colitis with fish oil n-3 omega fatty acid: an open trial. Journal of Clinical Gastroenterology, Vol. 12, April 1990, pp. 157-61
36. Siguel, E.N. and Lerman, R.H. Prevalence of essential fatty acid deficiency in patients with chronic gastrointestinal disorders. Metabolism, Vol. 45, January 1996, pp. 12-23
37. Simonsen, Neal, et al. Adipose tissue omega-3 and omega-6 fatty acid content and breast cancer in the EURAMIC Study. American Journal of Epidemiology, Vol. 147, No. 4, 1998, pp. 342-52
38. Cave, W.T. Jr. Dietary omega-3 polyunsaturated fats and breast cancer. Nutrition, Vol. 12 (suppl), January 1996, pp. S39-42
39. Fernandez-Banares, F., et al. Changes of the mucosal n3 and n6 fatty acid status occur early in the colorectal adenoma-carcinoma sequence. Gut, Vol. 38, 1996, pp. 254-59
40. Anti, M., et al. Effects of different doses of fish oil on rectal cell proliferation in patients with sporadic colonic adenomas. Gastroenterology, Vol. 107, December 1994, pp. 1709-18
41. Saynor, R. and Gillott, T. Changes in blood lipids and fibrinogen with a note on safety in a long term study on the effects of n-3 fatty acids in subjects receiving fish oil supplements and followed for seven years. Lipids, Vol. 27, July 1992, pp. 533-38
42. Eritsland, Jan. Safety considerations of polyunsaturated fatty acids. American Journal of Clinical Nutrition, Vol. 71 (suppl), January 2000, pp. 197S-201S

43. Nair, Padmanabhan P., et al. Dietary fish oil-induced changes in the distribution of alpha-tocopherol, retinol, and beta-carotene in plasma, red blood cells, and platelets: modulation by vitamin E. American Journal of Clinical Nutrition, Vol. 58, July 1993, pp. 98-102
44. Sanders, T.A.B. and Hinds, Allison. The influence of a fish oil high in docosahexaenoic acid on plasma lipoprotein and vitamin E concentrations and haemostatic function in healthy male volunteers. British Journal of Nutrition, Vol. 68, July 1992, pp. 163-73

Soy Products
1. Walsh, Patrick C. and Janet Farrar Worthington. Dr. Patrick Walsh's Guide to Surviving Prostate Cancer. NY, Time Warner Books, 2001, pp: 52-56
2. Campbell's Urology, 8th edition, 2002, Saunders, Philadelphia, PA, pp. 3003-04, 3017-18
3. Gronberg, Henrik. Prostate cancer epidemiology. The Lancet, Vol. 361, March 8, 2003, pp. 859-64
4. Adlercreutz, Herman, et al. Plasma concentrations of phyto-oestrogens in Japanese men. The Lancet, Vol. 342, November 13, 1993, pp. 1209-10
5. Holzbeierlein, JM, et al. The role of soy phytoestrogens in prostate cancer. Current Opinion in Urology, Vol. 15, 2005, pp. 17-22
6. Sonoda, T, et al. A case-control study of diet and prostate cancer in Japan: possible protective effect of traditional Japanese diet. Cancer Sci, Vol. 95, March 2004, pp. 238-42
7. Jacobsen, BK, et al. Does high soy milk reduce prostate cancer incidence? The Adventist Health Study (United States). Cancer Causes and Control, Vol. 9, 1998, pp. 553-57
8. Zhou, JR, et al. Soy phytochemicals and tea bioactive components synergistically inhibit androgen-sensitive human prostate tumors in mice. Journal of Nutrition, Vol. 133, February 2003, pp. 516-21
9. Nagata, C, et al. Soy product intake and hot flashes in Japanese women: results from a community-based prospective study. American Journal of Epidemiology, Vol. 153, April 15, 2001, pp. 790-93
10. Nagata, C, et al. Decreased serum total cholesterol concentration is associated with high intake of soy products in Japanese men and women. Journal of Nutrition, Vol. 128, 1998, pp. 209-13
11. Ozasa, K, et al. Serum phytoestrogens and prostate cancer risk in a nested case-control study among Japanese men. Cancer Sci, Vol. 95, January 2004, pp. 65-71
12. Geller, J, et al. Genistein inhibits the growth of human-patient BPH and prostate cancer in histoculture. Prostate, Vol. 34, No. 2, February 1, 1998, pp. 75-79
13. Brossner, C, et al. Phytoestrogen tissue levels in benign prostatic hyperplasia and prostate cancer and their association with prostatic diseases. Urology, Vol. 64, No. 4, October 2004, pp. 707-11
14. Ishizuki, Y, et al. The effects on the thyroid gland of soybeans administered experimentally in healthy subjects. Nippon Naibunpi Gakkai Zasshi, Vol. 67, No. 5, May 20, 1991, pp. 622-29 [article in Japanese]
15. Doerge, DR and Sheehan, DM. Goitrogenic and estrogenic activity of soy isoflavones. Environ Health Perspect, Vol. 110, Suppl 3, June 2002, pp. 349-53
16. White, LR, et al. Brain aging and midlife tofu consumption. Journal of the American College of Nutrition, Vol. 19, No. 2, 2000, pp. 242-55
17. Grodstein, F, et al. Tofu and cognitive function: food for thought. Journal of the American College of Nutrition, Vol. 19, No. 2, 2000, pp. 207-09
18. Sacks, FM, et al. Soy protein, isoflavones, and cardiovascular health. Circulation, Vol. 113, February 21, 2006

Garlic, Green Tea, and Flaxseed
1. Key, TJ, et al. A case-control study of diet and prostate cancer. British Journal of Cancer, Vol. 76, No. 5, 1997, pp. 678-87
2. Fleischauer, AT and Arab, L. Garlic and cancer: a critical review of the epidemiologic literature. Journal of Nutrition, Vol. 131, 2001, pp. 1032S-40S
3. Hsing, AW, et al. Allium vegetables and risk of prostate cancer: a population-based study. Journal of the National Cancer Institute, Vol. 94, November 6, 2002, pp. 1648-51

4. Pinto, JT, et al. Effects of garlic thioallyl derivatives on growth, glutathione concentration, and polyamine formation of human prostate carcinoma cells in culture. American Journal of Clinical Nutrition, Vol. 66, August 1997, pp. 398-405

5. Heber, David. The stinking rose: organosulfur compounds and cancer. American Journal of Clinical Nutrition, Vol. 66, August 1997, pp. 425-6

6. Yu Tang Gao, JL, et al. Reduced risk of esophageal cancer associated with green tea consumption. Journal of the National Cancer Institute, Vol. 86, No. 11, June 1, 1994, pp. 855-58

7. Jian, L, et al. Protective effect of green tea against prostate cancer: a case-control study in southeast China. International Journal of Cancer, Vol. 108, January 1, 2004, pp. 130-35

8. Bettuzi, S, et al. Green tea shown to prevent prostate cancer. Presentation to the American Association for Cancer Research, April 19, 2005, Anaheim, CA
http://www.eurekalert.org/pub_releases/2005-04/aafc-gts041205.php

9. Paschka, AG, et al. Induction of apoptosis in prostate cancer cell lines by the green tea component, (-)epigallocatechin-3-gallate. Cancer Lett., Vol. 130, August 14, 1998, pp. 1-7

10. Hussain, T., et al. Green tea constituent epigallocatechin-3-gallate selectively inhibits COX-2 without affecting COX-1 expression in human prostate carcinoma cells. International Journal of Cancer, September 28, 2004

11. Adhami, VM, et al. Oral consumption of green tea polyphenols inhibits insulin-like growth factor-I-induced signalling in an autochthonous mouse model of prostate cancer. Cancer Research, Vol. 64, No. 23, December 1, 2004, pp. 8715-22

12. Liao, S and Hiipakka, RA. Selective inhibition of steroid 5 alpha-reductase isozymes by tea epicatechin-3-gallate and epigallocatechin-3-gallate. Biochem Biophys Res Commun, Vol. 214, No. 3, September 25, 1995, pp. 833-38

13. Oguri, A, et al. Inhibitory effects of antioxidants on formation of heterocyclic amines. Mutat Res, Vol. 402, No. 1-2, June 18, 1998, pp. 237-45

14. Pezzato, E., et al. Prostate carcinoma and green tea: PSA-triggered basement membrane degradation and MMP-2 activation are inhibited by (-)epigallochetchin-3-gallate. International Journal of Cancer, Vol. 112, No. 5, 2004, pp. 787-92

15. Patel, SP, et al. The protective effects of green tea in prostate cancer. BJU International, Vol. 96, No. 9, December 2005, pp. 1212-14

16. Choan, E, et al. A prospective clinical trial of green tea for hormone refractory prostate cancer: an evaluation of the complementary/alternative therapy approach. Urol Oncol, Vol. 23, No. 2, March-April 2005, pp. 108-13

17. Trevisanato, SI and Kim, YI. Tea and health. Nutrition Reviews, Vol. 58, January 2000, pp. 1-10

18. Demark-Wahnefried, W, et al. Pilot study of dietary fat restriction and flaxseed supplementation in men with prostate cancer before surgery: exploring the effects on hormonal levels, prostate-specific antigen, and histopathologic features. Urology, Vol. 58, No.1, July 2001, pp. 47-52

19. Demark-Wahnefried, W, et al. Pilot study to explore effects of low-fat, flaxseed-supplemented diet on proliferation of benign prostatic epithelium and prostate-specific antigen. Urology, Vol. 63, No. 5, 2004, pp. 900-04

Lifestyle Factors

1. Oliveria, Susan A., et al. The association between cardiorespiratory fitness and prostate cancer. Medicine & Science in Sports & Exercise, Vol. 28, January 1996, pp. 97-104

2. Giovannucci, E, et al. A prospective study of physical activity and prostate cancer in male health professionals. Cancer Research, Vol. 58, No. 22, November 15, 1998, pp. 5117-22

3. Patel, AV, et al. Recreational physical activity and risk of prostate cancer in a large cohort of US men. Cancer Epidemiology, Biomarkers and Prevention, Vol. 14, January 2005, pp. 275-79

4. Zeegers, MP, et al. Physical activity and the risk of prostate cancer in the Netherlands cohort study, results after 9.3 years of follow-up. Cancer Epidemiology, Biomarkers and Prevention, Vol. 14, June 2005, pp. 1490-95

5. Pierotti, B, et al. Lifetime physical activity and prostate cancer risk. International Journal of Cancer, Vol. 114, April 2005, pp. 639-42

6. Bairati, I, et al. Lifetime occupational physical activity and incidental prostate cancer (Canada). Cancer Causes and Control, Vol. 11, No. 8, September 2000, pp. 759-64
7. Torti, DC and Matheson, GO. Exercise and prostate cancer, Sports Medicine, Vol. 34, No. 6, 2004, pp. 363-69
8. Luscombe, CJ, et al. Exposure to ultraviolet radiation: association with susceptibility and age at presentation with prostate cancer. The Lancet, Vol. 358, August 25, 2001, pp. 641-42
9. Bodiwala, D, et al. Associations between prostate cancer susceptibility and parameters of exposure to ultraviolet radiation. Cancer Lett, Vol. 200, No. 2, October 28, 2003, pp. 141-48
10. John, EM, et al. Residential sunlight exposure is associated with a decreased risk of prostate cancer. J Steroid Biochem Mol Biol., Vol. 89-90, No. 1-5, May 2004, pp. 549-52

Vitamin A and Beta-Carotene

1. Willett, WC. Micronutrients and cancer risk. American Journal of Clinical Nutrition, Vol. 59, Suppl, May 1994, pp. 1162S-65S
2. Steck-Scott, S., et al. Carotenoids, vitamin A and risk of adenomatous polyp recurrence in the Polyp Prevention Trial. International Journal of Cancer, Vol. 112, No. 2, 2004, pp. 295-305
3. Pasquali, Daniela, et al. Abnormal level of retinoic acid in prostate cancer tissues. Journal of Clinical Endocrinology and Metabolism, Vol. 81, No. 6, June 1996, pp. 2186-91
4. Giovannucci, E., et al. Intake of carotenoids and retinol in relation to risk of prostate cancer. Journal of the National Cancer Institute, Vol. 87, December 6, 1995, pp. 1767-76
5. Andersson, SO, et al. Energy, nutrient intake and prostate cancer risk: a population-based case-control study in Sweden. International Journal of Cancer, Vol. 68, No. 6, December 11, 1996, pp. 716-22
6. Kristal, AR. Vitamin A, retinoids and carotenoids as chemopreventive agents for prostate cancer. Journal of Urology, Vol. 1171, Pt. 2, February 2004, pp. S54-S58
7. Bosetti, C, et al. Retinol, carotenoids and the risk of prostate cancer: a case-control study from Italy. International Journal of Cancer, Vol. 112, No. 4, November 20, 2004, pp. 689-92
8. West, Clive E. Meeting requirements for vitamin A. Nutrition Reviews, Vol. 58, November 2000, pp. 341-45
9. Melhus, Hakan, et al. Excessive dietary intake of vitamin A is associated with reduced bone mineral density and increased risk for hip fracture. Annuals of Internal Medicine, Vol. 19, November 15, 1998, pp. 770-78
10. Peto, R., et al. Can dietary beta-carotene materially reduce human cancer rates? Nature, Vol. 290, March 19, 1981, pp. 201-08
11. Ziegler, Regina G., et al. Carotenoid intake, vegetables, and the risk of lung cancer among white men in New Jersey. American Journal of Epidemiology, Vol. 123, No. 6, 1986, pp. 1080-93
12. Ziegler, Regina G. Vegetables, fruits, and carotenoids and the risk of cancer. American Journal of Clinical Nutrition, Vol. 53, 1991, pp. 251S-59S
13. Mayne, Susan Taylor, et al. Dietary beta carotene and lung cancer risk in U.S. nonsmokers. Journal of the National Cancer Institute, Vol. 86, No. 1, January 5, 1994, pp. 33-8
14. Ferraroni, M., et al. Selected micronutrient intake and the risk of colorectal cancer. British Journal of Cancer, Vol. 70, December 1994, pp. 1150-55
15. Yuan, J.M., et al. Diet and breast cancer in Shanghai and Tianjin, China. British Journal of Cancer, Vol. 71, June 1995, pp. 1353-58
16. Pandey, Dilip K., et al. Dietary vitamin C and beta-carotene and risk of death in middle-aged men. American Journal of Epidemiology, Vol. 142, No. 12, December 15, 1995, pp. 1269-78
17. Freudenheim, Jo L., et al. Premenopausal breast cancer risk and intake of vegetables, fruits, and related nutrients. Journal of the National Cancer Institute, Vol. 88, No. 6, March 20, 1996, pp. 340-48
18. Menkes, Marilyn S., et al. Serum beta-carotene, vitamins A and E, selenium, and the risk of lung cancer. The New England Journal of Medicine, Vol. 315, No. 20, November 13, 1986, pp. 1250-54
19. Diplock, Anthony T. Antioxidant nutrients and disease prevention: an overview. American Journal of Clinical Nutrition, Vol. 53, 1991, pp. 189S-93S

20. Stahelin, Hannes B., et al. Plasma antioxidant vitamins and subsequent cancer mortality in the 12-year follow-up of the prospective Basel study. American Journal of Epidemiology, Vol. 133, No. 8, 1991, pp. 766-75

21. Kardinaal, A.F.M., et al. Antioxidant in adipose tissue and risk of myocardial infarction: the EURAMIC study. The Lancet, Vol. 342, December 4, 1993, pp. 1379-84

22. Street, Debra A., et al. Serum antioxidants and myocardial infarction. Circulation, Vol. 90, No. 3, September 1994, pp. 1154-61

23. Morris, Dexter L., et al. Serum carotenoids and coronary heart disease. Journal of the American Medical Association, Vol. 272, No. 18, November 9, 1994, pp. 1439-41

24. Ames, Bruce N. Dietary carcinogens and anticarcinogens. Science, Vol. 221, September 23, 1983, pp. 1256-64

25. Burton, G.W. and Ingold, K.U. Beta-carotene: an unusual type of lipid antioxidant. Science, Vol. 224, May 11, 1984, pp. 569-73

26. Halliwell, Barry. Free radicals and antioxidants: a personal view. Nutrition Reviews, Vol. 52, No. 8, August 1994, pp. 253-65

27. Frei, Balz. Reactive oxygen species and antioxidant vitamins: mechanisms of action. American Journal of Medicine, Vol. 97 (suppl 3A), September 26, 1994, pp. 5S-13S

28. Halliwell, Barry. Free radicals, antioxidants, and human disease: curiosity, cause, or consequence? The Lancet, Vol. 344, September 10, 1994, pp. 721-24

29. Cerutti, Peter A. Oxy-radicals and cancer. The Lancet, Vol. 344, September 24, 1994, pp. 862-63

30. Tribble, Diane L. and Frank, Erica. Dietary antioxidants, cancer, and atherosclerotic heart disease. Western Journal of Medicine, Vol. 161, No. 6, December 1994, pp. 605-13

31. Sies, Helmut and Stahl, Wilhelm. Vitamins E and C, beta-carotene, and other carotenoids as antioxidants. American Journal of Clinical Nutrition, Vol. 62 (suppl), 1995, pp. 1315S-21S

32. Hankinson, Susan E. and Stampfer, Meir J. All that glitters is not beta carotene. Journal of the American Medical Association, Vol. 272, No. 18, November 9, 1994, pp. 1455- 56

33. Johnson, Elizabeth J., et al. Relation between beta-carotene intake and plasma and adipose tissue concentrations of carotenoids and retinoids. American Journal of Clinical Nutrition, Vol. 62, September 1995, pp. 598-603

34. Khachik, F., et al. Lutein, lycopene, and their oxidative metalbolites in chemoprevention of cancer. Journal of Cellular Biochemistry, Vol. 22 (suppl), 1995, pp. 236-46

35. Di Mascio, Paolo, et al. Lycopene as the most efficient biological carotenoid singlet oxygen quencher. Archives of Biochemistry and Biophysics, Vol. 274, No. 2, November 1, 1989, pp. 532-38

36. Niki, Etsuo, et al. Interaction among vitamin C, vitamin E, and beta-carotene. American Journal of Clinical Nutrition, Vol. 62 (suppl), 1995, pp. 1322S-26S

37. Gaziano, J. Michael, et al. Discrimination in absorption or transport of beta- carotene isomers after oral supplementation with either all-trans- or 9-cis-beta-carotene. American Journal of Clinical Nutrition, Vol. 61, 1995, pp. 1248-52

38. Handelman, Garry J., et al. Destruction of tocopherols, carotenoids, and retinol in human plasma by cigarette smoke. American Journal of Clinical Nutrition, Vol. 63, April 1996, pp. 559-65

39. Ben-Amotz, Ami and Levy, Yishai. Bioavailability of a natural isomer mixture compared with synthetic all-trans beta-carotene in human serum. American Journal of Clinical Nutrition, Vol. 63, No. 5, May 1996, pp. 729-34

40. Heinonen, Olli P. and Albanes, Demetrius. The effect of vitamin E and beta carotene on the incidence of lung cancer and other cancers in male smokers. The New England Journal of Medicine, Vol. 330, April 14, 1994, pp. 1029-35

41. Smigel, Kara. Beta carotene fails to prevent cancer in two major studies; CARET intervention stopped. Journal of the National Cancer Institute, Vol. 88, No. 3/4, February 21, 1996, p. 145

42. Omenn, Gilbert S., et al. Effects of a combination of beta carotene and vitamin A on lung cancer and cardiovascular disease. The New England Journal of Medicine, Vol. 334, May 2, 1996, pp. 1150-55

43. Hennekens, Charles H., et al. Lack of effect of long-term supplementation with beta carotene on the incidence of malignant neoplasms and cardiovascular disease. The New England Journal of Medicine, Vol. 334, May 2, 1996, pp. 1145-49

44. Wu, K., et al. Plasma and dietary carotenoids, and the risk of prostate cancer: a nested case-control study. Cancer Epidemiol Biomarkers Prev., Vol. 13, February 2004, pp. 260-69

45. Subar, Amy F., et al. Fruit and vegetable intake in the United States. American Journal of Health Promotion, Vol. 9, May/June 1995, pp. 352-60

46. Martin, Simon. Is this the most powerful antioxidant yet found? International Journal of Alternative and Complementary Medicine, Vol. 14, No. 5, May 1996, pp. 11-12

B-Vitamins and Vitamin C

1. Pelucchi, C, et al. Dietary folate and risk of prostate cancer in Italy. Cancer Epidemiology, Biomarkers and Prevention, Vol. 14, April 2005, pp. 944-98

2. Hultdin, J, et al. Plasma folate, vitamin B12, and homocysteine and prostate cancer risk: a prospective study. International Journal of Cancer, Vol. 113, No. 5, February 20, 2005, pp. 819-24

3. Kim, YI. Will mandatory folic acid fortification prevent or promote cancer? American Journal of Clinical Nutrition, Vol. 80, November 2004, pp. 1123-28

4. Block, Gladys. Vitamin C and cancer prevention: the epidemiologic evidence. American Journal of Clinical Nutrition, Vol. 53, 1991, pp. 270S-82S

5. Block, Gladys. Vitamin C, cancer and aging. Age and Ageing, Vol. 16, 1993, pp. 55-58

6. Howe, GR, et al. Dietary factors and risk of breast cancer: combined analysis of 12 case control studies. Journal of the National Cancer Institute, Vol. 82, 1990, pp. 561-69

7. Wassertheil-Smoller, S, et al. Dietary vitamin C and uterine cervical dysplasia. American Journal of Epidemiology, Vol. 114, 1981, pp. 714-24

8. Romney, S, et al. Plasma vitamin C and uterine cervical dysplasia. American Journal of Obstetrics and Gynaecology, Vol. 151, 1985, pp. 978-80

9. Schiffman, MH. Diet and faecal genotoxicity, Cancer Surv., Vol. 6, 1987, pp. 653-672

10. Block, Gladys. The data support a role for antioxidants in reducing cancer risk. Nutrition Review, Vol. 50, July 1992, pp. 207-13

11. Frei, Balz. Reactive oxygen species and antioxidant vitamins: mechanisms of action. American Journal of Medicine, Vol. 97, Suppl. 3A, September 26, 1994, pp. 5S-13S

12. Block, Gladys. Epidemiologic evidence regarding vitamin C and cancer. American Journal of Clinical Nutrition, Vol. 54, December 1991, pp. 1310S-14S

13. Uddin, S. and Ahmad, S. Antioxidants protection against cancer and other human diseases. Comprehensive Therapy, Vol. 21, No. 1, 1995, pp. 41-45

14. Block, Gladys. Micronutrients and cancer: Time for action? Journal of the National Cancer Institute, Vol. 85, No. 11, June 2, 1993, pp. 846-47

15. Ferraroni, M, et al. Selected micronutrient intake and the risk of colorectal cancer. British Journal of Cancer, Vol. 70, December 1994, pp. 1150-55

16. Stahelin, H.B., et al. Plasma antioxidant vitamins and subsequent cancer mortality in the 12-year follow-up of the prospective Basel Study. American Journal of Epidemiology, Vol. 133, No. 8, April 15, 1991, pp. 766-75

17. Blot, William J., et al. Nutrition intervention trials in Linxian, China: Supplementation with specific vitamin/mineral combinations, cancer incidence, and disease-specific mortality in the general population. Journal of the National Cancer Institute, Vol. 85, No. 18, September 15, 1993, pp. 1483-91

18. Blot, William J., et al. Lung cancer and vitamin supplementation. New England Journal of Medicine, Vol. 331, No. 9, September 1, 1994, p. 614

19. Han, Jui. Highlights of the cancer chemoprevention studies in China. Preventive Medicine, Vol. 22, September 1993, pp. 712-22

20. Loria, CM, et al. Vitamin C status and mortality in US adults. American Journal of Clinical Nutrition, Vol. 72, July 2000, pp. 139-45

21. Khaw, KT, et al. Relation between plasma ascorbic acid and mortality in men and women in EPIC-Norfolk prospective study. The Lancet, Vol. 357, March 3, 2001, pp. 657-63

22. Daviglus, ML, et al. Dietary beta-carotene, vitamin C, and risk of prostate cancer: results from the Western Electric Study. Epidemiology, Vol. 7, No. 5, September 1996, pp. 472-77

23. Huang, HY, et al. Prospective study of antioxidant micronutrients in the blood and the risk of developing prostate cancer. American Journal of Epidemiology, Vol. 157, February 15, 2003, pp. 335-44

24. Kristal, AR, et al. Vitamin and mineral supplement use is associated with reduced risk of prostate cancer. Cancer Epidemiology, Biomarkers and Prevention, Vol. 8, October 1999, pp. 887-92

25. Berndt, SI, et al. Prediagnostic plasma vitamin C levels and the subsequent risk of prostate cancer. Nutrition, Vol. 21, June 2005, pp. 686-90

26. Deneo-Pellegrini, H., et al. Foods, nutrients and prostate cancer: a case-control study in Uruguay. British Journal of Cancer, Vol. 80, No. ¾, May 1999, pp. 591-97

27. Cameron, Ewan and Linus Pauling. Cancer and Vitamin C. Camino Books, Philadelphia, PA, 1993

28. Jamison, JM, et al. Evaluation of the invitro and in vivo antitumor activities of vitamin C and K-3 combination against human prostate cancer. Journal of Nutrition (American Society for Nutritional Sciences), Vol. 131, 2001, pp. 158S-60S

29. Levine, Mark, et al. Determination of optimal vitamin C requirements in humans. American Journal of Clinical Nutrition, Vol. 62, 1995, pp. 1347S-56S

30. Levine, Mark, et al. Vitamin C pharmacokinetics in healthy volunteers: Evidence for a recommended dietary allowance. Proceedings of the National Academy of Sciences USA, Vol. 93, No. 8, April 16, 1996, pp. 3704-09

31. Bruemmer,B, et al. Nutrient intake in relation to bladder cancer among middle-aged men and women. American Journal of Epidemiology, Vol. 144, No. 5, September 1, 1996, pp. 485-95

32. Malins, DC, et al. Progression of human breast cancers to the metastatic state is linked to hydroxyl radical-induced DNA damage. Proceedings of the National Academy of Sciences USA, Vol. 93, No. 6, March 19, 1996, pp. 2557-63

33. DeCosse, JJ, et al. Surgical and medical measures in prevention of large bowel cancer. Cancer, Vol. 40, November 1977, pp. 2549-52

34. Schwartz, JL. The dual roles of nutrients as antioxidants and pooxidants: their effects on tumor cell growth. Journal of Nutrition, Vol. 126, April 1996, pp. 1221S-27S

35. Voelker, Rebecca. Recommendations for antioxidants: How much evidence is enough? Journal of the American Medical Association, Vol. 271, No. 15, April 20, 1994, pp. 1148-49

36. Diplock, Anthony T. Safety of antioxidant vitamins and beta-carotene. American Journal of Clinical Nutrition, Vol. 62, December 1995, pp. 1510S-16S

37. Meyers, David G., et al. Safety of antioxidant vitamins. Archives of Internal Medicine, Vol. 156, May 13, 1996, pp. 925-35

38. Institute of Medicine.
    http://www4.nationalacademies.org/news.nsf/isbn/0309069351?OpenDocument

Vitamin D

1. Stewart, LV and Weigel, NL. Vitamin D and prostate cancer. Experimental Biology and Medicine, Vol. 229, 2004, pp. 277-84

2. Chen, TC and Holick, MF. Vitamin D and prostate cancer prevention and treatment. Trends in Endocrinol. Metab, Vol. 14, No. 9, November 2003, pp. 423-30

3. Gross, C, et al. Treatment of early recurrent prostate cancer with 1,25-dihydroxyvitamin D3 (calcitriol). Journal of Urology, Vol. 159, June 1998, pp. 2035-40

4. Beer, TM and Myrthue, A. Calcitriol in cancer treatment: From the lab to the clinic. Molecular Cancer Therapeutics, Vol. 3, No. 3, 2004, pp. 373-81

5. Gavrilov, V, et al. The combined treatment of 1,25-dihydroxyvitamin D3 and a non-steroid anti-inflammatory drug is highly effective in suppressing prostate cancer cell line (LNCaP) growth. Anticancer Research, Vol. 25, No. 5, September-October 2005, pp. 3425-29

6. Beer, TM, et al. Rationale for the development and current status of calcitriol in androgen-independent prostate cancer. World Journal of Urology, Vol. 23, No. 1, February 2005, pp. 28-32

7. Vieth, Reinhold. Vitamin D supplementation, 25-hydroxyvitamin D concentrations, and safety. American Journal of Clinical Nutrition, Vol. 69, May 1999, pp. 842-56

8. Heaney, Robert P. Lessons for nutritional science from vitamin D. American Journal of Clinical Nutrition, Vol. 69, May 1999, p. 825 (editorial)

Vitamin E

1. Eichholzer, M, et al. Prediction of male cancer mortality by plasma levels of interacting vitamins. International Journal of Cancer, Vol. 66, No. 2, April 10, 1996, pp. 145-50
2. Heinonen, OP, et al. Prostate cancer and supplementation with alpha-tocopherol and beta-carotene. Journal of the National Cancer Institute, Vol. 90, No. 6, March 18, 1998, pp. 440-46
3. Chan, JM, et al. Supplemental vitamin E intake and prostate cancer risk in a large cohort of men in the United States. Cancer Epidemiology, Biomarkers & Prevention, Vol. 8, No. 10, October 1999, pp. 893-99
4. Kristal, AR, et al. Vitamin and mineral supplement use is associated with reduced risk of prostate cancer. Cancer Epidemiology, Biomarkers & Prevention, Vol. 8, No. 10, October 1999, pp. 887-92
5. Helzlsouer, KJ, et al. Association between alpha-tocopherol, gamma-tocopherol, selenium, and subsequent prostate cancer. Journal of the National Cancer Institute, Vol. 92, No. 24, December 20, 2000, pp. 2018-23
6. Galli, F, et al. The effect of alpha- and gamma-tocopherol and their carboxyethyl hydroxychroman metabolites on prostate cancer cell proliferation. Arch Biochem Biophys, Vol. 423, No. 1, March 1, 2004, pp. 97-102
7. Jiang, Q, et al. Gamma-tocopherol induces apoptosis in androgen-responsive LNCaP prostate cancer cells via caspases-dependent and independent mechanisms. Annals of the New York Academy of Sciences, No. 1031, December 2004, pp. 399-400
8. Burton, Graham W., et al. Human plasma and tissue alpha-tocopherol concentrations in response to supplementation with deuterated natural and synthetic vitamin E. American Journal of Clinical Nutrition, Vol. 67, 1998, pp. 669-84
9. Jiang, Qing, et al. Gamma-tocopherol, the major form of vitamin E in the US diet, deserves more attention. American Journal of Clinical Nutrition, Vol. 74, December 2001, pp. 714-22
10. Packer, Lester. Protective role of vitamin E in biological systems. American Journal of Clinical Nutrition, Vol. 53 (suppl), 1991, pp. 1050S-55S
11. Jiang, Qing, et al. Gamma-tocopherol and its major metabolite, in contrast to alpha-tocopherol, inhibit cyclooxygenase activity in macrophages and epithelial cells. Proceedings of the National Academy of Sciences USA, Vol. 97, No. 21, October 10, 2000, pp. 11494-99
12. Cooney, Robert V., et al. Gamma-tocopherol detoxification of nitrogen dioxide: superiority to alpha-tocopherol. Proceedings of the National Academy of Sciences USA, Vol. 90, March 1993, pp. 1771-75
13. Christen, Stephan, et al. Gamma-tocopherol traps mutagenic electrophiles such as NOx and complements alpha-tocopherol: physiological implications. Proceedings of the National Academy of Sciences USA, Vol. 94, April 1997, pp. 3217-22
14. Helzlsouer, Kathy J., et al. Association between alpha-tocopherol, gamma-tocopherol, selenium, and subsequent prostate cancer. Journal of the National Cancer Institute, Vol. 92, No. 24, December 20, 2000, pp. 2018-23
15. Ford, Earl S. and Sowell, Anne. Serum alpha-tocopherol status in the United States population: findings from the Third National Health and Nutrition Examination Survey. American Journal of Epidemiology, Vol. 150, August 1, 1999, pp. 290-300
16. Handelman, Garry J., et al. Human adipose alpha-tocopherol and gamma-tocopherol kinetics during and after 1 year of alpha-tocopherol supplementation. American Journal of Clinical Nutrition, Vol. 59, 1994, pp. 1025-32
17. Burton, G.W. et al. (1988) Comparison of Free Alpha-tocopherol and Alpha- tocopheryl Acetate as Sources of Vitamin E in Rats and Humans. LIPIDS 23: 834-40
18. Horwitt, M.K. (1974) Status of human requirements for vitamin E. Am. J. Clin. Nutr. 27: 1182-93
19. Zhang, Y, et al. Vitamin E succinate inhibits the function of androgen receptor and the expression of prostate-specific antigen in prostate cancer cells. Proceedings of the National Academy of Sciences USA, Vol. 99, No. 11, May 28, 2002, pp. 7408-13

20. Zhang, M, et al. RRR-alpha-tocopheryl succinate inhibits human prostate cancer cell invasiveness. Oncogene, Vol. 23, No. 17, April 15, 2004, pp. 3080-88
21. Yu, A, et al. Vitamin E and the Y4 agonist BA-129 decrease prostate cancer growth and production of vascular endothelial growth factor. J. Surg Res, Vol. 105, No. 1, June 1, 2002, pp. 65-68
22. Prasad, KN, et al. Alpha-tocopheryl succinate, the most effective form of vitamin E for adjuvant cancer treatment: a review. Journal of the American College of Nutrition, Vol. 22, No. 2, 2003, pp. 108-17
23. Lippman, SM, et al. Designing the Selenium and Vitamin E Cancer Prevention Trial (SELECT). Journal of the National Cancer Institute, Vol. 97, January 19, 2005, pp. 94-102
24. Russell, RM. New micronutrient dietary reference intakes from the National Academy of Sciences. Nutrition Today, Vol. 36, May/June 2001, pp. 163-71

Coenzyme Q10 and Alpha-Lipoic Acid
1. Greenberg, Steven and Frishman, William H. Co-enzyme Q10: A new drug for cardiovascular disease. Journal of Clinical Pharmacology, Vol. 30, 1990, pp. 596-608
2. Lockwood, K., et al. Partial and complete regression of breast cancer in patients in relation to dosage of coenzyme Q10. Biochemical and Biophysical Research Communications, Vol. 199, 1994, pp. 1504-08
3. Lockwood, K, et al. Apparent partial remission of breast cancer in high risk patients supplemented with nutritional antioxidants, essential fatty acids and coenzyme Q10. Mol Aspects Med, Vol. 15 (suppl), 1994, pp. S231-S240
4. Lockwood, K, et al. Progress on therapy of breast cancer with vitamin Q10 and the regression of metastases. Biochem Biophys Res Commun, Vol. 212, No. 1, July 6, 1995, pp. 172-77
5. Judy, W.V., et al. Coenzyme Q10 reduction of adriamycin cardiotoxicity. In Biomedical and Clinical Aspects of Coenzyme Q, Vol. 4, eds. Folkers, K. and Yamamura, Y., Amsterdam, Elsevier, 1984, pp. 231-41
6. Portakal, O., et al. Coenzyme Q10 concentrations and antioxidant status in tissues of breast cancer patients. Clin Biochem, Vol. 33, No. 4, June 2000, pp. 279-84
7. Quiles, JL, et al. Coenzyme Q differentially modulates phospholipid hydroperoxide glutathione peroxidase gene expression and free radicals production in malignant and non-malignant prostate cells. Biofactors, Vol. 18, No. 1-4, 2003, pp. 265-70
8. Larsen, HR. Coenzyme Q10 – The Wonder Nutrient. International Journal of Alternative and Complementary Medicine, Vol. 16, February 1998, pp. 11-12 www.yourhealthbase.com/coenzyme_Q10.htm
9. Marincola, Rodolfo. Neurobiology and quantified pharmaco EEG of coenzyme Q10. Journal of Orthomolecular Medicine, Vol. 12, No. 2, Second Quarter, 1997, pp. 87-95
10. Murray, Michael T. Encyclopedia of Nutritional Supplements, Rocklin, CA, Prima Publishing, 1996, pp. 296-308
11. Earl Mindell's Vitamin Bible. Warner Books, NY, 1991, p. 289
12. Disease Prevention and Treatment. Life Extension Foundation, Hollywood, FL, 4th edition, 2003, p. 1377
13. Cadenas, Enrique and Packer, Lester, eds. Handbook of Antioxidants, NY, Marcel Dekker, Inc., 1996, pp. 545-91
14. Murray, Michael T. Encyclopedia of Nutritional Supplements, Rocklin, CA, Prima Publishing, 1996, pp. 343-46
15. Han, D, et al. Lipoic acid increases de novo synthesis of cellular glutathione by improving cysteine utilization. Biofactors, Vol. 6, No. 3, 1997, pp. 321-38
16. Bounous, G and Beer, D. Molecular pathogenesis and prevention of prostate cancer. Anticancer Research, Vol. 24, No. 2B, March/April 2004, pp. 553-54
17. Sen, CK and Packer, L. Thiol homeostasis and supplements in physical exercise. American Journal of Clinical Nutrition, Vol. 72 (suppl), August 2000, pp. 653S-69S

Boron and Magnesium
1. Travers, RL, et al. Boron and arthritis: the results of a double-blind pilot study. J Nutr Med, Vol. 1, 1990, pp. 127-32

2. Newnham, RE. Arthritis or skeletal fluorosis and boron. Int. Clin Nutr Rev, Vol. 11, 1991, pp. 68-70
3. Cui, Y, et al. Dietary boron intake and prostate cancer risk. Oncol Rep, Vol. 11, April 2004, pp. 887-92
4. Gallardo-Williams, MT, et al. Boron supplementation inhibits the growth and local expression of IGF-1 in human prostate adenocarcinoma (LNCaP) tumors in nude mice. Toxicol Pathol, Vol. 32, January/February 2004, pp. 73-78
5. Gallardo-Williams, MT, et al. Inhibition of the enzymatic activity of prostate-specific antigen by boric acid and 3-nitrophenyl boronic acid. The Prostate, Vol. 54, 2003, pp. 44-49
6. Murray, Michael T. Encyclopedia of Nutritional Supplements. Prima Publishing, Rocklin, CA, 1996, p.190-92
7. Yang, CY, et al. Calcium and magnesium in drinking water and risk of death from prostate cancer. J Toxicol Environ Health A., Vol. 60, No. 1, May 12, 2000, pp. 17-26
8. Klevay, L.M. and Milne, D.B. Low dietary magnesium increases supraventricular ectopy. American Journal of Clinical Nutrition, Vol. 75, March 2002, pp. 550-54
9. Firoz, M. and Graber, M. Bioavailability of US commercial magnesium preparations. Magnesium Research, Vol. 14, No. 4, December 2001, pp. 257-62
10. Martynov., A.I., et al. New approaches to the treatment of patients with idiopathic mitral valve prolapse. Ter Arkh, Vol. 72, No. 9, 2000, pp. 67-70 [English abstract of Russian article]
11. Geiss, K.R., et al. Effects of magnesium orotate on exercise tolerance in patients with coronary heart disease. Cardiovascular Drugs Therapy, Vol. 12, suppl 2, September 1998, pp. 153-56
12. Golf, S.W., et al. On the significance of magnesium in extreme physical stress. Cardiovascular Drugs Therapy, Vol. 12, Suppl 2, September 1998, pp. 197-202
13. Lindberg, J.S., et al. Magnesium bioavailability from magnesium citrate and magnesium oxide. Journal of the American College of Nutrition, Vol. 9, No. 1, February 1990, pp. 48-55
14. Lindberg, J., et al. Effect of magnesium citrate and magnesium oxide on the crystallization of calcium salts in urine: changes produced by food-magnesium interaction. Journal of Urology, Vol. 143, February 1990, pp. 248-51
15. Sabatier, M., et al. Meal effect on magnesium bioavailability from mineral water in healthy women. American Journal of Clinical Nutrition, Vol. 75, January 2002, pp. 65-71

Selenium

1. Willett, WC, et al. Prediagnostic serum selenium and risk of cancer. Lancet, July 16, 1983, pp. 130-34
2. Knekt, Paul, et al. Is low selenium status a risk factor for lung cancer? American Journal of Epidemiology, Vol. 148, November 15, 1998, pp. 975-82
3. Mark, Steven D., et al. Prospective study of serum selenium levels and incident esophageal and gastric cancers. Journal of the National Cancer Institute, Vol. 92, November 1, 2000, pp. 1753-63
4. Yoshizawa, K, et al. Study of prediagnostic selenium level in toenails and the risk of advanced prostate cancer. Journal of the National Cancer Institute, Vol. 90, No. 16, August 19, 1998, pp. 1219-24
5. Giovannucci, Edward. Selenium and risk of prostate cancer. The Lancet, Vol. 352, September 5, 1998, pp. 755-56
6. Brooks, James D., et al. Plasma selenium level before diagnosis and the risk of prostate cancer development. Journal of Urology, Vol. 166, December 2001, pp. 2034-38
7. Vogt, TM, et al. Serum selenium and risk of prostate cancer in US blacks and whites. International Journal of Cancer, Vol. 103, No. 5, February 20, 2003, pp. 664-70
8. Li, H, et al. A prospective study of plasma selenium levels and prostate cancer risk. Journal of the National Cancer Institute, Vol. 96, May 5, 2004, pp. 696-703
9. Taylor, PR, et al. Science peels the onion of selenium effects on prostate carcinogenesis. Journal of the National Cancer Institute, Vol. 96, May 5, 2004, pp. 645-47
10. van den Brandt, PA, et al. Toenail selenium levels and the subsequent risk of prostate cancer. Cancer Epidemiology, Biomarkers & Prevention, Vol. 12, September 2003, pp. 866-71

11. Combs, GF. Selenium in global food systems. British Journal of Nutrition, Vol. 85, May 2001, pp. 517-47

12. El-Bayoumy, K. The protective role of selenium on genetic damage and on cancer. Mutat Res, Vol. 475, No. 1-2, April 18, 2001, pp. 123-39

13. Oldfield, JE. Some implications of selenium for human health. Nutrition Today, July/August 1991, pp. 6-11

14. Sinha, R and El-Bayoumy, K. Apoptosis is a critical cellular event in cancer chemoprevention and chemotherapy by selenium compounds. Curr Cancer Drug Targets, Vol. 4, No. 1, February 2004, pp. 13-28

15. Clark, Larry C., et al. Effects of selenium supplementation for cancer prevention in patients with carcinoma of the skin. Journal of the American Medical Association, Vol. 276, No. 24, December 25, 1996, pp. 1957-63

16. Colditz, Graham A. Selenium and cancer prevention - promising results indicate further trials required. Journal of the American Medical Association, Vol. 276, No. 24, December 25, 1996, pp. 1984-85

17. Etminan, M, et al. Intake of selenium in the prevention of prostate cancer: a systematic review and meta-analysis. Cancer Causes and Control, Vol. 16, 2005, 1125-31

18. Kiremidjian-Schumacher, L and Roy, M. Selenium and immune function. Z Ernahrungswiss, Vol. 37, Suppl 1, 1998, pp. 50-56

19. Beck, MA, et al. Selenium deficiency and viral infection. Journal of Nutrition, Vol. 133, No. 5, Suppl 1, May 2003, pp. 1463S-67S

20. Gianduzzo, TRJ, et al. Prostatic and peripheral blood selenium levels after oral supplementation. Journal of Urology, Vol. 170, September 2003, pp. 870-73

21. Russell, RM. New micronutrient dietary reference intakes from the National Academy of Sciences. Nutrition Today, Vol. 36, May/June 2001, pp. 163-71

22. Thomson, CD, et al. Long-term supplementation with selenate and selenomethionine: selenium and glutathione peroxidase in blood components of New Zealand women. British Journal of Nutrition, Vol. 69, 1993, pp. 577-88

23. Murray, Michael T. Encyclopedia of Nutritional Supplements. Prima Publishing, Rocklin, CA, 1996, p. 223

24. Lippman, SM, et al. Designing the Selenium and Vitamin E Cancer Prevention Trial (SELECT). Journal of the National Cancer Institute, Vol. 97, January 19, 2005, pp. 94-102

Zinc

1. Russell, RM. New micronutrient dietary reference intakes from the National Academy of Sciences. Nutrition Today, Vol. 36, May/June 2001, pp. 163-71

2. Sandstead, HH. Requirement of zinc in human subjects. Journal of the American College of Nutrition, Vol. 4, No. 1, 1985, pp. 73-82

3. Costello, LC and Franklin, RB. Novel role of zinc in the regulation of prostate citrate metabolism and its implications in prostate cancer. Prostate, Vol. 35, No. 4, June 1, 1998, pp. 285-96

4. Costello, LC, et al. Zinc and prostate cancer: a critical scientific, medical, and public interest issue (USA). Cancer Causes and Control, Vol. 16, 2005, pp. 901-15

5. Tiwari, VS, et al. Comparative study of zinc levels in benign and malignant lesions of prostate. Indian Journal of Surgery, Vol. 66, No. 6, November-December 2004, pp. 352-55

6. Vartsky, D, et al. Prostatic zinc and prostate specific antigen: an experimental evaluation of their combined diagnostic value. Journal of Urology, Vol. 170, December 2003, pp. 2258-62

7. Li, XM, et al. Measurement of serum zinc improves prostate cancer detection efficiency in patients with PSA levels between 4 ng/mL and 10 ng/mL. Asian J Androl, Vol. 7, No. 3, September 2005, pp. 323-28

8. Iguchi, K, et al. Induction of necrosis by zinc in prostate carcinoma cells and identification of proteins increased in association with this induction. European Journal of Biochemistry, Vol. 253, No. 3, May 1, 1998, pp. 766-70

9. Liang, JY, et al. Inhibitory effect of zinc on human prostatic carcinoma cell growth. Prostate, Vol. 40, No. 3, August 1, 1999, pp. 200-07

10. Feng, P, et al. Effect of zinc on prostatic tumorigenicity of nude mice. Annals of the New York Academy of Sciences, No. 1010, December 2003, pp. 316-20

11. Ishii, K, et al. Evidence that the prostate-specific antigen (PSA)/Zn2+ axis may play a role in human prostate cancer cell invasion. Cancer Lett, Vol. 207, No. 1, April 15, 2004, pp. 79-87

12. Key, TJ, et al. A case-control study of diet and prostate cancer. British Journal of Cancer, Vol. 76, No. 5, 1997, pp. 678-87

13. Kristal, AR, et al. Vitamin and mineral supplement use is associated with reduced risk of prostate cancer. Cancer Epidemiology, Biomarkers and Prevention, Vol. 8, October 1999, pp. 887-92

14. Netter, A, et al. Effect of zinc administration on plasma testosterone, dihydrotestosterone, and sperm count. Arch Androl, Vol. 7, No. 1, August 1981, pp. 69-73

15. Leitzmann, MF, et al. Zinc supplement use and risk of prostate cancer. Journal of the National Cancer Institute, Vol. 95, No. 13, July 2, 2003, pp. 1004-07

16. Moyad, MA. Zinc for prostate disease and other conditions: a little evidence, a lot of hype, and a significant potential problem. Urol Nurs, Vol. 24, No. 1, February 2004, pp. 49-52

17. Encyclopedia of Natural Healing. Alive Books, Vancouver, Canada, 1998, p. 208

Plant Extracts

1. Kampa, M, et al. Wine antioxidant polyphenols inhibit the proliferation of human prostate cancer cell lines. Nutr Cancer, Vol. 37, No. 2, 2000, pp. 223-33

2. Rannikko, A, et al. Plasma and prostate phytoestrogen concentrations in prostate cancer patients after oral phytoestrogen supplementation. The Prostate, Vol. 66, 2006, pp. 82-87

3. Hong, SJ, et al. Comparative study of concentration of isoflavones and lignans in plasma and prostatic tissues of normal control and benign prostatic hyperplasia. Yonsei Medical Journal, Vol. 43, No. 2, 2002, pp. 236-41

4. Risbridger, GP, et al. The in vivo effect of red clover diet on ventral prostate growth in adult male mice. Reprod Fertil Dev, Vol. 13, No. 4, 2001, pp. 325-29

5. Jarred, RA, et al. Anti-androgenic action by red clover-derived dietary isoflavones reduces non-malignant prostate enlargement in aromatase knockout (ArKO) mice. The Prostate, Vol. 56, 2003, pp. 54-64

6. http://www.Trinovin.com

7. Wilt, TJ, et al. Saw palmetto extracts for treatment of benign prostatic hyperplasia. Journal of the American Medical Association, Vol. 280, November 11, 1998, pp. 1604-09

8. Goldmann, WH, et al. Saw palmetto berry extract inhibits cell growth and COX-2 expression in prostatic cancer cells. Cell Biol Int, Vol. 25, No. 11, 2001, pp. 1117-24

9. Hill, B and Kyprianou, N. Effect of Permixon on human prostate cell growth: lack of apoptotic action. Prostate, Vol. 61, No. 1, September 15, 2004, pp. 73-80

10. Habib, FK, et al. Serenoa repens (Permixon) inhibits the 5-alpha-reductase activity of human prostate cancer cell lines without interfering with PSA expression. International Journal of Cancer, Vol. 114, No. 2, March 20, 2005, pp. 190-94

11. Whitaker, Julian. The Prostate Report: Prevention and Healing. Phillips Publishing, Potomac, MD, 1996

12. Santa Maria Margalef, A, et al. Antimitogenic effect of Pygeum africanum extracts on human prostatic cancer cell lines and explants from benign prostatic hyperplasia. Arch Esp Urol, Vol. 56, No. 4, May 2003, pp. 369-78 [abstract only – article in Spanish]

13. Dorai, T, et al. Therapeutic potential of curcumin in human prostate cancer. I. Curcumin induces apoptosis in both androgen-dependent and androgen-independent prostate cancer cells. Prostate Cancer Prostatic Dis, Vol. 3, No. 2, August 2000, pp. 84-93

14. Dorai, T, et al. Therapeutic potential of curcumin in human prostate cancer. II. Curcumin inhibits tyrosine kinase activity of epidermal growth factor receptor and depletes the protein. Mol Urol, Vol. 4, No. 1, Spring 2000, pp. 1-6

15. Dorai, T, et al. Therapeutic potential of curcumin in human prostate cancer. III. Curcumin inhibits proliferation, induces apoptosis, and inhibits angiogenesis of LNCaP prostate cancer cells in vivo. Prostate, Vol. 47, No. 4, June 1, 2001, pp. 293-303

16. Leal, PF, et al. Functional properties of spice extracts obtained via supercritical fluid extraction. Journal of Agricultural and Food Chemistry, Vol. 51, No. 9, 2003, pp. 2520-25

17. Vimala, S., et al. Anti-tumour promoter activity in Malaysian ginger rhizobia used in traditional medicine. British Journal of Cancer, Vol. 80, No. ½, April 1999, pp. 110-16

18. Berges, RR, et al. Randomised, placebo-controlled, double-blind clinical trial of beta-sitosterol in patients with benign prostatic hyperplasia. Lancet, Vol. 345, June 17, 1995, pp. 1592-32

19. Berges, RR, et al. Treatment of symptomatic benign prostatic hyperplasia with beta-sitosterol: an 18-month follow-up. BJU International, Vol. 85, No. 7, May 2000, pp. 842-46

20. Klippel, KF, et al. A multicentric, placebo-controlled, double-blind clinical trial of beta-sitosterol (phytosterol) for the treatment of benign prostatic hyperplasia. British Journal of Urology, Vol. 80, No. 3, September 1997, pp. 427-32

21. Wilt, TJ, et al. Beta-sitosterol for the treatment of benign prostatic hyperplasia: a systematic review. BJU International, Vol. 83, No. 9, June 1999, pp. 976-83

22. Awad, AB, et al. In vitro and in vivo (SCID mice) effects of phytosterols on the growth and dissemination of human prostate cancer PC-3 cells. European Journal of Cancer Prevention, Vol. 10, No. 6, December 2001, pp. 507-13

23. von Holtz, RL, et al. Beta-sitosterol activates the sphingomyelin cycle and induces apoptosis in LNCaP human prostate cancer cells. Nutr Cancer, Vol. 32, No. 1, 1998, pp. 8-12

24. Awad, AB, et al. Effect of resveratrol and beta-sitosterol in combination on reactive oxygen species and prostaglandin release by PC-3 cells. Prostaglandins Leukot Essent Fatty Acids, Vol. 72, March 2005, pp. 219-26

25. Awad, AB, et al. Peanuts as a source of beta-sitosterol, a sterol with anticancer properties. Nutr Cancer, Vol. 36, No. 2, 2000, pp. 238-41

26. Flora, K, et al. Milk thistle (*Silybum marianum*) for the therapy of liver disease. American Journal of Gastroenterology, Vol. 93, February 1998, pp. 139-43

27. Zi, X and Agarwal, R. Silibinin decreases prostate-specific antigen with cell growth inhibition via G_1 arrest, leading to differentiation of prostate carcinoma cells: implications for prostate cancer intervention. Proceedings of the National Academy of Sciences USA, Vol. 96, June 1999, pp. 7490-95

28. Singh, RP and Agarwal, R. Prostate cancer prevention by silibinin. Current Cancer Drug Targets, Vol. 4, No. 1, February 2004, pp. 1-11

29. Singh, RP and Agarwal, R. A cancer chemopreventive agent silibinin, targets mitogenic and survival signalling in prostate cancer. Mutat Research, Vol. 555, No. 1-2, November 2004, pp. 21-32

30. Davis-Searles, PR, et al. Milk thistle and prostate cancer: differential effects of pure flavonolignans from *Silybum marianum* on antiproliferative end points in human prostate carcinoma cells. Cancer Research, Vol. 65, No. 10, May 15, 2005, pp. 4448-57

31. Deep, G, et al. Silymarin and silibinin cause G1 and G2-M cell sycle arrest via distinct circuitries in human prostate cancer PC3 cells: a comparison of flavanone silibinin with flavanolignan mixture silymarin. Oncogene, October 3, 2005 [Epub ahead of print]

32. Life Extension Foundation, http://www.lef.org

Polyphenols
1. Nair, HK, et al. Inhibition of prostate cancer cell colony formation by the flavonoid quercetin correlates with modulation of specific regulatory genes. Clin Diagn Lab Immunol, Vol. 11, January 2004, pp. 63-69

2. Murray, Michael T. Encyclopedia of Nutritional Supplements. Prima Publishing, Rocklin, CA, 1996, p. 330

3. Jang, M, et al. Cancer chemopreventive activity of resveratrol, a natural product derived from grapes. Science, Vol. 275, January 10, 1997, pp. 218-20

4. Jang, M and Pezzuto, JM. Cancer chemopreventive activity of resveratrol. Drugs Exp Clin Res, Vol. 25, No. 2-3, 1999, pp. 65-77

5. Sgambato, A, et al. Resveratrol, a natural phenolic compound, inhibits cell proliferation and prevents oxidative DNA damage. Mutat Res, Vol. 496, No. 1-2, September 20, 2001, pp. 171-80

6. Kim, YA, et al. Antiproliferative effect of resveratrol in human prostate carcinoma cells. J Med Food, Vol. 6, No. 4, Winter 2003, pp. 273-80

7. Schoonen, WM, et al. Alcohol consumption and risk of prostate cancer in middle-aged men. International Journal of Cancer, 113, No. 1, January 1, 2005, pp. 133-40

8. Damianaki, A, et al. Potent inhibitory action of red wine polyphenols on human breast cancer cells. J Cell Biochem, Vol. 78, No. 3, June 6, 2000, pp. 429-41

9. Agarwal, C, et al. Grape seed extract induces apoptotic death of human prostate carcinoma DU145 cells via caspases activation accompanied by dissipation of mitochondrial membrane potential and cytochrome C release. Carcinogenesis, Vol. 23, November 2002, pp. 1869-76

10. Singh, RP, et al. Grape seed extract inhibits advanced human prostate tumor growth and angiogenesis and upregulates insulin-like growth factor binding protein-3. International Journal of Cancer, Vol. 108, No. 5, February 20, 2004, pp. 733-40

11. Huynh, HT and Teel, RW. Selective induction of apoptosis in human mammary cancer cells (MCF-7) by pycnogenol. Anticancer Research, Vol. 20, No. 4, July-August, 2000, pp. 2417-20

Conclusion

1. Byers, T, et al. American Cancer Society guidelines on nutrition and physical activity for cancer prevention: reducing the risk of cancer with healthy food choices and physical activity. CA Cancer Journal for Clinicians, Vol. 52, No. 2, March/April 2002, pp. 92-119

CHAPTER 6 – Treatment of Localized Prostate Cancer

1. Whitmore WF, Jr., 1990. Natural history of low-stage prostatic cancer and the impact of early detection. Urol Clin North Am. 17(4):689-697.

2. Holmberg L et al., 2002. A randomized trial comparing radical prostatectomy with watchful waiting in early prostate cancer. N Engl J Med. 347(11):781-789.

3. Bill-Axelson A et al., 2005. Radical prostatectomy versus watchful waiting in early prostate cancer. N Engl J Med. 352(19):1977-1984.

4. Chodak GW, Warren KS, 2006. Watchful waiting for prostate cancer: a review article. Prostate Cancer Prostatic.Dis. 9(1):25-29.

5. Walsh PC, 2005. Radical prostatectomy versus watchful waiting in early prostate cancer. J Urol. 174(4 Pt 1):1291-1292.

6. Mitchell RE et al., 2006. Does year of radical prostatectomy independently predict outcome in prostate cancer? Urology. 67(2):368-372.

7. Nicholson PW, Harland SJ, 2002. Survival prospects after screen-detection of prostate cancer. BJU Int. 90(7):686-693.

8. Albertsen PC et al., 1995. Long-term survival among men with conservatively treated localized prostate cancer. JAMA: The Journal of the American Medical Association. 274(8):626-631.

9. Parker CC, 2003. Survival prospects after screen-detection of prostate cancer. BJU Int. 91(6):585.

10. Carter HB et al., 2002. Expectant management of nonpalpable prostate cancer with curative intent: preliminary results. J Urol. 167(3):1231-1234.

11. Walsh PC, 2002. Surgery and the reduction of mortality from prostate cancer. N Engl J Med. 347(11):839-840.

12. Choo R et al., 2002. Feasibility study: watchful waiting for localized low to intermediate grade prostate carcinoma with selective delayed intervention based on prostate specific antigen, histological and/or clinical progression. J Urol. 167(4):1664-1669.

13. Schroder FH, de Vries SH, Bangma CH, 2003. Watchful waiting in prostate cancer: review and policy proposals. BJU Int. 92(8):851-859.

14. Gann PH, Han M, 2005. The natural history of clinically localized prostate cancer. JAMA: The Journal of the American Medical Association. 293(17):2149-2151.

15. Walsh PC, 2005. 20-year outcomes following conservative management of clinically localized prostate cancer. J Urol. 174(4 Pt 1):1292-1293.

16. Johansson JE et al., 2004. Natural history of early, localized prostate cancer. JAMA: The Journal of the American Medical Association. 291(22):2713-2719.

17. Neugut AI, Grann VR, 2004. Waiting time in prostate cancer. JAMA: The Journal of the American Medical Association. 291(22):2757-2758.

18. Ohori M, Scardino PT, 2002. Localized prostate cancer. Curr Probl.Surg. 39(9):833-957.

19. Bahnson RR et al., 2000. NCCN Practice Guidelines for Prostate Cancer. Oncology (Williston.Park). 14(11A):111-119.

20. Clinical Practice Guidelines, Version 2.2005. www.nccn.org. accessed October 10, 2005 . 2005.

21. Walter LC, Covinsky KE, 2001. Cancer Screening in Elderly Patients: A Framework for Individualized Decision Making. JAMA: The Journal of the American Medical Association. 285(21):2750-2756.

22. Khan MA et al., 2004. Impact of surgical delay on long-term cancer control for clinically localized prostate cancer. J Urol. 172(5 Pt 1):1835-1839.

23. Boorjian SA et al., 2005. Does the time from biopsy to surgery affect biochemical recurrence after radical prostatectomy? BJU Int. 96(6):773-776.

24. Gwede CK et al., 2005. Treatment decision-making strategies and influences in patients with localized prostate carcinoma. Cancer. 104(7):1381-1390.

25. Allaf ME, Carter HB, 2004. Update on watchful waiting for prostate cancer. Curr Opin.Urol. 14(3):171-175.

26. Epstein JI et al., 2005. Utility of saturation biopsy to predict insignificant cancer at radical prostatectomy. Urology. 66(2):356-360.

27. Scardino PTKJ, Dr. Peter Scardino's Prostate Book. Avery/Penguin Group, New York, 2005.

28. Patel MI et al., 2004. An analysis of men with clinically localized prostate cancer who deferred definitive therapy. J Urol. 171(4):1520-1524.

29. Khatami A et al., 2003. Does initial surveillance in early prostate cancer reduce the chance of cure by radical prostatectomy?--A case control study. Scand.J Urol Nephrol. 37(3):213-217.

30. Carter CA et al., 2003. Temporarily deferred therapy (watchful waiting) for men younger than 70 years and with low-risk localized prostate cancer in the prostate-specific antigen era. Journal of Clinical Oncology. 21(21):4001-4008.

31. Harlan SR et al., 2003. Time trends and characteristics of men choosing watchful waiting for initial treatment of localized prostate cancer: results from CaPSURE. J Urol. 170(5):1804-1807.

32. Zietman AL et al., 2001. Conservative management of prostate cancer in the prostate specific antigen era: the incidence and time course of subsequent therapy. J Urol. 166(5):1702-1706.

33. Talcott JA, 2005. How could getting screened for prostate cancer hurt you? Urol Oncol. 23(5):374-375.

34. Walsh PC, Worthington Jf, Dr Patrick Walsh's Guide to Surviving Prostate Cancer. Warner Books, New York, 2001.

35. Swanson GP, Riggs MW, Earle JD, 2004. Long-term follow-up of radiotherapy for prostate cancer. International Journal of Radiation Oncology*Biology*Physics. 59(2):406-411.

36. Lepor H, 2004. Radical prostatectomy: status and opportunities for improving outcomes. Cancer Invest. 22(3):435-444.

37. Alibhai SM et al., 2005. 30-day mortality and major complications after radical prostatectomy: influence of age and comorbidity. JNCI Cancer Spectrum. 97(20):1525-1532.

38. Ward JF, Zincke H, 2003. Radical prostatectomy for the patient with locally advanced prostate cancer. Curr Urol Rep. 4(3):196-204.

39. Ohori M et al., 2004. Radical prostatectomy for carcinoma of the prostate. Mod.Pathol. 17(3):349-359.

40. Scardino PT, 2005. Continuing refinements in radical prostatectomy: more evidence that technique matters. J Urol. 173(2):338-339.

41. Ward JF et al., 2005. Radical prostatectomy for clinically advanced (cT3) prostate cancer since the advent of prostate-specific antigen testing: 15-year outcome. BJU Int. 95(6):751-756.

42. Barry MJ et al., 2001. Outcomes for men with clinically nonmetastatic prostate carcinoma managed with radical prostactectomy, external beam radiotherapy, or expectant management: a retrospective analysis. Cancer. 91(12):2302-2314.

43. Meltzer D, Egleston B, Abdalla I, 2001. Patterns of prostate cancer treatment by clinical stage and age. Am.J Public Health. 91(1):126-128.

44. Meng MV et al., 2003. Predictors of treatment after initial surveillance in men with prostate cancer: results from CaPSURE. J Urol. 170(6 Pt 1):2279-2283.

45. Yao SL, Lu-Yao G, 1999. Population-based study of relationships between hospital volume of prostatectomies, patient outcomes, and length of hospital stay. JNCI Cancer Spectrum. 91(22):1950-1956.

46. Van Poppel H, Boulanger SF, Joniau S, 2005. Quality assurance issues in radical prostatectomy. Eur.J Surg.Oncol. 31(6):650-655.

47. Birkmeyer JD et al., 2002. Hospital volume and surgical mortality in the United States. N Engl J Med. 346(15):1128-1137.

48. Begg CB, Scardino PT, 2003. Taking stock of volume-outcome studies. Journal of Clinical Oncology. 21(3):393-394.

49. Walsh PC, Marschke PL, 2002. Intussusception of the reconstructed bladder neck leads to earlier continence after radical prostatectomy. Urology. 59(6):934-938.

50. Poon M et al., 2000. Radical retropubic prostatectomy: bladder neck preservation versus reconstruction. J Urol. 163(1):194-198.

51. Gaker DL, Steel BL, 2004. Radical prostatectomy with preservation of urinary continence: pathology and long-term results. J Urol. 172(6 Pt 2):2549-2552.

52. Bianco J et al., 2003. Radical Prostatectomy with Bladder Neck Preservation: Impact of a Positive Margin. European Urology. 43(5):461-466.

53. Carlson KV, Nitti VW, 2001. Prevention and management of incontinence following radical prostatectomy. Urol Clin North Am. 28(3):595-612.

54. Kundu SD et al., 2004. Potency, continence and complications in 3,477 consecutive radical retropubic prostatectomies. J Urol. 172(6, Part 1 of 2):2227-2231.

55. Walsh PC, 2000. Radical prostatectomy for localized prostate cancer provides durable cancer control with excellent quality of life: a structured debate. J Urol. 163(6):1802-1807.

56. Lepor H, Kaci L, Xue X, 2004. Continence following radical retropubic prostatectomy using self-reporting instruments. J Urol. 171(3):1212-1215.

57. Bianco FJ, Jr., Scardino PT, Eastham JA, 2005. Radical prostatectomy: long-term cancer control and recovery of sexual and urinary function ("trifecta"). Urology. 66(5 Suppl):83-94.

58. Saranchuk JW et al., 2005. Achieving optimal outcomes after radical prostatectomy. Journal of Clinical Oncology. 23(18):4146-4151.

59. Walsh PC, 2001. Nerve grafts are rarely necessary and are unlikely to improve sexual function in men undergoing anatomic radical prostatectomy. Urology. 57(6):1020-1024.

60. Scardino PT, Kim ED, 2001. Rationale for and results of nerve grafting during radical prostatectomy. Urology. 57(6):1016-1019.

61. Han M et al., 2003. Biochemical (prostate specific antigen) recurrence probability following radical prostatectomy for clinically localized prostate cancer. J Urol. 169(2):517-523.

62. Gretzer MB et al., 2002. Substratification of stage T1C prostate cancer based on the probability of biochemical recurrence. Urology. 60(6):1034-1039.

63. Swindle P et al., 2005. Do margins matter? The prognostic significance of positive surgical margins in radical prostatectomy specimens. J Urol. 174(3):903-907.

64. Han M et al., 2004. An evaluation of the decreasing incidence of positive surgical margins in a large retropubic prostatectomy series. J Urol. 171(1):23-26.

65. Hernandez DJ et al., 2005. Radical retropubic prostatectomy. How often do experienced surgeons have positive surgical margins when there is extraprostatic extension in the region of the neurovascular bundle? J Urol. 173(2):446-449.

66. Andriole GL, 2001. Laparoscopic radical prostatectomy: CON. Urology. 58(4):506-507.

67. Bollens R et al., 2005. Laparoscopic radical prostatectomy: the learning curve. Curr Opin.Urol. 15(2):79-82.

68. Bhayani SB et al., 2004. Laparoscopic radical prostatectomy: a multi-institutional study of conversion to open surgery. Urology. 63(1):99-102.

69. Trabulsi EJ, Guillonneau B, 2005. Laparoscopic radical prostatectomy. J Urol. 173(4):1072-1079.

70. Dillenburg W et al., 2005. Laparoscopic radical prostatectomy: the value of intraoperative frozen sections. Eur.Urol. 48(4):614-621.

71. Patel VR et al., 2005. Robotic radical prostatectomy in the community setting–the learning curve and beyond: initial 200 cases. J Urol. 174(1):269-272.

72. Menon M, Shrivastava A, Tewari A, 2005. Laparoscopic radical prostatectomy: conventional and robotic. Urology. 66(5 Suppl):101-104.

73. Menon M et al., 2004. Vattikuti Institute prostatectomy, a technique of robotic radical prostatectomy for management of localized carcinoma of the prostate: experience of over 1100 cases. Urol Clin North Am. 31(4):701-717.

74. Perrotti M, Moran ME, 2005. Robotic prostatectomy outcomes. Urol Oncol. 23(5):341-345.

75. Herrell SD, Smith JA, Jr., 2005. Laparoscopic and robotic radical prostatectomy: what are the real advantages? BJU Int. 95(1):3-4.

76. Pisansky TM, 2005. External beam radiotherapy as curative treatment of prostate cancer. Mayo Clin Proc. 80(7):883-898.

77. Eng TY, Luh JY, Thomas CR, Jr., 2005. The efficacy of conventional external beam, three-dimensional conformal, intensity-modulated, particle beam radiation, and brachytherapy for localized prostate cancer. Curr Urol Rep. 6(3):194-209.

78. Zelefsky MJ et al., 1998. Dose escalation with three-dimensional conformal radiation therapy affects the outcome in prostate cancer. Int.J Radiat.Oncol Biol.Phys. 41(3):491-500.

79. Zelefsky MJ et al., 2001. High dose radiation delivered by intensity modulated conformal radiotherapy improves the outcome of localized prostate cancer. J Urol. 166(3):876-881.

80. Zelefsky MJ et al., 2002. High-dose intensity modulated radiation therapy for prostate cancer: early toxicity and biochemical outcome in 772 patients. Int.J Radiat.Oncol Biol.Phys. 53(5):1111-1116.

81. Morris DE et al., 2005. Evidence-based review of three-dimensional conformal radiotherapy for localized prostate cancer: an ASTRO outcomes initiative. Int.J Radiat.Oncol Biol.Phys. 62(1):3-19.

82. Zelefsky MJ, 2004. Three-dimensional conformal brachytherapy for prostate cancer. Curr Urol Rep. 5(3):173-178.

83. Zelefsky MJ et al., 2003. Improved conformality and decreased toxicity with intraoperative computer-optimized transperineal ultrasound-guided prostate brachytherapy. Int.J Radiat.Oncol Biol.Phys. 55(4):956-963.

84. Hollenbeck BK et al., 2004. Sexual health recovery after prostatectomy, external radiation, or brachytherapy for early stage prostate cancer. Curr Urol Rep. 5(3):212-219.

85. Miller NL, Theodorescu D, 2004. Health-related quality of life after prostate brachytherapy. BJU Int. 94(4):487-491.

86. Baxter NN et al., 2005. Increased risk of rectal cancer after prostate radiation: a population-based study. Gastroenterology. 128(4):819-824.

87. Grady WM, Russell K, 2005. Ionizing radiation and rectal cancer: victims of our own success. Gastroenterology. 128(4):1114-1117.

88. Morton GC, 2005. The emerging role of high-dose-rate brachytherapy for prostate cancer. Clin Oncol (R.Coll.Radiol.). 17(4):219-227.

89. Akimoto T et al., 2005. Acute genitourinary toxicity after high dose rate (HDR) brachytherapy combined with hypofractionated external-beam radiation therapy for localized prostate cancer: Second analysis to determine the correlation between the urethral dose in HDR brachytherapy and the severity of acute genitourinary toxicity. Int.J Radiat.Oncol Biol.Phys. 63(2):472-478.

90. Mahmoudieh A et al., 2005. Anatomy-based inverse planning dose optimization in HDR prostate implant: a toxicity study. Radiother.Oncol. 75(3):318-324.

91. Pinkawa M et al., 2005. Dose-volume impact in high-dose-rate Iridium-192 brachytherapy as a boost to external beam radiotherapy for localized prostate cancer- a phase II study. Radiother.Oncol.

92. Martin T et al., 2004. 3-D conformal HDR brachytherapy as monotherapy for localized prostate cancer. A pilot study. Strahlenther.Onkol. 180(4):225-232.

93. Galalae RM et al., 2004. Long-term outcome by risk factors using conformal high-dose-rate brachytherapy (HDR-BT) boost with or without neoadjuvant androgen suppression for localized prostate cancer. Int.J Radiat.Oncol Biol.Phys. 58(4):1048-1055.

94. Astrom L et al., 2005. Long-term outcome of high dose rate brachytherapy in radiotherapy of localised prostate cancer. Radiother.Oncol. 74(2):157-161.

95. Deger S et al., 2005. High dose rate (HDR) brachytherapy with conformal radiation therapy for localized prostate cancer. Eur.Urol. 47(4):441-448.

96. Sathya JR et al., 2005. Randomized trial comparing iridium implant plus external-beam radiation therapy with external-beam radiation therapy alone in node-negative locally advanced cancer of the prostate. Journal of Clinical Oncology. 23(6):1192-1199.
97. Brenner DJ et al., 2002. Direct evidence that prostate tumors show high sensitivity to fractionation (low alpha/beta ratio), similar to late-responding normal tissue. Int.J Radiat.Oncol Biol.Phys. 52(1):6-13.
98. Vicini FA et al., 2003. The role of high-dose rate brachytherapy in locally advanced prostate cancer. Semin.Radiat.Oncol. 13(2):98-108.
99. Vicini F et al., 2003. High dose rate brachytherapy in the treatment of prostate cancer. World J Urol. 21(4):220-228.
100. Grills IS et al., 2004. High dose rate brachytherapy as prostate cancer monotherapy reduces toxicity compared to low dose rate palladium seeds. J Urol. 171(3):1098-1104.
101. Cooperberg MR et al., 2004. The changing face of low-risk prostate cancer: trends in clinical presentation and primary management. Journal of Clinical Oncology. 22(11):2141-2149.
102. Akaza H et al., 2004. Characteristics of Patients with Prostate Cancer Who Have Initially been Treated by Hormone Therapy in Japan: J-CaP Surveillance. Japanese Journal of Clinical Oncology. 34(6):329-336.
103. Chodak GW, Keane T, Klotz L, 2002. Critical evaluation of hormonal therapy for carcinoma of the prostate. Urology. 60(2):201-208.
104. Janoff DM et al., 2005. Clinical outcomes of androgen deprivation as the sole therapy for localized and locally advanced prostate cancer. BJU Int. 96(4):503-507.
105. Aus G et al., 2005. EAU guidelines on prostate cancer. Eur.Urol. 48(4):546-551.
106. Merrick GS, Wallner KE, Butler WM, 2005. Prostate cryotherapy: more questions than answers. Urology. 66(1):9-15.
107. Long JP et al., 2001. Five-year retrospective, multi-institutional pooled analysis of cancer-related outcomes after cryosurgical ablation of the prostate. Urology. 57(3):518-523.
108. Pareek G, Nakada SY, 2005. The current role of cryotherapy for renal and prostate tumors. Urol Oncol. 23(5):361-366.
109. Vestal JC, 2005. Critical review of the efficacy and safety of cryotherapy of the prostate. Curr Urol Rep. 6(3):190-193.
110. Bahn DK et al., 2002. Targeted cryoablation of the prostate: 7-year outcomes in the primary treatment of prostate cancer. Urology. 60(2 Suppl 1):3-11.
111. Donnelly BJ et al., 2002. Prospective trial of cryosurgical ablation of the prostate: five-year results. Urology. 60(4):645-649.
112. Izawa JI et al., 2003. Incomplete glandular ablation after salvage cryotherapy for recurrent prostate cancer after radiotherapy. Int.J Radiat.Oncol Biol.Phys. 56(2):468-472.
113. Shuman BA et al., 1997. Histological presence of viable prostatic glands on routine biopsy following cryosurgical ablation of the prostate. J Urol. 157(2):552-555.

CHAPTER 7 – Treatment of Residual, Recurrent and Advanced Prostate Cancer

1. Pound CR et al., 1999. Natural History of Progression After PSA Elevation Following Radical Prostatectomy. JAMA: The Journal of the American Medical Association. 281(17):1591-1597.
2. Swindle PW, Kattan MW, Scardino PT, 2003. Markers and meaning of primary treatment failure. Urol Clin North Am. 30(2):377-401.
3. Freedland SJ et al., 2005. Risk of prostate cancer-specific mortality following biochemical recurrence after radical prostatectomy. JAMA: The Journal of the American Medical Association. 294(4):433-439.
4. Freedland SJ et al., 2003. Defining the ideal cutpoint for determining PSA recurrence after radical prostatectomy. Prostate-specific antigen. Urology. 61(2):365-369.
5. Shen S et al., 2005. Ultrasensitive serum prostate specific antigen nadir accurately predicts the risk of early relapse after radical prostatectomy. J Urol. 173(3):777-780.
6. Doherty AP et al., 2000. Undetectable ultrasensitive PSA after radical prostatectomy for prostate cancer predicts relapse-free survival. Br.J Cancer. 83(11):1432-1436.
7. Ellis WJ et al., 1997. Early detection of recurrent prostate cancer with an ultrasensitive chemiluminescent prostate-specific antigen assay. Urology. 50(4):573-579.

8. Vassilikos EJ et al., 2000. Relapse and cure rates of prostate cancer patients after radical prostatectomy and 5 years of follow-up. Clin Biochem. 33(2):115-123.

9. Ward JF, Moul JW, 2005. Biochemical recurrence after definitive prostate cancer therapy. Part I: defining and localizing biochemical recurrence of prostate cancer. Curr Opin.Urol. 15(3):181-186.

10. Djavan B et al., 2003. PSA progression following radical prostatectomy and radiation therapy: new standards in the new Millennium. Eur.Urol. 43(1):12-27.

11. Scardino PTKJ, Dr. Peter Scardino's Prostate Book. Avery/Penguin Group, New York, 2005.

12. Thames H et al., 2003. Comparison of alternative biochemical failure definitions based on clinical outcome in 4839 prostate cancer patients treated by external beam radiotherapy between 1986 and 1995. Int.J Radiat.Oncol Biol.Phys. 57(4):929-943.

13. Hanlon AL, Diratzouian H, Hanks GE, 2002. Posttreatment prostate-specific antigen nadir highly predictive of distant failure and death from prostate cancer. Int.J Radiat.Oncol Biol.Phys. 53(2):297-303.

14. Ray ME et al., 2005. PSA nadir predicts biochemical and distant failures after external beam radiotherapy for prostate cancer: A multi-institutional analysis. Int.J Radiat.Oncol Biol.Phys.

15. DeWitt KD et al., 2003. What does postradiotherapy PSA nadir tell us about freedom from PSA failure and progression-free survival in patients with low and intermediate-risk localized prostate cancer? Urology. 62(3):492-496.

16. Wallner K et al., 2005. 20 Gy versus 44 Gy supplemental beam radiation with Pd-103 prostate brachytherapy: preliminary biochemical outcomes from a prospective randomized multi-center trial. Radiother.Oncol. 75(3):307-310.

17. Ragde H et al., 2000. Modern prostate brachytherapy. Prostate specific antigen results in 219 patients with up to 12 years of observed follow-up. Cancer. 89(1):135-141.

18. Davis BJ, Pisansky TM, Leibovich BC, 2003. Adjuvant external radiation therapy following radical prostatectomy for node-negative prostate cancer. Curr Opin.Urol. 13(2):117-122.

19. Skinner EC, Glode LM, 2003. High-risk localized prostate cancer: primary surgery and adjuvant therapy. Urol Oncol. 21(3):219-227.

20. Gomella LG, Zeltser I, Valicenti RK, 2003. Use of neoadjuvant and adjuvant therapy to prevent or delay recurrence of prostate cancer in patients undergoing surgical treatment for prostate cancer. Urology. 62 Suppl 1:46-54.

21. Bolla M et al., 2005. Postoperative radiotherapy after radical prostatectomy: a randomised controlled trial (EORTC trial 22911). Lancet. 366(9485):572-578.

22. Hocht S, Hinkelbein W, 2005. Postoperative radiotherapy for prostate cancer. Lancet. 366(9485):524-525.

23. Vargas C et al., 2005. Improved biochemical outcome with adjuvant radiotherapy after radical prostatectomy for prostate cancer with poor pathologic features. Int.J Radiat.Oncol Biol.Phys. 61(3):714-724.

24. Tsien C et al., 2003. Long-term results of three-dimensional conformal adjuvant and salvage radiotherapy after radical prostatectomy. Urology. 62(1):93-98.

25. Taylor N et al., 2003. Adjuvant and salvage radiotherapy after radical prostatectomy for prostate cancer. Int.J Radiat.Oncol Biol.Phys. 56(3):755-763.

26. Kalapurakal JA et al., 2002. Biochemical disease-free survival following adjuvant and salvage irradiation after radical prostatectomy. Int.J Radiat.Oncol Biol.Phys. 54(4):1047-1054.

27. Catton C et al., 2001. Adjuvant and salvage radiation therapy after radical prostatectomy for adenocarcinoma of the prostate. Radiother.Oncol. 59(1):51-60.

28. Eggener SE et al., 2005. Contemporary survival results and the role of radiation therapy in patients with node negative seminal vesicle invasion following radical prostatectomy. J Urol. 173(4):1150-1155.

29. Stephenson AJ et al., 2004. Salvage radiotherapy for recurrent prostate cancer after radical prostatectomy. JAMA: The Journal of the American Medical Association. 291(11):1325-1332.

30. Hayes SB, Pollack A, 2005. Parameters for treatment decisions for salvage radiation therapy. Journal of Clinical Oncology. 23(32):8204-8211.

31. Khan MA, Partin AW, 2004. Management of patients with an increasing prostate-specific antigen after radical prostatectomy. Curr Urol Rep. 5(3):179-187.

32. Ward JF, Moul JW, 2005. Biochemical recurrence after definitive prostate cancer therapy. Part II: treatment strategies for biochemical recurrence of prostate cancer. Curr Opin.Urol. 15(3):187-195.

33. Ryan CJ, Small EJ, 2005. Progress in detection and treatment of prostate cancer. Curr Opin.Oncol. 17(3):257-260.

34. Macdonald OK, Schild SE, 2004. Radiotherapy for a rising PSA following radical prostatectomy. Urol Oncol. 22(1):57-61.

35. Brooks JP et al., 2005. Long-term salvage radiotherapy outcome after radical prostatectomy and relapse predictors. J Urol. 174(6):2204-2208.

36. Cheung R et al., 2005. Outcome of salvage radiotherapy for biochemical failure after radical prostatectomy with or without hormonal therapy. Int.J Radiat.Oncol Biol.Phys. 63(1):134-140.

37. Patel R et al., 2005. Prostate-specific antigen velocity accurately predicts response to salvage radiotherapy in men with biochemical relapse after radical prostatectomy. Urology. 65(5):942-946.

38. Jemal A et al., 2005. Cancer statistics, 2005. CA Cancer J Clin. 55(1):10-30.

39. Lee WR, Hanks GE, Hanlon A, 1997. Increasing prostate-specific antigen profile following definitive radiation therapy for localized prostate cancer: clinical observations. Journal of Clinical Oncology. 15(1):230-238.

40. Stephenson AJ, Eastham JA, 2005. Role of Salvage Radical Prostatectomy for Recurrent Prostate Cancer After Radiation Therapy. Journal of Clinical Oncology. 23(32):8198-8203.

41. Eastham JA, DiBlasio CJ, Scardino PT, 2003. Salvage radical prostatectomy for recurrence of prostate cancer after radiation therapy. Curr Urol Rep. 4(3):211-215.

42. Touma NJ, Izawa JI, Chin JL, 2005. Current status of local salvage therapies following radiation failure for prostate cancer. J Urol. 173(2):373-379.

43. Catton C et al., 2003. Recurrent prostate cancer following external beam radiotherapy: follow-up strategies and management. Urol Clin North Am. 30(4):751-763.

44. Ward JF et al., 2005. Salvage surgery for radiorecurrent prostate cancer: contemporary outcomes. J Urol. 173(4):1156-1160.

45. Amling CL et al., 1999. Deoxyribonucleic acid ploidy and serum prostate specific antigen predict outcome following salvage prostatectomy for radiation refractory prostate cancer. J Urol. 161(3):857-862.

46. Bianco FJ, Jr. et al., 2005. Long-term oncologic results of salvage radical prostatectomy for locally recurrent prostate cancer after radiotherapy. Int.J Radiat.Oncol Biol.Phys. 62(2):448-453.

47. Rogers E et al., 1995. Salvage radical prostatectomy: outcome measured by serum prostate specific antigen levels. J Urol. 153(1):104-110.

48. Horwitz EM et al., 2003. Brachytherapy for prostate cancer: follow-up and management of treatment failures. Urol Clin North Am. 30(4):737-7ix.

49. Beyer DC, 2004. Salvage brachytherapy after external-beam irradiation for prostate cancer. Oncology (Williston.Park). 18(2):151-158.

50. Niehoff P et al., 2005. Feasibility and preliminary outcome of salvage combined HDR brachytherapy and external beam radiotherapy (EBRT) for local recurrences after radical prostatectomy. Brachytherapy. 4(2):141-145.

51. Izawa JI et al., 2003. Incomplete glandular ablation after salvage cryotherapy for recurrent prostate cancer after radiotherapy. Int.J Radiat.Oncol Biol.Phys. 56(2):468-472.

52. Touma NJ, Izawa JI, Chin JL, 2005. Current status of local salvage therapies following radiation failure for prostate cancer. J Urol. 173(2):373-379.

53. Ahmed S, Lindsey B, Davies J, 2005. Salvage cryosurgery for locally recurrent prostate cancer following radiotherapy. Prostate Cancer Prostatic.Dis. 8(1):31-35.

54. Han KR et al., 2003. Treatment of organ confined prostate cancer with third generation cryosurgery: preliminary multicenter experience. J Urol. 170(4 Pt 1):1126-1130.

55. Chin JL et al., 2001. Results of salvage cryoablation of the prostate after radiation: identifying predictors of treatment failure and complications. J Urol. 165(6 Pt 1):1937-1941.

56. Bahn DK et al., 2003. Salvage cryosurgery for recurrent prostate cancer after radiation therapy: a seven-year follow-up. Clin Prostate Cancer. 2(2):111-114.

57. Ghafar MA et al., 2001. Salvage cryotherapy using an argon based system for locally recurrent prostate cancer after radiation therapy: the Columbia experience. J Urol. 166(4):1333-1337.

58. Shuman BA et al., 1997. Histological presence of viable prostatic glands on routine biopsy following cryosurgical ablation of the prostate. J Urol. 157(2):552-555.

59. Stephenson AJ et al., 2004. Salvage therapy for locally recurrent prostate cancer after external beam radiotherapy. Curr Treat.Options.Oncol. 5(5):357-365.

60. Satariano WA, Ragland KE, Van Den Eeden SK, 1998. Cause of death in men diagnosed with prostate carcinoma. Cancer. 83(6):1180-1188.

61. Loblaw DA et al., 2004. American Society of Clinical Oncology recommendations for the initial hormonal management of androgen-sensitive metastatic, recurrent, or progressive prostate cancer. Journal of Clinical Oncology. 22(14):2927-2941.

62. Caubet JF et al., 1997. Maximum androgen blockade in advanced prostate cancer: a meta-analysis of published randomized controlled trials using nonsteroidal antiandrogens. Urology. 49(1):71-78.

63. Oh WK et al., 2003. Finasteride and flutamide therapy in patients with advanced prostate cancer: response to subsequent castration and long-term follow-up. Urology. 62(1):99-104.

64. Ryan CJ, Small EJ, 2005. Early versus delayed androgen deprivation for prostate cancer: new fuel for an old debate. Journal of Clinical Oncology. 23(32):8225-8231.

65. Studer UE et al., 2004. Immediate versus deferred hormonal treatment for patients with prostate cancer who are not suitable for curative local treatment: results of the randomized trial SAKK 08/88. Journal of Clinical Oncology. 22(20):4109-4118.

66. Bhandari MS, Crook J, Hussain M, 2005. Should intermittent androgen deprivation be used in routine clinical practice? Journal of Clinical Oncology. 23(32):8212-8218.

67. Peyromaure M et al., 2005. Intermittent androgen deprivation for biologic recurrence after radical prostatectomy: long-term experience. Urology. 65(4):724-729.

68. Chen AC, Petrylak DP, 2005. Complications of androgen-deprivation therapy in men with prostate cancer. Curr Urol Rep. 6(3):210-216.

69. McLeod DG, Iversen P, 2000. Gynecomastia in patients with prostate cancer: a review of treatment options. Urology. 56(5):713-720.

70. Boccardo F et al., 2005. Evaluation of tamoxifen and anastrozole in the prevention of gynecomastia and breast pain induced by bicalutamide monotherapy of prostate cancer. Journal of Clinical Oncology. 23(4):808-815.

71. Dobs A, Darkes MJ, 2005. Incidence and management of gynecomastia in men treated for prostate cancer. J Urol. 174(5):1737-1742.

72. Malkin CJ et al., 2003. Testosterone as a protective factor against atherosclerosis–immunomodulation and influence upon plaque development and stability. J Endocrinol. 178(3):373-380.

73. Smith JC et al., 2001. The effects of induced hypogonadism on arterial stiffness, body composition, and metabolic parameters in males with prostate cancer. J Clin Endocrinol Metab. 86(9):4261-4267.

74. McLeod DG, 2003. Hormonal therapy: historical perspective to future directions. Urology. 61(2 Suppl 1):3-7.

75. Sharifi N, Gulley JL, Dahut WL, 2005. Androgen deprivation therapy for prostate cancer. JAMA: The Journal of the American Medical Association. 294(2):238-244.

76. Gottschalk AR, Roach M, III, 2004. The use of hormonal therapy with radiotherapy for prostate cancer: analysis of prospective randomised trials. Br.J Cancer. 90(5):950-954.

77. Bolla M et al., 2002. Long-term results with immediate androgen suppression and external irradiation in patients with locally advanced prostate cancer (an EORTC study): a phase III randomised trial. Lancet. 360(9327):103-106.

78. Bolla M et al., 1997. Improved survival in patients with locally advanced prostate cancer treated with radiotherapy and goserelin. N Engl J Med. 337(5):295-300.

79. D'amico AV et al., 2004. 6-month androgen suppression plus radiation therapy vs radiation therapy alone for patients with clinically localized prostate cancer: a randomized controlled trial. JAMA: The Journal of the American Medical Association. 292(7):821-827.

80. DeWeese TL, 2004. Radiation Therapy and Androgen Suppression as Treatment for Clinically Localized Prostate Cancer: The New Standard? JAMA: The Journal of the American Medical Association. 292(7):864-866.

81. D'Amico AV et al., 2004. Androgen Suppression Plus Radiation Therapy for Prostate Cancer--Reply. JAMA: The Journal of the American Medical Association. 292(17):2085.

82. Denham JW et al., 2005. Short-term androgen deprivation and radiotherapy for locally advanced prostate cancer: results from the Trans-Tasman Radiation Oncology Group 96.01 randomised controlled trial. Lancet Oncol. 6(11):841-850.

83. Hanks GE et al., 2003. Phase III trial of long-term adjuvant androgen deprivation after neoadjuvant hormonal cytoreduction and radiotherapy in locally advanced carcinoma of the prostate: the Radiation Therapy Oncology Group Protocol 92-02. Journal of Clinical Oncology. 21(21):3972-3978.

84. Roach M et al., 2000. Four prognostic groups predict long-term survival from prostate cancer following radiotherapy alone on Radiation Therapy Oncology Group clinical trials. Int.J Radiat.Oncol Biol.Phys. 47(3):609-615.

85. Roach M et al., 2000. Predicting long-term survival, and the need for hormonal therapy: a meta-analysis of RTOG prostate cancer trials. Int.J Radiat.Oncol Biol.Phys. 47(3):617-627.

86. Clinical Practice Guidelines, Version 2.2005. www.nccn.org. accessed October 10, 2005 . 2005.

87. Syed S, Petrylak DP, Thompson IM, 2003. Management of high-risk localized prostate cancer: the integration of local and systemic therapy approaches. Urol Oncol. 21(3):235-243.

88. Messing EM et al., 1999. Immediate hormonal therapy compared with observation after radical prostatectomy and pelvic lymphadenectomy in men with node-positive prostate cancer. N Engl J Med. 341(24):1781-1788.

89. Kaisary AV, 2005. Evaluating the use of early hormonal therapy in patients with localised or locally advanced prostate cancer. Prostate Cancer Prostatic.Dis. 8(2):140-151.

90. Zincke H et al., 2001. Role of early adjuvant hormonal therapy after radical prostatectomy for prostate cancer. J Urol. 166(6):2208-2215.

91. Laverdiere J et al., 2004. The efficacy and sequencing of a short course of androgen suppression on freedom from biochemical failure when administered with radiation therapy for T2-T3 prostate cancer. J Urol. 171(3):1137-1140.

92. Pilepich MV et al., 2001. Phase III radiation therapy oncology group (RTOG) trial 86-10 of androgen deprivation adjuvant to definitive radiotherapy in locally advanced carcinoma of the prostate. Int.J Radiat.Oncol Biol.Phys. 50(5):1243-1252.

93. Pilepich MV et al., 1997. Phase III trial of androgen suppression using goserelin in unfavorable-prognosis carcinoma of the prostate treated with definitive radiotherapy: report of Radiation Therapy Oncology Group Protocol 85-31. Journal of Clinical Oncology. 15(3):1013-1021.

94. Tay MH et al., 2004. Finasteride and bicalutamide as primary hormonal therapy in patients with advanced adenocarcinoma of the prostate. Ann.Oncol. 15(6):974-978.

95. Andriole G et al., 1995. Treatment with finasteride following radical prostatectomy for prostate cancer. Urology. 45(3):491-497.

96. Wang LG et al., 2004. The biological basis for the use of an anti-androgen and a 5-alpha-reductase inhibitor in the treatment of recurrent prostate cancer: Case report and review. Oncol Rep. 11(6):1325-1329.

97. Brufsky A et al., 1997. Finasteride and flutamide as potency-sparing androgen-ablative therapy for advanced adenocarcinoma of the prostate. Urology. 49(6):913-920.

98. Strum SaPD, A Primer on Prostate Cancer. Life Extension Media, Hollywoiod FL, 2005.

99. Leibowitz RL, Tucker SJ, 2001. Treatment of localized prostate cancer with intermittent triple androgen blockade: preliminary results in 110 consecutive patients. The Oncologist. 6(2):177-182.

100. Debes JD, Tindall DJ, 2004. Mechanisms of androgen-refractory prostate cancer. N Engl J Med. 351(15):1488-1490.

101. Shulman MJ, Benaim EA, 2004. The natural history of androgen independent prostate cancer. J Urol. 172(1):141-145.

102. Small EJ et al., 2004. Antiandrogen withdrawal alone or in combination with ketoconazole in androgen-independent prostate cancer patients: a phase III trial (CALGB 9583). Journal of Clinical Oncology. 22(6):1025-1033.
103. Moore CN, George DJ, 2005. Update in the management of patients with hormone-refractory prostate cancer. Curr Opin.Urol. 15(3):157-162.
104. Tannock IF et al., 2004. Docetaxel plus prednisone or mitoxantrone plus prednisone for advanced prostate cancer. N Engl J Med. 351(15):1502-1512.
105. Petrylak DP et al., 2004. Docetaxel and estramustine compared with mitoxantrone and prednisone for advanced refractory prostate cancer. N Engl J Med. 351(15):1513-1520.
106. Agell M, The Truth About the Drug Companies. Random House, New York, 2004.
107. Saad F, Schulman CC, 2004. Role of bisphosphonates in prostate cancer. Eur.Urol. 45(1):26-34.
108. Saad F, Karakiewicz P, Perrotte P, 2005. The role of bisphosphonates in hormone-refractory prostate cancer. World J Urol. 23(1):14-18.
109. Coxon JP et al., 2004. Advances in the use of bisphosphonates in the prostate cancer setting. Prostate Cancer Prostatic.Dis. 7(2):99-104.
110. Parker CC, 2005. The role of bisphosphonates in the treatment of prostate cancer. BJU Int. 95(7):935-938.
111. Saad F et al., 2002. A randomized, placebo-controlled trial of zoledronic acid in patients with hormone-refractory metastatic prostate carcinoma. JNCI Cancer Spectrum. 94(19):1458-1468.
112. Saad F et al., 2004. Long-term efficacy of zoledronic acid for the prevention of skeletal complications in patients with metastatic hormone-refractory prostate cancer. JNCI Cancer Spectrum. 96(11):879-882.
113. Smith MR et al., 2003. Randomized controlled trial of zoledronic acid to prevent bone loss in men receiving androgen deprivation therapy for nonmetastatic prostate cancer. J Urol. 169(6):2008-2012.
114. Yau V et al., 2004. Pain management in cancer patients with bone metastases remains a challenge. J Pain Symptom.Manage. 27(1):1-3.
115. Anderson KO et al., 2004. Pain education for underserved minority cancer patients: a randomized controlled trial. Journal of Clinical Oncology. 22(24):4918-4925.

CHAPTER 8 – Alternative and Complementary Therapies

Alternative Medicine – An Overview

1. Eisenberg, David M., et al. Trends in alternative medicine use in the United States, 1990-1997. Journal of the American Medical Association, Vol. 280, November 11, 1998, pp. 1569-75
2. Bensoussan, Alan. Complementary medicine - where lies its appeal? Medical Journal of Australia, Vol. 170, March 15, 1999, pp. 247-48 (editorial)
3. Fisher, Peter and Ward, Adam. Complementary medicine in Europe. British Medical Journal, Vol. 309, July 9, 1994, pp. 107-11
4. Hussain, Ghazala and Manyam, Bala V. Mucuna pruriens proves more effective than l-dopa in Parkinson's disease animal model. Phytotherapy Research, Vol. 11, 1997, pp. 419-23
5. Ernst, Edzard. Harmless herbs? A review of the recent literature. American Journal of Medicine, Vol. 104, February 1998, pp. 170-78
6. Anderson, Ian. Hospital errors are number three killer in Australia. New Scientist, June 10, 1995, p. 5
7. Cordner, Stephen M. Australia's preventable hospital deaths. The Lancet, Vol. 345, June 17, 1995, p. 1562
8. Bates, David W., et al. Incidence of adverse drug events and potential adverse drug events. Journal of the American Medical Association, Vol. 274, July 5, 1995, pp. 29-34
9. Pittet, Didier and Wenzel, Richard P. Nosocomial bloodstream infections. Archives of Internal Medicine, Vol. 155, June 12, 1995, pp. 1177-84
10. Roach, Gary W., et al. Adverse cerebral outcomes after coronary bypass surgery. New England Journal of Medicine, Vol. 335, December 19, 1996, pp. 1857-63

11. Lazarou, Jason, et al. Incidence of adverse drug reactions in hospitalized patients. Journal of the American Medical Association, Vol. 279, April 15, 1998, pp. 1200-05 and pp. 1216-17

Alternative Therapies

1. Cameron, E and Pauling, L. Cancer and Vitamin C, Camino Books Inc., Philadelphia, PA, 1993, p. xxiii
2. Woo, TCS, et al. Pilot study: potential role of vitamin D (cholecalciferol) in patients with PSA relapse after definitive therapy. Nutrition and Cancer, Vol. 51, No. 1, 2005, pp. 32-36
3. Hussain, M, et al. Soy isoflavones in the treatment of prostate cancer. Nutr Cancer, Vol. 47, No. 2, 2003, pp. 111-17
4. Li, Y, et al. Regulation of gene expression and inhibition of experimental prostate cancer bone metastasis by dietary genistein. Neoplasia, Vol. 6, No. 4, July-August 2004, pp. 354-63
5. Kumar, NB, et al. The specific role of isoflavones in reducing prostate cancer risk. Prostate, Vol. 59, No. 2, May 1, 2004, pp. 141-47
6. Dalais, FS, et al. Effects of a diet rich in phytoestrogens on prostate-specific antigen and sex hormones in men diagnosed with prostate cancer. Urology, Vol. 64, No. 3, September 2004, pp. 510-15
7. Kucuk, O, et al. Phase II randomized clinical trial of lycopene supplementation before radical prostatectomy. Cancer Epidemiology, Biomarkers & Prevention, Vol. 10, August 2001, pp. 861-68
8. Kucuk, O, et al. Effects of lycopene supplementation in patients with localized prostate cancer. Experimental Biology and Medicine, Vol. 227, 2002, pp. 881-85
9. Chen, Longwen, et al. Oxidative DNA damage in prostate cancer patients consuming tomato sauce-based entrees as a whole-food intervention. Journal of the National Cancer Institute, Vol. 93, December 19, 2001, pp. 1872-79
10. van Breemen, RB, et al. Liquid chromatography-mass spectrometry of cis- and all-trans-lycopene in human serum and prostate tissue after dietary supplementation with tomato sauce. J Agric Food Chem, Vol. 50, No. 8, April 10, 2002, pp. 2214-19
11. Rannikko, A, et al. Plasma and prostate phytoestrogen concentrations in prostate cancer patients after oral phytoestrogen supplementation. The Prostate, Vol. 66, 2006, pp. 82-87
12. Hong, SJ, et al. Comparative study of concentration of isoflavones and lignans in plasma and prostatic tissues of normal control and benign prostatic hyperplasia. Yonsei Medical Journal, Vol. 43, No. 2, 2002, pp. 236-41
13. Risbridger, GP, et al. The in vivo effect of red clover diet on ventral prostate growth in adult male mice. Reprod Fertil Dev, Vol. 13, No. 4, 2001, pp. 325-29
14. Jarred, RA, et al. Anti-androgenic action by red clover-derived dietary isoflavones reduces non-malignant prostate enlargement in aromatase knockout (ArKO) mice. The Prostate, Vol. 56, 2003, pp. 54-64
15. Stephens, Frederick O. Phytoestrogens and prostate cancer: possible preventive role. Medical Journal of Australia, Vol. 167, August 4, 1997, pp. 138-40
16. Jarred, RA, et al. Induction of apoptosis in low to moderate-grade human prostate carcinoma by red clover-derived dietary isoflavones. Cancer Epidemiology Biomarkers & Prevention, Vol. 11, December 2002, pp. 1689-96
17. http://www.Trinovin.com
18. Pezzato, E., et al. Prostate carcinoma and green tea: PSA-triggered basement membrane degradation and MMP-2 activation are inhibited by (-)epigallochetchin-3-gallate. International Journal of Cancer, Vol. 112, No. 5, 2004, pp. 787-92
19. Kaegi, E. Unconventional therapies for cancer: 2. Green tea. Canadian Medical Association Journal, Vol. 158, April 21, 1998, pp. 1033-35
20. Aviram, M, et al. Pomegranate juice consumption for 3 years by patients with carotid artery stenosis reduces common carotid intima-media thickness, blood pressure and LDL oxidation. Clin Nutr, Vol. 23, No. 3, June 2004, pp. 423-33
21. Azadzoi, KM, et al. Oxidative stress in arteriogenic erectile dysfunction: prophylactic role of antioxidants. Journal of Urology, Vol. 174, No. 1, July 2005, pp. 386-93
22. Albrecht, M, et al. Pomegranate extracts potently suppress proliferation, xenografts growth, and invasion of human prostate cancer cells. J Med Food, Vol. 7, No. 3, Fall 2004, pp. 274-83

23. Lansky, EP, et al. Pomegranate (Punica granatum) pure chemicals show possible synergistic inhibition of human PC-3 prostate cancer cell invasion across Matrigel.

24. Malik, A, et al. Pomegranate fruit juice for chemoprevention and chemotherapy of prostate cancer. Proceedings of the National Academy of Sciences (USA), Vol. 102, No. 41, October 11, 2005, pp. 14813-18

25. Pantuck, AJ, et al. Phase II study of pomegranate juice for men with rising PSA following surgery or radiation for prostate cancer. American Urological Association Annual Meeting, San Antonio, TX, 2005, Abstract #831.
http://professional.cancerconsultants.com/print.aspx?id=34168

26. Hoenjet, KMJLF, et al. Effect of a nutritional supplement containing vitamin E, selenium, vitamin C and coenzyme Q10 on serum PSA in patients with hormonally untreated carcinoma of the prostate: a randomised placebo-controlled study. European Urology, Vol. 47, 2005, pp. 433-40

27. Schroder, FH, et al. Randomized, double-blind, placebo-controlled crossover study in men with prostate cancer and rising PSA: effectiveness of a dietary supplement. European Urology, Vol. 48, 2005, pp. 922-31

28. DiPaola, RS, et al. Clinical and biologic activity of an estrogenic herbal combination (PC-SPES) in prostate cancer. New England Journal of Medicine, Vol. 339, No. 12, September 17, 1998, pp. 785-91

29. Pirani, John F. The effects of phytotherapeutic agents on prostate cancer: an overview of recent clinical trials of PC SPES. Urology, Vol. 58, suppl. 2A, August 2001, pp. 36-38

30. Weinrobe, Mark C. and Bruce Montgomery. Acquired bleeding diathesis in a patient taking PC-SPES. New England Journal of Medicine, Vol. 345, October 18, 2001, pp. 1213-14

31. California Department of Health Services, Office of Public Affairs, Press Release 02-03, February 7, 2002

32. Sovak, Milos, et al. Herbal composition PC-SPES for management of prostate cancer: identification of active principles. Journal of the National Cancer Institute, Vol. 94, September 4, 2002, pp. 1275-81

33. White, Jeffrey. PC-SPES: a lesion for future dietary supplement research. Journal of the National Cancer Institute, Vol. 94, September 4, 2002, pp. 1261-63

34. Oh, WK, et al. Prospective, multicenter, randomized phase II trial of the herbal supplement, PC-SPES, and diethylstilbestrol in patients with androgen-independent prostate cancer. Journal of Clinical Oncology, Vol. 22, No. 18, September 15, 2004, pp. 3705-12

35. Williams, David G. Alternatives for the Health-Conscious Individual, Vol. 9, No. 24, June 2003, pp. 185-89

36. Goldman, Erik L. Columbia's Center for Holistic Urology tests botanicals for prostate disease. Holistic Primary Care, Vol. 4, No. 3, July 2003, pp. 1-2

37. Leal, PF, et al. Functional properties of spice extracts obtained via supercritical fluid extraction. Journal of Agricultural and Food Chemistry, Vol. 51, No. 9, 2003, pp. 2520-25

38. Ornish, Dean, et al. Intensive lifestyle changes may affect the progression of prostate cancer. Journal of Urology, Vol. 174, September 2005, pp. 1065-70

39. Hildenbrand, GL, et al. Five-year survival rates of melanoma patients treated by diet therapy after the manner of Gerson: a retrospective review. Altern Ther Health Med, Vol. 1, No. 4, September 1995, pp. 29-37

40. Walters, R. Options: The Alternative Cancer Therapy Book. Avery Publishing Group, Garden City Park, NY, 1993, pp. 95-104

41. Walters, R. Options: The Alternative Cancer Therapy Book. Avery Publishing Group, Garden City Park, NY, 1993, pp. 59-81

42. Walters, R. Options: The Alternative Cancer Therapy Book. Avery Publishing Group, Garden City Park, NY, 1993, pp. 17-27

43. Breuss, Rudolph. The Breuss Cancer Cure, Alive Books, Vancouver, Canada, 1995

Complementary Therapies

1. Wilkinson, S, et al. Attitudes and use of complementary medicine in men with prostate cancer. Journal of Urology, Vol. 168, December 2002, pp. 2505-09

2.   Cameron, E and Pauling, L. Supplemental ascorbate in the supportive treatment of cancer: reevaluation of prolongation of survival times in terminal human cancer. Proceedings of the National Academy of Sciences USA, Vol. 75, No. 9, September 1978, pp. 4538-42
3.   Cameron, E and Pauling, L. Cancer and Vitamin C. Camino Books Inc., Philadelphia, PA, 1993, pp. 108-19
4.   Cameron, E and Pauling, L. Cancer and Vitamin C. Camino Books Inc., Philadelphia, PA, 1993, pp. 242-55
5.   Lamm, DL, et al. Megadose vitamins in bladder cancer: a double-blind clinical trial. Journal of Urology, Vol. 151, January 1994, pp. 21-26
6.   Creagan, ET, et al. Failure of high-dose vitamin C (ascorbic acid) therapy to benefit patients with advanced cancer: a controlled trial. New England Journal of Medicine, Vol. 301, September 27, 1979, pp. 687-90
7.   Moertel, CG, et al. High-dose vitamin C versus placebo in the treatment of patients with advanced cancer who have had no prior chemotherapy: a randomized double-blind comparison. New England Journal of Medicine, Vol. 312, January 17, 1985, pp. 137-41
8.   Padayatty, SJ, et al. Vitamin C pharmacokinetics: implications for oral and intravenous use. Annals of Internal Medicine, Vol. 140, April 6, 2004, pp. 533-37
9.   Drisko, JA, et al. The use of antioxidants with first-line chemotherapy in two cases of ovarian cancer. Journal of the American College of Nutrition, Vol. 22, No. 2, 2003, pp. 118-23
10. Padayatty, SJ, et al. Intravenously administered vitamin C as cancer therapy: three cases. Canadian Medical Association Journal, Vol. 174, No. 7, March 28, 2006, pp. 937-42
11. Assouline, S. and Miller, WH. High-dose vitamin C therapy: renewed hope or false promise? Canadian Medical Association Journal, Vol. 174, No. 7, March 28, 2006, pp. 956-57
12. Drisko, JA, et al. The use of antioxidants with first-line chemotherapy in two cases of ovarian cancer. Journal of the American College of Nutrition, Vol. 22, No. 2, 2003, pp. 118-23
13. Prasad, KN, et al. Scientific rationale for using high-dose multiple micronutrients as an adjunct to standard and experimental cancer therapies. Journal of the American College of Nutrition, Vol. 20 (suppl), 2001, pp. 450S-63S
14. Weijl, NI, et al. Free radicals and antioxidants in chemotherapy induced toxicity. Cancer Treat Res, Vol. 23, 1997, pp. 209-40
15. Lamson, DW, et al. Antioxidants in cancer therapy: their actions and interactions with oncologic therapies. Alt Med Rev, Vol. 4, 1999, pp. 304-29
16. Prasad, KN, et al. High doses of multiple antioxidant vitamins: essential ingredients in improving the efficacy of standard cancer therapy. Journal of the American College of Nutrition, Vol. 18, 1999, pp. 13-25
17. Chinery, R, et al. Antioxidants enhance the cytotoxicity of chemotherapeutic agents in colorectal cancer. Nat Med, Vol. 3, 1997, pp. 1233-41
18. Prasad, KN, et al. Pros and cons of antioxidant use during radiation therapy. Cancer Treat Rev, Vol. 28, April 2002, pp. 79-91
19. Weijl, NI, et al. Supplementation with antioxidant micronutrients and chemotherapy-induced toxicity in cancer patients treated with cisplatin-based chemotherapy. European Journal of Cancer, Vol. 40, No. 11, July 2004, pp. 1713-23
20. Prasad, KN. Multiple dietary antioxidants enhance the efficacy of standard and experimental cancer therapies and decrease their toxicity. Integr Cancer Ther, Vol. 3, No. 4, December 2004, pp. 310-22
21. The use of vitamin C and other antioxidants with chemotherapy and radiotherapy in cancer treatment. Journal of Orthomolecular Medicine, Vol. 19, No. 4, 4th Quarter 2004 (special issue)
22. Traxer, O, et al. Effect of ascorbic acid consumption on urinary stone risk factors. Journal of Urology, Vol. 170, August 2003, pp. 397-401
23. Prasad, KN, et al. Alpha-tocopheryl succinate, the most effective form of vitamin E for adjuvant cancer treatment: a review. Journal of the American College of Nutrition, Vol. 22, No. 2, 2003, pp. 108-17
24. Kumar, B, et al. d-alpha-tocopheryl succinate (vitamin E) enhances radiation-induced chromosomal damage levels in human cancer cells, but reduces it in normal cells. Journal of the American College of Nutrition, Vol. 21, No. 4, 2002, pp. 339-43

25. Shiau, CW, et al. Alpha-tocopheryl succinate induces apoptosis in prostate cancer cells in part through inhibition of BCL-XL/BCL-2 function. J Biol Chem, March 6, 2006

26. Munstedt, K, et al. Oncologic mistletoe therapy: physician's use and estimation of efficiency. Dtsch Med Wochenschr, Vol. 125, 2000, pp. 1222-26

27. Beuth, Josef and Moss, Ralph W. Complementary Oncology. Georg Thieme Verlag, Stuttgart, Germany, 2006, pp. 189-96

28. Augustin, M, et al. Safety and efficacy of the long-term adjuvant treatment of primary intermediate- to high-risk malignant melanoma with a standardized fermented European mistletoe (*Viscum album L.*) extract. Arzneimittelforschung, Vol. 55, No. 1, 2005, pp. 38-49

29. Bock, PR, et al. Efficacy and safety of long-term complementary treatment with standardized European mistletoe extract (Viscum album L.) in addition to the conventional adjuvant oncologic therapy in patients with primary non-metastasized mammary carcinoma. Results of a multi-center, comparative, epidemiological cohort study in Germany and Switzerland. Arzneimittelforschung, Vol. 54, 2004, pp. 456-66

30. Piao, BK, et al. Impact of complementary mistletoe extract treatment on quality of life in breast, ovarian and non-small cell lung cancer patients. A prospective randomized, controlled clinical trial. Anticancer Research, Vol. 24, 2004, pp. 303-09

31. Kaegi, E. Unconventional therapies for cancer: 3 – Iscador. Canadian Medical Association Journal, Vol. 158, May 5, 1998, pp. 1157-59

32. Beuth, Josef and Moss, Ralph W. Complementary Oncology. Georg Thieme Verlag, Stuttgart, Germany, 2006, pp. 171-82

33. Beuth, Josef and Moss, Ralph W. Complementary Oncology. Georg Thieme Verlag, Stuttgart, Germany, 2006, pp. 183-88

34. Pfeifer, BL and Aeikens, B. Complementary therapies for hormone refractory prostate cancer. Positive Health, Issue 120, February 2006, pp. 19-25
http://www.clearfeed.com/pfeifer/docs/Positive_Health_0206.pdf

35. Pfeifer, BL. Phytotherapy and immune system support for prostate cancer patients. Presentation given at the Complementary & Natural Healthcare Expo, London, UK, October 23, 2005 http://www.clearfeed.com/pfeifer/05excel-transcript.html

36. Barber, M.D., et al. The effect of an oral nutritional supplement enriched with fish oil on weight-loss in patients with pancreatic cancer. British Journal of Cancer, Vol. 81, No. 1, September 1999, pp. 80-86

37. Kaegi, Elizabeth. Unconventional therapies for cancer: 4. Hydrazine sulfate. Canadian Medical Association Journal, Vol. 158, May 19, 1998, pp. 1327-30

38. Beuth, Josef and Moss, Ralph W. Complementary Oncology. Georg Thieme Verlag, Stuttgart, Germany, 2006, pp. 207-20

39. Nanba, H. Activity of Maitake D-fraction to inhibit carcinogenesis and metastasis. Annals of the NY Academy of Sciences, Vol. 768, 1995, pp. 243-45

40. Blaylock, Russell L. Natural Strategies for Cancer Patients. Kensington Publishing Corp., NY, 2003, pp. 210-12

41. Blaylock, Russell L. Natural Strategies for Cancer Patients. Kensington Publishing Corp., NY, 2003, pp. 221-22

42. Lamson, DW and Brignall, MS. Antioxidants and cancer, part 3: quercetin. Altern Med Rev, Vol. 5, No. 3, June 2000, pp. 196-208

43. Cui, Y, et al. Association of ginseng use with survival and quality of life among breast cancer patients. American Journal of Epidemiology, Vol. 163, April 1, 2006, pp. 645-53

44. Beer, TM, et al. Randomized study of high-dose pulse calcitriol or placebo prior to radical prostatectomy. Cancer Epidemiology, Biomarkers and Prevention, Vol. 13, No. 12, 2004, pp. 2225-32

45. Keedwell, RG, et al. A retinoid-related molecule that does not bind to classical retinoid receptors potently induces apoptosis in human prostate cancer cells through rapid caspases activation. Cancer Research, Vol. 64, May 1, 2004, pp. 3302-12

CHAPTER 9 – The Future: Diagnosis, Staging, Novel Therapies

1. Chuang YC, Giannantoni A, Chancellor MB, 2006. The potential and promise of using botulinum toxin in the prostate gland. BJU Int.

2. Maria G et al., 2003. Relief by botulinum toxin of voiding dysfunction due to benign prostatic hyperplasia: results of a randomized, placebo-controlled study. Urology. 62(2):259-264.

3. Apostolidis A, Dasgupta P, Fowler CJ, 2006. Proposed mechanism for the efficacy of injected botulinum toxin in the treatment of human detrusor overactivity. Eur.Urol. 49(4):644-650.

4. Deutsch E et al., 2004. Environmental, genetic, and molecular features of prostate cancer. Lancet Oncol. 5(5):303-313.

5. Gsur A, et al. 2004. Genetic polymorphisms & prostate cancer risk. World J Urol. 21(6):414-23

6. Cancel-Tassin G, Cussenot O, 2005. Genetic susceptibility to prostate cancer. BJU Int. 96(9):1380-1385.

7. Saad F, 2005. UPM3: review of a new molecular diagnostic urine test for prostate cancer. Can.J Urol. 12 Suppl 1:40-43.

8. Fradet Y et al., 2004. uPM3, a new molecular urine test for the detection of prostate cancer. Urology. 64(2):311-315.

9. Hessels D et al., 2003. DD3(PCA3)-based molecular urine analysis for the diagnosis of prostate cancer. Eur.Urol. 44(1):8-15.

10. Henrique R, Jeronimo C, 2004. Molecular detection of prostate cancer: a role for GSTP1 hypermethylation. Eur.Urol. 46(5):660-669.

11. Crocitto LE et al., 2004. Prostate cancer molecular markers GSTP1 and hTERT in expressed prostatic secretions as predictors of biopsy results. Urology. 64(4):821-825.

12. Zhou M et al., 2004. Quantitative GSTP1 methylation levels correlate with Gleason grade and tumor volume in prostate needle biopsies. J Urol. 171(6 Pt 1):2195-2198.

13. Warlick CA, Allaf ME, Carter HB, 2006. Expectant treatment with curative intent in the prostate-specific antigen era: triggers for definitive therapy. Urol Oncol. 24(1):51-57.

14. Warlick C et al., 2006. Delayed versus immediate surgical intervention and prostate cancer outcome. JNCI Cancer Spectrum. 98(5):355-357.

15. Epstein JI et al., 2005. Utility of saturation biopsy to predict insignificant cancer at radical prostatectomy. Urology. 66(2):356-360.

16. Datta S, Datta MW, 2006. Sonic Hedgehog signaling in advanced prostate cancer. Cell Mol.Life Sci. 63(4):435-48.

17. Sanchez P, Clement V, Altaba A, 2005. Therapeutic targeting of the Hedgehog-GLI pathway in prostate cancer. Cancer Res. 65(8):2990-2992.

18. Karhadkar SS et al., 2004. Hedgehog signalling in prostate regeneration, neoplasia and metastasis. Nature. 431(7009):707-712.

19. Panakova D et al., 2005. Lipoprotein particles are required for Hedgehog and Wingless signalling. Nature. 435(7038):58-65.

20. Beachy PA, Karhadkar SS, Berman DM, 2004. Tissue repair and stem cell renewal in carcinogenesis. Nature. 432(7015):324-331.

21. Beachy PA, et al. 2004. Mending and malignancy. Nature. 431(7007):402.

22. Essand M, 2005. Gene therapy and immunotherapy of prostate cancer: adenoviral-based strategies. Acta Oncol. 44(6):610-627.

23. Dilley J et al., 2005. Oncolytic adenovirus CG7870 in combination with radiation demonstrates synergistic enhancements of antitumor efficacy without loss of specificity. Cancer Gene Ther. 12(8):715-722.

24. Morgan G, Ward R, Barton M, 2004. The contribution of cytotoxic chemotherapy to 5-year survival in adult malignancies. Clin Oncol (R.Coll.Radiol.). 16(8):549-560.

25. Clarke NW, Wylie JP, 2004. Chemotherapy in hormone refractory prostate cancer: where do we stand? Eur.Urol. 46(6):709-711.

26. Slater JD et al., 2004. Proton therapy for prostate cancer: the initial Loma Linda University experience. Int.J Radiat.Oncol Biol.Phys. 59(2):348-352.

27. Scardino PTKJ, Dr. Peter Scardino's Prostate Book. Avery/Penguin Group, New York, 2005.

28. Moore CM et al., 2005. Does photodynamic therapy have the necessary attributes to become a future treatment for organ-confined prostate cancer? BJU Int. 96(6):754-758.

29. Muschter R, 2003. Photodynamic therapy: a new approach to prostate cancer. Curr Urol Rep. 4(3):221-228.

30. Jankun J et al., 2005. Diverse optical characteristic of the prostate and light delivery system: implications for computer modelling of prostatic photodynamic therapy. BJU Int. 95(9):1237-1244.

31. Moore CM et al., 2006. Photodynamic therapy using meso tetra hydroxy phenyl chlorin (mTHPC) in early prostate cancer. Lasers Surg Med.

32. Colombel M, Gelet A, 2004. Principles and results of high-intensity focused ultrasound for localized prostate cancer. Prostate Cancer Prostatic.Dis. 7(4):289-294.

33. Uchida T et al., 2006. Treatment of localized prostate cancer using high-intensity focused ultrasound. BJU Int. 97(1):56-61.

34. Blana A et al., 2004. High-intensity focused ultrasound for the treatment of localized prostate cancer: 5-year experience. Urology. 63(2):297-300.

35. Vallancien Guy et al., 2004. Transrectal focused ultrasound combined with transurethral resection of the prostate for the treatment of localized prostate cancer: feasibility study. The Journal of Urology. 171(6, Part 1):2265-2267.

36. Thuroff S et al., 2003. High-intensity focused ultrasound and localized prostate cancer: efficacy results from the European multicentric study. J Endourol. 17(8):673-677.

37. Chaussy C, Thuroff S, 2003. The status of high-intensity focused ultrasound in the treatment of localized prostate cancer and the impact of a combined resection. Curr Urol Rep. 4(3):248-252.

38. Gianduzzo TR, Eden CG, Moon DA, 2006. Treatment of localised prostate cancer using high-intensity focused ultrasound. BJU Int. 97(4):867-868.

39. Randal J, 2002. High-intensity focused ultrasound makes its debut. JNCI Cancer Spectrum. 94(13):962-964.

40. Sherar MD et al., 2001. Interstitial microwave thermal therapy for prostate cancer: method of treatment and results of a phase I/II trial. J Urol. 166(5):1707-1714.

41. Sherar MD et al., 2003. Interstitial microwave thermal therapy for prostate cancer. J Endourol. 17(8):617-625.

42. Huidobro C et al., 2004. Evaluation of microwave thermotherapy with histopathology, magnetic resonance imaging and temperature mapping. J Urol. 171(2 Pt 1):672-678.

43. Sherar MD et al., 2004. Interstitial microwave thermal therapy and its application to the treatment of recurrent prostate cancer. Int.J Hyperthermia. 20(7):757-768.

44. Larson BT et al., 2003. Histological changes of minimally invasive procedures for the treatment of benign prostatic hyperplasia and prostate cancer: clinical implications. J Urol. 170(1):12-19.

45. Tucker RD et al., 2000. Use of permanent interstitial temperature self-regulating rods for ablation of prostate cancer. J Endourol. 14(6):511-517.

46. Tucker RD et al., 2002. Interstitial thermal therapy in patients with localized prostate cancer: histologic analysis. Urology. 60(1):166-169.

47. Tucker RD, 2003. Use of interstitial temperature self-regulating thermal rods in the treatment of prostate cancer. J Endourol. 17(8):601-607.

48. Ryu S et al., 1996. Preferential radiosensitization of human prostatic carcinoma cells by mild hyperthermia. Int.J Radiat.Oncol Biol.Phys. 34(1):133-138.

49. Deger S et al., 2004. Thermoradiotherapy using interstitial self-regulating thermoseeds: an intermediate analysis of a phase II trial. Eur.Urol. 45(5):574-579.

50. Van Vulpen M et al., 2004. Radiotherapy and hyperthermia in the treatment of patients with locally advanced prostate cancer: preliminary results. BJU Int. 93(1):36-41.

51. Kalapurakal JA et al., 2003. Efficacy of irradiation and external hyperthermia in locally advanced, hormone-refractory or radiation recurrent prostate cancer: a preliminary report. Int.J Radiat.Oncol Biol.Phys. 57(3):654-664.

52. Tucker RD, Huidobro C, Larson T, 2005. Ablation of stage T1/T2 prostate cancer with permanent interstitial temperature self-regulating rods. J Endourol. 19(7):865-867.

53. Johannsen M et al., 2005. Clinical hyperthermia of prostate cancer using magnetic nanoparticles: presentation of a new interstitial technique. Int.J Hyperthermia. 21(7):637-647.

54. Prasad KN et al., 2003. Alpha-tocopheryl succinate, the most effective form of vitamin E for adjuvant cancer treatment: a review. J Am.Coll.Nutr. 22(2):108-117.

55. Asea A et al., 2001. Effects of the flavonoid drug quercetin on the response of human prostate tumours to hyperthermia in vitro and in vivo. Int.J Hyperthermia. 17(4):347-356.

Subject Index

Flaxseed
    cholesterol and, 163
    prostate cancer prevention and, 80,
    163-64
    PSA level and, 163
Flomax. See Tamsulosin
Floppy iris syndrome, tamsulosin and, 45
Fluoroquinolones, 9-10
Flutamide, 269, 280
Folic acid, prostate cancer prevention
and, 170-71
Fruits and vegetables, prostate cancer
prevention and, 147-51

G
Gabapentin, CPPS treatment and, 23
Gamma-tocopherol (vitamin E), 174-77
Garlic, prostate cancer prevention and,
159-60
Gene expression, prostate cancer and,
318-19
Genetic contribution, BPH and, 31
Genistein
    BPH and, 35-36, 55
    prostate cancer and, 158, 295
Gerson Institute, 313
Gerson therapy, 303
GH enhancers, prostate cancer risk and,
87
Ginger
    Aeskulap protocol and, 309
    prostate cancer prevention and, 186
Ginseng, Aeskulap protocol and, 309
Glandular cells, 2
Gleason score, 128-31
    accuracy of, 129-31, 141
    cancer severity and, 129
    definition of, 103
    interpretation of, 128-31
    PSA and, 103
    PSA cut-off and, 104
GLUT-4 transporters, 93
Glutathione
    alpha-lipoic acid and, 178, 179
    prostate cancer prevention and, 178-
    79
    selenium and, 83, 84
Glutathione peroxidase, selenium and,
181
Glutathione-S-transferase, prostate
cancer and, 70, 71

Glycemic loads, 150, 345-46
Gold, Dr. Joseph, 310-11
Goserelin, 269
Grape seed extract, prostate cancer
prevention and, 189
Green tea, prostate cancer and, 160-63,
298
Gynecomastia, hormone therapy and,
273

H
Hager, Dr. Dieter, 312
HDR. See High dose radiation
Heart disease. See Cardiovascular
disease
Hedgehog pathway, prostate cancer and,
322-24
Herbal medicine, 291
Hereditary factors, prostate cancer risk
and, 73-75, 318-19
Heterocyclic amines, prostate cancer risk
and, 76
HIFU, 330-31
    BPH and, 60
    TURP and, 331
High dose radiation (HDR), brachytherapy
and, 234-36
High frequency electrostimulation, CPPS
treatment and, 21
High-intensity focused ultrasound. See
HIFU
Histamine, CPPS and, 14
Hoffer, Dr. Abram, 294
Homeopathy, 291
Hormone involvement, BPH and, 28-29
Hormone therapy, 267-82
    action of LHRH agonists, 269
    adverse effects of, 272-75
    anemia and, 274
    bone loss and, 274
    cardiovascular disease and, 274
    cognitive problems and, 274
    erectile dysfunction and, 273
    finasteride and, 279-81
    guidelines for, 268-69
    gynecomastia and, 273
    hot flashes and, 273
    intermittent vs continuous, 272
    localized prostate cancer and, 237-38
    loss of libido and, 273
    options for, 271-72, 288-89

About the Authors

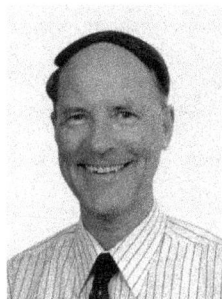

Hans Larsen is a Professional Engineer and holds a Master's degree in Chemical Engineering from the Technical University of Denmark. He developed a lifelong interest in biochemistry and nutrition through his early studies with Professor Henrik Dam, the Nobel Prize-winning discoverer of vitamin K. Later he honed his technical writing skills by abstracting for *Chemical Abstracts* then the world's largest abstracting service. After a rewarding career in research and management in the oil and petrochemicals industry, Hans Larsen retired and in 1992 began publishing *International Health News,* first in printed form and then exclusively on the Internet. He later did extensive research into lone atrial fibrillation, a disorder now reaching epidemic proportions, and in December 2002 published his first book *Lone Atrial Fibrillation: Towards A Cure.* This book was followed by *Thrombosis and Stroke Prevention* – a layman's guide to the causes and prevention of ischemic strokes. Both books have achieved great popularity among atrial fibrillation patients. Hans resides in Victoria, British Columbia with Judi, his wife of 35 years, and keeps his prostate healthy through hiking, cycling (with a soft cut-out saddle), and good nutrition.

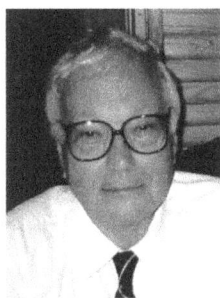

The co-author of this book, **William Ware**, is an emeritus professor of chemistry at the University of Western Ontario in London. He received a Ph.D. in nuclear chemistry and physical chemistry from the University of Rochester and subsequently held academic positions at San Diego State University and the University of Minnesota. He was enticed to move to Canada in 1971 to join five other senior professors in forming the Photochemistry Unit, a research institute within the Chemistry Department of the University of Western Ontario devoted to basic research in photochemistry, photophysics, photobiology and spectroscopy.

His research was mainly concentrated in the fields of fast reactions of excited molecules and time-resolved fluorescence spectroscopy. He was also involved as principal investigator in the clinical testing of a novel fluorescent technique for the diagnosis of cancer. In 1980 he served on the faculty of the NATO Advanced Study Institute at St. Andrews, Scotland, which was devoted to time-resolved fluorescence spectroscopy in biology and biochemistry. He has authored over one hundred scientific papers and reviews and edited three volumes of the series *Creation and Detection of the Excited State,* a series published by Marcel Dekker.

Retirement provided an opportunity to devote considerable time to another interest, preventive and complementary medicine, approached from an evidence-based point of view. Access to the world's medical literature through the University Library, coupled with the background derived from a career in basic research, enabled this interest to flourish and eventually led to the writing of a number of research reviews for *International Health News.* Bill resides in London, Ontario with his wife Hannah. When not researching and writing about health issues he collects, restores and deals in both antique and modern stringed instruments and their bows.

www.ingramcontent.com/pod-product-compliance
Lightning Source LLC
Chambersburg PA
CBHW061741210326
41599CB00034B/6756